Pulmonary Hypertension

LUNG BIOLOGY IN HEALTH AND DISEASE

Executive Editor

Claude Lenfant

Former Director, National Heart, Lung, and Blood Institute
National Institutes of Health
Bethesda, Maryland

1. Immunologic and Infectious Reactions in the Lung, *edited by C. H. Kirkpatrick and H. Y. Reynolds*
2. The Biochemical Basis of Pulmonary Function, *edited by R. G. Crystal*
3. Bioengineering Aspects of the Lung, *edited by J. B. West*
4. Metabolic Functions of the Lung, *edited by Y. S. Bakhle and J. R. Vane*
5. Respiratory Defense Mechanisms (in two parts), *edited by J. D. Brain, D. F. Proctor, and L. M. Reid*
6. Development of the Lung, *edited by W. A. Hodson*
7. Lung Water and Solute Exchange, *edited by N. C. Staub*
8. Extrapulmonary Manifestations of Respiratory Disease, *edited by E. D. Robin*
9. Chronic Obstructive Pulmonary Disease, *edited by T. L. Petty*
10. Pathogenesis and Therapy of Lung Cancer, *edited by C. C. Harris*
11. Genetic Determinants of Pulmonary Disease, *edited by S. D. Litwin*
12. The Lung in the Transition Between Health and Disease, *edited by P. T. Macklem and S. Permutt*
13. Evolution of Respiratory Processes: A Comparative Approach, *edited by S. C. Wood and C. Lenfant*
14. Pulmonary Vascular Diseases, *edited by K. M. Moser*
15. Physiology and Pharmacology of the Airways, *edited by J. A. Nadel*
16. Diagnostic Techniques in Pulmonary Disease (in two parts), *edited by M. A. Sackner*
17. Regulation of Breathing (in two parts), *edited by T. F. Hornbein*
18. Occupational Lung Diseases: Research Approaches and Methods, *edited by H. Weill and M. Turner-Warwick*
19. Immunopharmacology of the Lung, *edited by H. H. Newball*
20. Sarcoidosis and Other Granulomatous Diseases of the Lung, *edited by B. L. Fanburg*
21. Sleep and Breathing, *edited by N. A. Saunders and C. E. Sullivan*
22. *Pneumocystis carinii* Pneumonia: Pathogenesis, Diagnosis, and Treatment, *edited by L. S. Young*
23. Pulmonary Nuclear Medicine: Techniques in Diagnosis of Lung Disease, *edited by H. L. Atkins*
24. Acute Respiratory Failure, *edited by W. M. Zapol and K. J. Falke*

For information on volumes 25–182 in the *Lung Biology in Health and Disease* series, please visit www.informahealthcare.com

183. Acute Exacerbations of Chronic Obstructive Pulmonary Disease, *edited by N. M. Siafakas, N. R. Anthonisen, and D. Georgopoulos*

184. Lung Volume Reduction Surgery for Emphysema, *edited by H. F. Fessler, J. J. Reilly, Jr., and D. J. Sugarbaker*

185. Idiopathic Pulmonary Fibrosis, *edited by J. P. Lynch III*

186. Pleural Disease, *edited by D. Bouros*

187. Oxygen/Nitrogen Radicals: Lung Injury and Disease, *edited by V. Vallyathan, V. Castranova, and X. Shi*

188. Therapy for Mucus-Clearance Disorders, *edited by B. K. Rubin and C. P. van der Schans*

189. Interventional Pulmonary Medicine, *edited by J. F. Beamis, Jr., P. N. Mathur, and A. C. Mehta*

190. Lung Development and Regeneration, *edited by D. J. Massaro, G. Massaro, and P. Chambon*

191. Long-Term Intervention in Chronic Obstructive Pulmonary Disease, *edited by R. Pauwels, D. S. Postma, and S. T. Weiss*

192. Sleep Deprivation: Basic Science, Physiology, and Behavior, *edited by Clete A. Kushida*

193. Sleep Deprivation: Clinical Issues, Pharmacology, and Sleep Loss Effects, *edited by Clete A. Kushida*

194. Pneumocystis Pneumonia: Third Edition, Revised and Expanded, *edited by P. D. Walzer and M. Cushion*

195. Asthma Prevention, *edited by William W. Busse and Robert F. Lemanske, Jr.*

196. Lung Injury: Mechanisms, Pathophysiology, and Therapy, *edited by Robert H. Notter, Jacob Finkelstein, and Bruce Holm*

197. Ion Channels in the Pulmonary Vasculature, *edited by Jason X.-J. Yuan*

198. Chronic Obstructive Pulmonary Disease: Cellular and Molecular Mechanisms, *edited by Peter J. Barnes*

199. Pediatric Nasal and Sinus Disorders, *edited by Tania Sih and Peter A. R. Clement*

200. Functional Lung Imaging, *edited by David Lipson and Edwin van Beek*

201. Lung Surfactant Function and Disorder, *edited by Kaushik Nag*

202. Pharmacology and Pathophysiology of the Control of Breathing, *edited by Denham S. Ward, Albert Dahan, and Luc J. Teppema*

203. Molecular Imaging of the Lungs, *edited by Daniel Schuster and Timothy Blackwell*

204. Air Pollutants and the Respiratory Tract: Second Edition, *edited by W. Michael Foster and Daniel L. Costa*

205. Acute and Chronic Cough, *edited by Anthony E. Redington and Alyn H. Morice*

206. Severe Pneumonia, *edited by Michael S. Niederman*

207. Monitoring Asthma, *edited by Peter G. Gibson*

208. Dyspnea: Mechanisms, Measurement, and Management, Second Edition, *edited by Donald A. Mahler and Denis E. O'Donnell*

209. Childhood Asthma, *edited by Stanley J. Szefler and Søren Pedersen*

210. Sarcoidosis, *edited by Robert Baughman*

211. Tropical Lung Disease, Second Edition, *edited by Om Sharma*

212. Pharmacotherapy of Asthma, *edited by James T. Li*

213. Practical Pulmonary and Critical Care Medicine: Respiratory Failure, *edited by Zab Mosenifar and Guy W. Soo Hoo*

214. Practical Pulmonary and Critical Care Medicine: Disease Management, *edited by Zab Mosenifar and Guy W. Soo Hoo*

215. Ventilator-Induced Lung Injury, *edited by Didier Dreyfuss, Georges Saumon, and Rolf D. Hubmayr*

216. Bronchial Vascular Remodeling in Asthma and COPD, *edited by Aili Lazaar*

217. Lung and Heart–Lung Transplantation, *edited by Joseph P. Lynch III and David J. Ross*

218. Genetics of Asthma and Chronic Obstructive Pulmonary Disease, *edited by Dirkje S. Postma and Scott T. Weiss*

219. *Reichman and Hershfield's* Tuberculosis: A Comprehensive, International Approach, Third Edition (in two parts), *edited by Mario C. Raviglione*

220. Narcolepsy and Hypersomnia, *edited by Claudio Bassetti, Michel Billiard, and Emmanuel Mignot*

221. Inhalation Aerosols: Physical and Biological Basis for Therapy, Second Edition, *edited by Anthony J. Hickey*

222. Clinical Management of Chronic Obstructive Pulmonary Disease, Second Edition, *edited by Stephen I. Rennard, Roberto Rodriguez-Roisin, Gérard Huchon, and Nicolas Roche*

223. Sleep in Children, Second Edition: Developmental Changes in Sleep Patterns, *edited by Carole L. Marcus, John L. Carroll, David F. Donnelly, and Gerald M. Loughlin*

224. Sleep and Breathing in Children, Second Edition: Developmental Changes in Breathing During Sleep, *edited by Carole L. Marcus, John L. Carroll, David F. Donnelly, and Gerald M. Loughlin*

225. Ventilatory Support for Chronic Respiratory Failure, *edited by Nicolino Ambrosino and Roger S. Goldstein*

226. Diagnostic Pulmonary Pathology, Second Edition, *edited by Philip T. Cagle, Timothy C. Allen, and Mary Beth Beasley*

227. Interstitial Pulmonary and Bronchiolar Disorders, *edited by Joseph P. Lynch III*

228. Chronic Obstructive Pulmonary Disease Exacerbations, *edited by Jadwiga A. Wedzicha and Fernando J. Martinez*

229. Pleural Disease, Second Edition, *edited by Demosthenes Bouros*

230. Interventional Pulmonary Medicine, Second Edition, *edited by John F. Beamis, Jr., Praveen Mathur, and Atul C. Mehta*

231. Sleep Apnea: Implications in Cardiovascular and Cerebrovascular Disease, Second Edition, *edited by Douglas T. Bradley and John Floras*

232. Respiratory Infections, *edited by Sanjay Sethi*

233. Acute Respiratory Distress Syndrome, *edited by Augustine M. K. Choi*

234. Pharmacology and Therapeutics of Airway Disease, *edited by Kian Fan Chung and Peter J. Barnes*

235. Sleep Apnea: Pathogenesis, Diagnosis, and Treatment, Second Edition, *edited by Allan I. Pack*

236. Pulmonary Hypertension, *edited by Marc Humbert and Joseph P. Lynch III*

The opinions expressed in these volumes do not necessarily represent the views of the National Institutes of Health.

Pulmonary Hypertension

edited by

Marc Humbert
Université Paris Sud 11
Hôpital Antoine Béclère, Assistance Publique Hôpitaux de Paris
Clamart, France

Joseph P. Lynch III
David Geffen School of Medicine at UCLA
Los Angeles, California, USA

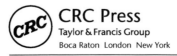

CRC Press
Taylor & Francis Group
Boca Raton   London   New York

CRC Press is an imprint of the
Taylor & Francis Group, an **informa** business

CRC Press
Taylor & Francis Group
6000 Broken Sound Parkway NW, Suite 300
Boca Raton, FL 33487-2742

First issued in paperback 2019

© 2009 by Taylor & Francis Group, LLC
CRC Press is an imprint of Taylor & Francis Group, an Informa business

No claim to original U.S. Government works

ISBN-13: 978-1-4200-9475-6 (hbk)
ISBN-13: 978-0-367-38542-2 (pbk)

A CIP record for this book is available from the British Library.

Library of Congress Cataloging-in-Publication Data available on application

**Visit the Taylor & Francis Web site at
http://www.taylorandfrancis.com**

**and the CRC Press Web site at
http://www.crcpress.com**

Introduction

The journey of pulmonary artery hypertension began on the eve of the previous century, in 1881, when E. von Romberg published a report titled "About sclerosis of the pulmonary artery" (1). Later, in 1907, J. G. Monckeberg corroborated Romberg's description with his paper titled "Genuine arterio-sclerosis of the pulmonary artery" (2). O. Brenner in 1935 described what he named "primary pulmonary vascular sclerosis," and he emphasized that "before the diagnosis of primary pulmonary arteriosclerosis is made, all the factors commonly (though perhaps erroneously) thought to cause secondary pulmo-nary vascular sclerosis must be absent and there must be marked hypertrophy of the right ventricle" (3). A few years later, in 1940, De Navasquez et al. described cases "further defining the condition that has been termed primary pulmonary arteriosclerosis"; the title of this report introduced the name of "so-called pulmonary hypertension" (4). Successive publications included the term "pulmonary hypertension" in the title or text.

The introduction of cardiac catheterization (5) justified Brinton's state-ment in 1950 that "until recently pulmonary hypertension was an assumption from physical signs and morbid anatomy, but in the last few years, evidence has accrued from cardiac catheterization that it does in fact exist ..." (6). After half a century, this disease of the small pulmonary arteries characterized by obstructive remodeling leading to progressive pulmonary vascular resistance had found its name!

In the following years, the clinical community continued to work on this disease that was then, and to a point continues to be, relatively rare. However, the "epidemic" of cases in the 1960s to 1970s due to the appetite reducer *aminorex* initiated considerable interest in pulmonary hypertension, be it idiopathic (formerly primary pulmonary hypertension), familial, anorexigen associated, or associated with other conditions such as HIV and COPD. The research and clinical communities have risen to the huge, but fascinating, challenges to understand and treat this disease. The advances have stimulated the pharmaceutical industry to respond in a productive way.

However, pulmonary hypertension remains a relatively rare disease, but it is serious and often fatal. The idiopathic form affects young individuals and more women than men. It has been reported by the U.S. Center for Disease Control and Prevention that in 2002 there were 15,666 deaths from pulmonary hypertension and 260,000 hospital visits for pulmonary hypertension by 160,000 women and 100,000 men.

Twelve years ago, the series of monographs *Lung Biology in Health and Disease* published volume 99 titled *Primary Pulmonary Hypertension*, edited by Lewis J. Rubin and Stuart Rich; this book energized the interest in research on this disease. Today, we take pride to present volume 236 titled *Pulmonary Hypertension*, edited by Marc Humbert and Joseph P. Lynch III, with contributions by globally recognized experts. This comprehensive volume has two distinct goals: one is to bring the medical community up-to-date on what is known about pulmonary hypertension and how physicians can approach and treat this disease and its varieties. The second feature of the volume is to bring forth ideas and directions that will undoubtedly stimulate the research community. Much work is needed to decipher the many remaining secrets of this disease, and the editors and authors open the door to new hypotheses and investigations. Ultimately, it will be the patients who will benefit from this book and from the new work it is certain to stimulate.

The series *Lung Biology in Health and Disease* is privileged to introduce this volume. As the executive editor of the series, I want to thank the editors and authors for giving the series the opportunity to present their work.

Claude Lenfant, MD
Vancouver, Washington, U.S.A.

References

1. von Romberg E. Ueber Sklerose der Lungenarterie. Deutsches Arch Klin Med 1891; 48: 197–206.
2. Monckeberg JG. Ueber die genuine Arteriosklerose der Lungenarterie. Dtsch Med Wochenschr 1907; 33:1243–1246.
3. Brenner O. Pathology of the vessels of the pulmonary circulation. Arch Intern Med 1935; 56(pt 1–4):211–237, 457–497, 724–753, 976–1014, 1190–1241.
4. De Navasquez S, Forbes JP, and Holling HE. Right ventricular hypertrophy of unknown origin: so-called pulmonary hypertension. Br Heart J 1940; 2:177–188.
5. Cournand A. Recent observations on the dynamics of the pulmonary circulation. Bull N Y Acad Med 1947; 23:27–50.
6. Brinton WD. Primary pulmonary hypertension. Br Heart J 1950; 12:305–311.

Preface

Pulmonary Hypertension will provide a comprehensive review of *clinical and investigative* aspects of pulmonary hypertension including idiopathic (primary) and secondary forms. Management of pulmonary arterial hypertension (PAH) is difficult and has generally been managed by a few cardiologists or pulmonologists. Given the rarity of PAH and the need for right-heart catheterization (RHC) to substantiate the diagnosis (i.e., a mean pulmonary artery pressure above 25 mmHg), most practicing clinicians have inadequate personal experience to deal with these diverse disorders. This book enlists internationally recognized experts to discuss controversies and evolving concepts in the diagnosis and management of pulmonary hypertension. The first nine chapters provide an overview of PAH, including classification and epidemiology, pathology, pathogenesis, genetics, and diagnosis. Chapters 10 through 21 discuss the most important causes of pulmonary hypertension, starting with idiopathic pulmonary arterial hypertension (IPAH). Individual chapters review PAH complicating connective tissue diseases (CTD), congenital heart diseases, human immunodeficiency virus (HIV) infection, and a host of other disorders. Chapters 22 through 32 discuss treatment. Separate chapters are included for each of the pharmacological and surgical therapies [including lung transplantation (LT)] for PAH. Importantly, separate chapters are devoted to each of the pharmacological agents (or classes of agents) used to treat PAH. This provides a detailed understanding of mechanisms, toxicities, and efficacy of each of these agents. A separate chapter by Drs. Rubin and Gaine addresses in detail the role of combination therapies, novel agents, and future directions. Additionally, the management of PAH in *specific patient populations* (e.g., pregnancy, the pediatric population, and critically ill patients in intensive care units) is discussed in chapters 31–33. The final chapter by Dr. Peacock discusses appropriate end points and designs for future therapeutic trials.

PAH is a disease of the small pulmonary arteries characterized by vascular proliferation and remodeling. Progressive increase in pulmonary vascular resistance ultimately leads to right ventricular failure and death. In the 1970s, major causes of pulmonary hypertension are recognized including the so-called "secondary" causes [e.g., congenital heart disease, collagen vascular disease (typically scleroderma), chronic pulmonary thromboembolism, or end-stage lung disease] and IPAH. In the 1960s, a link between PAH and the appetite suppressant aminorex fumarate was established in Europe. Subsequent studies implicated other toxic agents (e.g., fenfluramine, toxic rapeseed oil) in some patients with PAH. Within the past two decades, it has increasingly been recognized that PAH may complicate diverse diseases such as HIV infection, hepatic cirrhosis, hemolytic anemia, interstitial lung disorders, etc. In 1998, the World Symposium on Primary Pulmonary Hypertension proposed a classification schema and definition for PAH. Within the past few years, further insights into familial cases of PAH were gained, when mutations in the coding region of the gene for bone morphogenetic protein receptor type 2 (BMPPR2) were discovered.

Most of the data on treatment of PAH has been gleaned from studies in IPAH, a rare disorder (with an incidence of only two cases per million) that predominantly affects women in the prime of life. In the 1980s, median survival after diagnosis was 2.8 years. The use of intravenous (IV) epoprostenol in the mid-1990s led to improvements in clinical outcomes, quality of life (QoL), and survival. Within the past decade, several additional agents have been added to the therapeutic armamentarium for IPAH. However, these therapies are not curative. Further, the relevance and application of these agents for causes of PAH other than IPAH have not been rigorously studied.

Given the devastating nature of the disease, initial treatment in the 1970s and 1980s involved the use of vasodilators, diuretics, and anticoagulants, with limited efficacy. A small subset of patients responded to vasodilators (principally calcium channel blockers), but for most patients, the course was inexorable, leading to death within two to five years of onset. By the 1990s, it was clear that vasoconstriction is only one component of this disease. Vascular remodeling is a cardinal feature and may lead to irreversible destruction and distortion of pulmonary vessels. The pathogenesis of PAH reflects deficiencies of pulmonary vasodilators (particularly nitric oxide and prostacyclin) with overexpression of endothelin-1, a potent vasoconstrictor and mitogen. Novel therapeutic strategies targeting vascular remodeling have improved the prognosis of this once inevitably fatal disorder. IV epoprostenol (prostacyclin) was first used to treat PAH in the early 1980s and approved for use in the United States and several European agencies in the mid-1990s. IV prostacyclin remain the gold standard for severe PAH. However, IV epoprostenol is logistically difficult (requires a central line and continuous infusion) and expensive (>$60,000 annually) and has potentially serious adverse effects. Subsequently, additional agents were developed, including subcutaneous treprostinil, inhaled iloprost, endothelin-1 receptor antagonists (e.g., bosentan, sitaxsentan, and ambrisentan), and phosphodiesterase type 5 inhibitors (e.g., sildenafil, tadalafil). These agents are expensive and are associated with significant adverse effects. Importantly, optimal therapy has not yet been established; randomized studies comparing one agent versus another are lacking. Further, clinical trials comprised primarily patients with IPAH and (in some studies) associated PAH such as patients with systemic sclerosis.

Whether conclusions from these pivotal studies can be extrapolated to PAH from diverse other causes (e.g., HIV infections, congenital heart diseases, portopulmonary hypertension, etc.) has not been well established. Currently, prostacyclin derivatives have a central role in treating patients with severe PAH. Phosphodiesterase type 5 inhibitors and endothelin-1 receptor antagonists may be of value in patients with less severe disease or to augment the effects of prostacyclin. However, responses to these diverse pharmacological agents are incomplete and may not be sustained. Combinations of therapies have been used, with some successes, but are very expensive and require additional studies to demonstrate that they affect mortality. Additionally, each of these agents is expensive (typically >$40,000 annually), so irresponsible or inappropriate use will lead to escalating health care costs. Patients failing medical therapy may be candidates for LT. However, LT has significant morbidity and mortality. Who to list for LT and when to list are difficult decisions. Delays in listing may result in severe, even fatal, right-heart failure. Additional surgical techniques such as pulmonary endarterectomy are curative for the subset of patients with proximal chronic thromboembolic disease.

Given the rarity of IPAH, many physicians have limited experience with this disease, and appropriate management remains controversial. Further, optimal techniques to diagnose PAH have not been clarified. Right-heart catheterization is the "gold standard" but is invasive. Echocardiography is of major interest to screen for pulmonary hypertension. It gives an estimate of pulmonary arterial pressure and assesses right ventricular function, but it has several limitations. Additional diagnostic studies include magnetic resonance imaging, blood tests (e.g., brain natriuretic peptide), and physiological tests (e.g., six-minute walk tests, cardiopulmonary exercise tests, etc.). Further, optimal tests or markers to monitor response to therapy or the course of the disease have not been well defined. Each of these questions and issues will be addressed in this comprehensive book.

This book will provide a global perspective of the current and future management of these diverse pulmonary vascular disorders. The book will be of great interest to pulmonologists, cardiologists, intensivists (physicians and nurses), pathologists, radiologists, and basic scientists with an interest in the pulmonary vasculature and PAH.

Marc Humbert
Joseph P. Lynch III

Contributors

Jamil Aboulhosn David Geffen School of Medicine at UCLA, Los Angeles, California, U.S.A.

William R. Auger University of California, San Diego, California, U.S.A.

Eric D. Austin Vanderbilt University School of Medicine, Nashville, Tennessee, U.S.A.

Maurice Beghetti University Children's Hospital, Geneva, Switzerland

John A. Belperio David Geffen School of Medicine at UCLA, Los Angeles, California, U.S.A.

Herman Bogaard Virginia Commonwealth University, Richmond, Virginia, U.S.A.

Ari Chaouat Service des Maladies Respiratoires et de Réanimation Respiratoire, Centre Hospitalier Universitaire Nancy, Vandoeuvre les Nancy, France

Paul A. Corris Institute of Cellular Medicine, Newcastle University and Freeman Hospital, Newcastle upon Tyne, U.K.

Philippe G. Dartevelle Marie Lannelongue Hospital, Université Paris Sud 11, Le Plessis Robinson, France

Bruno Degano CHU Rangueil-Larrey, Toulouse; and Hôpital Antoine Béclère, Clamart, France

Laurence Dewachter Free University of Brussels, Brussels, Belgium

Peter Dorfmüller Université Paris Sud 11, Service de Pneumologie et Réanimation Respiratoire, Hôpital Antoine Béclère, Assistance Publique Hôpitaux de Paris, Clamart, France

Dominique Fabre Marie Lannelongue Hospital, Université Paris Sud 11, Le Plessis Robinson, France

Elie Fadel Marie Lannelongue Hospital, Université Paris Sud 11, Le Plessis Robinson, France

Peter F. Fedullo University of California, San Diego, California, U.S.A.

Caio J. C. S. Fernandes University of São Paulo Medical School, São Paulo, Brazil

Anna Fijałkowska Institute of Tuberculosis and Lung Diseases, Warsaw, Poland

Michael C. Fishbein David Geffen School of Medicine at UCLA, Los Angeles, California, U.S.A.

Paul R. Forfia University of Pennsylvania, Philadelphia, Pennsylvania, U.S.A.

Sean P. Gaine Mater Misericordiae University Hospital, University College Dublin, Dublin, Ireland

Nazzareno Galiè University of Bologna, Bologna, Italy

Jorge Gaspar Instituto Nacional de Cardiologia, Ignacio Chavez, Mexico

Mark T. Gladwin University of Pittsburgh Medical Center, Pittsburgh, Pennsylvania, U.S.A.

Paul M. Hassoun Johns Hopkins University, Baltimore, Maryland, U.S.A.

Marius M. Hoeper Hannover Medical School, Hannover, Germany

Marc Humbert Université Paris Sud 11, Service de Pneumologie et Réanimation Respiratoire, Hôpital Antoine Béclère, Assistance Publique Hôpitaux de Paris, Clamart, France

Carlos Jardim University of São Paulo Medical School, São Paulo, Brazil

Xavier Jaïs Université Paris Sud 11, Service de Pneumologie et Réanimation Respiratoire, Hôpital Antoine Béclère, Assistance Publique Hôpitaux de Paris, Clamart, France

Kristina Kemp   Université Paris Sud 11, Service de Pneumologie et Réanimation Respiratoire, Hôpital Antoine Béclère, Assistance Publique Hôpitaux de Paris, Clamart, France

Michael J. Krowka   Mayo Clinic, Rochester, Minnesota, U.S.A.

Jerome Le Pavec   Université Paris Sud 11, Service de Pneumologie et Réanimation Respiratoire, Hôpital Antoine Béclère, Assistance Publique Hôpitaux de Paris, Clamart, France

Daniel S. Levi   Mattel Children's Hospital at UCLA, Los Angeles, California, U.S.A.

James E. Loyd   Vanderbilt University School of Medicine, Nashville, Tennessee, U.S.A.

Joseph P. Lynch III   David Geffen School of Medicine at UCLA, Los Angeles, California, U.S.A.

Sophie Maître   Université Paris-Sud 11, UPRES EA 2705, Centre National de Référence de l'Hypertension Artérielle Pulmonaire, Service de Radiologie, Hôpital Antoine Béclère, Assistance Publique Hôpitaux de Paris, Clamart, France

Vallerie V. McLaughlin   University of Michigan Health System, Ann Arbor, Michigan, U.S.A.

Olaf Mercier   Marie Lannelongue Hospital, Université Paris Sud 11, Le Plessis Robinson, France

David Montani   Université Paris Sud 11, Service de Pneumologie et Réanimation Respiratoire, Hôpital Antoine Béclère, Assistance Publique Hôpitaux de Paris, Clamart, France

Dominique Musset   Université Paris-Sud 11, UPRES EA 2705, Centre National de Référence de l'Hypertension Artérielle Pulmonaire, Service de Radiologie, Hôpital Antoine Béclère, Assistance Publique Hôpitaux de Paris, Clamart, France

Sacha Mussot   Marie Lannelongue Hospital, Université Paris Sud 11, Le Plessis Robinson, France

Robert Naeije   Free University of Brussels, Brussels, Belgium

Florence Parent   Université Paris Sud 11, Service de Pneumologie et Réanimation Respiratoire, Hôpital Antoine Béclère, Assistance Publique Hôpitaux de Paris, Clamart, France

Andrew J. Peacock   Golden Jubilee National Hospital, Glasgow, U.K.

Dante Penaloza   University Cayetano Heredia, Lima, Peru

John A. Phillips III   Vanderbilt University School of Medicine, Nashville, Tennessee, U.S.A.

Laura Claire Price   Université Paris Sud 11, Service de Pneumologie et Réanimation Respiratoire, Hôpital Antoine Béclère, Assistance Publique Hôpitaux de Paris, Clamart, France

Tomás Pulido   Instituto Nacional de Cardiologia, Ignacio Chavez, Mexico

Ivan M. Robbins   Vanderbilt University Medical Center, Nashville, Tennessee, U.S.A.

Lewis J. Rubin   University of California, San Diego School of Medicine, La Jolla, California, U.S.A.

Rajan Saggar   David Geffen School of Medicine at UCLA, Los Angeles, California, U.S.A.

Rajeev Saggar   David Geffen School of Medicine at UCLA, Los Angeles, California, U.S.A.

Julio Sandoval   Instituto Nacional de Cardiologia, Ignacio Chavez, Mexico

Victoria Scott   David Geffen School of Medicine at UCLA, Los Angeles, California, U.S.A.

Francisco Sime   University Cayetano Heredia, Lima, Peru

Gérald Simonneau   Université Paris Sud 11, Service de Pneumologie et Réanimation Respiratoire, Hôpital Antoine Béclère, Assistance Publique Hôpitaux de Paris, Clamart, France

Olivier Sitbon Université Paris Sud 11, Service de Pneumologie et Réanimation Respiratoire, Hôpital Antoine Béclère, Assistance Publique Hôpitaux de Paris, Clamart, France

Rogério Souza University of São Paulo Medical School, São Paulo, Brazil

Lori Sweeney Virginia Commonwealth University, Richmond, Virginia, U.S.A.

Benjamin Sztrymf Université Paris Sud 11, Service de Pneumologie et Réanimation Respiratoire, Hôpital Antoine Béclère, Assistance Publique Hôpitaux de Paris, Clamart, France

Cecile Tissot University Children's Hospital, Geneva, Switzerland

Adam Torbicki Institute of Tuberculosis and Lung Diseases, Warsaw, Poland

Norbert F. Voelkel Virginia Commonwealth University, Richmond, Virginia, U.S.A.

Emmanuel Weitzenblum Service de Pneumologie, Nouvel Hôpital Civil, Strasbourg, France

David A. Zisman David Geffen School of Medicine at UCLA, Los Angeles, California, U.S.A.

Contents

Introduction   Claude Lenfant   . . . .   *vii*
Preface   . . . .   *ix*
Contributors   . . . .   *xiii*

**Section 1: Classification, Epidemiology, Pathology, Pathogenesis
and Genetics**

1. **Updated Clinical Classification of Pulmonary Hypertension** . . .   *1*
   Ivan M. Robbins and Gérald Simonneau

2. **Epidemiology of Pulmonary Arterial Hypertension** *10*
   Marc Humbert

3. **Pathology of Pulmonary Hypertension** *20*
   Peter Dorfmüller

4. **Pathogenesis of Pulmonary Hypertension** *40*
   Norbert F. Voelkel, Lori Sweeney, and Herman Bogaard

5. **Animal Models of Pulmonary Hypertension** *59*
   Laurence Dewachter and Robert Naeije

6. **Genetics of PAH** *83*
   Eric D. Austin, James E. Loyd, and John A. Phillips III

Section 2: Imaging and Diagnosis of Pulmonary Hypertension

7. **Imaging of Pulmonary Hypertension** *95*
   Dominique Musset and Sophie Maître

8. **Echocardiography of Pulmonary Arterial Hypertension** . . .   *122*
   Adam Torbicki and Anna Fijałkowska

9. **Diagnosis and Hemodynamic Assessment of
    Pulmonary Arterial Hypertension** *132*
    *Rajan Saggar, Rajeev Saggar, John A. Belperio, David A. Zisman,
    Joseph P. Lynch III, and Jamil Aboulhosn*

Section 3: Clinical Variants of Pulmonary Hypertension

10. **Idiopathic, Familial, and Anorexigen-Associated
    Pulmonary Arterial Hypertension** *150*
    Jerome Le Pavec and Marc Humbert

11. **Pulmonary Arterial Hypertension Complicating Connective
    Tissue Diseases** *161*
    Paul M. Hassoun

12. **Pulmonary Arterial Hypertension in Congenital
    Heart Disease** *176*
    Daniel S. Levi, Victoria Scott, and Jamil Aboulhosn

13. **Pulmonary Arterial Hypertension and
    Human Immunodeficiency Virus Infection** *196*
    Bruno Degano and Olivier Sitbon

14. **Portopulmonary Hypertension** *207*
    Michael J. Krowka

15. **Pulmonary Hypertension Complicating Schistosomiasis** *214*
    Caio J. C. S. Fernandes, Carlos Jardim, and Rogério Souza

16. **Pulmonary Hypertension in Sickle Cell Disease** *222*
    Mark T. Gladwin

17. **Pulmonary Veno-occlusive Disease and Pulmonary
    Capillary Hemangiomatosis** *237*
    David Montani

18. **Pulmonary Hypertension in Chronic Obstructive
    Pulmonary Disease** *250*
    Emmanuel Weitzenblum and Ari Chaouat

19. **Pulmonary Hypertension Complicating
    Interstitial Lung Disease** *264*
    *David A. Zisman, John A. Belperio, Rajan Saggar, Rajeev Saggar,
    Michael C. Fishbein, and Joseph P. Lynch III*

20. **Pulmonary Hypertension in Chronic Mountain Sickness** ... *292*
    Dante Penaloza and Francisco Sime

21. **Chronic Thromboembolic Pulmonary Hypertension** *305*
    William R. Auger and Peter F. Fedullo

Section 4: Medical Treatment of Pulmonary Arterial Hypertension

22. **Pulmonary Arterial Hypertension: Conventional Therapy** ... *325*
    Olivier Sitbon

23. **Medical Treatment of PAH: Prostacyclins** *338*
    Paul R. Forfia and Vallerie V. McLaughlin

24. **Phosphodiesterase Type 5 Inhibitors** *350*
    Nazzareno Galiè

25. **Medical Treatment of Pulmonary Arterial Hypertension:**
    Endothelin Receptor Antagonists *355*
    Kristina Kemp and Marc Humbert

26. **Medical Treatment of PAH: Combination Therapy,**
    Novel Agents, Future Directions, and
    Current Recommendations *367*
    Lewis J. Rubin and Sean P. Gaine

27. **Goal-Oriented Therapy in Pulmonary Arterial**
    Hypertension *377*
    Marius M. Hoeper

Section 5: Atrioseptostomy and Surgery for Pulmonary Hypertension

28. **Atrial Septostomy for the Treatment of Severe**
    Pulmonary Hypertension *388*
    Julio Sandoval, Jorge Gaspar, and Tomás Pulido

29. **Surgical Management of Pulmonary Hypertension** *401*
    Philippe G. Dartevelle, Elie Fadel, Sacha Mussot,
    Dominique Fabre, Olaf Mercier, Marc Humbert, and
    Gérald Simonneau

30. **The Selection and Timing of Transplantation for Patients**
    with Pulmonary Arterial Hypertension *412*
    Paul A. Corris

Section 6: Difficult Pulmonary Hypertension

31. **Pulmonary Arterial Hypertension and Pregnancy** **422**
    Xavier Jaïs, Laura Claire Price, Florence Parent,
    and Marc Humbert

32. **Pediatric Pulmonary Hypertension** **434**
    Cecile Tissot and Maurice Beghetti

33. **Practical Management of Pulmonary Arterial Hypertension**
    in the Intensive Care Unit **455**
    Benjamin Sztrymf and Marc Humbert

Section 7: Endpoints and Clinical Trials

34. **End Points and Clinical Trial Design in Pulmonary Arterial**
    Hypertension: Clinical and Regulatory Perspectives **462**
    Andrew J. Peacock

Index *477*

1

Updated Clinical Classification of Pulmonary Hypertension

IVAN M. ROBBINS
Vanderbilt University Medical Center, Nashville, Tennessee, U.S.A.

GÉRALD SIMONNEAU
Université Paris Sud 11, Service de Pneumologie et Réanimation Respiratoire, Hôpital Antoine Béclère, Assistance Publique Hôpitaux de Paris, Clamart, France

I. Introduction

The classification of pulmonary hypertension (PH) has gone through a series of changes since the first classification was proposed in 1973 (1). During the Fourth World Symposium on Pulmonary Hypertension held in 2008 in Dana Point, California, the consensus of an international group of experts was to maintain the general philosophy and organization of the previous Venice classification held in 2003 (2). Although the five major categories of PH were retained in the Dana Point classification, a number of important modifications were made to accurately reflect the information published over the past five years as well as to clarify some areas that were unclear in the previous classification. The Venice classification is listed in Table 1 and the new Dana Point classification is listed in Table 2.

II. Group 1: Pulmonary Arterial Hypertension

Idiopathic and Heritable PAH

Idiopathic pulmonary arterial hypertension (PAH) corresponds to sporadic disease in which there is neither a family history of PAH nor an identified risk factor. When PAH occurs in a familial context, germline mutations in the bone morphogenetic protein receptor 2 (*BMPR2*) gene, a member of the transforming growth factor β (TGF-β) signaling family, can be detected in about 70% of cases (3). More rarely, mutations in activin receptor-like kinase 1 (*ALK 1*) or endoglin, also members of the TGF-β signaling family, have been identified in patients with PAH, predominantly with coexistent hereditary hemorrhagic telangiectasia (HHT).

BMPR2 mutations have also been detected in 11% to 40% of apparently idiopathic cases with no family history (4); therefore, the distinction between idiopathic and familial BMPR2 mutations is artificial as all patients with a BMPR2 mutation have heritable disease. Thus, it was decided to replace the term "familial PAH" with "heritable PAH" in the new classification.

Table 1 Venice Clinical Classification of Pulmonary Hypertension (2003)

1. Pulmonary arterial hypertension (PAH)
    Idiopathic (IPAH)
    Familial (FPAH)
    Associated with (APAH)
        Collagen vascular disease
        Congenital systemic to pulmonary shunts
        Portal hypertension
        HIV infection
        Drugs and toxins
        Other (thyroid disorders, glycogen storage disease, Gaucher disease, hereditary hemor-
            rhagic telangiectasia, hemoglobinopathies, myeloproliferative disorders, splenectomy)
    Associated with significant venous or capillary involvement
        Pulmonary veno-occlusive disease (PVOD)
        Pulmonary capillary hemangiomatosis (PCH)
    Persistent pulmonary hypertension of the newborn
2. Pulmonary hypertension with left-heart disease
    Left-sided atrial or ventricular heart disease
    Left-sided valvular heart disease
3. Pulmonary hypertension associated with lung diseases and/or hypoxemia
    Chronic obstructive pulmonary disease
    Interstitial lung disease
    Sleep-disordered breathing
    Alveolar hypoventilation disorders
    Chronic exposure to high altitude
    Developmental abnormalities
4. Pulmonary hypertension due to chronic thrombotic and/or embolic disease
    Thromboembolic obstruction of proximal pulmonary arteries
    Thromboembolic obstruction of distal pulmonary arteries
    Nonthrombotic pulmonary embolism (tumor, parasites, foreign material)
5. Miscellaneous
    Sarcoidosis, histiocytosis X, lymphangiomatosis, compression of pulmonary vessels
    (adenopathy, tumor, fibrosing mediastinitis)

Drug- and Toxin-Induced PAH

A number of risk factors for the development of PAH have been identified and were
included in previous classifications (2). Updated risk factors and associated conditions
for PAH are presented in Table 3. The use of methamphetamine is now considered a
"very likely" risk factor for the development of PAH (5), and use of selective serotonin
reuptake inhibitors in pregnant women has been reclassified as a "possible" risk factor,
in offspring, for the development of persistent PH of the newborn, a form of PAH (6).

PAH Associated with Connective Tissue Disease

PAH associated with connective tissue disease (CTD) represents an important clinical
subgroup. The prevalence of PAH in systemic sclerosis is between 7% and 12% (7,8).
Importantly, there are other causes of PH in systemic sclerosis, including associated lung
fibrosis and diastolic left-heart dysfunction (8,9).

Table 2 Dana Point Clinical Classification of Pulmonary Hypertension (2008)

1. Pulmonary arterial hypertension (PAH)
    Idiopathic PAH
    Heritable
    BMPR2
    ALK 1, endoglin (with or without hereditary hemorrhagic telangiectasia)
    Unknown
    Drug and toxin induced
    Associated with
       Connective tissue diseases
       HIV infection
       Portal hypertension
       Congenital heart diseases
       Schistosomiasis
       Chronic hemolytic anemia
    Persistent pulmonary hypertension of the newborn
1'. Pulmonary veno-occlusive disease (PVOD) and pulmonary capillary hemangiomatosis (PCH)
2. Pulmonary hypertension due to left-heart disease
    Systolic dysfunction
    Diastolic dysfunction
    Valvular disease
3. Pulmonary hypertension due to lung diseases and/or hypoxia
    Chronic obstructive pulmonary disease
    Interstitial lung disease
    Other pulmonary diseases with mixed restrictive and obstructive pattern
    Sleep-disordered breathing
    Alveolar hypoventilation disorders
    Chronic exposure to high altitude
    Developmental abnormalities
4. Chronic thromboembolic pulmonary hypertension (CTEPH)
5. PH with unclear multifactorial mechanisms
    Hematologic disorders: myeloproliferative disorders, splenectomy
    Systemic disorders, sarcoidosis, pulmonary Langerhans cell histiocytosis,
       lymphangioleiomyomatosis, neurofibromatosis, vasculatis
    Metabolic disorders: glycogen storage disease, Gaucher disease, thyroid disorders
    Others: tumor obstruction, fibrosing mediastinitis, chronic renal failure on dialysis

In systemic lupus erythematosis (10) and mixed CTD (11), the prevalence of PAH remains unknown but likely occurs less frequently than in systemic sclerosis. In the absence of fibrotic lung disease, PAH has been reported infrequently in other CTDs.

PAH Associated with HIV Infection

PAH is a well-established complication of HIV infection. Epidemiologic data, prior to, as well as with the use of, highly active antiretroviral therapy indicate a stable prevalence of about 0.5% (12,13). HIV-associated PAH has clinical, hemodynamic, and histologic characteristics similar to those seen in IPAH.

Table 3 Updated Risk Factors and Associated Conditions for PAH

Definite	Likely	Possible	Unlikely
Aminorex	Amphetamines	Cocaine	Oral contraceptives
Fenfluramine	L-Tryptophan	Phenylpropanolamine	Estrogen
Dexfenfluramine	Methamphetamines	St. John's wort	Cigarette smoking
Toxic rapeseed oil		Chemotherapeutic agents	
		SSRIs	

A "definite" association is defined as an epidemic or large, multicenter epidemiologic studies demonstrating an association between a drug and PAH. A "likely" association is defined as a single center case control study demonstrating an association, or a multiple-case series. "Possible" is defined as drugs with similar mechanisms of action as those in the definite or likely categories, but which have not yet been studied. An "unlikely" association is defined as one in which a drug has been studied in epidemiologic studies and an association with PAH has not been demonstrated.

PAH Associated with Portopulmonary Hypertension

The development of PAH in association with elevated pressure in the portal circulation is known as portopulmonary hypertension (POPH) (14). Prospective hemodynamic studies have shown that up to 7% of patients with portal hypertension have PH (15). However, several factors, other than pulmonary vascular disease, may increase pulmonary artery pressure in the setting of advanced liver disease. These include high flow associated with the hyperdynamic circulatory state and increased pulmonary wedge pressure (PWP) due to fluid overload and/or diastolic dysfunction (14).

PAH Associated with Congenital Heart Disease

A significant proportion of patients with congenital heart disease (CHD), in particular those with relevant systemic to pulmonary shunts, will develop PAH if left untreated. Persistent exposure of the pulmonary vasculature to increased pressure and/or blood flow may result in pulmonary obstructive arteriopathy, which leads to increased pulmonary vascular resistance that will result in shunt reversal and central cyanosis: Eisenmenger syndrome (16). Approximately 8% of this population is affected by Eisenmenger syndrome, although the incidence varies according to the type of CHD (16,17). The classification of CHD with systemic to pulmonary shunts has been updated and expanded in the current classification to provide a more detailed description of each condition.

PAH Associated with Schistosomiasis

Another important modification of the new classification is the inclusion of PH associated with schistosomiasis in group 1. Recent publications indicate that PH associated with schistosomiasis can have a similar clinical presentation to IPAH (18), with similar histologic findings, including the development of plexiform lesions (19). Data from studies in which hemodynamics were measured directly indicate that up to 1% of all patients with schistosomiasis may develop PH (20).

PAH Associated with Chronic Hemolytic Anemia

The chronic hemolytic anemias represent a new subcategory of PAH. Since the Venice classification, there has been increasing evidence that PAH is a complication of chronic hereditary and acquired hemolytic anemias (21,22). PH has been described most frequently in patients with sickle cell disease (SCD) who may develop histologic lesions similar to those found in IPAH, including plexiform lesions in one case series (22). The prevalence of PAH in SCD is not clearly established but one large study, using primarily echocardiographic estimates, reported elevated systolic pulmonary artery pressure (PAP) in 32% of patients (21). A substantial proportion of SCD patients, however, have pulmonary venous hypertension; 46% in one study of patients with SCD and PH (23).

III. Group 1' : Pulmonary Veno-occlusive Disease and Pulmonary Capillary Hemangiomatosis

Pulmonary veno-occlusive disease (PVOD) and pulmonary capillary hemangiomatosis (PCH) are uncommon conditions that were placed together as a subgroup of PAH in the Venice classification. Their continued classification together is supported by a recent clinicopathologic study showing overlap of many of the pathologic findings of these two entities (24). The clinical presentation of PVOD/PCH and PAH is often indistinguishable and unrecognized antemortem, and mutations in BMPR2 have been identified in patients with PVOD (25). However, there are a number of important differences on examination, chest computed tomography, and gas exchange between patients with PAH and those with PVOD/PCH (25). In addition, the response to medical therapy and the prognosis in PVOD/PCH are worse than in PAH (25). Given the current evidence, it was decided that PVOD/PCH should be a distinct category but not completely separated from PAH, and they are designated as 1' in the Dana Point classification.

IV. Group 2: PH Due To Left-Heart Disease

PH is commonly observed in patients with left-heart disease, which represents a frequent cause of PH (26). Left-sided ventricular or valvular diseases may produce an increase of left atrial pressure (LAP), with passive backward transmission of the pressure leading to increased PAP. In this situation, PVR is normal or near normal (<3.0 Wood units), and there is no gradient between mean PAP and PWP (transpulmonary gradient <12 mmHg) (26). The subcategories of group 2 have been modified from the Venice classification and now include three distinct etiologies (Tables 1 and 2). Importantly, in some patients with left-heart disease, the elevation of PAP is out of proportion to that expected from the elevation of LAP (transpulmonary gradient >12 mmHg), and PVR is increased to >3.0 Wood units. This has been reported in 17% to 36% of patient referred to cardiac transplant centers (27,28). Some patients with left-heart valvular disease or even left-heart dysfunction can develop severe PH of the same magnitude as that seen in PAH (29).

V.   Group 3: PH Due To Lung Diseases and/or Hypoxia

The predominant cause of PH in this category is alveolar hypoxia as a result of lung disease, impaired control of breathing, or residence at high altitude. The prevalence of PH in all of these conditions remains largely unknown and is generally modest (meant PAP of 25–35 mmHg) (30). The primary modification in this group was the addition of a category of lung disease characterized by a mixed obstructive and restrictive pattern. This new subgroup includes chronic bronchiectasis, cystic fibrosis, and a newly identified syndrome characterized by the combination of pulmonary fibrosis, mainly of the lower zones of the lung, and emphysema, mainly of the upper zones of the lung, with a prevalence of PH of almost 50% (31). In a small group of patients, particularly those with only moderate pulmonary mechanical impairment, the PH is considered "out-of-proportion" to the degree of lung disease. In a recent retrospective study of 998 patients with chronic obstructive pulmonary disease who underwent right-heart catheterization, only 1% had a mean PAP >40 mmHg (32).

VI.   Group 4: Chronic Thromboembolic PH

In the Venice classification, group 4 was very heterogeneous and included obstruction of pulmonary arterial vessels by thromboemboli, tumors, or foreign bodies. Chronic thromboembolic pulmonary hypertension (CTEPH) represents a frequent cause of PH. CTEPH occurs in up to 4% of patients after an acute pulmonary embolism (33). In contrast, other obstructive etiologies are very rare. It was decided, therefore, to maintain only CTEPH in group 4. Since there is no consensus on the definition of proximal, operable disease and distal, inoperable disease (34), it was further decided to maintain only a single category of CTEPH.

VII.   Group 5: PH with Unclear or Multifactorial Etiologies

1. The first subgroup comprises several hematologic disorders. PH has been reported in myeloproliferative disorders (35) and in association with splenectomy (36).
2. The second subgroup includes systemic disorders that are associated with an increased risk of developing PH. These include Sarcoidosis in which PH has been reported in 74% in patients referred for lung transplantation (37). The severity of PH does not always correlate well with the degree of parenchymal lung disease and blood gas abnormalities (38). Other mechanisms have been reported including extrinsic compression of large pulmonary arteries by mediastinal and hilar adenopathy and direct granulomatous infiltration of the pulmonary vasculature (39). Pulmonary Langerhans cell histiocytosis is an uncommon cause of infiltrative lung disease. Severe PH is a common feature in patients with end-stage disease (40). PH has recently been reported in patients with neurofibromatosis type 1 (41). Lung fibrosis and CTEPH are thought to play a role in the development of PH in this disorder (41).

3. The third subgroup comprises metabolic disorders. PH has been reported in type 1a glycogen storage disease (42). The mechanism of PH is uncertain but has been associated with portocaval shunts, atrial septal defects, severe restrictive pulmonary defects and possibly thrombosis. PH has also been observed in Gaucher's discase (43). Several potential mechanisms for PH have been suggested, including interstitial lung disease, chronic hypoxemia, capillary plugging by Gaucher cells and splenectomy. The association between thyroid disease and PH has been reported in a number of studies (44).

4. The last subgroup in category 5 includes a number of miscellaneous conditions. Tumor obstruction has rarely been reported due, principally, to pulmonary artery sarcomas (45) and the differential diagnosis with CTEPH can be difficult. Occlusion of the microvasculature by metastatic tumor emboli represents another rare cause of rapidly progressive PH (46) often associated with marked hypoxemia. Patients with mediastinal fibrosis may present with severe PH due to compression of both pulmonary arteries and veins (47). Lastly, PH has been reported in patients with end-stage renal disease (ESRD) maintained on long-term hemodialysis. The prevalence of PH in this patient population is estimated at up to 40% by echocardiogram (48). There are several potential mechanisms including high cardiac output (resulting from the arteriovenous access itself and often concomitant anemia), fluid overload, and systolic or diastolic left-heart dysfunction (49).

VIII. Conclusion

The changes in the Dana Point classification of PH are based on new findings over the last five years, and attempts to clarify areas of ambiguity. The current classification is more comprehensive and better reflects our current understanding of the pathogenesis and treatment of the different forms of PH. We hope that this will provide better guidance in the management of this heterogenous group of disorders.

References

1. Hatano S, Strasser T. Primary pulmonary hypertension. Report on a WHO meeting, October 15–17, 1973. Geneva: WHO, 1975.
2. Simonneau G, Galie N, Rubin LJ, et al. Clinical classification of pulmonary hypertension. J Am Coll Cardiol 2004; 43:5S–12S.
3. Cogan JD, Pauciulo MW, Batchman AP, et al. High frequency of BMPR2 exonic deletions/duplications in familial pulmonary arterial hypertension. Am J Respir Crit Care Med 2006; 174: 590–598.
4. Machado RD, Aldred MA, James V, et al. Mutations of the TGF-beta type II receptor BMPR2 in pulmonary arterial hypertension. Hum Mutat 2006; 27:121–132.
5. Chin KM, Channick RN, Rubin LJ. Is methamphetamine use associated with idiopathic pulmonary arterial hypertension? Chest 2006; 130:1657–1663.
6. Chambers CD, Hernandez-Diaz S, Van Marter LJ, et al. Selective serotonin-reuptake inhibitors and risk of persistent pulmonary hypertension of the newborn. N Engl J Med 2006; 354:579–587.

7. Hachulla E, Gressin V, Guillevin L, et al. Early detection of pulmonary arterial hypertension in systemic sclerosis: a French nationwide prospective multicenter study. Arthritis Rheum 2005; 52:3792–3800.
8. Mukerjee D, St George D, Coleiro B, et al. Prevalence and outcome in systemic sclerosis associated pulmonary arterial hypertension: application of a registry approach. Ann Rheum Dis 2003; 62:1088–1093.
9. de Groote P, Gressin V, Hachulla E, et al. Evaluation of cardiac abnormalities by Doppler echocardiography in a large nationwide multicentric cohort of patients with systemic sclerosis. Ann Rheum Dis 2008; 67:31–36.
10. Tanaka E, Harigai M, Tanaka M, et al. Pulmonary hypertension in systemic lupus erythematosus: evaluation of clinical characteristics and response to immunosuppressive treatment. J Rheumatol 2002; 29:282–287.
11. Jais X, Launay D, Yaici A, et al. Immunosuppressive therapy in lupus- and mixed connective tissue disease-associated pulmonary arterial hypertension: a retrospective analysis of twenty-three cases. Arthritis Rheum 2008; 58:521–531.
12. Opravil M, Pechere M, Speich R, et al. HIV-associated primary pulmonary hypertension. A case control study. Swiss HIV cohort study. Am J Respir Crit Care Med 1997; 155:990–995.
13. Sitbon O, Lascoux-Combe C, Delfraissy JF, et al. Prevalence of HIV-related pulmonary arterial hypertension in the current antiretroviral therapy era. Am J Respir Crit Care Med 2008; 177:108–113.
14. Rodriguez-Roisin R, Krowka MJ, Herve P, et al. On behalf of the ERS Task Force Pulmonary-Hepatic Vascular Disorders Scientific Committee ERS Task Force PHD Scientific Committee. Pulmonary-hepatic vascular disorders (PHD). Eur Respir J 2004; 24:861–880.
15. Krowka MJ, Swanson KL, Frantz RP, et al. Portopulmonary hypertension: results from a 10-year screening algorithm. Hepatology 2006; 44:1502–1510.
16. Wood P. The Eisenmenger syndrome or pulmonary hypertension with reversed central shunt. I. Br Med J 1958; 2:701–709.
17. Galie N, Manes A, Palazzini M, et al. Management of pulmonary arterial hypertension associated with congenital systemic-to-pulmonary shunts and Eisenmenger's syndrome. Drugs 2008; 68:1049–1466.
18. Lapa MS, Ferreira EV, Jardim C, et al. Clinical characteristics of pulmonary hypertension patients in two reference centers in the city of Sao Paulo. Rev Assoc Med Bras 2006; 52:139–143.
19. Chaves E. The pathology of the arterial pulmonary vasculature in manson's schistosomiasis. Dis Chest 1966; 50:72–77.
20. Dias B, Lapa M, Figueiredo M, et al. Prevalence of pulmonary hypertension in hepatosplenic schistosomiasis. Am J Respir Crit Care Med 2008; 177:A443 (abstr).
21. Gladwin MT, Sachdev V, Jison ML, et al. Pulmonary hypertension as a risk factor for death in patients with sickle cell disease. N Engl J Med 2004; 350:886–895.
22. Haque AK, Gokhale S, Rampy BA, et al. Pulmonary hypertension in sickle cell hemoglobinopathy: a clinicopathologic study of 20 cases. Hum Pathol 2002; 33:1037–1043.
23. Anthi A, Machado RF, Jison ML, et al. Hemodynamic and functional assessment of patients with sickle cell disease and pulmonary hypertension. Am J Respir Crit Care Med 2007; 175:1272–1279.
24. Lantuejoul S, Sheppard MN, Corrin B, et al. Pulmonary veno-occlusive disease and pulmonary capillary hemangiomatosis: a clinicopathologic study of 35 cases. Am J Surg Pathol 2006; 30: 850–857.
25. Montani D, Achouh L, Dorfmuller P, et al. Pulmonary veno-occlusive disease: clinical, functional, radiologic, and hemodynamic characteristics and outcome of 24 cases confirmed by histology. Medicine (Baltimore) 2008; 87:220–233.

26. Oudiz RJ. Pulmonary hypertension associated with left-sided heart disease. Clin Chest Med 2007; 28:233–241.
27. Chen JM, Levin HR, Michler RE, et al. Reevaluating the significance of pulmonary hypertension before cardiac transplantation: determination of optimal thresholds and quantification of the effect of reversibility on perioperative mortality. J Thorac Cardiovasc Surg 1997; 114:627–634.
28. Delgado JF, Gomez-Sanchez MA, Saenz de la Calzada C, et al. Impact of mild pulmonary hypertension on mortality and pulmonary artery pressure profile after heart transplantation. J Heart Lung Transplant 2001; 20:942–948.
29. Braunwald E, Braunwald NS, Ross J Jr., et al. Effects of mitral-valve replacement on the pulmonary vascular dynamics of patients with pulmonary hypertension. N Engl J Med 1965; 273:509–514.
30. Weitzenblum E, Hirth C, Ducolone A, et al. Prognostic value of pulmonary artery pressure in chronic obstructive pulmonary disease. Thorax 1981; 36:752–758.
31. Cottin V, Nunes H, Brillet PY, et al. Combined pulmonary fibrosis and emphysema: a distinct underrecognised entity. Eur Respir J 2005; 26:586–593.
32. Chaouat A, Bugnet AS, Kadaoui N, et al. Severe pulmonary hypertension and chronic obstructive pulmonary disease. Am J Respir Crit Care Med 2005; 172:189–194.
33. Tapson VF, Humbert M. Incidence and prevalence of chronic thromboembolic pulmonary hypertension: from acute to chronic pulmonary embolism. Proc Am Thorac Soc 2006; 3:564–567.
34. Kim NH. Assessment of operability in chronic thromboembolic pulmonary hypertension. Proc Am Thorac Soc 2006; 3:584–588.
35. Dingli D, Utz JP, Krowka MJ, et al. Unexplained pulmonary hypertension in chronic myeloproliferative disorders. Chest 2001; 120:801–808.
36. Peacock AJ. Pulmonary hypertension after splenectomy: a consequence of loss of the splenic filter or is there something more? Thorax 2005; 60:983–984.
37. Shorr AF, Helman DL, Davies DB, et al. Pulmonary hypertension in advanced sarcoidosis: epidemiology and clinical characteristics. Eur Respir J 2005; 25:783–788.
38. Handa T, Nagai S, Miki S, et al. Incidence of pulmonary hypertension and its clinical relevance in patients with sarcoidosis. Chest 2006; 129:1246–1252.
39. Nunes H, Humbert M, Capron F, et al. Pulmonary hypertension associated with sarcoidosis: mechanisms, haemodynamics and prognosis. Thorax 2006; 61:68–74.
40. Fartoukh M, Humbert M, Capron F, et al. Severe pulmonary hypertension in histiocytosis X. Am J Respir Crit Care Med 2000; 161:216–223.
41. Samuels N, Berkman N, Milgalter E, et al. Pulmonary hypertension secondary to neurofibromatosis: intimal fibrosis versus thromboembolism. Thorax 1999; 54:858–859.
42. Humbert M, Labrune P, Sitbon O, et al. Pulmonary arterial hypertension and type-I glycogen-storage disease: the serotonin hypothesis. Eur Respir J 2002; 20:59–65.
43. Elstein D, Klutstein MW, Lahad A, et al. Echocardiographic assessment of pulmonary hypertension in Gaucher's disease. Lancet 1998; 351:1544–1546.
44. Li JH, Safford RE, Aduen JF, et al. Pulmonary hypertension and thyroid disease. Chest 2007; 132:793–797.
45. Kim HK, Choi YS, Kim K, et al. Surgical treatment for pulmonary artery sarcoma. Eur J Cardiothorac Surg 2008; 33:712–716.
46. Roberts KE, Hamele-Bena D, Saqi A, et al. Pulmonary tumor embolism: a review of the literature. Am J Med 2003; 115:228–232.
47. Davis AM, Pierson RN, Loyd JE. Mediastinal fibrosis. Semin Respir Infect 2001; 16:119–130.
48. Yigla M, Nakhoul F, Sabag A, et al. Pulmonary hypertension in patients with end-stage renal disease. Chest 2003; 123:1577–1582.
49. Nakhoul F, Yigla M, Gilman R, et al. The pathogenesis of pulmonary hypertension in haemodialysis patients via arterio-venous access. Nephrol Dial Transplant 2005; 20:1686–1692.

2

Epidemiology of Pulmonary Arterial Hypertension

MARC HUMBERT
Université Paris Sud 11, Service de Pneumologie et Réanimation Respiratoire, Hôpital Antoine Béclère, Assistance Publique Hôpitaux de Paris, Clamart, France

I. Introduction

Pulmonary arterial hypertension (PAH) is a rare disease that affects 15 to 50 subjects/ million inhabitants in the Western world (1). PAH corresponds to a group of pulmonary vascular diseases characterized by remodeling of the small pulmonary arteries leading to progressive vascular obstruction, causing breathlessness, loss of exercise capacity, and death due to elevated pulmonary artery pressure and subsequent right-heart failure (2–4). A definite diagnosis of PAH requires strict right-heart catheter criteria (2,3). PAH is defined by an elevation of the mean pulmonary artery pressure above 25 mmHg at rest without elevation of the pulmonary capillary wedge pressure (less than 15 mmHg), and elimination of frequent causes of so-called "secondary" pulmonary hypertension due to left-heart diseases, chronic hypoxia, obstructive and restrictive respiratory diseases, and chronic thromboembolic pulmonary disease (2,3).

Right-heart catheterization is a safe diagnostic tool mandatory in all patients with PAH (2,5). Less invasive tools such as cardiac echo-Doppler are of interest for screening, but one has to bear in mind that a significant proportion of patients with echocardiography parameters compatible with a diagnosis of PAH may have normal pulmonary hemodynamics and/or another condition mimicking PAH, such as left-heart diastolic dysfunction (6). This was well emphasized in a recent multicenter cross-sectional analysis of 599 patients with systemic sclerosis, where only 18 out of 33 patients with an echo-Doppler compatible with PAH had confirmation of PAH after right-heart catheterization, while 3 out of 33 had diastolic left-heart dysfunction and 12 normal or near-normal values (6). These data explain why epidemiological PAH studies should be based on gold standard confirmation of the diagnosis by means of invasive measurements.

II. The French PAH Registry

The natural history of PAH has been described in a pioneer national registry conducted in the United States in the early 1980s, where 187 patients with "primary" pulmonary hypertension (corresponding to idiopathic and familial PAH in the recent classification) were described and followed for up to five years (7,8). More recently, the French PAH Registry has collected data on PAH patients in the modern management era (5,9,10), and studied survival during a three-year follow-up. In this recent registry established in 2002 to 2003, 674 patients were included with a strict catheter diagnosis of PAH in a network of 17 university pulmonary vascular centers spread throughout the country (5).

In the French PAH Registry, the female to male sex ratio was 1.9 confirming the female predominance in most PAH subtypes, including idiopathic, familial, and PAH associated with anorexigen use, connective tissue diseases (CTD), and congenital heart diseases (5). PAH associated with portal hypertension or human immunodeficiency virus (HIV) infection was characterized by a moderate male predominance, presumably reflecting the epidemiology of portal hypertension and HIV infection in France. This registry also noted that PAH may develop at all ages, with a quarter of cases occurring after the age of 60, and that the condition may be first detected in patients in their 80s (5). The mean ($\pm$SD) age of PAH patients enrolled was 50 $\pm$ 15 years and was the same for females and males. A significant proportion of the population was older than 70 years at the time of diagnosis (9.1%). Body mass index was normal (24.4 $\pm$ 5.5 kg/m^2) and a value above 30 was observed in 14.8% of the cases, a proportion similar to that of the adult French population (5).

More than half of enrolled patients (52.6%) presented with idiopathic (39.2%), familial (3.9%), or anorexigen-associated PAH (9.5%). The remaining patients had PAH associated with another disease such as CTD, congenital heart diseases, portal hypertension, or HIV infection (Fig. 1). Of note, 29 patients (4.3%) displayed two coexisting conditions known to be associated with PAH (Fig. 1), HIV infection and portal hypertension being the most common coexisting conditions.

Idiopathic PAH corresponds to sporadic disease, without any familial history of PAH or known trigger (2–4). In the French Registry, idiopathic PAH was seen more commonly in women, with a female to male ratio of 1.6:1; the mean age at diagnosis

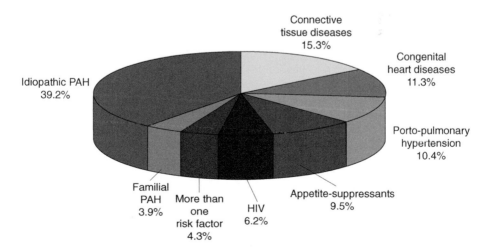

Figure 1 (*See color insert*) Distribution of patients with PAH in the 2002 to 2003 French Registry. *Abbreviations*: HIV, human immunodeficiency virus. *Source*: From Ref. 5.

was 52 years, older than in prior series (5), and 80% of patients presented with New York Heart Association (NYHA) functional class III or IV at diagnosis, a situation that has not improved since the 1980s (5,7). Familial PAH represented 3.9% of the whole population of the French Registry (5). Interestingly, familial PAH has a similar female predominance with a female to male ratio of 2.2:1, but occurs earlier than idiopathic PAH (mean age at diagnosis was 37 years) (5). Nearly 70% of familial PAH cases presented with a NYHA functional class III or IV at diagnosis (5). Germline mutations in the bone morphogenetic protein receptor 2 (*BMPR2*) gene are detected in at least 70% of familial PAH cases and *BMPR2* mutations can also be detected in 11% to 40% of apparently sporadic cases (11). Interestingly, it was recently shown that, as compared with noncarriers, *BMPR2* mutation carriers were younger at diagnosis of PAH, had worse hemodynamic parameters, shorter time to death or lung transplantation, younger age at death, but similar overall survival (11). *BMPR2* mutants were also less likely to respond to acute vasodilator challenge and by inference responded poorly to chronic calcium-channel blocker therapy (11–13).

The use of anorexigens (mainly aminorex and fenfluramine derivatives) was associated with an increased risk of PAH in Europe and North America (14–17). Interestingly, 11.4% of patients included in the French Registry in 2002 to 2003 had a history of anorexigen intake (alone or in the context of another condition known to be associated with PAH), a majority of cases being related to fenfluramine derivatives (5). This proportion was still 3% in incident cases in 2002 to 2003, more than five years after fenfluramine derivatives were withdrawn from the French market. As previously indicated by Abenhaim and colleagues (16), obesity was not a confounding factor explaining appetite-suppressant exposure in our population, as distribution of body mass index was similar in idiopathic and anorexigen-associated PAH patients, a proportion similar to that of the adult French population (5). Duration of exposure and delay between last anorexigen intake and the first symptoms of PAH varied markedly between cases, indicating that anorexigen-associated PAH could be described even after short exposures of less than three months and a long time after last anorexigen intake (5). A history of anorexigen exposure in the absence of associated conditions was found in 9.5% of patients of the registry (77% of exposure to fenfluramine derivatives). Duration of exposure to fenfluramine derivatives ranged from 1 to 300 months, 15.3% being exposed for less than 3 months, 19.4% from 3 to 6 months, 36.1% from 6 to 12 months, and 29.2% more than 12 months. Delay between last appetite suppressant intake and the first PAH symptoms was within two years of exposure in 24.2% of cases, two to five years in 32.3%, and more than five years in 43.5% (5). In this registry, anorexigen-associated PAH occurred mostly in females, with a women to men ratio of 14.9:1, a mean age of 57 years, and in NYHA functional class III or IV in 81% of cases (17). More recently, we retrospectively studied the records of all patients with the diagnosis of fenfluramine-associated PAH evaluated at our center from 1986 to 2004. This analysis indicated that fenfluramine-associated PAH shares clinical, functional, hemodynamic, and genetic features with idiopathic PAH, as well as the same overall survival (17), therefore indicating that fenfluramine exposure characterizes a potent trigger for PAH without influencing its clinical course (17).

PAH may complicate the course of CTD, such as systemic sclerosis, systemic lupus erythematosus, mixed CTD, dermatomyositis and polymyositis, primary Sjögren's syndrome, or rheumatoid arthritis (3,5). In the French Registry, 15.3% of patients had CTD, systemic sclerosis and systemic lupus erythematosus representing 76% and 15% of these cases, respectively (5). Two-thirds of systemic sclerosis patients had limited forms (5). Systemic sclerosis–associated PAH has a poor outcome and represents a leading cause of death in this patient population (18). Similarly, PAH complicating other CTD has historically had a poor prognosis (18). A recent study investigated the survival and characteristics of all patients diagnosed with CTD-associated PAH in the U.K. Pulmonary Hypertension Service between 2001 and 2006 (18). Survival in systemic sclerosis–associated PAH in the modern treatment era is better than in the historical series with one- and three-year survival rates of 78% and 47%, respectively, in patients without significant pulmonary fibrosis (18). In contrast, survival was much worse in systemic sclerosis patients with interstitial lung disease and pulmonary hypertension, with a three-year survival of 28%, highlighting the dismal prognosis of this subset of patients (18). Survival rates were better in PAH patients with systemic lupus erythematosus, mixed CTD, and dermatomyositis or polymyositis (18). PAH is a very rare complication of primary Sjögren's syndrome, since fewer than 50 cases have been reported to date (3).

In systemic sclerosis, the occurrence of PAH is known to have a major impact on outcome and survival (18). As more than 10% of patients with systemic sclerosis will develop PAH, echocardiography-based screening program is recommended (6). If such strategies are widely applied, it is likely that larger numbers of PAH will be reported, thus increasing the prevalence of this condition (see the following text). Similarly, congenital heart diseases were certainly underrepresented in the French Registry performed in pulmonary vascular centers (5). This presumably reflects the fact that these patients have a relatively stable course and are rarely referred to pulmonary vascular centers, unless they need to be listed on a lung/heart-lung transplantation program or treated with complex specific PAH therapies such as continuous intravenous epoprostenol. Thus, we assume that only a subset of patients with systemic sclerosis or congenital heart diseases with PAH were followed-up in pulmonary vascular centers in France in 2002 to 2003. The most common congenital heart diseases associated with PAH were atrial and ventricular septal defects, and patent ductus arteriosus.

In the whole cohort of PAH patients, delay between onset of symptoms and diagnosis was 27 months, and most patients had severe symptoms at presentation, with 75% in NYHA functional class III or IV (1% in class I, 24% in class II, 63% in class III, and 12% in class IV) (Fig. 2). Exercise capacity was evaluated at the time of diagnosis

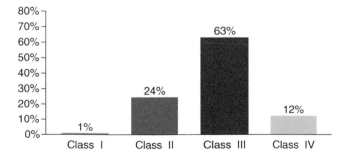

Figure 2 (*See color insert*) NYHA functional class at diagnosis in 674 patients with PAH from the French Registry. *Abbreviation*: NYHA, New York Heart Association. *Source*: From Ref. 5.

Table 1   Pulmonary Hemodynamics at Diagnosis in Patients with PAH from the French Registry

NYHA functional class	I/II	III	IV	Total
Catheter data available (%)	94	96	93	95
RAP (mmHg)	6 ± 4	9 ± 5	11 ± 7	8 ± 5
mPAP (mmHg)	51 ± 17	56 ± 15	57 ± 13	55 ± 15
Cardiac output (l/min)	5.0 ± 1.6	4.2 ± 1.4	3.5 ± 1.5	4.3 ± 1.5
SvO$_2$ (%)	67 ± 8	62 ± 8	54 ± 9	63 ± 9
TPR (Wood units)	9.5 ± 6.8	13.0 ± 6.9	16.2 ± 8.2	12.5 ± 7.3

Abbreviations: I/II, III, IV, New York Heart Association functional class I/II, III, and IV; mPAP, mean pulmonary artery pressure; RAP, right atrial pressure; SvO$_2$, mixed venous oxygen saturation; TPR, total pulmonary resistance.
Source: From Ref. 5.

through a six-minute walk test that was abnormal in most patients, as low as 60% and 55% of reference values for men and women, respectively (19). Six-minute walk distance correlated with NYHA functional class in PAH (5). Right-heart catheterization demonstrated a severe hemodynamic compromise, which correlated with clinical severity assessed by NYHA functional class (Table 1). Acute vasodilator challenge was performed either with inhaled nitric oxide (95.8%), intravenous prostacyclin (2.4%), or both (1.8%). As previously described (20,21), the rate of acute vasodilator response was low (5.8%). Acute vasodilator response was more likely in patients with idiopathic and anorexigen-associated PAH (5).

On the basis of the 674 PAH cases in our registry, the low estimate of prevalence in France is of 15.0 cases/million of adult inhabitants (5). The low estimate of prevalence for idiopathic PAH is 5.9 cases/million of inhabitants. Regional prevalence was evaluated according to the region where the patients lived. A wide range of PAH regional prevalence was observed from 5 to 25 cases/million of adult inhabitants (Fig. 3). In 2002 and 2003, the low estimate of PAH incidence was 2.4 cases/million of adult inhabitants per year. Recent studies have allowed novel estimates of the prevalence and incidence of PAH. When analyzing data from the Scottish Morbidity Record Scheme, a prevalence of 52 PAH cases/million was obtained (22). However, this number may overestimate the true prevalence of the disease, because PAH was not confirmed by right-heart catheterization in many cases (22). Conversely, it is likely that the expert data based on gold standard procedures from the reference center (Scottish Pulmonary Vascular Unit) might underestimate the true frequency of the disease. On the basis of this expert center experience, the corresponding prevalence was 26 cases/million in Scotland (22). Therefore, it is likely that the prevalence of PAH in Western Europe lies between 25 and 50/million inhabitant (1,4,22).

One-year survival exceeded 85% in the whole PAH group as well as in patients with idiopathic, familial, and anorexigen-associated PAH from the French Registry (5). Although preliminary unpublished analysis of the three-year survival of idiopathic PAH demonstrates that PAH remains a severe life-threatening condition, this one-year survival data compared favorably with the estimated one-year survival calculated with the National Institutes of Health (NIH) equation (71.8%) (8).

A U.S.-based registry from a single large referral center in Chicago established that PAH patients are also referred late to specialized centers in the United States, with

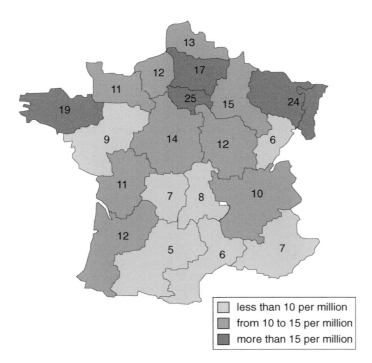

Figure 3   (*See color insert*) Regional prevalence of PAH in France in 2002 to 2003 from the French Registry. Prevalence less than 10 per million inhabitants (*light gray*). Prevalence between 10 and 15 per million (*darker gray*). Prevalence above 15 per million (*most dark area*). *Source*: From Ref. 5.

80% in NYHA class III or IV (23). This registry also emphasized that medical management is often inappropriate with an excessive use of oral calcium channel blockers in PAH patients showing no acute vasodilator response (23). Finally, it was apparent from this registry that referral of PAH patients with CTDs (mainly systemic sclerosis) was increasing, while referral of HIV-infected patients remained low (23). This latter feature is markedly different from the French Registry (5) and may indicate the under-appreciation of PAH in HIV-infected patients in the United States at the time of recruitment in this center. This single tertiary center registry may not reflect the U.S. national trends, which might be better evaluated by the REVEAL Registry (Registry to Evaluate Early and Long-term PAH Disease Management), a multicenter, observational, industry-sponsored U.S.-based registry currently enrolling patients in the United States.

III.   Screening Programs

PAH is a condition that is notoriously difficult to diagnose (2,6). In the early stages of disease, patients are generally asymptomatic. Initial symptoms, including dyspnea, exercise intolerance, and fatigue, are often rather unspectacular, and may lead patients, relatives, and physicians to assume that they are simply "out of shape." Later, the described symptoms are often attributed to a more common cardiorespiratory disease. As a result, there is commonly a substantial delay of two or more years in the diagnosis and initiation of treatment of PAH (5). Thus, early detection of PAH is still inadequate. The implementation of screening programs targeting high-risk patient groups should help in identifying patients earlier. Recent screening programs (based on cardiac echo-Doppler evaluation followed by right-heart catheterization if PAH is suspected) have demonstrated that early diagnosis of PAH is possible in patients displaying HIV infection (24), systemic sclerosis (6), and sickle cell disease (25). These screening programs have allowed diagnosis of patients with markedly lower mean pulmonary artery pressure and pulmonary vascular resistance, as compared with patients diagnosed with symptomatic PAH (5–8,24,25).

These screening programs have also demonstrated that left-heart disease is common in some patient populations at risk of PAH, emphasizing the importance of a complete evaluation including right-heart catheterization to properly distinguish patients with precapillary from those with postcapillary pulmonary hypertension (6,25). For instance, in a prospective multicenter study of 599 patients with systemic sclerosis, PAH was confirmed in 8%, while left-ventricle diastolic dysfunction was found in 18% (6,26). In this study, approximately 10% of systemic sclerosis patients with peak velocity of tricuspid regurgitation greater than 2.5 m/sec had evidence of diastolic left-heart dysfunction and postcapillary pulmonary hypertension (6). Systemic sclerosis patients from this study were followed for a median duration of 37 months, representing 1547 patient-years (27). In total, 47 patients died, giving a three-year survival of 91.1% and cumulative mortality of 3.04 deaths per 100 patient-years; 17 deaths (32.2%) resulted from PAH and 8 (17.1%) from cancer. Of 47 patients with PAH at baseline, 20 died during follow-up, giving a three-year survival of 56.3%. In a multivariate analysis, PAH [hazard ratio (HR) 7.246], age at first symptom (HR 1.052), duration of systemic sclerosis (HR 1.047/yr), and Rodnan skin score (HR 1.045) were associated with increased mortality (27). In the same cohort, 384 patients were followed for a mean duration of 41.03 ± 5.66 months to estimate the incidence of PAH in this patient population with no evidence for PAH at baseline (28). Patients with suspected PAH due to a velocity of tricuspid regurgitation 2.8 to 3.0 m/sec and unexplained dyspnea, or >3.0 m/sec underwent right-heart catheterization to confirm diagnosis. PAH was diagnosed in eight patients, postcapillary pulmonary hypertension due to diastolic left-heart disease in eight patients, and pulmonary hypertension due to rapidly progressive severe pulmonary fibrosis in two patients (28). The incidence of PAH was estimated to be 0.61 cases per 100 patient-years, and the possible occurrence of postcapillary pulmonary hypertension further highlighted the value of right-heart catheterization in investigating suspected PAH (28).

Hemodynamics and cardiopulmonary function was recently described in 43 patients with sickle cell disease, including 26 patients with a mean pulmonary artery pressure of 25 mmHg or greater (pulmonary hypertension group) (29). Upon catheterization, 54% of the patients with pulmonary hypertension had PAH, while 46% had postcapillary pulmonary hypertension (29). Thus, evaluating the mechanisms of pulmonary hypertension in patients with sickle cell disease also requires a complete evaluation, including right-heart catheterization. In sickle cell patients with PAH, mean pulmonary artery pressure was moderately elevated, and the cardiac output was high, contrasting to what is usually found in idiopathic PAH (5). Further investigation is warranted to assess the potential benefits and risks of using PAH-specific therapies in sickle cell disease–related pulmonary hypertension (29).

IV. PAH in Developing Countries

Pulmonary hypertension is certainly much more prevalent than reported in developing countries where relatively common diseases such as schistosomiasis, sickle cell disease, HIV infection, liver cirrhosis, and others including autoimmune and congenital heart diseases may trigger pulmonary vascular disease (1,3,30,31). In addition, hypoxia is a major risk factor for pulmonary hypertension with more than 140 million individuals living above 2500 m worldwide, including 80 millions in Asia and 35 millions in South America (32). Of note, chronic mountain sickness is a public health problem in the Andean mountains and other mountainous regions around the world (30–32). Improving awareness, diagnosis, prevention, and treatment of pulmonary hypertension in developing countries are currently supported by a WHO program of the Global Alliance Against Chronic Respiratory Diseases (GARD) (33). Pulmonary hypertension is now being formally studied in developing countries such as China and Brazil (31,33–35).

V. Conclusion: The Global Burden of Pulmonary Hypertension

It remains widely believed that pulmonary hypertension is a rare condition (1). Although true for PAH (1,5,7,22,23), the global burden of pulmonary hypertension as a whole is currently unknown and largely underestimated. In the developing world, highly prevalent diseases such as schistosomiasis in parts of South America, Asia, and Africa, or sickle cell disease in populations of African origin are associated with a marked risk of pulmonary hypertension (31). In addition, hypoxia is a major worldwide risk factor for pulmonary hypertension (32,36). Last, up to 4% of all patients with acute pulmonary embolism may develop chronic thromboembolic disease and pulmonary hypertension (37–40). Altogether pulmonary hypertension is certainly underestimated both in developing and in developed countries, and further well-designed studies are mandatory to better approach the burden of the disease in populations exposed to different risk factors (1).

References

1. Humbert M. The burden of pulmonary hypertension. Eur Respir J 2007; 30:1–2.
2. Runo JR, Loyd JE. Primary pulmonary hypertension. Lancet 2003; 361:1533–1544.
3. Simonneau G, Galie N, Rubin LJ, et al. Clinical classification of pulmonary hypertension. J Am Coll Cardiol 2004; 43:5S–12S.
4. Chin KM, Rubin LJ. Pulmonary arterial hypertension. J Am Coll Cardiol 2008; 51: 1527–1538.
5. Humbert M, Sitbon O, Chaouat A, et al. Pulmonary arterial hypertension in France: results from a national registry. Am J Respir Crit Care Med 2006; 173:1023–1030.
6. Hachulla E, Gressin V, Guillevin L, et al. Early detection of pulmonary arterial hypertension in systemic sclerosis: a French nationwide prospective multicenter study. Arthritis Rheum 2005; 52:3792–3800.

7. Rich S, Danzker DR, Ayres SM, et al. Primary pulmonary hypertension: a national prospective study. Ann Int Med 1987; 107:216–223.
8. D'Alonzo GE, Barst RJ, Ayres SM, et al. Survival in patients with primary pulmonary hypertension. Ann Int Med 1991; 115:343–349.
9. Humbert M, Sitbon O, Simonneau G. Treatment of pulmonary arterial hypertension. N Engl J Med 2004; 351:1425–1436.
10. Barst RJ, Mc Goon M, Torbicki A, et al. Diagnosis and differential assessment of pulmonary arterial hypertension. J Am Coll Cardiol 2004; 43:40S–47S.
11. Sztrymf B, Coulet F, Girerd B, et al. Clinical outcomes of pulmonary arterial hypertension in carriers of BMPR2 mutation. Am J Respir Crit Care Med 2008; 177:1377–1383.
12. Sztrymf B, Yaïci A, Girerd B, et al. Genes and pulmonary arterial hypertension. Respiration 2007; 74:123–132.
13. Elliott CG, Glissmeyer EW, Havlena GT, et al. Relationship of *BMPR2* mutations to vasoreactivity in pulmonary arterial hypertension. Circulation 2006; 113:2509–2515.
14. Gurtner HP. Pulmonary hypertension, (plexogenic pulmonary arteriopathy) and the appetite depressant drug aminorex: post or propter? Bull Eur Physiopathol Respir 1979; 15:897–923.
15. Simonneau G, Fartoukh M, Sitbon O, et al. Primary pulmonary hypertension associated with the use of fenfluramine derivatives. Chest 1998; 114:195S–199S.
16. Abenhaim L, Moride Y, Brenot F, et al. Appetite-suppressant drugs and the risk of primary pulmonary hypertension. N Engl J Med 1996; 335:609–616.
17. Souza R, Humbert M, Sztrymf B, et al. Pulmonary arterial hypertension associated with fenfluramine exposure: report of 109 cases. Eur Respir J 2008; 31:343–348.
18. Condliffe R, Kiely DG, Peacock AJ, et al. Connective tissue disease-associated pulmonary arterial hypertension in the modern treatment era. Am J Respir Crit Care Med 2009; 179: 151–157.
19. Enright PL, Sherrill DL. Reference equations for the six-minute walk in healthy adults. Am J Respir Crit Care Med 1998; 158:1384–1387.
20. Sitbon O, Humbert M, Jagot JL, et al. Inhaled nitric oxide as a screening agent for safely identifying responders to oral calcium-channel blockers in primary pulmonary hypertension. Eur Respir J 1998; 12:265–270.
21. Sitbon O, Humbert M, Jais X, et al. Long-term response to calcium-channel blockers in idiopathic pulmonary arterial hypertension. Circulation 2005; 111:3105–3111.
22. Peacock A, Murphy NF, McMurray JJV, et al. An epidemiological study of pulmonary arterial hypertension in Scotland. Eur Respir J 2007; 30:104–109.
23. Thenappan T, Shah SJ, Rich S, et al. A USA-based registry for pulmonary arterial hypertension: 1982 to 2006. Eur Respir J 2007; 30:1103–1110.
24. Sitbon O, Lascoux-Combe C, Delfraissy JF, et al. Prevalence of HIV-related pulmonary arterial hypertension in the current antiretroviral therapy era. Am J Respir Crit Care Med 2008; 177:108–113.
25. Gladwin MT, Sachdev V, Jison ML, et al. Pulmonary hypertension as a risk of death in patients with sickle cell disease. N Engl J Med 2004; 350:886–895.
26. de Groote P, Gressin V, Hachulla E, et al. Evaluation of cardiac abnormalities by Doppler echocardiography in a large nationwide multicentric cohort of patients with systemic sclerosis. Ann Rheum Dis 2008; 67:31–36.
27. Hachulla E, Carpentier P, Gressin V, et al. Risk factors for death and the 3-year survival of patients with systemic sclerosis: the French ItinerAIR-Sclerodermie study. Rheumatology (Oxford) 2009; 48:304–308.
28. Hachulla E, de Groote P, Gressin V, et al. The 3-year incidence of pulmonary arterial hypertension associated with systemic sclerosis in a multicenter nationwide longitudinal study (ItinérAIR-Sclérodermie Study). Arthritis Rheum 2009; 60:1831–1839.

29. Anthi A, Machado RF, Jison ML, et al. Hemodynamic and functional assessment of patients with sickle cell disease and pulmonary hypertension. Am J Respir Crit Care Med 2007; 175: 1272–1279.
30. Humbert M, Khaltaev N, Bousquet J, et al. Pulmonary hypertension: from an orphan disease to a public health problem. Chest 2007; 132:365–367.
31. Lapa M, Dias B, Jardim C, et al. Cardio-pulmonary manifestations of hepatosplenic schistosomiasis. Circulation 2009; 119:1518–1523.
32. Penaloza D, Arias-Stella J. The heart and pulmonary circulation at high altitudes: healthy highlanders and chronic mountain sickness. Circulation 2007; 115:1132–1146.
33. Bousquet J, Dahl R, Khaltaev N. Global alliance against chronic respiratory diseases. Allergy 2007; 62:216–222.
34. Jing ZC, Xu XQ, Han ZY, et al. Registry and survival study in Chinese patients with idiopathic and familial pulmonary arterial hypertension. Chest 2007; 132:373–379.
35. Souza R, Jardim C, Carvalho C. The need for national registries in rare diseases. Am J Respir Crit Care Med 2006; 174:228.
36. Chaouat A, Naeije R, Weitzenblum E. Pulmonary hypertension in COPD. Eur Respir J 2008; 32:1371–1385.
37. Fedullo PF, Auger WR, Kerr KM, et al. Chronic thromboembolic pulmonary hypertension. N Engl J Med 2001; 345:1465–1472.
38. Pengo V, Lensing AW, Prins MH, et al. Incidence of chronic thromboembolic pulmonary hypertension after pulmonary embolism. N Engl J Med 2004; 350:2257–2264.
39. Hoeper MM, Mayer E, Simonneau G, et al. Chronic thromboembolic pulmonary hypertension. Circulation 2006; 113:2011–2020.
40. Tapson VF, Humbert M. Incidence and prevalence of chronic thromboembolic pulmonary hypertension: from acute to chronic pulmonary embolism. Proc Am Thorac Soc 2006; 3: 564–567.

3
Pathology of Pulmonary Hypertension

PETER DORFMÜLLER
Université Paris Sud 11, Service de Pneumologie et Réanimation Respiratoire, Hôpital Antoine Béclère, Assistance Publique Hôpitaux de Paris, Clamart, France

I. Vascular Lesions In Pulmonary Hypertension—Overview

Vascular lesions found in lungs of patients suffering from pulmonary hypertension (PH) are classically considered as responsible for the increase of pulmonary arterial pressures and share some characteristic peculiarities, but should not be regarded as specific or even pathognomonic. These fibrotic and proliferative lesions concern the small lung vessels; arterial lesions are typically located in muscular arteries of less than 500 μm diameter in patients with pulmonary arterial hypertension (PAH), while septal veins and preseptal venules are affected in patients with pulmonary veno-occlusive disease (PVOD). And finally the exceptional entity known as pulmonary capillary hemangiomatosis (PCH) concerns alveolar septal capillaries within the lung parenchyma. Previously integrated into the group 1 of PH during the consensus meeting in Venice in 2003, the latter two entities were assigned to a novel category of pulmonary venous hypertension (group 1') after the World Symposium in Dana Point, California, in 2008 (1) (Gérald Simonneau, personal communication).

II. Pathological Anatomy of PH—the Descriptive Work in Time

PH due to pulmonary arterial "sclerosis" was described for the first time in 1891 by Ernst von Romberg, a German internal medicine physician (2). After several case reports, Dresdale and colleagues in 1951 published clinical and hemodynamic data of 39 patients displaying severe precapillary PH of unknown cause and the term primary pulmonary hypertension was coined (3). The first histological classification of hypertensive pulmonary vascular disease among patients with congenital heart disease was proposed by Heath and Edwards in 1958 (4). The grading relies on six grades of "severity": The authors designated arterial muscular hypertrophy, arteriolar muscularization, and subintimal fibrosis into a category of potentially reversible lesions, whereas angiomatoid lesions, plexiform lesions, and necrotizing arteritis were considered irreversible. However, this classification addressed a subgroup of patients with PH and included some peculiarities, e.g., necrotizing arteritis, a lesion uncommon in other forms of PH. In 1970, the pathologists Wagenvoort and Wagenvoort retrospectively examined histological material from 156 patients from 51 medical centers with a diagnosis of primary PH (5). In 1973, the World Health Organization (WHO) presented a first definition of the disease, which relied on morphological and etiological criteria (6). Over the next decade, a few retrospective studies were published, comprising a limited number of patients. In 1987, the National Institutes of Health (NIH) initiated a large prospective study (American National Register) to better understand the epidemiology, pathogenesis, and possible therapy of this disease (7). In 1997, Pietra proposed a revised histological classification, roughly based on the observations made by Wagenvoort and Wagenvoort (8). This assessment of typical pathological lesions in PH was the foundation for expert meetings within the pathobiology group during three world symposia held in Evian (France, 1998), Venice (Italy, 2003), and Dana Point (United States, 2008) (findings are discussed later in this chapter).

III. PH and Its Correlate In Histopathology—Snapshots in Disease Evolution

The pathobiology of PH will be addressed in the appropriate chapters elsewhere in this book, but a few remarks on the pondering question of what all this diversity of vascular lesions has to mean should be made. The descriptive approach to pulmonary arteries in PAH and their histological phenotype is based on the different vascular compartments affected and different cell types involved in this pathological anatomy. As we lack longitudinal temporal information of histological changes in most cases, observations and hypotheses are based on transversal time points of different subjects. In addition, most PAH cases are diagnosed initially on clinical grounds; histological confirmation is often achieved preterminally via analysis of the lung explants at the time of lung transplantation (best case scenario) or by autopsy (worse case). In the actual diagnostic setting, lung biopsy is contraindicated for the vast majority of patients suffering from PAH and so the morphological correlate will be a tardy one, possibly skipping important levels of disease evolution.

A. Arterial Lesions

As mentioned in the introduction, characteristic arterial lesions in lungs of patients with PAH do not involve the larger pulmonary arteries of the elastic type; intimal and medial lesions on this level may be found in patients with chronically increased pulmonary arterial pressures, but mainly correspond to nonobstructing atherosclerotic lesions as are typically found in the systemic vasculature (8). Typical obliterating PAH lesions are found in pre- and intra-acinar arteries with a muscular medial layer. Different vessel wall compartments may contribute to the thickening of the arterial wall, and hence various histological patterns may occur (presented below).

Isolated Medial Hypertrophy

This abnormality of the vessel wall can be observed in all subgroups of PAH and may even be encountered in other forms of PH, e.g., mitral valve stenosis. The lesion corresponds to a proliferation of smooth muscle cells within the tunica media. The

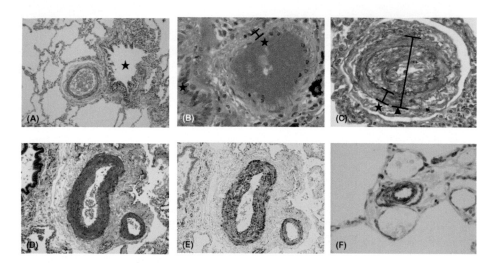

Figure 1   (*See color insert*) Remodelling of the media with proliferation of smooth muscle-cells in pulmonary arteries and arterioles of patients suffering from IPAH and controls. (**A**) Normal muscular pulmonary artery with adjacent bronchiole (asterisk) lacking any signs of remodelling. WHPS (Weigert-Hematoxylin-Phloxin-Saffron) staining, magnification ×40. (**B**) Unaffected, slender medial layer in a congestive pulmonary artery (asterisk). WHPS staining, magnification ×200. (**C**) Medial hypertrophy (and intimal thickening) of a pulmonary artery: the medial thickness is defined as the distance between internal and external elastic lamina (asterisk). Medial hypertrophy is defined as the exceeding of 10 per cent of the arterial cross-sectional diameter (triangle). WHPS staining, magnification ×200. (**D**) Pulmonary artery and a smaller branch, both with hypertrophy of the tunica media, WHPS staining, magnification ×100. (**E**) Same arteries after immunohistochemical reaction with an antibody directed against smooth muscle cell actin highlighting the tunica media. Magnification ×100. (**F**) Muscularized arteriole (<100 µm) with anti-smooth muscle cell actin staining. Magnification ×200.

histological criterion of medial hypertrophy (which corresponds more precisely to hypertrophy and hyperplasia, i.e., increase in volume and number of smooth muscle cells, respectively) is fulfilled when the diameter of a single medial layer, delineated by its internal and external elastic lamina, exceeds 10% of the artery's cross-sectional diameter. Isolated hypertrophy of the medial layer may be considered as an early and even reversible event, as has been shown for PH due to hypoxia at high altitude (9). However, medial hypertrophy is usually associated with other PAH lesions (Fig. 1).

Analogy and Significance: Medial Hypertrophy Is Reversible in High-Altitude PH

It is widely accepted that an early phase of pulmonary arterial pressure elevation in PAH patients is reflected by the thickening of the medial layer by hyperplasia and hypertrophy of smooth muscle cells. This process is present in reversible forms of PH, e.g., high-altitude PH and chronic mountain sickness. In a recent study and review of the literature, Penaloza and Arias-Stella noted that healthy natives of high-altitude regions over 3500 m above sea level have PH, right ventricular hypertrophy, and increased amount of smooth muscle cells in the distal pulmonary arterial branches (10). These investigators examined clinical and histological findings from 30 healthy high-altitude natives and 30 sea level natives. The main factor responsible for PH in healthy high-landers is the increased amount of smooth muscle cells in the distal pulmonary arteries and arterioles, which increases pulmonary vascular resistance. Vasoconstriction is a secondary factor because the administration of oxygen decreases the pulmonary arterial pressure only by 15% to 20%. This adaptive increase in cardiac and smooth muscle cell mass reverses after a prolonged residence at sea level (10).

Concentric and Eccentric Nonlaminar Intimal Fibrosis

Fibrotic lesions of the intimal layer are frequent in PAH-diseased lungs. The intima may be thickened by proliferation and recruitment of fibroblasts, myofibroblasts and other connective tissue cells, and consequently by the interstitial deposition of collagen. In a purely descriptive approach, this thickening may be uniform and concentric, or focally predominating and eccentric. Both forms can lead to a complete occlusion of the artery. In fact, the eccentric intimal thickening is frequently observed in cases with thrombotic events and probably represents residues of wall-adherent, organized thrombi. Thrombotic lesions, or so-called in situ thrombosis, are a frequent pattern in different PAH subgroups: Organization and recanalization of totally occluding thrombotic material may lead to bizarre, fibrotic multichannel lesions (so-called "colander-like" lesions), which can easily be confounded with proliferative complex lesions (see the following text). Nonetheless, thrombotic or thromboembolic events are not a necessary precondition of intimal fibrosis; the gain in intimal cellularity is generally understood as a reaction of the inner arterial layer to a luminal stimulus, e.g., chronic pressure and shear stress (11). In many cases, adventitial fibrosis is associated with intimal changes, but remains difficult to evaluate due to the lack of a clear anatomical delimitation (Fig. 2).

Concentric Laminar Intimal Fibrosis

This morphologically conspicuous phenotype of intimal fibrosis is also known as "onion-skin" or "onion-bulb" lesion. Numerous concentrically arranged fibrotic layers occlude the arterial lumen of small (diameter: 100–200 µm) arteries. The scary, cell-lacking morphology of this lesion may be found in lungs of patients suffering from all different forms of PAH, including PAH associated with connective tissue disease (12). Nevertheless, the observation that intimal thickening proximal to plexiform lesions in supernumerary arteries usually displays a concentric laminar phenotype seems to closely associate these two lesions. Immunohistochemical analysis reveals fibroblasts, myofibroblasts, and smooth muscle cells (Fig. 3).

Analogy and Significance: Intimal Fibrosis in Idiopathic Spontaneous Pneumothorax and Idiopathic Pulmonary Fibrosis

As mentioned earlier, intimal thickening with concentric laminar and/or nonlaminar fibrosis is a striking abnormality and a regular feature in severe forms of PAH. Interestingly, alterations of the tunica intima, which physiologically consists of a single endothelial layer and a basal membrane, can be observed in other pulmonary diseases without PH. Cyr and coworkers described medial and intimal thickening in 20 cases of

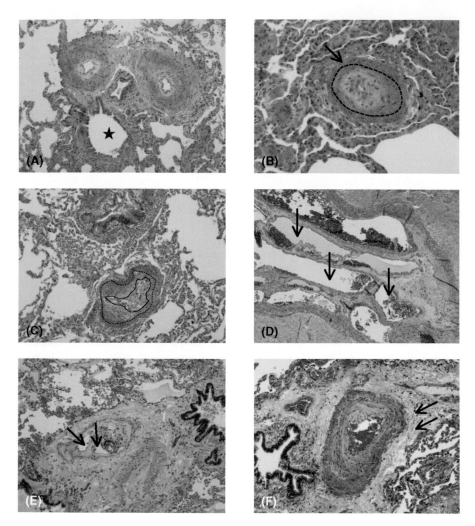

Figure 2   (*See color insert*) Concentric and eccentric remodelling, thrombotic lesions and adventitial fibrosis in pulmonary arteries of patients suffering from IPAH. (**A**) Pulmonary artery (2 branches) and their adjacent bronchiole (asterisk): the arterial lumina are narrowed by intimal concentric non-laminar fibrosis. HES (Hematoxylin-Eosin-Saffron) staining, magnification ×40 (**B**) Another artery with intimal concentric non-laminar fibrosis. The internal elastic lamina (iel, dashed line) delimits the inner boundary of the medial layer and emphasizes the extensive intimal thickening, as compared to the discrete medial hypertrophy (arrow). HES staining, magnification ×100. (**C**) Pulmonary artery with eccentric intimal fibrosis: note the uneven thickening of the intimal layer, which is delimited by the internal elastic lamina (dashed line) and by the lumen (continuous line). HES staining, magnification ×40. (**D**) Large pulmonary artery with remodeled thrombus/embolus in a patient with thromb-embolic disease: note the wide lumina of newly developed vessels within the occlusion (arrows) in an attempt to recanalize the obstructed artery. WHPS staining, magnification ×40. (**E**) Small pulmonary artery with thrombotic lesion, or "colander lesion" in a patient with IPAH: same recanalization phenomenon (arrows) leading sometimes to confusion with plexiform lesions (see beneath). WHPS staining, magnification ×40. (**F**) Pulmonary artery with occluding intimal fibrosis and associated excessive adventitial fibrosis (arrows). WHPS staining, magnification ×40.

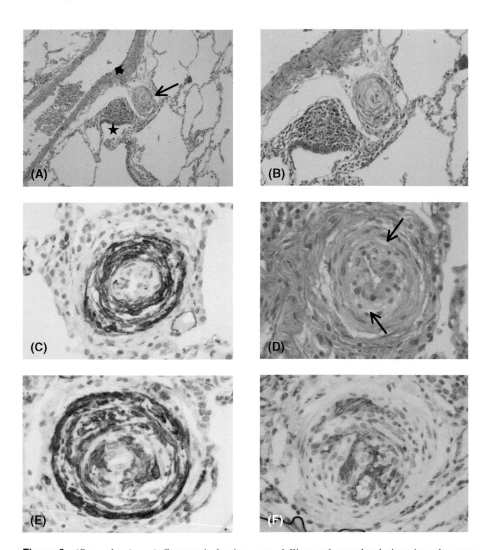

Figure 3 (*See color insert*) Concentric laminar remodelling and complex lesions in pulmonary arteries of patients suffering from IPAH. (**A**) Longitudinally sectioned larger pulmonary artery (arrowhead) with small branch displaying concentric laminar fibrosis (arrow) and adjacent bronchiole (asterisk). HES staining, magnification ×40. (**B**) Magnification of same arterial lesion: note the concentric and laminar arrangement of fibrous layers with a decrease of cellular density in the periphery of the lesion. HES staining, magnification ×100. (**C**) Smooth muscle cell staining in a concentric laminar fibrosis: smooth muscle elements are present within this intimal lesion. Note negativity of the inner, endothelial layer. Magnification ×200. (**D**) Concentric laminar "onion-skin" lesion with near arterial occlusion. This lesion was adjacent to a plexiform lesion and small channels within the occlusion are faintly perceivable (arrows). HES staining, magnification ×200. (**E**) Same lesion after immunohistochemical reaction with an antibody directed against smooth muscle cell actin. Note negativity of the mentioned channels. Magnification ×200. (**F**) Same lesion after immunohistochemical reaction with an antibody directed against endothelial cells. Note the staining of endothelium-lined channels within the occlusion, probably the "beginning" of a plexiform lesion. Magnification ×200.

idiopathic spontaneous pneumothorax. They identified pulmonary vasculopathy in 18 out of 20 cases (90%). The most frequent lesion was intimal fibrosis of the small pulmonary arteries and veins. In 6 cases (30%), pulmonary arterial intimal fibrosis was graded as severe because the mean intimal thickness exceeded 20% of the internal diameter (distance from one elastic internal lamina to the diametrically opposite elastic internal lamina). In 19 cases (95%), the lungs revealed some histological features of fibrosis and chronic inflammation, with a significant positive correlation between mean pulmonary artery medial thickness and lung fibrosis/chronic inflammation scores, linking arterial remodeling and inflammatory activity in the absence of elevated pulmonary arterial pressures (13).

Another frequent lung disease combining alterations of different vascular compartments is idiopathic pulmonary fibrosis (IPF) (synonym: usual interstitial pneumonia). This condition is marked by interstitial collagen deposition and so-called fibroblastic foci, probably the stigma of an ongoing aggressive fibrosing process. Moreover, interstitial smooth muscle proliferation may be observed. Typically, fibrotic remodeled areas within the pulmonary parenchyma closely alternate with unremodeled areas in a patchy pattern. Pulmonary arterial adventitial thickening can be seen and is due to an increase of fibroblasts, myofibroblasts, and extracellular matrix deposition. Smooth muscle cell hypertrophy and proliferation and collagen accumulation occur in the media of the small muscular pulmonary arteries, and distal pulmonary arterioles become muscularized. In addition, there may be extensive intimal hyperplasia, fibrosis, and reduplication of the inner elastic lamina in the small muscular pulmonary arteries in IPF (14). Vascular changes may occur in unaffected parenchyma but are more consistently confined to the patchy fibrotic areas, frequently displaying inflammatory pattern with lymphocytic infiltration. However, PH in those patients is only present in 20% to 40% before lung transplantation, hence in a terminal phase. This lack of correlation between quality of vascular lesions and hemodynamic changes could be explained by the typical persistence of nonfibrotic areas in IPF: it underscores that the installation of high pulmonary arterial pressures probably requires a more or less constant fraction of obstructed lung vessels, or in other words a threshold in vascular overall-diameter reduction. Recently, Colombat and coworkers documented intimal proliferation and fibrosis in the pulmonary veins and venules of patients with IPF. Arterial lesions and occlusive veins were observed in fibrotic areas but venular lesions were equally present in architecturally preserved lung zones in 65% of the patients, compared with only mild changes of muscular pulmonary arteries in normal areas (15). Interestingly, the authors found a significant positive correlation between the macroscopic extent of lung fibrosis and mean pulmonary artery pressure, supporting the concept of a quantitative threshold in arterial obstruction leading to relevant PH (Fig. 4A–D).

Complex Lesions

The pathological classification of the World Symposium meeting in Venice comprises three lesion entities:

- The *plexiform lesion* probably represents the most illustrious form of vascular lesions in PAH: it was considered for a long time as a pathognomonic pattern of idiopathic PAH (formerly known as primary PH) (5). Hitherto, this

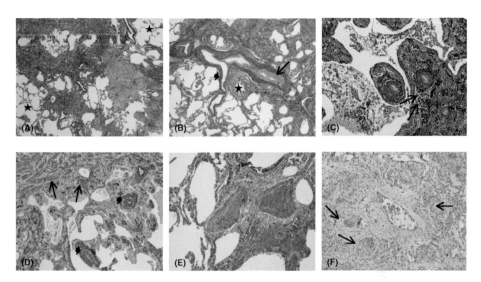

Figure 4 (*See color insert*) Pulmonary vascular lesions in other pathologies of the lung. (**A**) Histological aspect of lungs from a patient with interstitial pulmonary fibrosis (IPF). Note the patchy distribution of parenchymal fibrotic lesions with alternating unaffected parenchyma (asterisks). Elastica van Gieson staining (EvG), magnification ×20. (**B**) Transition zone between diseased and preserved pulmonary parenchyma. Note the pulmonary artery and the adjacent bronchiole (asterisk): Arterial intimal thickening is present within the zone of IPF typical parenchymal remodelling (arrow), while absent in the arterial branch leaving the main artery into the preserved area (arrowhead). EvG staining, magnification ×20. (**C**) Small pulmonary arteries of the same lung displaying concentric intimal fibrosis. Note the close association to inflammatory cells mainly consisting of lymphocytes (arrows). EvG staining, magnification ×40. (**D**) Same lung with smooth muscle actin staining: Smooth muscle cell hyperplasia is present in a remodeled arteries (arrowheads) and in the pulmonary inter-stitium (arrows). Magnification ×20. (**E**) Pulmonary arteries in a lung resection specimen of a patient with spontaneous idiopathic pneumothorax: intimal thickening is present in the absence of pulmonary hypertension. HES staining, magnification ×40. (**F**) Pulmonary arterial remodeling in a patient with pulmonary hypertension associated with sarcoidosis. The arterial wall displays intense inflammatory infiltrate and numerous epitheloid granulomas with giant cells (arrows), narrowing the arterial lumen considerably. CD68 (macrophages) stain, magnification ×40.

presumption has been revised, as plexiform lesions have been shown to occur in other PAH subgroups like congenital heart disease-associated PAH or porto-PH. The peculiar lesion affects various vascular compartments: A focal intimal thickening of small pulmonary arteries, preferably beyond branching points, is followed by an exuberant endothelial cell proliferation, leading to the formation of capillary-like sinusoidal channels on a smooth muscle cell and collagen-rich matrix within the native arterial lumen and resulting in obstruction (1,16). This glomerular-like arterial zone feeds into dilated vein-like congestive vessels, which are perceivable at low magnification and may be helpful as sentinel lesions when tracing plexiform lesions.

- The latter vein-like congestive pulmonary vessels, also known as *dilation lesions*, may predominate the histological pattern, but are most frequently associated with plexiform lesions. Pulmonary hemorrhage in PAH patients could be a consequence of the unstable aneurysm-like vessel wall structure.

- Classical *arteritis* with transmural inflammation and fibrinoid necrosis, as first described by Heath and Edwards, has become a rather infrequent phenomenon in PAH, possibly due to the prolonged survival of patients (4). Nevertheless, perivascular inflammatory infiltrates of diseased pulmonary arteries in PAH patients can be found regularly. Infiltrates mainly consisting of T lymphocytes and macrophages, as well as scattered mast cells are frequently associated with plexiform or other intimal lesions. This inflammatory phenotype, in most cases, is evaluated as "mild" to "moderate" (Figs. 3 and 5).

Analogy and Significance: Plexiform Lesions—an Intriguing Phenomenon and Still a Matter of Interpretation

The complex lesion is generally regarded as a peculiar, if not unique, lesion occurring in PAH. It was first described in patients with congenital cardiac left to right shunts (4), and eventually in other forms of PAH, all belonging to the group 1 of the Venice and Dana Point classification. In a 1993 publication (17), plexiform lesions were detected in 20 out of 31 patients with confirmed chronic major vessel thrombembolic PH, suggesting a possible relation between organizing thrombembolic and complex lesions, which mirrors an old theory first inspired by Harrison in 1958 (18). Another historic hypothesis explaining the pathogenesis of the glomerular-like exuberant endothelial cell proliferation within the affected pulmonary artery is the formation of arteriovenous shunts (19). Wagenvoort and Wagenvoort explained the generation of plexiform lesions in cardiac left to right shunting by an increased blood flow eliciting reflective vaso-constriction with subsequent development of endothelial alteration (5). More interestingly, they speculated that vascular necrosis with arteritis might result from intense vasospasm, as seen in the systemic circulation. The pathogenetic plot, here, is that plexiform lesions develop in the focal areas of fibrinoid necrosis by active cellular reorganization and recanalization of the thrombus composed of fibrin and platelets, usually present in this setting and observed within plexiform lesions. In fact, the only animal model leading to obvious plexiform lesions was achieved by producing necrosis of pulmonary arterioles in dogs after two weeks of severe PH due to the creation of a shunt between pulmonary and systemic circulations (20). This explanation would take into consideration that elements of inflammation are consistently present in the range of plexiform and other vascular lesions in PAH (21,22). On the other hand, Tuder and coworkers have proposed a neoplastic approach to the hardly understandable proliferation of intraluminal neovessels at the core of plexiform lesions: they found that a large proportion of the endothelial cells in this area show monoclonality, raising the question of possible tumor-like growth (23). These different observations of arterial wall alteration within plexiform lesions are probably connected in a temporary line. However, they could feed into a broader concept of pathogenesis, first mentioned by Wagenvoort, but interestingly developed by Yaginuma and coworkers (24). They submitted histological data from 11 patients with PH due to congenital heart disease to a computer-based three-dimensional image reconstruction and found that plexiform lesions mostly occurred in supernumerary arteries branching apart from larger pulmonary arteries,

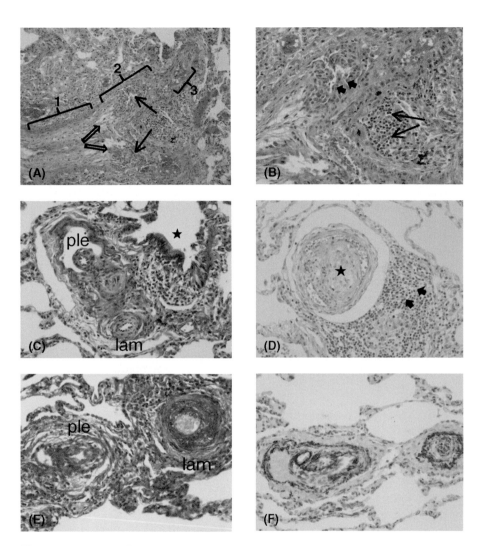

Figure 5 (*See color insert*) Complex lesions in pulmonary arteries of patients suffering from IPAH. (**A**) Branching point of a pulmonary artery (bold arrows) with 2 complex lesions developing on each of the successive branches (arrows). Typical constellation with 3 segments: 1 = intimal thickening; 2 = plexiform lesion with exuberant endothelial cell proliferation; 3 = dilation lesion. HES staining, magnification ×40. (**B**) Magnification of the upper plexiform lesion (arrowheads): note the perivascular lymphocytic infiltrate at the arterial bifurcation (arrows). HES staining, magnification ×100. (**C**) Another small "developing" plexiform lesion forming sinusoidal channels within the original arterial lumen (ple). Note the regular association with concentric laminar intimal thickening (lam). WHPS staining, magnification ×100. (**D**) Fibrous, scarred aspect of a plexiform lesion (asterisk) surrounded by inflammatory, round cells, corresponding to lymphocytes (arrowheads). HES staining, magnification ×100. (**E**) Close association of a plexiform and a concentric laminar intimal lesion. WHPS staining, magnification ×100. (**F**) Same lesions with smooth muscle cell staining: smooth muscle cells/myofibroblasts nicely highlight the remodelling process in both lesions. Magnification ×100.

proximal to arterial lesions with intimal fibrosis and medial hypertrophy. They also gathered evidence for generation of indirect anastomoses between the post-plexiform arterial segment and bronchial arteries running along the close bronchiole, passing via arterioles and the capillary bed and thereby creating the thin-walled congestive dilation lesions (24). In this view, the generation of proximal complex lesions might be the mere attempt of the pulmonary vasculature to bypass the primary downstream obstruction and to ensure capillary oxygenation through overt contact with arterial blood from proximal pulmonary and distal bronchial arteries. On the other hand, plexiform lesions are not restricted to supernumerary branching and can be observed after distal dichotomous branching of pulmonary arteries. Cool and coworkers have come to different con- clusions after a computerized three-dimensional study on five patients with severe PH of different cause. In their view, plexiform lesions are functionally important because blood flow is severely obstructed along the entire length of a vessel affected by a single lesion (25). This, in fact, puts at least a working shunt concept into question. They hypothesize that the plexiform lesion could be an early vascular alteration in severe PH, independent of a component of medial smooth muscle cell hypertrophy. At a later time point in disease evolution, the plexiform lesion could transform into an intraluminal concentric obstruction composed of endothelial cells and recruited myofibroblasts, following the path of the plexiform lesion and thus representing a fibrous scar of the latter (25). The close association that can be observed between concentric laminar intimal fibrosis and plexiform lesions in lungs of patients suffering from PAH, indeed, makes this thought a tempting assumption. Nevertheless, a shunt hypothesis would not be contradictory if seen in the light of a failed attempt to shortcut other correlates of obstruction such as medial hypertrophy, intimal nonlaminar fibrosis, and thrombotic lesions.

Analogy and Significance: Inflammation is Frequently Observed in the Range of Vascular Lesions in PH

It has not yet been elucidated whether the inflammatory pattern seen in plexiform lesions and other intimal lesions is of pathogenetic importance or it represents a pure epi- phenomenon within disease evolution. The reported evidence of proinflammatory mediators, so-called chemokines, released by altered endothelial cells of PAH lungs strongly indicates a self-supporting and self-amplifying process (26,27). As elements of inflammation seem to be present in affected arteries of patients displaying PAH in various associated disease conditions, as well as in idiopathic PAH, the specific role of immune cells within installation and/or maintenance of obstructive lesions remains unclear. It seems unlikely that intimal proliferation and medial hypertrophy of pulmo- nary arteries could be the sole result of "scarring" vasculitis-like lesions, because lymphocytic and macrophagic infiltrates observed in the setting of PAH remain peri- vascular and are less abundant than in pulmonary forms of vasculitis, e.g., as seen in Wegener's granulomatosis (28). Nonetheless, Wagenvoort and coworkers had discussed such a possibility 40 years ago, and it cannot be excluded that a phase of intense inflammatory activity precedes a clinically symptomatic arterial remodeling with pro- liferation and recruitment of smooth muscle cells, endothelial cells, and fibroblasts/ myofibroblasts. This straight inflammatory involvement can be observed in cases of PH due to sarcoidosis, with typical epithelioid and histiocytic granulomas directly participating in vessel wall remodeling (Fig. 4E). In fact, latest investigations provide evidence that chemokines with specific chemotactic activity for T lymphocytes and macrophages can increase smooth muscle proliferation (29). A link between inflammatory components and growth-stimulating factors would be of great interest in inflammatory diseases with vast proliferation of fibrotic and myofibroblastic elements, as it can be seen in highly active forms of IPF, for example (see the preceding text), presenting fibroblastic foci and interstitial smooth muscle proliferation (30).

B. Venous and Venular Lesions

During the Dana Point meeting in 2008 a consensus was reached, formally separating group 1 (PAH) of the classification of PH from the rare entities of PVOD and PCH, now categorized as the new group 1′ (one prime): pulmonary venous hypertension. This differentiation seemed necessary because of particularities regarding therapeutic strategies and the cautious, if not restrictive, use of potent vasodilating drugs, such as intravenous epoprostenol, in the case of pulmonary venous involvement. From the pathologist's standpoint, this separation is comprehensible, but not ideal: in fact some cases of PAH (group 1) show PVOD-like pattern (see the following section), and the vast majority of PVOD and PCH cases (group 1′) present at least mild arterial alteration. The frequent occurrence of mixed vascular involvement seems to demand a less absolutistic evaluation into pulmonary vascular lesions either predominating the arterial or the venous system.

Pulmonary Veno-Occlusive Disease

PVOD is a rare pulmonary vascular disease causing PH and has been considered together with PCH, a subgroup of PAH until recently, according to the Venice classification of 2003. It shows an estimated prevalence of 0.1 to 0.2 per million persons per year (31). Historical reports and large case studies have extrapolated a proportion of PVOD in PAH ranging from 5% to 25% (8,31). In PVOD as in PCH, vascular lesions predominate on the postcapillary level of pulmonary vasculature. However, lesions frequently involve both veins and arteries in lungs of patients with PVOD. Interestingly, a recent report indicates that certain subgroups of PAH regarded as precapillary forms simultaneously display a PVOD-like pattern (see the following text). In PVOD the observed postcapillary lesions involve septal veins and preseptal venules and frequently consist of loose fibrous remodeling of the intima, which may totally occlude the lumen. The involvement of preseptal venules should be considered as necessary for the histological diagnosis of PVOD; fibrous occlusion of large septal veins may be seen in many forms of pulmonary venous hypertension, including a frequently reported obstruction of large pulmonary veins following catheter ablation for cardiac atrial fibrillation (32). While septal veins usually display a paucicellular, cushion-like fibrous obstruction, intimal thickening of preseptal venules can present with a dense pattern and increased cellularity. Anti-α-actin staining may reveal involvement of smooth muscle cells and/or myofibroblasts within such venular lesions. Also, thrombotic occlusion of small postcapillary microvessels has been observed, corresponding to "colander-like" lesions, which can be seen otherwise in small pulmonary arteries. The tunica media may be muscularized in both septal veins and preseptal venules. Pleural and pulmonary lymphatic vessels are usually dilated (4). The presence of calcium-encrusting elastic fibers

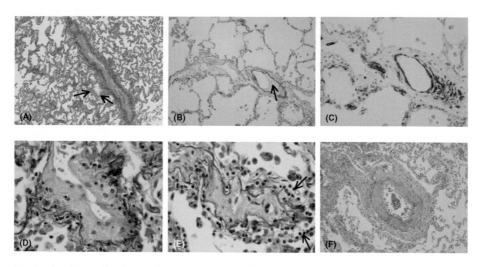

Figure 6 (*See color insert*) Remodeling of pulmonary septal veins and pre-septal venules in patients suffering from PVOD. (**A**) Fibrous intimal thickening in a large septal vein. Note the adjacent broad alveolar septa with capillary multiplication (arrows). WHPS staining, magnification ×20. (**B**) Smaller septal vein with loose intimal fibrosis, partially occluding the lumen (arrow). WHPS staining, magnification ×40. (**C**) Same vein with smooth muscle cell staining, highlighting partial muscularization. Magnification ×100. (**D**) Small pre-septal venule displaying occlusive intimal fibrosis. Note the paucicellular aspect of the occluded venule. WHPS staining, magnification ×200. (**E**) Small pulmonary vein with near occlusion and inflammatory lymphocytic infiltrate (arrows). WHPS staining, magnification ×200. (**F**) Pulmonary artery in a patient with PVOD with medial hypertrophy and adventitial fibrosis: note the typical broadening of alveolar septa and intra-alveolar macrophages. HE (Hematoxylin-Eosin) staining, magnification ×40.

in the vessel wall or the perivascular space and inflammatory activation through a foreign body giant-cell response are considered as an argument in favor of PVOD compared with secondary venous hypertension (1). Importantly, occult pulmonary hemorrhage regularly occurs in patients displaying PVOD. This particularity, which is certainly due to the postcapillary block, is of diagnostic interest, as bronchoalveolar lavage can reveal occult hemorrhage. The degree of hemorrhage can be evaluated semiquantitatively and qualitatively using the Golde score, which assesses intra-alveolar siderin-laden macrophages by Perls Prussian blue staining (33,34). In addition to an increased number of siderophages, large amounts of hemosiderin can be found in type II pneumocytes and within the interstitial space. Moreover, postcapillary obstruction may frequently lead to capillary angiectasia and even capillary angioproliferation; in PVOD cases, doubling and tripling of the alveolar septal capillary layers may be focally present. Lately, this histological peculiarity has raised questions concerning a possible overlap between PVOD and cases of PCH, a disease classically characterized by an aggressive patch-like angioproliferation of capillaries; indeed, Lantuejoul and coworkers recently reported 35 cases of PVOD and PCH with more or less similar pattern and evoke the possibility of a same disease entity (35) (Figs. 6 and 7).

Pulmonary Capillary Hemangiomatosis

Wagenvoort and colleagues were the first to describe this lesion as an entity of its own within the pulmonary capillary bed in a 71-year-old woman with progressive dyspnea, hemoptysis, and hemorrhagic pleural effusions. They found a distinctive "atypical proliferation of capillary-like channels" in the lung tissue and compared it with angiomatous growth (36). This rare cause of PH has recently been regrouped into group 1′ (pulmonary venous hypertension). Histologically, an aggressive capillary proliferation with patchy to nodular distribution can be observed in the pulmonary parenchyma: early lesions demonstrate several rows of capillaries along alveolar walls. Eventually, this feature progresses to nodules and sheets of back-to-back capillaries in advanced lesions (37). Alveolar septa are thickened by three to four capillary layers, and this multiplication leads to the histological appearance of densely cellular alveolar walls. A malignant disorder is unlikely as cytological atypia and mitoses are usually absent. Proliferating capillaries surround and compress walls of pulmonary venules and veins, causing intimal fibrosis and secondary vein occlusion. An infiltration of bronchiolar structures has also been described. It is thought that a clinically relevant postcapillary block causes this angiomatoid expansion. Occult hemorrhage or hemosiderosis, therefore, is frequently found (37). As in PVOD, these characteristics lead to compensatory muscularization of arterioles and medial hypertrophy. As mentioned earlier, the similarities in clinical and histological presentation have recently led to the assumption that PVOD and PCH might be a same disease entity with a vein- or a capillary-predominating phenotype (35) (Fig. 7).

C. Forms of PH with Significant Arterial and Venous Remodeling

PAH Associated with Connective Tissue Disease

Connective tissue diseases (CTD) such as systemic sclerosis and systemic lupus erythematosus (SLE) can be complicated by severe PH, a condition that dramatically worsens prognosis (38). Indeed, systemic sclerosis represents one of the leading pathological conditions associated with PH, and CTD-associated PH belongs to group 1 (PAH) as defined by the World Symposium in Dana Point. Prevalence of PAH in certain forms of CTD has been estimated to up to 50% of cases (39). In a recent cross-sectional national screening, at least 8% of scleroderma patients displayed moderate to severe PAH (40). In patients with CTD, PAH is the leading cause of mortality and necessitates intensive medical treatment, which frequently proves difficult and with mixed results (41). Treatment with vasodilators like continuous intravenous epoprostenol has shown improvement of exercise capacity and cardiopulmonary hemodynamics, but the response is less effective than in IPAH and survival remains poor among patients with associated CTD (42,43). Equally, endothelin receptor antagonists seem to show less impressive effects in systemic sclerosis patients than in other forms of PAH (44). In addition, adverse effects of vasoactive treatment in PAH associated with CTD can occur and may lead to severe pulmonary edema (45). Noteworthy, in small series of patients suffering from SLE with PAH, beneficial effects were cited with immunosuppressive therapy (46,47), highlighting a possible link between systemic inflammatory condition and pulmonary vascular disease. Until now, lesions of the pulmonary arterial system,

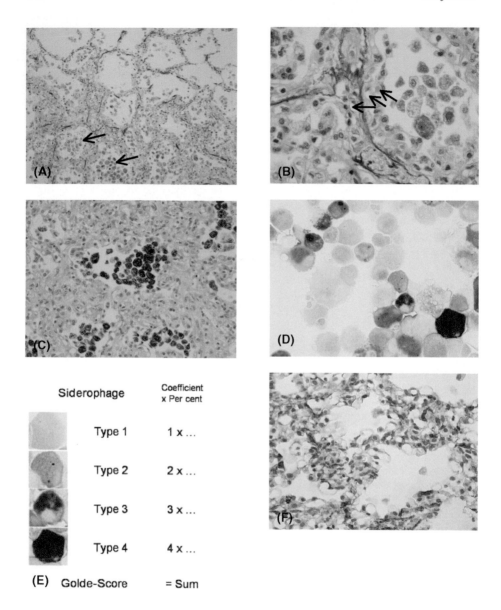

Figure 7 (*See color insert*) Remodeling of alveolar septa and alveolar hemorrhage in patients suffering from PVOD. (**A**) Patchy distribution of alveolar septal thickening. Alveoli within this remodeled area contain numerous macrophages (arrows). HES staining, magnification ×40. (**B**) Capillary multiplication leading to alveolar septal thickening with doubling or even trebling of the capillary lumina (arrows). Note the pigment-rich macrophages to the left of the marked alveolar septum. HES staining, magnification ×400. (**C**) Same area with Perls Prussian Blue staining, revealing siderin-laden macrophages within the alveoli, the morphologic equivalent of persistent hemorrhage. Magnification ×200. (**D**) Broncho-alveolar lavage: numerous siderin-laden macrophages

more or less similar to those occurring in idiopathic PAH, have been held responsible for PH in these patients. In a recently published analysis of eight patients suffering from CTD-associated PAH, we observed that six out of eight patients (75%) exhibited occlusive lesions of pulmonary veins and venules, as it can be typically seen in PVOD. In contrast, only 5 out of 29 non-CTD control patients with the primary diagnosis PAH displayed venous involvement (48). Though all investigated CTD-PAH patients exhibited pulmonary arterial changes, venous and venular fibrous remodeling, when present, was more pronounced than arterial changes, concerning the quantity of affected vessels. All cases of CTD-associated PAH revealed pulmonary arterial lesions, involving small muscular vessels on the pre- and intra-acinar level. The vessel wall remodeling corresponded to arterial changes found in PAH, ranging from intimal constrictive and nonconstrictive lesions to associated medial hypertrophy and adventitial thickening. Inflammatory infiltrates were observed in six patients. Besides interstitial involvement, immunostaining experiments revealed the importance of perivascular lymphocytic infiltrates involving both pulmonary arteries and veins. The role of inflammatory cells and their mediators in the evolution of PAH has been widely discussed over the years and seems, in particular, noteworthy in PAH associated with systemic inflammatory disease (21,22,49). However, the described findings of a PVOD-like setting in CTD-associated PAH highlight the important hemodynamic effect of postcapillary occlusion on the pulmonary vasculature. Resistance of CTD-associated PAH to common vasodilator therapies and complications such as pulmonary edema could be the mere consequence of a higher prevalence of veno-occlusive remodeling in these patients, compared with other forms of PAH (Fig. 8).

New Perspectives: Are Venous Lesions Underestimated in IPAH?

As PVOD seems to be frequently concomitant with pulmonary arterial lesions on the one hand and venous remodeling is present in some forms of PAH on the other, the question may be raised whether mild venous remodeling occurs in IPAH. In a recent retrospective analysis of the author's study group, five cases of IPAH and five cases of PVOD (9 lung transplant explants, 1 autopsy) confirmed by a first histopathological analysis were reviewed in a double-blind mode (unpublished data). Lesions were semiquantified using a four-level score system (0 = no, 1 = some, 2 = numerous, 3 = plentiful). Assessment of venous lesions in IPAH lungs underwent secondary regrouping into a three-level score (arterial lesions, venous lesions, both) with a cutoff for venous involvement <2 (numerous) to avoid overestimation. The reanalysis of this small collective confirmed the primary histological findings that all IPAH patients had arterial complex lesions.

(or siderophages) are present, displaying different degrees of Prussian Blue staining. Magnification ×400. (**E**) Siderophages isolated from figure 6D: typing of macrophagic Prussian Blue staining is performed in order to assess the degree of alveolar hemorrhage: a Golde score above 100 is considered as occult alveolar hemorrhage. (**F**) Pulmonary parenchyma of a patient suffering from PCH: note the capillary proliferation within the alveolar septa leading to a histological pattern very similar to PVOD. Smooth-muscle staining, magnification ×200.

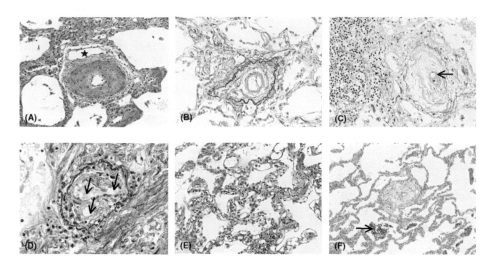

Figure 8 (*See color insert*) Pulmonary vascular lesions found in patients suffering from PAH associated to connective tissue disease. (**A**) Intimal concentric non-laminar fibrosis of a small pulmonary artery. Note the dilated lymphatic vessel adjacent to the artery (asterisk). HE staining, magnification ×100. (**B**) Pre-septal venule with loose occlusive intimal fibrosis. WHPS staining, magnification ×100. (**C**) Occlusive loose fibrotic remodeling of a pre-septal venule (arrow) with peri-vascular lymphocytic infiltrate. WHPS staining, magnification ×100. (**D**) Thrombotic lesion of a pre-septal venule with recanalization channels within the occluded vessel (arrows). WHPS staining, magnification ×200. (**E**) Capillary angiectasia and alveolar septal thickening similar to the histological pattern seen in PVOD (see above). HE staining, magnification ×100. (**F**) Occluded vein (center) and signs of occult alveolar hemorrhage: note the stained siderin-laden macrophages within the adjacent alveoli. Perls Prussian Blue staining, magnification ×40.

Interestingly, two out of five lungs of IPAH displayed both arterial and venous lesions with loose fibrous remodeling of small preseptal venules. The same two IPAH patients displayed patchy capillary proliferation, as can be found in PVOD, but also in CTD-associated PAH. With respect to the clinical data, three of five IPAH patients including the two patients with PAH-VOD pattern exhibited a survival time (time to trans-plantation) less than the mean of the IPAH group (35.3 months). Of course, further histological studies of larger numbers of patients are required to confirm the trend for an unfavorable clinical outcome among IPAH patients with venous involvement. As expected, all lungs of PVOD patients presented with arterial remodeling and three out of five PVOD patients displayed patchy capillary proliferation. Noteworthy, the two PVOD cases without capillary proliferation displayed the lowest venous remodeling score (≤2) in the PVOD group, linking these two phenomena typically seen in PVOD. Even if this preanalysis is very restricted due to the small sample size, it can nevertheless serve as a probe and should incite further exploration of this intriguing question: Can a different equilibrium of lesions within the integrality of the pulmonary vascular system lead to a different clinical phenotype of PH?

IV. Conclusion

In conclusion, characteristic vascular lesions in PH may involve the lung vasculature and microvasculature from the pre- to the postcapillary level. In addition to clinical differentiation, histological resemblance or difference has led to the categorization of PH into different groups, now summed up under the 2008 Dana Point classification. It is important to stress that the differentiation of lesions and their localization might be of importance in the outcome and therapeutic strategies. However, a clear cut separation of different forms of PH through recognition of a histological phenotype will always be difficult or even impossible: different etiological factors (e.g., hypoxia vs. anorexigen intake) may trigger a final common step in the cascade of pathological events (e.g., oxidative stress and consecutive growth factor expression) and finally lead to the same morphological pattern (e.g., medial hypertrophy). Nonetheless, the correct interpretation of the pathological vascular anatomy remains an important tool in the successful interplay of clinical, biological, and pharmaceutical research dedicated to PH.

References

1. Pietra GG, Capron F, Stewart S, et al. Pathological assessment of vasculopathies in pulmonary hypertension. J Am Coll Cardiol 2004; 43:25S–32S.
2. Romberg E. Über die Sklerose der Lungenarterien. Dtsch Arch Klin Med 1891; 48:197–206.
3. Dresdale DT, Schultz M, Mitchom RJ. Primary pulmonary hypertension: clinical and hemodynamic study. Am J Med 1951; 11:686–694.
4. Heath D, Edwards JE. The pathology of hypertensive pulmonary vascular disease. Circulation 1958; 18:533–547.
5. Waagenvoort CA, Waagenvoort N. Primary pulmonary hypertension: a pathological study of the lung vessels in 156 clinically diagnosed cases. Circulation 1970; 42:1163–1184.
6. Hatano S, Strasser T, eds. Primary pulmonary hypertension. Report on a WHO-meeting October 15–17, 1975; Geneva: WHO.
7. Rich S, Dantzer DR, Ayres SM, et al. Primary pulmonary hypertension: a national prospective study. Ann Intern Med 1987; 107:216–223.
8. Pietra GG. The pathology of primary pulmonary hypertension. In: Rubin L, Rich S, eds. Primary Pulmonary Hypertension. New York: Marcel Dekker, 1997:19–61.
9. Heath D, Williams DR. High-Altitude Medicine and Pathology. London: Butterworths, 1989:102–114.
10. Penaloza D, Arias-Stella J. The heart and pulmonary circulation at high altitudes: healthy highlanders and chronic mountain sickness. Circulation 2007; 115:1132–1146.
11. Voelkel NF, Tuder RM. Cellular and molecular mechanisms in the pathogenesis of severe pulmonary hypertension. Eur Respir J 1995; 8:2129–2138.
12. Cool CD, Kennedy D, Voelkel NF, et al. Pathogenesis and evolution of plexiform lesions in pulmonary hypertension associated with scleroderma and human immunodeficiency virus infection. Hum Pathol 1997; 28:434–442.
13. Cyr PV, Vincic L, Kay M. Pulmonary vasculopathy in idiopathic spontaneous pneumothorax in young subjects. Arch Pathol Lab Med 2000; 124:717–720.
14. Patel NM, Lederer DJ, Borczuk AC, et al. Pulmonary hypertension in idiopathic pulmonary fibrosis. Chest 2007; 132:998–1006.
15. Colombat M, Mal H, Groussard O, et al. Pulmonary vascular lesions in end-stage idiopathic pulmonary fibrosis: histopathologic study on lung explant specimens and correlations with pulmonary hemodynamics. Hum Pathol 2007; 38:60–65.

16. Bjornsson J, Edwards WD. Primary pulmonary hypertension: a histopathologic study of 80 cases. Mayo Clin Proc 1985; 60:16–25.

17. Moser KM, Bloor CM. Pulmonary vascular lesions occurring in patients with chronic major vessel thromboembolic pulmonary hypertension. Chest 1993; 103:685–692.

18. Harrison CV. The pathology of the pulmonary vessels in pulmonary hypertension. Br J Radiol 1958; 31:217–226.

19. Kucsko L. Arteriovenous communications in the human lung and their functional significance. Frankf Z Pathol 1953; 64:54–83.

20. Saldana ME, Harley RA, Liebow AA, et al. Experimental extreme pulmonary hypertension and vascular disease in relation to polycythemia. Am J Pathol 1968; 52:935–981.

21. Tuder RM, Groves B, Badesch DB, et al. Exuberant endothelial cell growth and elements of inflammation are present in plexiform lesions of pulmonary hypertension. Am J Pathol 1994; 144:275–285.

22. Dorfmüller P, Perros F, Balabanian K, et al. Inflammation in pulmonary arterial hypertension. Eur Respir J 2003; 22:358–363.

23. Lee SD, Shroyer KR, Markham NE, et al. Monoclonal endothelial cell proliferation is present in primary but not secondary pulmonary hypertension. J Clin Invest 1998; 101:927–934.

24. Yaginuma GY, Mohri H, Takahashi T. Distribution of arterial lesions and collateral pathways in the pulmonary hypertension of congenital heart disease: a computer aided reconstruction study. Thorax 1990; 45:586–590.

25. Cool CD, Stewart JS, Werahera P, et al. Three-dimensional reconstruction of pulmonary arteries in plexiform pulmonary hypertension using cell-specific markers. Am J Pathol 1999; 155:411–419.

26. Dorfmüller P, Zarka V, Durand-Gasselin I, et al. Chemokine RANTES in severe pulmonary arterial hypertension. Am J Respir Crit Care Med 2002; 165:534–539.

27. Balabanian K, Foussat A, Dorfmüller P, et al. CX$_3$C chemokine fractalkine in pulmonary arterial hypertension. Am J Respir Crit Care Med 2002; 165:1419–1425.

28. Dorfmüller P, Humbert M, Capron F, et al. Pathology and aspects of pathogenesis in pulmonary arterial hypertension. Sarcoidosis Vasc Diffuse Lung Dis 2003; 20:9–19.

29. Perros F, Dorfmüller P, Souza R, et al. Fraktalkine-induced smooth muscle cell proliferation in pulmonary hypertension. Eur Respir J 2007; 29:937–943.

30. Ohta K, Mortenson RL, Clark RA, et al. Immunohistochemical identification and characterzation of smooth-muscle-like cells in idiopathic pulmonary fibrosis. Am J Respir Crit Care Med 1995; 152:1659–1665.

31. Mandel J, Mark EJ, Hales CA. Pulmonary veno-occlusive disease. Am J Respir Crit Care Med 2000; 162:1964–1973.

32. Di Biase L, Fahmy TS, Wazni OM, et al. Pulmonary vein total occlusion following catheter ablation for atrial fibrillation: clinical implications after long-term follow-up. J Am Coll Cardiol 2006; 48:2493–2499.

33. Golde DW, Drew WL, Klein HZ, et al. Occult pulmonary haemorrhage in leukaemia. Br Med J 1975; 2:166–168.

34. Capron F. Bronchoalveolar lavage and alveolar hemorrhage. Ann Pathol 1999; 19:395–400.

35. Lantuejoul S, Sheppard MN, Corrin B, et al. Pulmonary veno-occlusive disease and pulmonary capillary hemangiomatosis: a clinicopathologic study of 35 cases. Am J Surg Pathol 2006; 30:850–857.

36. Wagenvoort CA, Beetstra A, Spijker J. Capillary haemangiomatosis of the lungs. Histopathology 1978; 2:401–406.

37. Tron V, Magee F, Wright JL, et al. Pulmonary capillary hemangiomatosis. Hum Pathol 1986; 17:1144–1150.

38. Simonneau G, Galie N, Rubin LJ, et al. Clinical classification of pulmonary hypertension. J Am Coll Cardiol 2004; 43:5S–12S.

39. Ungerer RG, Tashkin DP, Furst D, et al. Prevalence and clinical correlates of pulmonary arterial hypertension in progressive systemic sclerosis. Am J Med 1983; 75:65–74.
40. Hachulla E, Gressin V, Guillevin L, et al. Early detection of pulmonary arterial hypertension in systemic sclerosis: a French nationwide prospective multicenter study. Arthritis Rheum 2005; 52:3792–3800.
41. Sanchez O, Humbert M, Sitbon O, et al. Treatment of pulmonary hypertension secondary to connective tissue diseases. Thorax 1999; 54:273–277.
42. Badesch DB, Tapson VF, McGoon MD, et al. Continuous intravenous epoprostenol for pulmonary hypertension due to the scleroderma spectrum of disease. Ann Intern Med 2000; 132:425–434.
43. Ramirez A, Varga J. Pulmonary arterial hypertension in systemic sclerosis: clinical manifestations, pathophysiology, evaluation, and management. Treat Respir Med 2004; 3:339–352.
44. Humbert M, Simonneau G. Drug insight: endothelin-receptor antagonists for pulmonal arterial hypertension in systemic rheumatic diseases. Nat Clin Pract Rheum 2005; 1:93–101.
45. Humbert M, Sanchez O, Fartoukh M, et al. Short-term and long-term epoprostenol (prostacyclin) therapy in pulmonary hypertension secondary to connective tissue diseases: results of a pilot study. Eur Respir J 1999; 13:1351–1356.
46. Tanaka E, Harigai M, Tanaka M, et al. Pulmonary hypertension in systemic lupus erythematosus: evaluation of clinical characteristics and response to immunosuppressive treatment. J Rheumatol 2002; 29:282–287.
47. Sanchez O, Sitbon O, Jaïs X, et al. Immunosuppressive therapy in connective tissue diseases-associated pulmonary arterial hypertension. Chest 2006; 130:182–189.
48. Dorfmüller P, Humbert M, Perros F, et al. Fibrous remodelling of the pulmonary venous system in pulmonary arterial hypertension associated with connective diseases. Hum Pathol 2007; 38:893–902.
49. Humbert M, Monti G, Brenot F, et al. Increased interleukin-1 and interleukin-6 serum concentrations in severe primary pulmonary hypertension. Am J Respir Crit Care Med 1995; 151:1628–1631.

4

Pathogenesis of Pulmonary Hypertension

NORBERT F. VOELKEL, LORI SWEENEY, and HERMAN BOGAARD
Virginia Commonwealth University, Richmond, Virginia, U.S.A.

I. Introduction

Pulmonary hypertension and pulmonary vascular diseases have been reviewed for this *Lung Biology in Health and Diseases* series three times previously, in volumes 14, 28, and 99. The pathogenesis of pulmonary arterial hypertension (PAH) had been dissected each time, and it is tempting to look back and identify the key words and concepts that were emblematic of the state of knowledge at the time of writing these books in 1979, 1989, and 1997. To begin with volume 14, the term "primary" pulmonary hypertension was then used and also in the 1975 WHO definition of "unexplained pulmonary vascular disease." Wrestling with a large number of published reports, many anecdotal, the authors concluded: "In the naturally occurring disease not attributed to aminorex, primary pulmonary hypertension is by and large a disease of young women." Familial clusters of primary pulmonary hypertension were known at this time, but of course not the name of the gene. Factors associated with female maturation were considered as pathogenetically important, but "no specific hormone or endocrine factor had been identified in these patients." Autoimmune mechanisms were discussed and the authors concluded that "at least some occurrences of primary pulmonary hypertension show a common etiology with autoimmune disease processes." The first epidemic of diet drug–induced primary pulmonary hypertension was fresh in everyone's memory, yet the authors had to admit that "all the experimental work to demonstrate the effect of chronic (drug) application on pulmonary hemodynamics and morphology has failed to produce significant alterations." Wagenvoort favored vasoconstriction as important in the pathogenesis of primary pulmonary hypertension and a diagram illustrated the prevailing pathogenetic concept that connected "the dots" in the following fashion:

> Individual pulmonary vascular hyperreactivity (genetic disposition) → vasoconstriction → elevation of the pulmonary artery pressure → right ventricular hypertrophy.

The authors also connected vasoconstriction with "endothelial cell lesions" and "media hypertrophy" and speculated that "if vasoconstriction precedes the development of intimal lesions in lung arteries, then multiple etiologies of primary pulmonary hypertension are likely." Under "remaining problems" the authors stated, "we thus remain largely ignorant of the details of the changes in the intimal and smooth muscle cells, that is, if vasoconstriction is the initial event, what abnormalities in the contractile machinery are present? If the process originates in the intima, what are the ultrastructural changes early in the disease?" In addition, the authors found "no published reports bringing the methodology of immunopathology to bear on the disease" (1). In volume 28, the authors contemplated the following:

> The injured endothelium may either produce growth factors and proliferate to ultimately accomplish total or near lumen obliteration, or it may respond to factors like platelet-derived growth factor (PDGF) or even angiogenesis factors. Because the angioproliferative aspects of primary pulmonary hypertension cannot be overlooked, future work must focus on the role of the pulmonary vascular muscle cell and its cross talk with endothelial cell and fibroblasts.

The female factor of primary pulmonary hypertension was again discussed, quoting Folkman and Inger that "physiological angiogenesis seems to be a uniquely female affair, recurring during ovulation, repair of menstruating uterus and placentation." Folkman had described angiostatic steroids, and the authors of 1989 speculated "that overproduction of growth factors overpowering the prevailing angiostatic principles could act preferentially during the female reproductive life" (2). Volume 99 published in 1997 (3) began to prepare the grounds for the development of pathogenetic concepts, which considered vascular cell proliferation and inflammation as important primary or at least contributory events. Severe pulmonary hypertension was seen as the consequence of a vicious cycle of two principle components: vascular cell proliferation $\rightleftarrows$ shear stress.

An image of an "early plexiform lesion" was reproduced, and it was suggested that in collagen vascular disease–associated pulmonary hypertension, early lymphocytic cell inflammation could somehow lead to later pulmonary hypertension development. Human immunodeficiency virus (HIV)-related severe pulmonary hypertension, characterized by plexiform lesions, was discussed and endothelin and vascular endothelial growth factor (VEGF) entered the stage. Now, 10 years later, we believe that the term pathobiology is preferred over "pathophysiology" (2), the term "primary" pulmonary hypertension has given way to "pulmonary arterial" hypertension: this likely allows us to recognize which elements of the pathobiology of severe pulmonary hypertension forms are shared, and by now, we have begun appreciating the limited success of vasodilator therapy (4–7). Another very important new dimension—precisely because we now have been informed about two different pulmonary hypertension genes—is the interface between genes and epigenetic factors in the pathobiology of severe pulmonary hypertension (see the next section).

II. Severe Pulmonary Arterial Hypertension— Angioproliferation

There appears to be now an emerging consensus and an acceptance of a role of angiogenic mechanisms in the pathobiology of many forms of severe pulmonary hypertension (Fig. 1). With this acceptance comes the recognition that it is difficult to explain the spectrum of the vascular pathomorphology (8) with smooth muscle cell hypertrophy and hyperplasia, and endothelial cell growth becomes of central importance (9–13). This said, it is now equally clear that in the fully developed lesions we are confronted with a picture of multicellularity as is illustrated in Figure 2. The past discussions of the pathogenesis of primary pulmonary hypertension have been contentious, in particular

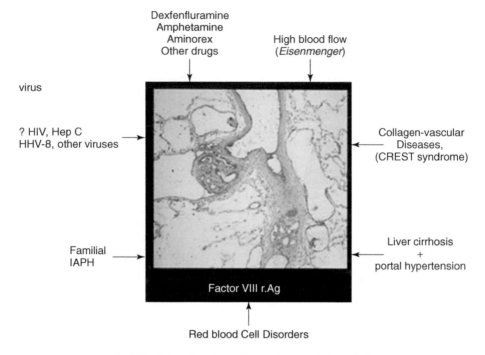

Dexfenfluramine
Amphetamine
Aminorex
Other drugs

High blood flow
(*Eisenmenger*)

virus

? HIV, Hep C
HHV-8, other viruses

Collagen-vascular
Diseases,
(CREST syndrome)

Familial
IAPH

Liver cirrhosis
+
portal hypertension

Factor VIII r.Ag

Red blood Cell Disorders

Endothelial cell proliferation and transdifferentiation

Figure 1 Remarkably a number of conditions and trigger factors converge on precapillary pulmonary arteriolar sites and—by using similar or different signal transducing pathways—generate lumen-obliterating angioproliferation.

when based on the examination of the plexiform lesions. Some investigators still maintain that plexiform lesions are end-stage, scar-like formations and that every attempt of a pathogenetic analysis based on an "archeological dig" of these "ancient sites" must fail. The work of many investigators during the last decade who have been using specific protein and gene-based probes has shown this not to be the case. Not only can cell types be identified and localized with great accuracy but also their state of activation and their gene expression. This allusion to archeology is not without a caveat. Although archeologists have carbon dating and a fossil record, their final results are often narrative, based more on contextual arguments than on a linear step-by-step analysis of sequence of events. Analyzing the complex pulmonary vascular lesions in PAH, let us ask not only what kind of cells are in and around the lesions but also where do they come from and how do they get there? And what are they doing there?

The following is guided both by the principle of "homeostasis" and by a teleological cell biological approach, hence pathobiology or vascular biology gone awry. We start with the homeostatic theory of a stable vascular wall that, in spite of hemodynamic stress, maintains an endothelial cell monolayer (14). It is intuitive that unbridled endothelial cell proliferation will lead to vessel lumen obliteration and violates vascular

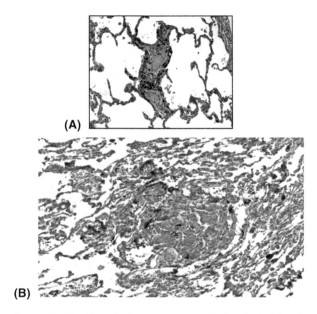

Figure 2 Plexiform lesions are composed of endothelial and smooth muscle cell, there are cells of the immune system (**A**) CD20+ B lymphocytes and (**B**) megakaryocytes, in and around these lesions.

homeostasis. An animal model of severe angioproliferative PAH in normal wild-type rats based on the combination of chronic VEGF receptor blockade (induction of pulmonary endothelial cell apoptosis) plus chronic hypoxia (high vascular shear stress that inhibits endothelial cell apoptosis) (15,16) (Fig. 3) allowed us to propose a pathobiological model of severe PAH. We found that VEGF receptor blockade alone did not cause angioproliferation, nor did chronic hypoxia alone, but when combined, angioproliferation resulted, which could be prevented by concomitant treatment with a broad-spectrum apoptosis inhibitor (14). A similar endothelial cell proliferation was induced with the combination of VEGF receptor blockade and high shear stress in an ex vivo system and prevented by caspase inhibition (Fig. 4) (17). These data led to the postulate that endothelial cell apoptosis precedes subsequent endothelial cell proliferation and that pulmonary vascular endothelial cell growth can be enforced in animals with no particular genetic predisposition, that is, endothelial cell apoptosis and high shear stress—when combined in vivo or in vitro—are sufficient to cause angio-obliterative lesions. This led to the question: what is the nature of the dying endothelial cell when compared to the nature of the surviving and proliferating cells? Likely the dying cells are highly dependent on autocrine and paracrine VEGF-dependent survival signals, which may involve prostacyclin (PGI2), nitric oxide (NO), and Akt-dependent regulation, whereas the surviving cells are apparently not. If so, then our model becomes Darwinistic in that endothelial cell death in the vessel wall selects cells that are characterized by a high proliferative potential (18). These highly proliferative (perhaps stem-like precursor) cells are liberated from the "no growth constraints" of the intact monolayer and perhaps activated by growth signals released from neighboring endothelial cells that are

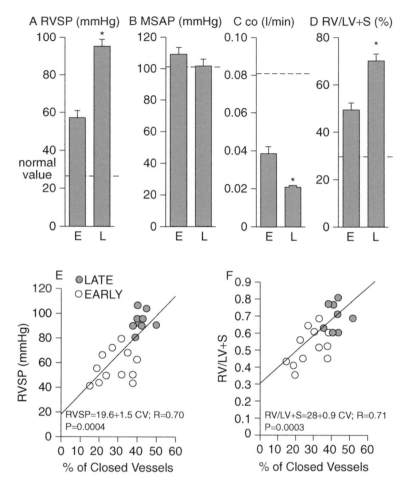

Figure 3 Hemodynamic profile of the angioproliferative pulmonary hypertension model. The degree of pulmonary hypertension (represented by the right ventricular systolic pressure, RVSP) is severe and the reduced CO documents RV failure. The CO reduction is even greater at the later time point (L) when compared to the earlier phase of the disease. The dotted line indicates normal values for rats living at the altitude of Denver. The data show also that the degree of pulmonary hypertension is related to the degree of small vessel lumen obliteration. *Abbreviation*: CO, cardiac output. *Source*: From Ref. 16.

undergoing apoptosis (19). Proof of this concept awaits the availability of specific markers that can identify lung vascular precursor cells. If we assume for the time being that this pathobiological model is indeed correct then the remaining questions are as follows: What causes the initial endothelial cell apoptosis? Why do the complex vascular lesions develop at particular sites of the precapillary arterioles? A number of noxious stimuli and even cell-cell interactions from drugs to infectious organisms and cytotoxic T lymphocytes can be imagined to induce endothelial cell apoptosis. However,

Caspase 3   PCNA

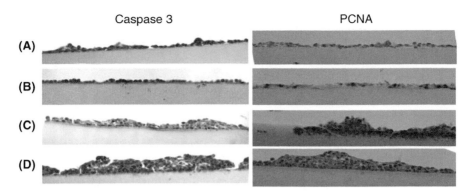

Figure 4 To determine whether initial apoptosis would be followed by cell proliferation, we explored the time course under high shear stress; (**A**) before SU5416 addition under high shear (day 0), (**B**) one day after SU5416 addition (day 1), (**C**) three days after SU5416 addition (day 3), and (**D**) seven days after SU5416 addition (day 7). Active caspase 3 immunostaining was detected in HPMVEC at day 1 (**B**) and day 3 (**C**) after SU5416 addition. There was a decrease in the number of cells staining for active caspase 3 but an increase in the number of PCNA staining cells at day 7 after SU5416 addition (**D**). The magnification is 200×.

exuberant endothelial cell growth (9) may require sites along the peripheral vascular tree where precursor cells are enriched. The group of Troy Stephens has described in the adult rat lung a border zone, or a seam, where macrovascular and microvascular endothelial cells join without any apparent overlap; the microvascular endothelial cell population contains highly proliferative precursor cells. Such a "seam" has recently been identified in the eye in the "limbus" (which is the zone at the junction of the cornea and the conjunctiva), which is a stem cell niche, where "by an elutriation-like cell sorting mechanism" stem cells from the conjunctival and corneal side accumulate (20). These sites in the lung vessels can be visualized as tectonic plates of vascular instability or sites that are particularly shear stress sensitive.

III. The Endothelial Cell Growth is Quasi-Neoplastic

Here we attempt to address the question: What is the nature of the surviving and proliferating endothelial cell? Lee et al. (21) conducted an analysis of plexiform lesion endothelial cells comparing lung tissue samples from patients with idiopathic pulmonary arterial hypertension (IPAH) with tissue samples from patients with associated forms and by assessing loss of heterozygosity. Lee et al. (21) found that the clusters of endothelial cells in the lesions from patients with IPAH had grown by monoclonal expansion, whereas the endothelial cells in the associated forms were polyclonal. Thus, clonal endothelial cell growth, since clonal cell growth characterizes cancer growth, is cancer-like. There are other strategies to further characterize the complex vascular lesion endothelial cells. One such strategy is to search for tumor markers, another strategy is to search for somatic endothelial cell mutations. Both of these strategies were applied and were productive (22,23). For example, plexiform lesion endothelial cells have lost the

Table 1 Immunohistochemical Characterization of the Plexiform Lesion Endothelial Cell
Phenotype in Severe Angioproliferative Pulmonary Hypertension (SAPPH)

Protein expressed or overexpressed			Protein expression diminished or lost
VEGF	++	Prostacyclin synthase	−
PDGF	++		−
KDR	++	Prostacyclin receptor	−
5-LO	+	P27	−
FLAP	+	PPAR-γ	−
RANTES	++		−
IL-32	++		−
Endothelin	+	ALCAM-1	−
HIF-1α	+	N-cadherin	−
ARNT	+	TGF-β RII	−
eNOS	+	Smad	−
Survivin	+	Caveolin-1	−
P16	+	Heme oxygenase	−
c-Myc	+		−
B-catenin	++	MDR	−
RANTES	++		
IL-32	++		

expression of tumor suppressor proteins like PPARγ and caveolin 1 and 2, and ALCAM-1
(22,24,25). Because endothelial cells in hemangiomata express the caveolin proteins
although they are not expressed in plexiform lesion cells, it was concluded that the
endothelial cell phenotype of the plexiform lesions does not resemble that of benign
hemangiomas. It is tempting to consider that the phenotype switch of the lesion endothelial cells, which is now well documented (14) (Table 1), is related to the angioproliferative growth of these cells. What has not been resolved is whether the phenotype
changes precede the growth or the phenotype is responsible for (causes) the endothelial
cell growth. As in many cancers, the transcription factor HIF-1α (hypoxia-inducible
factor 1α) (26,27) is expressed in the plexiform lesion cells (28), and mechanisms
dependent on HIF-1α-transcribed genes can cause the proliferation of the apoptosis-
resistant endothelial cells. To summarize, initial endothelial cell apoptosis could select
for endothelial cells with a robust growth potential, and the proliferation could be
maintained by HIF-1α-dependent regulated genes and proteins. We tend to believe that
the phenotypic changes of the endothelial cells can be acquired; for example, pulmonary
microvascular endothelial cells treated with apoptosis-inducing VEGF-R blockade and
exposed to shear stress expressed the antiapoptotic survivin (17) and lost expression of
the tumor suppressor protein PPARγ (25). Alterations in the expression of K+ channels
(29–34) may be part of the acquired phenotype switch. Yeager et al. (23) investigated
whether the monoclonal endothelial cell growth was accompanied by somatic endothelial cell mutations. Microdissected lesion cells were extracted and the DNA analyzed
with guidance from the colon cancer literature (35,36), which partially explains the luck
of finding the needle in the haystack. Myeroff et al. (37) had previously reported a
mutation in the transforming growth factor (TGF)-β RII gene in nearly 30% of colon

cancer tissue samples. Because TGF-β controls endothelial cell apoptosis (38–41), this gene was a reasonable candidate gene and the hypothesis became that a TGF-β RII gene mutation could result in a truncated TGF-β receptor, which was signaling impaired. Although methodological difficulties at the time precluded effective transfection of the mutated gene and expression in endothelial cells of the faulty receptor protein to formally prove that this mutant gene would code for endothelial cell apoptosis resistance, the concept that mutations of genes, which are members of the TGF-β superfamily, affect the pulmonary endothelial cell apoptosis control has survived (42,43). Subsequently, Richter et al. (44) followed this initial TGF-β RII workup and showed, using immunohistochemistry, that plexiform lesion cells displayed additional TGF-β receptor signaling defects, because they have lost expression of several of the Smad proteins. Taken together, the plexiform lesion endothelial cell phenotype appears to be reprogramed for growth; the cells express HIF-1α and VEGF, but the TGF-β receptor "brake" on endothelial cell growth is malfunctioning. Likely this concept applies to impaired signaling of the mutated bone morphogenetic protein receptor 2 (BMPR2) in the setting of familial IPAH (45,46). Still, to take all this information and embed it in a cancer paradigm of severe angioproliferative PAH (22) requires further explanation. If the concept of quasi-malignancy indeed apply then Harold Dvorak's characterization "cancer is the wound that never heals" comes also to mind.

The abnormally large size of the proliferating and lumen-obliterating endothelial cells and a shape reminiscent of the spindle cells of Kaposi sarcoma (C.D. Cool, personal communication) together with the resistance of these vascular lesions to pharmacological treatment [which is also applicable to the Su5416/chronic hypoxia rat model of severe pulmonary hypertension (47)] raise the question whether the angioproliferative component is part of a quasi-malignant pathobiology. The landmark article published by Hanahan and Weinberg in Cell in 2000 (48) titled "The Hallmarks of Cancer" can be used as a template when we ask whether severe angioproliferative PAH shares descriptors, in the words of the authors "hallmarks" of cancers. The Hallmarks of Cancer paper was written in the firm belief that all cancers, inspite of a large catalog of organ- and cell-specific presentations, metastatic patterns, cell growth kinetics, and different response to therapies, share a relatively small set of fundamental features or hallmarks, perhaps laws of cancer biology and rules of engagement. If this template of hallmarks is applied to severe angioproliferative pulmonary hypertension, the quasi-malignant nature of this group of disease becomes apparent (Table 2).

Table 2 Hanahan-Weinberg Cancer Criteria in Severe Angioproliferative PAH

	Cancer	PAH (Refs.)
Apoptosis evasion	+	+ (25,56)
Sustained angiogenesis	+	+ (28)
Self-sufficiency in growth signals	+	+ (28,57)
Insensitivity to antigrowth signals	+	+ (22)
Limitless replicative potential	+	?
Tissue invasion	+	–
Metastasis	+	?[a]

[a]See text.
Source: From Ref. 48.

Whether plexiform lesion endothelial cells have a limitless replicative potential (Table 2) is uncertain, because these cells have not been isolated and studied in culture. There is no tissue invasion as is typical for cancers, the lesion cells remain within the boundaries of the vessel wall, but whether or not there is a metastatic component to PAH is less clear. Angiogenic precursor cells can be released from the bone marrow—this likely occurs in sickle cell disease—and lodged in the lung circulation, and phenotypically altered lesion cells could be released and recirculated. Such a "seed and soil" hypothesis envisions that dislodged from the lesions, "wandering cancer-like cells" may return to a welcoming microenvironment in which they are first developed. Such "escape cells" would be predicted to form polyclonal lesions. Other cancer features, which did not make the short list of Hanahan and Weinberg, are loss of K+ channel expression in breast cancer (49) and ion channel disturbances in other cancers (50), presence of cells involved in immune surveillance, and anaerobic glycolysis of the cancer cells (51). Indeed the plexiform cells are associated with a variety of immune cells (52,53), and circulating endothelial cells, which are increased in PAH (54) when isolated from the blood of patients with IPAH, are glycolytically active and produce lactate (55).

Although a unifying hypothesis of severe angioproliferative PAH will need to incorporate and consider genetic and epigenetic factors, it is now reasonable to begin to propose that such a unifying hypothesis be formulated that can prove or disprove the pieces or elements of the hypothesis. In search of one particularly attractive organizer of pulmonary angioproliferation and the endothelial cell phenotype switch, one can settle on HIF-1α, the transcription factor described 15 years ago by Gregg Semenza (26,27). HIF-1α is likely involved in the pathogenesis of severe PAH as it links hypoxia, inflammation, innate immunity, and tumor angiogenesis (58,59). This protein not only controls the expression of VEGF but also the expression of a number of other angiogenesis-selected proteins like endothelin-1 (60), but is also involved in vascular smooth muscle cell (VSMC) migration, mobilization of bone marrow precursor cells (61,62), macrophage activation (59), and development of chemoresistance of cancer cells (63). Intriguingly human herpes virus 8 (HHV-8)-associated viral interferon (IFN)-regulatory factor 3 stabilizes HIF-1α and induces VEGF expression (64), and Epstein-Barr virus latent membrane protein-1 induces synthesis of HIF-1α (65). Furthermore, returning to the "cancer paradigm," virtually all of the proteins regulating anaerobic glycolysis of tumor cells are under HIF-1α transcriptional control (61). The schematic (Fig. 5) attempts to organize some of the known information.

IV. The Immune System Component of Severe Pulmonary Hypertension: The Tip of the Iceberg

The forms of PAH associated with immune disorders, which include autoimmune diseases as well as immune insufficiency, are particularly challenging because they are even more difficult to treat than other forms of PAH, have an overall worse survival (67), and are not associated with BMPR2 mutations (68). The lung vascular histology is identical with that of IAPH with the exception of a thicker, more sclerosed adventitia in patients with scleroderma. Nicolls et al. recently reviewed the topic of immune system involvement in severe PAH (69). Although antinuclear and antiphospholipid antibodies

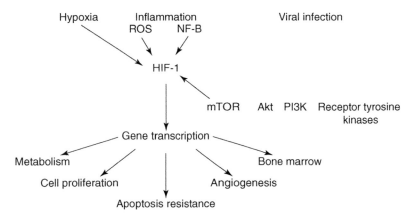

Figure 5 The transcription factor HIF-1 as the organizer or hub of the pathobiologically important components of angioproliferative PAH. The regulation of HIF-1 protein stability is very complex, as is the coordinated response triggered subsequent to the transcription of a large number of genes. This hub and spoke model of cellular and molecular biology of PAH can be probed with increasingly more specific tools. Whereas this model has been drawn scale-free, the relative weight or impact of individual interactions will likely vary between different forms of PAH. The model also leaves room for additional spokes like BMPRII and TGF, and dendritic cells and B lymphocytes. *Abbreviations*: HIF-1, hypoxia-inducible factor 1; PAH, pulmonary arterial hypertension; TGF, transforming growth factor. *Source*: From Refs. 53 and 66.

and anti-endothelial antibodies are shared between IPAH and collagen vascular disease–associated PAH, the exact pathobiological importance—disease marker or actor—remains elusive. This statement also holds true in regards to the presence of immune cells in the plexiform lesions (see chap. 3). Again, connecting the dots of experimental mouse antigen immunization data (70) and data obtained with immune compromised athymic rats (71), we wonder whether T lymphocytes monitor lung vascular stress and promote arteriolar muscularization (70), but prevent angioproliferative endothelial cell growth (71). Anti-endothelial cell antibodies may be involved, causing endothelial cell apoptosis; the dendritic cells (53) and perivascular lymphocytes may be part of a localized "tumor surveillance program." Whether pathogenetic T lymphocytes can transfer pulmonary angioproliferative disease to a naive animal has not been investigated, whereas transfer of wild-type T lymphocytes to athymic rats prevents angioproliferative PAH (71). This new branch of lung vascular remodeling, perhaps appropriately termed "lung vascular immunology," will need to grow further and stronger. The immune component in pulmonary hypertension needs to be examined in greater detail because immune responses could play a role in the initiation of PAH or in the maintenance and progression of the lung vascular disease. Lessons may also be learned from Castleman's lymphoma where HHV-8 infection and B lymphocytes play a role (72). Lenz et al. (73) conducted a gene profiling study of large B-cell lymphocytes and described a "stromal cell gene expression" signature representing markers of endothelial cells, angiogenesis factors (VEGFRII, TEK) and reflecting an increased capillary density of the lymphomas. Cool et al. described the presence of markers of

HHV-8 infection in plexiform lesions from patients with IPAH (72). This observation, although unconfirmed by a number of studies from around the world (74–77) remains intriguing as a conceptual bridge between latent viral infections, malignancy and PAH. Recently Bull et al. demonstrated that infection of cultured lung microvascular endothelial cells causes initial apoptosis followed by cell proliferation. Thus, HHV-8 virus can infect lung microvascular endothelial cells and induce an angiogenic gene expression profile (78), and Shan et al. (79) transfected human pulmonary arterial cells with the IIHV-8 vGPCR gene and described Src activation and angiogenic activity.

Certainly the most generally accepted form of viral infection–associated PAH is PAH developing subsequent to HIV infection (80–82). PAH develops in 1 in 200 HIV-infected patients (81), is not tightly coupled to the CD4+ lymphocyte count, and occurs in patients on highly active antiretroviral therapy (HAART) (82). Until recently, we had no pathogenetic concept of HIV-associated PAH. A multiteam effort of serendipity has now provided first insights (83). Comparative analysis of macaque lung tissue samples collected from two different primate research centers in the United States revealed that nonhuman primates infected with a chimeric viral construct containing the HIV nef gene in a simian immunoinsufficiency virus (SIV) backbone cause the development of complex pulmonary vascular lesions. Lung vascular cells and mononuclear cells expressed the HIV nef protein, consistent with viral replication (84). Importantly, the animals infected with SIV constructs not containing the human HIV nef gene did not develop plexiform lesions, and also of importance is the finding that lung vascular cells of patients with HIV-related PAH also expressed the nef protein (84). As these investigations have zoned in on the human nef gene, more recent studies have revealed nef gene mutations that have been detected in peripheral blood cell DNA samples (83). Thus, a molecular hypothesis of HIV-associated PAH has emerged, which links a mutated HIV gene product with angioproliferative PAH. Clearly the mechanism of mutated nef-induced pulmonary angiopathy deserves detailed investigation in primates and in cell culture systems.

Another area that is a fertile ground for investigations of a viral etiology of PAH is the co-existence of hepatitis B and C infections and pulmonary hypertension, with and without portal hypertension (85,86).

V.   Endocrine Factors and Pulmonary Hypertension

In addition to our recent knowledge about mutations of the *BMPR2* and *ALK-1* genes, we are beginning to gather information regarding epigenetic factors that are most likely involved in the pathogenesis of severe angioproliferative PAH. We postulate that there are at least three endocrine conditions or factors that need to be considered: estrogen as a known angiogenesis factor, thyroid disorders, and obesity.

Whereas it has been acknowledged for many decades that IPAH is a disease which affects more women than men and that collagen vascular disease–associated PAH is more frequently diagnosed in women, a review of a number of clinical studies and drug trials supports the notion that female predominance of PAH is far greater than previously appreciated. Recent data collected for the REVEAL (Registry to Evaluate Early and Long-Term PAH Disease Management) database indicate that 70% of patients with the diagnosis of IAPH ($n = 1394$) are women and 78% of 1483 patients with associated or secondary forms of PAH are female. If severe PAH has in recent years become more prevalent (87), then this increased prevalence may have occurred in older and likely postmenopausal women, of whom many did receive hormonal replacement therapy. Although estrogen-based birth control pills had been previously suspected as risk factors for PAH development, limited epidemiological studies apparently did not support this concept, and a WHO working group dismissed birth control pills as a risk factor. However, recently estrogen has appeared on the radar screen. West et al. (88) conducted a gene expression survey using B lymphocytes from patients with familial IPAH and BMPR2 mutation carriers, of whom only 20% developed IPAH and identified a decreased expression of the estrogen metabolizing Cyt P450 1B1 gene as a strong candidate for a modifier gene in female PAH patients. Estrogen affects pulmonary vascular tone (89). Beretta et al. (90) suggest that hormone replacement therapy may in postmenopausal women with systemic sclerosis prevent the development of PAH: Wu et al. (91) reported that intermittent hypoxia promoted in rat lungs the expression of the estrogen receptor 1 gene (see also Ref. 92). Like certain cancers with hormone dependency, PAH may be a hormonally influenced quasi-malignant group of diseases. Estrogen-triggered or -enhanced angioproliferation is most likely HIF-1 dependent (93–95); both HIF-1 and estrogen are strong promoters of VEGF gene expression and both estrogen receptor–dependent and -independent mechanisms could participate in the angioproliferative PAH (95). A large number of reports confirm the original observation of Badesch et al. (96) that many patients with PAH are hypothyroid (97–100). Taraseviciute et al. (101) found 23% to 25% of hypothyroid patients in a retrospective cohort analysis, and a recent survey found that close to 40% carried the diagnosis of a thyroid disease (102). Most likely the coexistence of PAH and thyroid diseases points to an autoimmune disease component that may be another epigenetic promoter of PAH. Again, as with estrogen, HIF-1 may be the bridge to pulmonary angioproliferation; it has been shown that thyroid hormone (T3) stimulates HIF-1 activation (103) and that hypoxia, via HIF-1-activated induction of the enzyme 3 deiodinase, reduces the thyroid hormone signaling (104). We propose that obesity is the third endocrine disorder to influence the genesis of PAH. Hypoxia has not been directly demonstrated in adipose tissues of obese mouse models (105), and it is increasingly accepted that adipose tissue releases inflammatory cytokines, including the angiogenic leptin and VEGF (106,107). As stated above, HIF-1 may be a critically important hub connecting hormonal influences, metabolism, and inflammation with angioproliferation; suffice it to say: HIF-1 plays a role in the inflamed hypoxic adipose tissue. Against this backdrop, the hypothesis that obesity is a risk factor for PAH, which had been entertained by Abenheim et al. (108), should be revisited, particularly in countries where obesity has become epidemic.

VI. Summary and Outlook

At this time—30 years after the pathogenesis of primary pulmonary hypertension had been reviewed in volume 14 of this series—we can say that genetic mutations are neither necessary nor sufficient to cause severe pulmonary hypertension; this has been illustrated by the development of angioproliferative PAH in rats and monkeys without a particular genetic background. The pathobiology of human severe angioproliferative PAH rests on genetic factors and environmental triggers (viral infection, anorexigen drugs) and on epigenetic (likely hormonal) influences. If the exploration of pathogenesis is more than l'art pour l'art, then it should serve the purpose of improvement of quality of life and prolongation of life of our patients (109). Whereas gene mutations may not be repairable for a long time, the autoimmune component of PAH and the hormonal modifiers may become treatable. In addition, the genetic data are only as good as the documentation and annotation of the clinical phenotype and outcome.

Great conceptual progress in the area of the pathobiology of severe PAH has been made, thanks to the work of a growing number of dedicated investigators. Some of us, given the age-dependent long view, remember—not so long ago—the statement and the question: "Surely pulmonary hypertension causes artherosclerosis, why should the lung circulation be different from the coronary or cerebral circulation?" Unfortunately, a quasi-malignant pathobiology is much worse than atherosclerosis; the difference is between a site-specific angioproliferation and a widely spread endothelial cell dysfunction. The pulmonary hypertension centers of the future may quickly apportion the various disease components as soon as the diagnosis of PAH has been established in each individual patient by assessment of the autoimmune component, the bone marrow component, and the response to antiproliferative drugs. Circulating endothelial cells (54) may be monitored as a marker of ongoing active vascular disease (110); circulating microparticles appear to correlate with the severity of PAH (111,112), and quantitative analysis data based on measurement of such particles may guide our therapeutic strategies. New imaging technology, for example, imaging of apoptotic cells and VEGF receptors, may become helpful diagnostic and therapy-monitoring tools (113).

References

1. Voelkel N, Revves JT. Primary pulmonary hypertension. In: Moser KM, ed. Lung Biology in Health and Disease. New York: Marcel Dekker, 1979:573–628.
2. Voelkel NF, Weir EK. Etiologic mechanisms in primary pulmonary hypertension in pulmonary vascular physiology and pathophysiology. In: Weir EK, Reeves JT, eds. Lung Biology in Health and Disease. New York: Marcel Dekker, 1989:513–540.
3. Voelkel NF, Tuder RM, Weir EK. Pathophysiology of primary pulmonary hypertension: from physiology to molecular mechanisms. In: Rubin LJ, Rich S, eds. Lung Biology in Health and Disease. New York: Marcel Dekker, 1997:83–130.
4. Macchia A, Marchioli R, Marfisi R, et al. A meta-analysis of trials of pulmonary hypertension: a clinical condition looking for drugs and research methodology. Am Heart J 2007; 153(6):1037–1047.
5. Chin KM, Rubin LJ. Pulmonary arterial hypertension. J Am Coll Cardiol 2008; 51(16): 1527–1538.
6. Sakuma M, Demachi J, Nawata J, et al. Epoprostenol infusion therapy changes angiographic findings of pulmonary arteries in patients with idiopathic pulmonary arterial hypertension. Circ J 2008; 72(7):1147–1151.
7. Benedict N, Seybert A, Mathier MA. Evidence-based pharmacologic management of pulmonary arterial hypertension. Clin Ther 2007; 29(10):2134–2153.
8. Humbert M, Morrell NW, Archer SL, et al. Cellular and molecular pathobiology of pulmonary arterial hypertension. J Am Coll Cardiol 2004; 43(12 suppl S):13S–24S.
9. Tuder RM, Groves B, Badesch DB, et al. Exuberant endothelial cell growth and elements of inflammation are present in plexiform lesions of pulmonary hypertension. Am J Pathol 1994; 144(2):275–285.

10. Tuder RM, Cool CD, Yeager M, et al. The pathobiology of pulmonary hypertension. Endothelium. Clin Chest Med 2001; 22(3):405–418.
11. Cool CD, Stewart JS, Werahera P, et al. Three-dimensional reconstruction of pulmonary arteries in plexiform pulmonary hypertension using cell-specific markers. Evidence for a dynamic and heterogeneous process of pulmonary endothelial cell growth. Am J Pathol 1999; 155(2):411–419.
12. Cool CD, Groshong SD, Oakey J, et al. Pulmonary hypertension: cellular and molecular mechanisms. Chest 2005; 128(6 suppl):565S–571S.
13. Stenmark KR, Davie N, Frid M, et al. Role of the adventitia in pulmonary vascular remodeling. Physiology (Bethesda) 2006; 21:134–145.
14. Voelkel NF, Nicolls MR. The central role of endothelial cells in severe angioproliferative pulmonary hypertension. In: Aird WC, ed. Endothelial Biomedicine. New York: Cambridge University Press, 2000:1193–1198.
15. Taraseviciene-Stewart L, Kasahara Y, Alger L, et al. Inhibition of the VEGF receptor 2 combined with chronic hypoxia causes cell death-dependent pulmonary endothelial cell proliferation and severe pulmonary hypertension. FASEB J 2001; 15(2):427–438.
16. Oka M, Homma N, Taraseviciene-Stewart L, et al. Rho kinase-mediated vasoconstriction is important in severe occlusive pulmonary arterial hypertension in rats. Circ Res 2007; 100(6): 923–929.
17. Sakao S, Taraseviciene-Stewart L, Lee JD, et al. Initial apoptosis is followed by increased proliferation of apoptosis-resistant endothelial cells. FASEB J 2005; 19(9):1178–1180.
18. Alvarez DF, Huang L, King JA, et al. Lung microvascular endothelium is enriched with progenitor cells that exhibit vasculogenic capacity. Am J Physiol Lung Cell Mol Physiol 2008; 294(3):L419–L430.
19. Golpon HA, Fadok VA, Taraseviciene-Stewart L, et al. Life after corpse engulfment: phagocytosis of apoptotic cells leads to VEGF secretion and cell growth. FASEB J 2004; 18(14): 1716–1718.
20. Majo F, Rochat A, Nicolas M, et al. Oligopotent stem cells are distributed throughout the mammalian ocular surface. Nature 2008; 456(7219):250–254.
21. Lee SD, Shroyer KR, Markham NE, et al. Monoclonal endothelial cell proliferation is present in primary but not secondary pulmonary hypertension. J Clin Invest 2008; 101(5): 927–934.
22. Rai PR, Cool CD, King JA, et al. The cancer paradigm of severe pulmonary arterial hypertension. Am J Respir Crit Care Med 2008; 178(6):558–564.
23. Yeager ME, Halley GR, Golpon HA, et al. Microsatellite instability of endothelial cell growth and apoptosis genes within plexiform lesions in primary pulmonary hypertension. Circ Res 2001; 88(1):E2–E11.
24. Ameshima S, Golpon H, Cool CD, et al. Peroxisome proliferator-activated receptor gamma (PPARgamma) expression is decreased in pulmonary hypertension and affects endothelial cell growth. Circ Res 2003; 92(10):1162–1169.
25. Achcar RO, Demura Y, Rai PR, ct al. Loss of caveolin and heme oxygenase expression in severe pulmonary hypertension. Chest 2006; 129(3):696–705.
26. Wang GL, Jiang BH, Rue EA, et al. Hypoxia-inducible factor 1 is a basic-helix-loop-helix-PAS heterodimer regulated by cellular O2 tension. Proc Natl Acad Sci U S A 1995; 92(12): 5510–5514.
27. Wang GL, Semenza GL. Purification and characterization of hypoxia-inducible factor 1. J Biol Chem 1995; 270(3):1230–1237.
28. Tuder RM, Chacon M, Alger L, et al. Expression of angiogenesis-related molecules in plexiform lesions in severe pulmonary hypertension: evidence for a process of disordered angiogenesis. J Pathol 2001; 195(3):367–374.

29. Archer SL, Huang JM, Hampl V, et al. Nitric oxide and cGMP cause vasorelaxation by activation of a charybdotoxin-sensitive K channel by cGMP-dependent protein kinase. Proc Natl Acad Sci U S A 1994; 91(16):7583–7587.

30. Ekhterae D, Platoshyn O, Krick S, et al. Bcl-2 decreases voltage-gated K+ channel activity and enhances survival in vascular smooth muscle cells. Am J Physiol Cell Physiol 2001; 281(1):C157–C165.

31. Platoshyn O, Zhang S, McDaniel SS, et al. Cytochrome c activates K+ channels before inducing apoptosis. Am J Physiol Cell Physiol 2002; 283(4):C1298–C1305.

32. Brevnova EE, Platoshyn O, Zhang S, et al. Overexpression of human KCNA5 increases IK V and enhances apoptosis. Am J Physiol Cell Physiol 2004; 287(3):C715–C722.

33. Pardo LA, Contreras-Jurado C, Zientkowska M, et al. Role of voltage-gated potassium channels in cancer. J Membr Biol 2005; 205(3):115–124.

34. Stuhmer W, Alves F, Hartung F, et al. Potassium channels as tumour markers. FEBS Lett 2006; 580(12):2850–2852.

35. Wang J, Sun L, Myeroff L, et al. Demonstration that mutation of the type II transforming growth factor beta receptor inactivates its tumor suppressor activity in replication error-positive colon carcinoma cells. J Biol Chem 1995; 270(37):22044–22049.

36. Grady WM, Rajput A, Myeroff L, et al. Mutation of the type II transforming growth factor-beta receptor is coincident with the transformation of human colon adenomas to malignant carcinomas. Cancer Res 1998; 58(14):3101–3104.

37. Myeroff LL, Parsons R, Kim SJ, et al. A transforming growth factor beta receptor type II gene mutation common in colon and gastric but rare in endometrial cancers with micro-satellite instability. Cancer Res 1995; 55(23):5545–5547.

38. Yan Q, Sage EH. Transforming growth factor-beta1 induces apoptotic cell death in cultured retinal endothelial cells but not pericytes: association with decreased expression of p21waf1/cip1. J Cell Biochem 1998; 70(1):70–83.

39. Mauro M, Kim J, Costello C, et al. Role of transforming growth factor beta1 in micro-vascular endothelial cell apoptosis associated with thrombotic thrombocytopenic purpura and hemolytic-uremic syndrome. Am J Hematol 2001; 66(1):12–22.

40. Lu Q. Transforming growth factor-beta1 protects against pulmonary artery endothelial cell apoptosis via ALK5. Am J Physiol Lung Cell Mol Physiol 2008; 295(1):L123–L133.

41. Cook BD, Ferrari G, Pintucci G, et al. TGF-beta1 induces rearrangement of FLK-1-VE-cadherin-beta-catenin complex at the adherens junction through VEGF-mediated signaling. J Cell Biochem 2008; 105(6):1367–1373.

42. Harrison RE, Flanagan JA, Sankelo M, et al. Molecular and functional analysis identifies ALK-1 as the predominant cause of pulmonary hypertension related to hereditary hae-morrhagic telangiectasia. J Med Genet 2003; 40(12):865–871.

43. Elliott CG. Genetics of pulmonary arterial hypertension: current and future implications. Semin Respir Crit Care Med 2005; 26(4):365–371.

44. Richter A, Yeager ME, Zaiman A, et al. Impaired transforming growth factor-beta signaling in idiopathic pulmonary arterial hypertension. Am J Respir Crit Care Med 2004; 170 (12):1340–1348.

45. Teichert-Kuliszewska K, Kutryk MJ, Kuliszewski MA, et al. Bone morphogenetic protein receptor-2 signaling promotes pulmonary arterial endothelial cell survival: implications for loss-of-function mutations in the pathogenesis of pulmonary hypertension. Circ Res 2006; 98(2):209–217.

46. Morty RE, Nejman B, Kwapiszewska G, et al. Dysregulated bone morphogenetic protein signaling in monocrotaline-induced pulmonary arterial hypertension. Arterioscler Thromb Vasc Biol 2007; 27(5):1072–1078.

47. Taraseviciene-Stewart L, Scerbavicius R, Choe KH, et al. Simvastatin causes endothelial cell apoptosis and attenuates severe pulmonary hypertension. Am J Physiol Lung Cell Mol Physiol 2006; 291(4):L668–L676.
48. Hanahan D, Weinberg RA. The hallmarks of cancer. Cell 2000; 100(1):57–70.
49. Brevet M, Ahidouch A, Sevestre H, et al. Expression of K+ channels in normal and cancerous human breast. Histol Histopathol 2008; 23(8):965–972.
50. Kunzelmann K. Ion channels and cancer. J Membr Biol 2005; 205(3):159–173.
51. Wallace DC. Mitochondria and cancer: Warburg address. Cold Spring Harb Symp Quant Biol 2005; 70:363–374.
52. Voelkel NF, Cool C, Lee SD, et al. Primary pulmonary hypertension between inflammation and cancer. Chest 1998; 114(3 suppl):225S–230S.
53. Perros F, Dorfmuller P, Souza R, et al. Dendritic cell recruitment in lesions of human and experimental pulmonary hypertension. Eur Respir J 2007; 29(3):462–468.
54. Bull TM, Golpon H, Hebbel RP, et al. Circulating endothelial cells in pulmonary hypertension. Thromb Haemost 2003; 90(4):698–703.
55. Xu W, Koeck T, Lara AR, et al. Alterations of cellular bioenergetics in pulmonary artery endothelial cells. Proc Natl Acad Sci U S A 2007; 104(4):1342–1347.
56. McMurtry MS, Archer SL, Altieri DC, et al. Gene therapy targeting survivin selectively induces pulmonary vascular apoptosis and reverses pulmonary arterial hypertension. J Clin Invest 2005; 115(6):1479–1491.
57. Perros F, Montani D, Dorfmuller P, et al. Platelet-derived growth factor expression and function in idiopathic pulmonary arterial hypertension. Am J Respir Crit Care Med 2008; 178(1):81–88.
58. Rius J, Guma M, Schachtrup C, et al. NF-kappaB links innate immunity to the hypoxic response through transcriptional regulation of HIF-1alpha. Nature 2008; 453(7196):807–811.
59. Kakinuma Y, Miyauchi T, Yuki K, et al. Novel molecular mechanism of increased myocardial endothelin-1 expression in the failing heart involving the transcriptional factor hypoxia-inducible factor-1{{alpha}} induced for impaired myocardial energy metabolism. Circulation 2001; 103(19):2387–2394.
60. Semenza GL. Hypoxia-inducible factor 1 (HIF-1) pathway. Sci STKE 2007; 2007(407):cm8.
61. Du R, Lu KV, Petritsch C, et al. HIF1alpha induces the recruitment of bone marrow-derived vascular modulatory cells to regulate tumor angiogenesis and invasion. Cancer Cell 2008; 13(3):206–220.
62. Sullivan R, Pare GC, Frederiksen LJ, et al. Hypoxia-induced resistance to anticancer drugs is associated with decreased senescence and requires hypoxia-inducible factor-1 activity. Mol Cancer Ther 2008; 7(7):1961–1973.
63. Oda S, Oda T, Nishi K, et al. Macrophage migration inhibitory factor activates hypoxia-inducible factor in a p53-dependent manner. PLoS ONE 2008; 3(5):e2215.
64. Shin YC, Joo CH, Gack MU, et al. Kaposi's sarcoma-associated herpesvirus viral IFN regulatory factor 3 stabilizes hypoxia-inducible factor-1 alpha to induce vascular endothelial growth factor expression. Cancer Res 2008; 68(6):1751–1759.
65. Wakisaka N, Kondo S, Yoshizaki T, et al. Epstein-Barr virus latent membrane protein 1 induces synthesis of hypoxia-inducible factor 1 alpha. Mol Cell Biol 2004; 24(12):5223–5234.
66. Tamby MC, Chanseaud Y, Humbert M, et al. Anti-endothelial cell antibodies in idiopathic and systemic sclerosis associated pulmonary arterial hypertension. Thorax 2005; 60(9):765–772.
67. Kawut SM, Taichman DB, rcher-Chicko CL, et al. Hemodynamics and survival in patients with pulmonary arterial hypertension related to systemic sclerosis. Chest 2003; 123(2):344–350.
68. Morse J, Barst R, Horn E, et al. Pulmonary hypertension in scleroderma spectrum of disease: lack of bone morphogenetic protein receptor 2 mutations. J Rheumatol 2002; 29(11):2379–2381.
69. Nicolls MR, Taraseviciene-Stewart L, Rai PR, et al. Autoimmunity and pulmonary hypertension: a perspective. Eur Respir J 2005; 26(6):1110–1118.

70. Daley E, Emson C, Guignabert C, et al. Pulmonary arterial remodeling induced by a Th2 immune response. J Exp Med 2008; 205(2):361–372.
71. Ulrich S, Nicolls MR, Taraseviciene L, et al. Increased regulatory and decreased CD8+ cytotoxic T cells in the blood of patients with idiopathic pulmonary arterial hypertension. Respiration 2008; 75(3):272–280.
72. Taraseviciene-Stewart L, Nicolls MR, Kraskauskas D, et al. Absence of T cells confers increased pulmonary arterial hypertension and vascular remodeling. Am J Respir Crit Care Med 2007; 175(12):1280–1289.
73. Lenz G, Wright G, Dave SS, et al. Stromal gene signatures in large-B-cell lymphomas. N Engl J Med 2008; 359(22):2313–2323.
74. Henke-Gendo C, Mengel M, Hoeper MM, et al. Absence of Kaposi's sarcoma-associated herpesvirus in patients with pulmonary arterial hypertension. Am J Respir Crit Care Med 2005; 172(12):1581–1585.
75. Bresser P, Cornelissen MI, van der BW, et al. Idiopathic pulmonary arterial hypertension in Dutch Caucasian patients is not associated with human herpes virus-8 infection. Respir Med 2007; 101(4):854–856.
76. Bendayan D, Sarid R, Cohen A, et al. Absence of human herpesvirus 8 DNA sequences in lung biopsies from Israeli patients with pulmonary arterial hypertension. Respiration 2008; 75(2):155–157.
77. Galambos C, Montgomery J, Jenkins FJ. No role for kaposi sarcoma-associated herpesvirus in pediatric idiopathic pulmonary hypertension. Pediatr Pulmonol 2006; 41(2):122–125.
78. Bull TM, Meadows CA, Coldren CD, et al. Human herpesvirus-8 infection of primary pulmonary microvascular endothelial cells. Am J Respir Cell Mol Biol 2008; 39(6):706–716.
79. Shan B, Morris CA, Zhuo Y, et al. Activation of proMMP-2 and Src by HHV8 vGPCR in human pulmonary arterial endothelial cells. J Mol Cell Cardiol 2007; 42(3):517–525.
80. Reinsch N, Buhr C, Krings P, et al. Effect of gender and highly active antiretroviral therapy on HIV-related pulmonary arterial hypertension: results of the HIV-HEART Study. HIV Med 2008; 9(7):550–556.
81. Sitbon O, Lascoux-Combe C, Delfraissy JF, et al. Prevalence of HIV-related pulmonary arterial hypertension in the current antiretroviral therapy era. Am J Respir Crit Care Med 2008; 177(1):108–113.
82. Opravil M, Sereni D. Natural history of HIV-associated pulmonary arterial hypertension: trends in the HAART era. AIDS 2008; 22(suppl 3):S35–S40.
83. Voelkel NF, Cool CD, Flores S. From viral infection to pulmonary arterial hypertension: a role for viral proteins? AIDS 2008; 22(suppl 3):S49–S53.
84. Marecki JC, Cool CD, Parr JE, et al. HIV-1 Nef is associated with complex pulmonary vascular lesions in SHIV-nef-infected macaques. Am J Respir Crit Care Med 2006; 174(4):437–445.
85. Sen S, Biswas PK, Biswas J, et al. Primary pulmonary hypertension in cirrhosis of liver. Indian J Gastroenterol 1999; 18(4):158–160.
86. Grander W, Eller P, Fuschelberger R, et al. Bosentan treatment of portopulmonary hypertension related to liver cirrhosis owing to hepatitis C. Eur J Clin Invest 2006; 36(suppl 3):67–70.
87. Hyduk A, Croft JB, Ayala C, et al. Pulmonary hypertension surveillance—United States, 1980–2002. MMWR Surveill Summ 2005; 54(5):1–28.
88. West J, Cogan J, Geraci M, et al. Gene expression in BMPR2 mutation carriers with and without evidence of Pulmonary Arterial Hypertension suggests pathways relevant to disease penetrance. BMC Med Genomics 2008; 1:45.
89. Lahm T, Crisostomo PR, Markel TA, et al. The effects of estrogen on pulmonary artery vasoreactivity and hypoxic pulmonary vasoconstriction: potential new clinical implications for an old hormone. Crit Care Med 2008; 36(7):2174–2183.

90. Beretta L, Caronni M, Origgi L, et al. Hormone replacement therapy may prevent the development of isolated pulmonary hypertension in patients with systemic sclerosis and limited cutaneous involvement. Scand J Rheumatol 2006; 35(6):468–471.

91. Wu W, Dave NB, Yu G, et al. Network Analysis of temporal effects of intermittent and sustained hypoxia on rat lungs. Physiol Genomics 2008; 36(1):24–34.

92. Cho J, Bahn JJ, Park M, et al. Hypoxic activation of unoccupied estrogen-receptor alpha is mediated by hypoxia-inducible factor-1 alpha. J Steroid Biochem Mol Biol 2006; 100(1–3): 18–23.

93. Kazi AA, Koos RD. Estrogen-induced activation of hypoxia-inducible factor-1alpha, vascular endothelial growth factor expression, and edema in the uterus are mediated by the phosphatidylinositol 3-kinase/Akt pathway. Endocrinology 2007; 148(5):2363–2374.

94. Yun SP, Lee MY, Ryu JM, et al. Role of HIF-1(alpha) and VEGF in human mesenchymal stem cell proliferation by estradiol17(beta): involvement of PKC, PI3K/Akt, and MAPKs. Am J Physiol Cell Physiol 2009(296):317–326.

95. Kazi AA, Jones JM, Koos RD. Chromatin immunoprecipitation analysis of gene expression in the rat uterus in vivo: estrogen-induced recruitment of both estrogen receptor alpha and hypoxia-inducible factor 1 to the vascular endothelial growth factor promoter. Mol Endocrinol 2005; 19(8):2006–2019.

96. Badesch DB, Wynne KM, Bonvallet S, et al. Hypothyroidism and primary pulmonary hypertension: an autoimmune pathogenetic link? Ann Intern Med 1993; 119(1):44–46.

97. Curnock AL, Dweik RA, Higgins BH, et al. High prevalence of hypothyroidism in patients with primary pulmonary hypertension. Am J Med Sci 1999; 318(5):289–292.

98. Ferris A, Jacobs T, Widlitz A, et al. Pulmonary arterial hypertension and thyroid disease. Chest 2001; 119(6):1980–1981.

99. Kashyap AS, Kashyap S. Hypothyroidism and primary pulmonary hypertension. Circulation 2001; 104(20):E103.

100. Ghamra ZW, Dweik RA, Arroliga AC. Hypothyroidism and pulmonary arterial hypertension. Am J Med 2004; 116(5):354–355.

101. Taraseviciute A, Voelkel NF. Severe pulmonary hypertension in postmenopausal obese women. Eur J Med Res 2006; 11(5):198–202.

102. Sweeney L, Voelkel NF. Estrogen exposure, obesity and thyroid disease in women with severe pulmonary hypertension. AJRCCM, 2009.

103. Otto T, Fandrey J. Thyroid hormone induces hypoxia-inducible factor 1alpha gene expression through thyroid hormone receptor beta/retinoid x receptor alpha-dependent activation of hepatic leukemia factor. Endocrinology 2008; 149(5):2241–2250.

104. Simonides WS, Mulcahey MA, Redout EM, et al. Hypoxia-inducible factor induces local thyroid hormone inactivation during hypoxic-ischemic disease in rats. J Clin Invest 2008; 118(3):975–983.

105. Wang B, Wood IS, Trayhurn P. Dysregulation of the expression and secretion of inflammation-related adipokines by hypoxia in human adipocytes. Pflugers Arch 2007; 455(3): 479–492.

106. Trayhurn P, Wang B, Wood IS. Hypoxia and the endocrine and signalling role of white adipose tissue. Arch Physiol Biochem 2008; 114(4):267–276.

107. Rega G, Kaun C, Demyanets S, et al. Vascular endothelial growth factor is induced by the inflammatory cytokines interleukin-6 and oncostatin m in human adipose tissue in vitro and in murine adipose tissue in vivo. Arterioscler Thromb Vasc Biol 2007; 27(7):1587–1595.

108. Abenhaim L, Moride Y, Brenot F, et al. Appetite-suppressant drugs and the risk of primary pulmonary hypertension. International Primary Pulmonary Hypertension Study Group. N Engl J Med 1996; 335(9):609–616.

109. Zlupko M, Harhay MO, Gallop R, et al. Evaluation of disease-specific health-related quality of life in patients with pulmonary arterial hypertension. Respir Med 2008; 102(10):1431–1438.

110. Del PN, Colombo G, Fracchiolla N, et al. Circulating endothelial cells as a marker of
      ongoing vascular disease in systemic sclerosis. Arthritis Rheum 2004; 50(4):1296–1304.
111. Bakouboula B, Morel O, Faure A, et al. Procoagulant membrane microparticles correlate
      with the severity of pulmonary arterial hypertension. Am J Respir Crit Care Med 2008;
      177(5):536–543.
112. Amabile N, Heiss C, Real WM, et al. Circulating endothelial microparticle levels predict
      hemodynamic severity of pulmonary hypertension. Am J Respir Crit Care Med 2008;
      177(11):1268–1275.
113. Rodriguez-Porcel M, Cai W, Gheysens O, et al. Imaging of VEGF receptor in a rat myo-
      cardial infarction model using PET. J Nucl Med 2008; 49(4):667–673.

5

Animal Models of Pulmonary Hypertension

LAURENCE DEWACHTER and ROBERT NAEIJE
Free University of Brussels, Brussels, Belgium

I. Introduction

Pulmonary hypertension may occur as "pulmonary arterial hypertension" (PAH), which is a rare dyspnea-fatigue syndrome with clear lungs and an isolated increase in pulmonary vascular resistance (PVR), or more commonly as a complication of chronic hypoxemic lung diseases, high-altitude exposure, left-heart conditions or pulmonary embolism (1). All these different types of pulmonary hypertension present with variable degrees of remodeling of the entire pulmonary arteriolar wall. Medial hypertrophy with variable adventitial changes dominates early PAH and purely hypoxic pulmonary hypertension. Intimal proliferation is prominent in chronic obstructive pulmonary disease (COPD). Plexiform lesions are pathognomonic of PAH but have been reported in some patients with chronic thromboembolic pulmonary hypertension (CTEPH). Proximal pulmonary arterial obstruction amenable to surgical endarteriectomy is an exclusive feature of CTEPH, which however also presents with peripheral arteriolar changes.

PAH has the clearest phenotype, very high pulmonary artery pressures, and a particularly poor prognosis (1). In spite of its relative rarity, PAH has attracted most of the attention, as it is the pulmonary hypertension subtype for which the most striking progresses, biological understanding, and treatment have been achieved (2). Experimental animal models of pulmonary hypertension are often used with the implicit assumption of translational value for PAH. However, the current classification of pulmonary hypertension is based on a clinical picture, histopathology, and known response to specific therapies, with no biological criteria.

The histopathology of pulmonary hypertension has been extensively documented. In the early years of corrective surgery for congenital cardiac shunts, lung biopsies were routinely performed to predict reversibility of PVR. Exclusive medial hypertrophy or medial hypertrophy with minimal intimal proliferation was shown to represent less advanced and reversible disease, while thickening of the three layers of the pulmonary arteriolar wall with concentric or eccentric laminar sclerosis, fibrinoid necrosis, and plexiform lesions were the signature of more advanced and irreversible disease (3). These aspects, illustrated in Figure 1, have also been described in the other PAH subcategories, including idiopathic PAH or PAH associated with conditions such as intake of anorexigens, portal hypertension, and connective tissue disease (4–6). It is interesting that prominent medial hypertrophy could also be shown to be associated with reversibility at vasodilator testing in idiopathic PAH (4). Plexiform lesions were thought

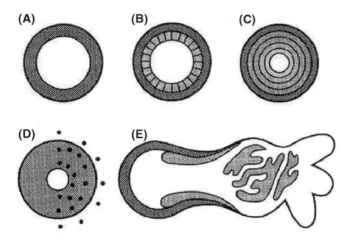

Figure 1 Progressive remodeling of the pulmonary arterioles in congenital heart disease–associated pulmonary arterial hypertension: (**A**) medial hypertrophy, (**B**) medial hypertrophy and intimal proliferation, (**C**) medial hypertrophy and concentric laminar sclerosis, (**D**) medial hypertrophy and fibrinoid necrosis, (**E**) plexiform lesion. Stages **A** and **B** are reversible after surgical closure of the shunt. *Source*: From Ref. 3.

to be pathognomonic of PAH but have been found in only 30% to 50% of the patients, leading to the notion of "plexogenic" PAH (6). Plexiform lesions reported in CTEPH may actually correspond to PAH with proximal thrombotic lesions (7). Microthrombotic lesions are part of the histopathological picture of PAH but found in only approximately one-third of the patients (4–6).

On the pathobiological side, pulmonary arterioles from PAH patients have been shown to present with an endothelial overexpression of vasoconstrictor endothelin-1 and decreased expressions of the vasodilatators nitric oxide (NO) and prostacyclin, a medial overexpression of serotonin transporter (5-HTT), and phosphodiesterase 5 (PDE-5), accompanied by a downregulation of voltage-gated potassium channels (Kv) and an adventitial overexpression of tenascin-C (1,8). Germline mutations in the gene encoding for bone morphogenetic protein receptor type 2 (BMPR2) with associated function loss have been identified in about 50% of patients with familial PAH and in 10% to 30% of sporadic idiopathic PAH patients (1,8). The pulmonary expression of BMPR2 has been shown to be reduced in PAH patients carrying BMPR2 mutations predicted to cause truncation of the protein, and also in PAH patients in whom no BMPR2 mutations could be identified (9). Disturbances in angiopoietin-1 and its tyrosine kinase Tie2 receptor pathway have also been reported (10–12), though not exclusively for PAH, and according to one study, possibly associated with abnormal BMPR2 function through the downregulation of BMPR1A (11). While the exact pathogenetic role of angiopoietin-1 may remain controversial (11,13), its interaction with the Tie2 receptor has been consistently shown to trigger the endothelial release of the pro-proliferative and vasoconstrictive mediators, serotonin and endothelin-1 (10,12).

A realistic model of pulmonary hypertension is expected to integrate clinical, histopathological, and pathobiological features reported in severe pulmonary hypertension, and more particularly PAH.

II. Hypoxia-Induced Pulmonary Hypertension

Chronic hypoxia induces pulmonary vasoconstriction followed by arteriolar remodeling (14). The hypoxia-induced pulmonary pressure response is intense in pig, horse, and cow; moderate in rodent and human; and very low in dog, guinea pig, yak, and lama (14). Chronic hypoxia induces pulmonary hypertension in proportion to initial vasoconstriction. Initial hypoxic vasoconstriction is induced by inhibition of voltage-gated potassium channels localized in smooth muscle cells, and the quasi-immediate response is modulated by endothelium-derived mediators (15). The temporal sequence of hypoxia-induced remodeling is less well known. In humans, chronic hypoxic exposure induces a rapid five-minute increase in PVR followed by a slower further increase, leading to a first stabilization in 2 hours (16) and a maximal response in approximately 24 hours (16,17). After 6 hours of hypoxic exposure, reoxygenation immediately decreases PVR without however a complete return to normal (16). The loss of reversibility of increased PVR is even more striking after 24- to 48-hour exposure to hypoxia (17,18). These data suggest that in the human species, hypoxic pulmonary hypertension evolves in approximately 24 hours from initial vasoconstriction to remodeling.

The temporal sequence of vasoconstriction rapidly followed by remodeling has been confirmed in a variety of experimental animal models. In addition, short-term hypoxic exposure studies in rodents have disclosed an important component of inflammation. Mice exposed to hypoxia for 24 to 48 hours present with medial hypertrophy, infiltrates of polynuclear neutrophils, and induction of proinflammatory cytokines and chemokines such as monocyte chemoattractant protein 1 (MCP-1), intercellular adhesion molecule 1 (ICAM-1), interleukin 6 (IL-6), tumor necrosis factor α (TNF-α), and endothelin-1 (19). Bronchoalveolar lavage studies in rats exposed to hypoxia during eight hours show an early extravasation of albumin, with increased NF-κB activity and increased expressions of TNF-α, hypoxia-inducible factor 1α (HIF-1α), MCP-1, and ICAM-1 (20). These observations explain the recent report of prevention of acute hypoxic hypertension by high doses of corticosteroids in normal subjects rapidly taken to the altitude of approximately 4500 m (21).

The most common hypoxic pulmonary hypertension model has been reported in small rodents, rats or mice, exposed during two to three weeks to 10% oxygen in nitrogen (or equivalent hypobaric hypoxia). These animals present with pulmonary arteriolar remodeling with medial hypertrophy and some adventitial proliferation, but minimal or no intimal thickening and no inflammatory infiltrates (Fig. 2) (22). The mean pulmonary artery pressure is increased, but moderately, reaching values of 20 to 35 mmHg in rats, and even more in mice, with subspecies variability. Neonatal hypoxic exposure in more reactive species, like newborn calves, is associated with more severe pulmonary hypertension, with right-heart failure, and sometimes systemic level pulmonary artery pressures. In these animals, there is a marked remodeling pattern, involving the three layers of the pulmonary arteriolar wall (23).

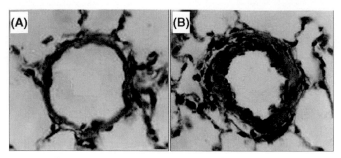

Ppa: 22 mmHg   Ppa: 36 mmHg

Figure 2   (*See color insert*) Pulmonary arterioles and pulmonary artery pressure (Ppa) of normal (**A**) and two-week chronic hypoxia (**B**) exposed rats. Chronic hypoxia induces medial hypertrophy, without any intimal or adventitial alterations. *Source*: From Ref. 22.

Aging animals are relatively preserved from hypoxic pulmonary hypertension (24). The same is true for monocrotaline-induced pulmonary hypertension (25). Newborn animals develop malignant forms of pulmonary hypertension when exposed to hypoxia (23,26) or monocrotaline (26). The fact that rapidly growing animals are also particularly susceptible to pulmonary hypertension is typically observed in the avian species. Broiler chicken are probably one of the fastest growing vertebrate species. A 37 g chick, just out of the egg, can weigh more then 3 kg in six weeks, which represents a 100-fold increase in initial weight (27). Fast-growing chicken are exquisitely sensitive to hypoxia and may develop pulmonary hypertension even in conditions of over-populated sea-level livestocks (28). Figure 3 illustrates remodeling of all three layers of the pulmonary arteriolar wall of young chicken exposed to chronic hypoxia (27). The fact that growth favors the development of pulmonary hypertension is illustrated by the fact that slowing of growth by a decreased food intake limits the increase in pulmonary artery pressures in chicken (27).

In spite of major interindividual and interspecies variations, hypoxia-induced pulmonary hypertension is essentially characterized by medial hypertrophy with adventitial more than intimal changes. No fibrinoid necrosis, plexiform lesions, or microthrombotic changes have been reported in hypoxic pulmonary hypertension.

Hypoxic pulmonary hypertension is associated with intimal overexpression of endothelin-1 and its B receptor (29,30), NO synthase (31), and prostacyclin synthase (32). There is also a medial overexpression of the serotonin transporter (33) and of phosphodiesterase 5 (34) and decreased expression of voltage-gated potassium channels (35). Exposure to hypoxia and subsequent development of pulmonary hypertension is associated with an adventitial overexpression of matrix metalloproteinases and tenascin-C (36). The expression of BMPR2 is decreased (37). Except for the intimal over-expressions of prostacyclin and NO synthases, the biology of experimental hypoxia-induced pulmonary hypertension is similar to that reported in human PAH.

Hypoxic pulmonary hypertension can be prevented and partially reversed by prolonged NO inhalation (38), soluble guanylate cyclase activators (39), phosphodiesterase 5 inhibitors (40,41), inhaled prostacyclin analogues (42), overexpression of

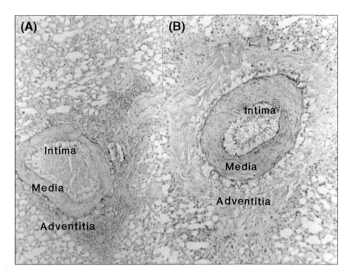

Figure 3 (*See color insert*) Pulmonary arterioles of normal-growing (**A**) and very fast-growing (**B**) chickens after two weeks of hypoxic exposure. There is a marked remodeling of the three layers of the vascular wall in fast-growing chickens. *Source*: From Ref. 27.

prostacyclin synthase (43), serotonin transporter inhibitors (44), potassium channel activators (45), selective (46) and nonselective (22) endothelin receptor antagonists, serine elastase inhibitors (47), and imatinib, a platelet-derived growth factor (PDGF) receptor antagonist (48). Inhibition of lung matrix metalloproteinases aggravates hypoxic pulmonary hypertension (49).

It is difficult to compare the merits of all these effective treatments of hypoxic pulmonary hypertension. In all cases, prevention is easier than reversal. Efficacy in reversing pulmonary hypertension is more appealing for clinical extrapolations. Prevention by targeting specific signaling pathways helps pathobiological understanding.

III. Monocrotaline-Induced Pulmonary Hypertension

Monocrotaline is a pyrrolizidine alkaloid present in the stems, leaves, and seeds of the *Crotalaria spectabilis*, an annual shrub that is distributed throughout tropical and subtropical regions of the world (50). The plant is believed to have originated in India and was introduced into the southern United States in 1921 for the use as cover crop and green manure in agricultural practice (50). The seeds of *C. spectabilis* contain 3% to 5% of monocrotaline. The toxicity of monocrotaline is essentially hepatic and pulmonary. Poisoning by *Crotalaria* has been reported in the veterinary literature for chicken, turkey, pig, cow, monkey, and rat. Like other toxic pyrrolizidine alkaloids, monocrotaline is present in all the *Crotalaria* sp. *C. sagittalis* has caused the equine "Missouri river bottom disease" reported in the southern United States, *C. retusa* and *crispata* the equine "walkabout disease" described in western and northern Australia, respectively, and *C. dura* the equine "jaagsiekte" observed in southern Africa. Animals intoxicated with monocrotaline present with hepatic necrotic lesions and cirrhosis, with variable degrees of pulmonary hemorrhagic edema and fibrosis. Cases of pulmonary hypertension with pulmonary and liver veno-occlusive disease have been reported in Jamaica after ingestion of "bush tea" prepared from different *Crotalaria* leaves including *C. fulva*. Fulvine has been used in the laboratory to induce experimental hepatic and pulmonary veno-occlusive diseases (50).

Young rats fed on a diet containing powdered *C. spectabilis* seeds present with reduced growth, dyspnea, cyanosis, and right-heart failure, leading to death in 30 to 60 days depending on the ingested dose (51). At autopsy, the animals present with cardiomegaly associated with right ventricular hypertrophy and dilatation, variable degrees of lung fibrosis with sometimes congestion and hepatic congestion with centrolobular necrosis. The only histopathological abnormality in the heart comprises small foci of myocarditis and remodeling of the right ventricle. The pulmonary arterioles present with medial hypertrophy, which is also observed in the pulmonary veins, and eventual adventitial inflammatory changes in a proportion of cases, with or without fibrinoid necrosis (Fig. 4). No plexiform lesions or intimal sclerosis have been reported in monocrotaline-induced pulmonary hypertension. It has been thought that a large part of these histopathological features were to be explained by the rapid increase of pulmonary venous pressures, much like in mitral stenosis (50,51). Monocrotaline-induced pulmonary hypertension is severe, with, in rats, increased systolic pulmonary artery pressure from 62 to 112 mmHg, compared to 22 to 36 mmHg in controls, and major right ventricular hypertrophy, with a twofold increase in the Fulton index (ratio of right ventricular free wall weight divided by the sum of the septum plus left ventricular free wall weight) (52).

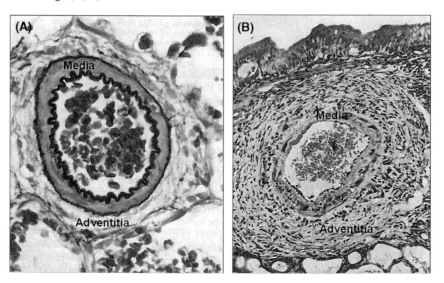

Figure 4 Pulmonary arterioles of monocrotaline-intoxicated rats. (**A**) Medial hypertrophy associated with little or no adventitial proliferation; (**B**) medial hypertrophy, fibrinoid necrosis, and inflammatory adventitial proliferation. *Source*: From Ref. 51.

The administration of monocrotaline induces an early endothelial cell injury associated with an acute lung edema, already prominent after 24 hours and persisting from two days to one week (52,53). Along with the regression of lung edema, there is a rapid arteriolar (and venous) remodeling and right-heart failure. The severity of pulmonary hypertension and subsequent mortality are decreased in older animals (25). After the initial endothelial cell injury, monocrotaline-induced pulmonary hypertension remains inflammatory all along its evolution. The major inflammatory component of this pulmonary hypertension model explains the preventive efficacy of corticosteroids (54,55).

Intoxication with monocrotaline is associated with increased venous plasma endothelin-1 concentrations preceding the development of pulmonary hypertension (56). The intimal expression of endothelin-1 is decreased (57) or increased (58,59), while the expressions of the endothelin receptor type B (60) and endothelial NO synthase (31) are decreased. The medial expressions of the serotonin transporter (61) and of survivin, an inhibitor of apoptosis (62), are increased, while there is a decreased expression of voltage-gated potassium channels, including Kv1.5 (62,63) and Kv2.1 (63) and the hepatocyte growth factor (HGF) (57). There is an adventitial increased production of extracellular matrix glycoproteins, like tropoelastin (64), fibronectin (64), collagen (57,64), and tenascin-C (65), with increased expression and activation of matrix metalloproteinases (66). Lungs from monocrotaline-intoxicated rats present increased expression of several pro-inflammatory cytokines such as IL-1β, IL-6, MCP1 (61), ICAM-1, E-selectin (67), and transforming growth factor β (TGF-β) (57). The expression of BMPR2 is decreased, but its restoration does not improve pulmonary hypertension (68). Thus, the pathobiology of monocrotaline-induced pulmonary hypertension presents similarities to that reported in PAH, with however no plexiform lesions, discordant endothelin-1 and endothelial NO synthase expressions, and an overabundant inflammatory reaction.

Monocrotaline-induced PH can be prevented and/or improved by a wide range of treatments including corticoids (54,55), hydralazine (54), sulfinpyrazone (54), nifedipine (69), prostacyclin analogues (70,71), soluble guanylate cyclase activators (39), continuous NO inhalation (67), phosphodiesterase 5 inhibitors (72), selective (71,73) and nonselective (73) endothelin receptor antagonists, serotonin transporter inhibitors (61), protein C inhibitors (74), anti-MCP1 gene therapy (75), serin elastase inhibitors (76), imatinib (48), mesenchymal stem cells (77), and endothelial progenitor cells, preferably NO synthase transduced (78). Selective endothelin B receptor antagonists aggravate monocrotaline-induced pulmonary hypertension (79). Overexpression of angiopoietin-1 improves survival and pulmonary hemodynamics in monocrotaline-induced pulmonary hypertension (13), which is intriguing as rats genetically manipulated to overexpress angiopoietin-1, develop severe pulmonary hypertension with striking medial hypertrophy (12). This apparent paradox may be explained by anti-apoptotic effects of angiopoietin-1 preventing early disappearance of the pulmonary vascular endothelium after administration of monocrotaline.

Monocrotaline-induced pulmonary hypertension is similar to PAH in terms of hemodynamic and histopathological severity and naturally high mortality. However, it differs from PAH by an initial permeability lung edema, with early loss of the endothelial barrier and striking inflammatory adventitial proliferation. Unlike PAH, monocrotaline-induced pulmonary hypertension can be cured by a variety of vasodilators and anti-inflammatory agents. Initial apoptosis of endothelial cells explains the favorable effects of angiogenic factors (angiopoietin-1) and stem cells, which are unlikely to be effective in more exclusively proliferative forms of the disease. An interesting feature of monocrotaline-induced pulmonary hypertension is that it allows an examination of the effects of interventions on survival. As the inflammatory component of PAH is becoming better understood, monocrotaline-induced pulmonary hypertension offers a model for the study of the signaling pathways involved.

IV. Overcirculation-Induced Pulmonary Hypertension

Pulmonary hypertension is a classically described complication of congenital cardiac malformations with left to right shunting (80). The severity of shunt-induced pulmonary hypertension depends on the amount of shunt flow and pressure. Pulmonary hypertension is an uncommon and late consequence of atrial septal defects, but an early and frequent complication of ventricular septal defects and persistent *ductus arteriosus*. Shunt-induced pulmonary hypertension is associated with adaptative right ventricular hypertrophy and eventual failure with increased atrial and/or ventricular pressures as a cause of shunt reversal. The pathology of this stage of congenital cardiac shunt–induced pulmonary hypertension was first reported by Viktor Eisenmenger in 1897 (81). The clinical and hemodynamic picture of congenital cardiac shunt–induced pulmonary hypertension with shunt reversal as a cause of profound hypoxemia, polycythemia, and digital clubbing was described more than half a century later by Paul Wood, who coined the term Eisenmenger syndrome (82).

Left to right shunt–induced pulmonary hypertension can be reproduced in animals. For this purpose, the pig is the preferred species as presenting with the most reactive and prone to remodeling pulmonary circulation, especially during the first weeks and months of life. It has been estimated that shunted piglets would reproduce, in a few months, a natural history of the disease that would require decades in the human species (83). A synthetic material aortapulmonary shunt in growing piglets induces severe pulmonary hypertension with medial hypertrophy in a few months (83). However, in this model, there has been disappointment because of a relatively limited increase in PVR disclosed after normalization for pulmonary flow (84). This is explained by the fact that synthetic material shunts are necessarily limited in size while a piglet is fast growing, thereby decreasing the mechanical stress on the pulmonary circulation over time. This is why the model was improved by the surgical anastomosis of the subclavian artery or the inno-minate artery to the pulmonary arterial trunk, which corresponds to the Blalock-Taussig operation for the reoxygenation of blue babies with complex cardiac malformations and underperfused lungs (85). The modified Blalock-Taussig shunt increases with the growth of the animals, maintaining a maximum mechanical stress as a cause of arteriolar remodeling and increased PVR. It has indeed been shown that three months of Blalock-Taussig shunting increases mean pulmonary artery pressure to 30 to 40 mmHg at a normalized cardiac output (measured after shunt closure) and produces a histopatho-logical picture of pronounced medial hypertrophy with or without some intimal remodeling (Fig. 5) (86). The correlation between the medial thickness of the smallest arterioles and the severity of pulmonary hypertension (Fig. 5) makes the model suitable for hemodynamic and pathobiological studies. An alternative to shunt is the ligation of a pulmonary artery in piglets, which doubles chronically the flow to the contralateral lung

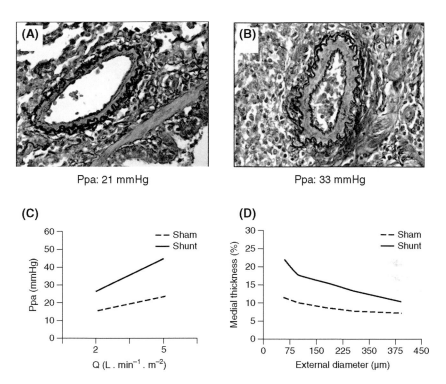

Figure 5 (*See color insert*) Pulmonary arterioles and pulmonary artery pressures (Ppa) of sham-operated (**A**) and shunted (**B**) piglets. Three months of shunting induces a shift of the pulmonary artery pressure (Ppa) versus flow curves (**Q**) to higher pressures (**C**) and an upward shift of medial thickness versus arteriolar diameter curves (**D**), mainly in smallest pulmonary resistive arterioles. *Source*: From Ref. 86.

(87), but this has been less well studied and is actually a less realistic reproduction of the congenital cardiac shunt–induced pulmonary hypertension.

Pulmonary hypertension due to congenital heart disease has also been reproduced in other animal species. An anastomosis between the inferior vena cava and the abdominal aorta has been reported in rats (88) and in utero aortapulmonary shunts in late gestation fetal lambs (89). Both models are associated with no or minimal increases in PVR. The aortocaval shunt has therefore been combined in rats with the injection of monocrotaline. However, the resulting pulmonary hypertension is not clearly different from that produced by monocrotaline alone (90). Another mode of mechanical stress on the pulmonary circulation is by the increase in pulmonary venous pressure, to mimic pulmonary hypertension on mitral stenosis or advanced left-heart failure. This has been successfully achieved in calves (91), but attempts in other animal species have generally failed to increase PVR.

Experimental shunt-induced pulmonary hypertension is generally limited to medial hypertrophy, which corresponds to the early stage of PAH (3). This is related to periods of observation necessarily limited to only a few months in rapidly growing large animals, like piglets and lambs, thereafter difficult to maintain for longer periods of time in most animal facilities. However, older previous studies had looked at the effects of several years of shunting in animal species with low pulmonary vascular reactivity, like dogs, and reported in a small number of these animals severe pulmonary hypertension with all the typical features of PAH, including fibrinoid necrosis and plexiform lesions (Fig. 6) (92,93). These experiments have not been repeated.

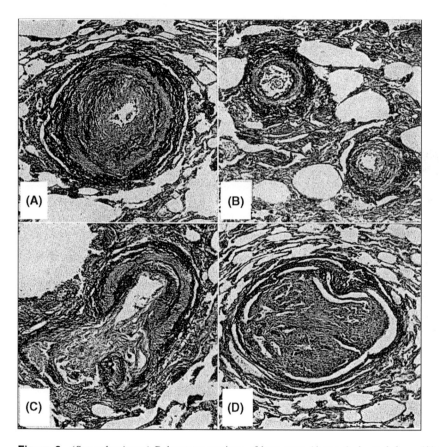

Figure 6 (*See color insert*) Pulmonary sections of long-term (4 years) shunted dogs. (**A**) Transverse section of a muscular pulmonary artery, with medial hypertrophy. The vessel is almost totally occluded by fibrous tissue, most of which is acellular. (**B**) Transverse section of two pulmonary arterioles. In both, there is a thick muscular media between distinct internal and external elastic laminae. The arteriole to the right is partially occluded by acellular fibrous tissue and the underlying muscular media is thinned. There is no intimal fibrosis and no thinning of the media in the arteriole to the left. (**C**) Transverse sections of a muscular pulmonary artery showing medial hypertrophy, severe acellular intimal fibrosis, and a dilated branch that forms a distented sac filled with proliferated cellular endothelium. The appearances are characteristic of those of a "plexiform dilatation" lesion. (**D**) Transverse section of a "plexiform dilatation" lesion that forms a distented sac containing proliferated cellular endothelium arranged in parts in a plexiform pattern. An arc of the remaining media of the parent muscular pulmonary artery can be seen at the periphery of the sac. *Source*: From Ref. 93.

The pathobiology of shunt-induced pulmonary hypertension is essentially known from experiments on piglets and lambs, with concordant results. In piglets, chronic systemic to pulmonary shunting increases the pulmonary expressions of endothelin-1 and endothelin B receptor, inducible NO synthase, vascular endothelial growth factor (VEGF), the serotonin receptor-1B, angiopoietin-1, angiotensin II and its AT1 and AT2 receptors, phosphodiesterase 5, and tenascin-C (86,94–97). In these studies, there were no changes in the expressions of the endothelin receptor type A, endothelin-converting enzyme 1, endothelial NO synthase, Tie2 receptor, angiopoietin-2, serotonin transporter, and serotonin receptor-2B (86,94–97). The expressions of BMPR2 and BMPR1A were decreased (94). In these piglet experiments, the expressions of endothelin-1, endothelin receptor type B, angiopoietin-1, angiotensin II, and phosphodiesterase 5 were directly correlated to the severity of induced pulmonary hypertension (86,94,95). The expression of BMPR2 was inversely correlated to the severity of pulmonary hypertension (94).

In in utero shunted lambs present with increased expressions in endothelial NO synthase (98), endothelin-1, and the endothelin receptor type A, while the endothelin receptor type B showed a biphasic evolution with a decrease and an increase respectively one month and two months after birth (99,100). There is also report of increased VEGF and its receptors, Flt-1 and Flt-1/KDR (101), transforming growth factor β (TGF-β) and its ALK1 receptor (102), phosphodiesterase 5 and soluble guanylate cyclase (103), and calcium-activated potassium channels, but not voltage-gated potassium channels, while pH-sensitive potassium channels pulmonary expressions are decreased (104). In aortocaval shunted rats, the expression of endothelial NO synthase expression has been found to be unchanged (105).

Shunt-induced pulmonary hypertension models have been used for the study of specific therapies. In piglets, prevention with a nonselective (bosentan) or selective (sitaxsentan) endothelin receptor antagonists, a phosphodiesterase 5 inhibitor (sildenafil), or an angiotensin II receptor blocker (losartan) all limit the increase in PVR and arteriolar remodeling to variable extents (86,94–96). An a posteriori comparison of these interventions show bosentan and sildenafil as most efficacious, closely followed by sitaxsentan, while the effects of losartan are more limited. In lambs born with in utero placed shunts, a selective endothelin receptor type A blockade decreases PVR but does not appear to limit pulmonary vascular remodeling (106). In rats with pulmonary hypertension on combined aortocaval shunting and monocrotaline injection, a prostacyclin analogue has been reported to improve the clinical course and to decrease pulmonary artery pressure, with however no significant effect on right ventricular hypertrophy or pulmonary arteriolar remodeling (90). In shunt-induced pulmonary hypertension, PVR remains generally reversible by inhaled NO or intravenous prostacyclin (85) or tezosentan, a nonselective endothelin receptor antagonist (85,107).

Left to right shunt–induced pulmonary hypertension is a realistic PAH model, which has been shown productive for the study of the signaling pathways involved in the most early stages of the disease, and thus for the search of its *primum movens*. It is most suitable for combined hemodynamic, morphometric, and biological approaches for the investigation of the pulmonary circulation and the right ventricle.

V. Persistent Pulmonary Hypertension of the Newborn

In utero ligation of the *ductus arteriosus* is a model of persistent pulmonary hypertension after birth (108). Persistent pulmonary hypertension (PPHN) of the newborn is characterized by persistent fetal morphology of the pulmonary circulation, associated with severe pulmonary hypertension, medial hypertrophy, peripheral extension of smooth muscle cell, and adventitial remodeling.

The pathobiology of experimental PPHN is characterized by impaired endothelium-dependent relaxation of the pulmonary arterioles (109), with decreased endothelial NO synthase expression (110) and depressed soluble guanylate cyclase activity (111). The expression of phosphodiesterase 5 is unchanged, but its activity is increased by 150% (112). The expression of preproendothelin-1 is increased, with no changes in the expressions of endothelin-converting enzyme 1 and the endothelin receptor type A (113) and a decreased expression of the endothelin receptor type B (114). The expression of VEGF is also decreased (115). In normal fetal lambs, the administration of a selective VEGF inhibitor mimics the structural and physiological changes of experimental PPHN, by elevating PVR by 50% and reducing endothelial NO synthase, together with an impaired endothelium-dependent relaxation (115). The expressions of the cGMP kinase 1α (PKG-1α), the α-chain of voltage-operated calcium channels, and the α-subunit of the calcium-sensitive potassium channels are decreased (114). This observation could be related to decreased contribution of calcium-sensitive potassium channels to the membrane potential and to decreased oxygen sensitivity of pulmonary artery smooth muscle cells (116). Impaired endothelium-dependent vasodilatation, related to decreased soluble guanylate cyclase and maintained phosphodiesterase 5 activities, has also been reported in an experimental model of severe PPHN consecutive to congenital diaphragmatic hernia in lambs (117).

Experimental PPHN models have also been used for the evaluation of therapeutic interventions. The infusion of phosphodiesterase 5 inhibitors, zaprinast and dipyridamole, has been shown to decrease PVR by 55% and 35%, respectively, in lambs with in utero ligation of the *ductus arteriosus* (112). The direct activator of soluble guanylate cyclase, BAY 41-2272, has been reported to cause a 60% fall in PVR, greater than sildenafil treatment alone in the same PPHN model (118). In PPHN induced by a surgically induced diaphragmatic hernia, the selective endothelin receptor type A antagonist, BQ-123, caused a greater pulmonary vasodilatation than acetylcholine, sodium nitroprusside, zaprinast, and dipyridamole (119). In diaphragmatic hernia PPHN, pinacidil, an ATP-dependent potassium-channel opener, has also been reported to decrease PVR (120).

Experimental PPHN models in fetal lambs show some histopathological and biological similarities with PAH, including very high pulmonary artery pressures, major medial hypertrophy and abnormal endothelium-dependent relaxation, associated with upregulated endothelin and downregulated NO/cGMP signaling pathways. However, the models differ from PAH by the absence of intimal proliferation and by the lack of alterations identified in the signaling pathways of prostacyclin, serotonin, angiopoietin-1, voltage-gated potassium channels, BMP, and tenascin-C. Therefore, as it stands, results are essentially transposable to real PPHN. The inclusion of PPHN into the PAH category of expert consensus classifications of pulmonary hypertension has remained a matter of debate.

VI. Genetic Manipulations

Pulmonary hypertension models have been conceived from manipulation of genes shown to be involved in up- or downregulation of signaling pathways involved in experimental or clinical pulmonary hypertension. An overexpression of angiopoietin-1 using adeno-associated virus vector has been shown to be the cause of severe pulmonary hypertension associated with striking medial hypertrophy (121). The gene transfer of a Tie2 receptor antagonist in rats prevented pulmonary hypertension induced by mono-crotaline or by angiopoietin-1 overexpression, but did not affect hypoxic pulmonary hypertension (122). Transgenic serotonin transporter–deficient mice have been shown to present with normal hemodynamics in normoxia but to develop less severe hypoxic pulmonary hypertension, vascular remodeling, and ventricle hypertrophy than wild-type mice in chronic hypoxia, despite a potentiation of hypoxic pulmonary vasoconstriction (123). Transgenic mice overexpressing the serotonin transporter under the control of the SM22 promoter spontaneously developed pulmonary hypertension with marked increases in right ventricular systolic pressure, pulmonary arteriolar remodeling, and Fulton index (right ventricle/left ventricle + septum ratio) in normoxia (Fig. 7). These SM22-5HTT+ mice showed depressed hypoxic pulmonary vasoconstriction when compared with wild-type mice, contrasting with greater severity of hypoxia- or mono-crotaline-induced pulmonary hypertension (124). The opposing effects of the serotonin transporter gene expression on hypoxic pulmonary vasoconstriction (acute) and remodeling (chronic) may be related to increased amounts of serotonin made available at the serotonin receptor-1B site.

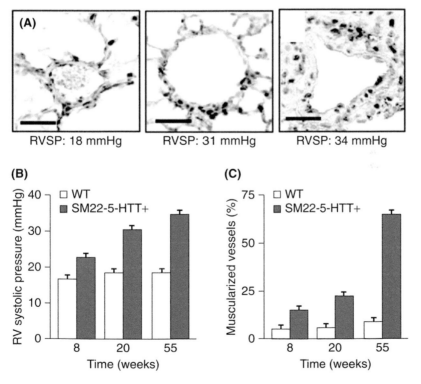

Figure 7 (*See color insert*) Pulmonary arterioles (**A**) and right ventricular (RV) systolic pressure curves (**B**) and morphometry (**C**) of wild-type and transgenic mice overexpressing serotonin transporter (5-HTT) under the control of the SM22 promoter (SM22–5-HTT+) at 20 and 55 weeks of age. *Source*: From Ref. 124.

Because the mutation of the BMPR2 receptor is a cause of inheritable PAH, but also, though less frequently, of sporadic idiopathic PAH, a lot of attention has been devoted to BMPR2 knockout mice. Mice with a homozygous *BMPR2* mutation, by lack of exons 4 and 5, actually die at a very early stage of in utero, before gastrulation (125). This observation underscores the critical role of the BMP pathway in early embryogenesis and vascular development. On the other hand, heterozygous BMPR2+/− mice survive to adulthood and breed normally with no readily discernable phenotype, and may or not spontaneously develop a mild form of pulmonary hypertension (126,127). However, in these BMPR2+/− mice, an overexpression of interleukin 1β (128), a chronic infusion of serotonin associated to chronic hypoxia (127), or combined monocrotaline injection with intratracheal instillation of 5-lipoxygenase adenovirus (129) induce greater increases in PVR and ventricular hypertrophy than in wild-type mice. Chronic hypoxia alone does not induce pulmonary hypertension in BMPR2+/− mice (127). Thus, transgenic BMPR2+/− mice mimic at genetic level of the haploinsufficiency underlying the pathogenesis of familial PAH and support the concept that BMPR2 dysfunction increases the susceptibility to pulmonary hypertension, without causing it. Furthermore, as already mentioned, an overexpression of BMPR2 does not ameliorate pulmonary hypertension induced by the injection of monocrotaline (68).

Like BMPR2−/− mice, homozygous null mice for BMPR1A die in utero because of defective mesoderm formation (130). To avoid this embryonic lethality, BMPR1A knockout mice with specific deletion (on tetracycline withdrawal) in vascular smooth muscle cells and cardiac myocytes have been constructed. These mice show similar chronic hypoxia-induced pulmonary hypertension compared with wild-type mice, but a decreased cardiac contractility (131). Transgenic BMP4 (132) or Smad4 (133) homozygous null mice die in utero by defective mesoderm formation.

Male insulin-resistant apoE-deficient mice present with an increased ventricular systolic pressure associated with right ventricular hypertrophy and increased peripheral pulmonary artery muscularization compared with corresponding female mice presenting insulin resistance and deficiency of apoE as risk factors for PAH (134). Whether this is clinically relevant remains to be explored.

Cyclooxygenase 2 (COX-2)-deficient mice with associated enhanced endothelin receptor type A expression develop severe pulmonary hypertension with exaggerated elevation of right ventricular systolic pressure, significant right ventricular hypertrophy, and striking vascular remodeling following chronic hypoxia (135). This observation may be related more to endothelin signaling than abnormal cyclooxygenase as a cause of decreased vasodilating prostanoids. Nonsteroidal anti-inflammatory drugs have not been found to be a risk factor for PAH (1).

Homozygous vasoactive intestinal peptide (VIP)-deficient mice develop spontaneously pulmonary hypertension (136). This observation opens the perspective of nonadrenergic, noncholinergic control of pulmonary vascular tone and structure and may perhaps lead to a new treatment of PAH by repeated inhalations of VIP (137). Mice with targeted disruption of eNOS (138), adrenomedullin (139), or the prostacyclin receptor (140) genes are more susceptible to develop pulmonary hypertension in chronic hypoxia. This is in keeping with the notion of a disequilibrium between endothelium released vasoconstrictors and vasodilators to cause and/or perpetuate PAH (1,2).

Transgenic mice expressing an inducible dominant negative mutation of the TGF-β type 2 receptor develop attenuated hypoxia-induced increases in right ventricular pressure, right ventricular hypertrophy, and pulmonary arterial remodeling compared with wild-type mice, underscoring the importance of TGF-β signaling in pulmonary hypertension (141). Knockout mice for the serotonin receptor-1B present with decreased pulmonary vasoreactivity to hypoxia and are relatively protected against hypoxic pulmonary hypertension (142). Hypoxia-induced pulmonary hypertension is attenuated in tryptophan hydroxylase-1 knockout mice characterized by very low serotonin synthesis in the gut and lung (143,144). These observations are in keeping with the notion of disturbed serotonin signaling in PAH. On the angiogenesis side, it has been shown that VEGF-B knockout mice are rather protected against pulmonary hypertension induced by chronic hypoxia, probably through indirect effects of associated increase in NO signaling (145). Pulmonary gene overexpression of inducible NO synthase (146) or downregulation of anti-apoptotic survivin (62) protect against pulmonary hypertension respectively induced by chronic hypoxic exposure and monocrotaline injection. Pulmonary overexpression of prostacyclin synthase protects against hypoxia- (43) and monocrotaline-induced (147) pulmonary hypertension. All these observations reinforce the notion of disrupted endothelial control of pulmonary vascular tone and structure as an important cause of pulmonary hypertension.

Genetic manipulations of the laboratory mouse has become a very powerful investigation tool. Simple transgenics and knockouts can potentially be useful for the "quick" determination as to whether a specific gene, when overexpressed or down-regulated, plays a role in the susceptibility to the development of pulmonary hypertension. The transgenic and knockout models can be crossed to produce mice carrying mutations in more than one gene, to examine the synergistic effects of certain combinations of mutations, to determine modifier gene effects. The transgenic approach to the study of pulmonary hypertension is clearly in its infancy. There are many models yet to be generated. Transgenic animal models have improved current understanding of the complex pathophysiology of pulmonary hypertension, but none of them has yet achieved a realistic reproduction of any various pulmonary hypertensive categories of the disease encountered in clinical practice.

VII. Cell Cultures

Primary cultures of human pulmonary artery smooth muscle cells have been used to investigate in vitro the effects of potential new antiproliferative therapies (148,149).

Pulmonary artery smooth muscle cells isolated from pulmonary hypertensive patients present with an in vitro proliferative phenotype, associated with abnormal responses to specific agents such as BMP and TGF-β (150,151). This proliferative phenotype is exaggerated in the presence of supernatant collected from cultured endothelial cells isolated from pulmonary hypertensive patients (152), suggesting a role for altered cross talk between these two vascular cell types in the pulmonary vascular remodeling. Main factors of this cross talk are smooth muscle-derived angiopoietin-1 and endothelial serotonin and endothelin-1, which are produced after the activation of Tie2 receptor by angiopoietin-1 (10,152).

An in vitro proliferative phenotype has also been described in pulmonary artery adventitial fibroblasts isolated from chronic hypoxic rodents. These fibroblasts present an enhanced proliferative response to serum compared with fibroblasts isolated from pulmonary or systemic arteries of normoxic rodents (153). This particular behavior could be related to abnormal serotonin signaling via the serotonin receptor-2A and the serotonin transporter (154).

Primary cultures of pulmonary artery cells are convenient for the study of specific or crossed signaling pathways. Whether the in vitro proliferative phenotype shown for pulmonary smooth muscle cells (PAH) or fibroblasts (hypoxic rats) represent realistic pulmonary hypertension models is an intriguing question; whether pulmonary endothelial cells from PAH patients or some animal models of pulmonary hypertension also present with specific proliferative characteristics in vitro is not yet exactly known. The in vitro persistence of abnormal growth patterns together with disturbed intra- or intercell signaling pathways needs to be further investigated to better define its translational relevance. Another yet unsolved issue is that of possibility of phenotypic variability from proximal versus distal pulmonary artery smooth muscle cells.

VIII. Conclusions

Research on the pathobiology of pulmonary hypertension will continue to use a variety of in vivo models of pulmonary hypertension, together with genetic manipulations and cell cultures. The choice and implementation of each model will depend on specific hypothesis. All models remain of limited translational relevance. The perfect animal model of pulmonary hypertension does not yet exist.

References

1. Farber HW, Loscalzo J. Pulmonary arterial hypertension. N Engl J Med 2004; 351: 1655–1665.
2. Humbert M, Sitbon O, Simonneau G. Treatment of pulmonary arterial hypertension. N Engl J Med 2004; 351:1425–1436.
3. Heath D, Edwards JE. The pathology of hypertensive pulmonary vascular disease; a description of six grades of structural changes in the pulmonary arteries with special reference to congenital cardiac septal defects. Circulation 1958; 18:533–547.
4. Palevsky HI, Schloo BL, Pietra GG, et al. Primary pulmonary hypertension. Vascular structure, morphometry, and responsiveness to vasodilator agents. Circulation 1989; 80:1207–1221.
5. Pietra GG, Capron F, Stewart S, et al. Pathologic assessment of vasculopathies in pulmonary hypertension. J Am Coll Cardiol 2004; 43:25S–32S.
6. Wagenvoort CA, Wagenvoort N. Primary pulmonary hypertension: a pathological study of the lung vessels in 156 clinically diagnosed cases. Circulation 1970; 42:1163–1184.
7. Moser KM, Bloor CM. Pulmonary vascular lesions occurring in patients with chronic major vessel thromboembolic pulmonary hypertension. Chest 1993; 103:685–692.
8. Humbert M, Morrell NW, Archer SL, et al. Cellular and molecular pathobiology of pulmonary arterial hypertension. J Am Coll Cardiol 2004; 43:13S–24S.
9. Atkinson C, Stewart S, Upton PD, et al. Primary pulmonary hypertension is associated with reduced pulmonary vascular expression of type II bone morphogenetic protein receptor. Circulation 2002; 105:1672–1678.

10. Dewachter L, Adnot S, Fadel E, et al. Angiopoietin/Tie2 pathway influences smooth muscle hyperplasia in idiopathic pulmonary hypertension. Am J Respir Crit Care Med 2006; 174:1025–1033.

11. Du L, Sullivan CC, Chu D, et al. Signaling molecules in nonfamilial pulmonary hypertension. N Engl J Med 2003; 348:500–509.

12. Sullivan CC, Du L, Chu D, et al. Induction of pulmonary hypertension by an angiopoietin 1/TIE2/serotonin pathway. Proc Natl Acad Sci U S A 2003; 100:12331–12336.

13. Zhao YD, Campbell AI, Robb M, et al. Protective role of angiopoietin-1 in experimental pulmonary hypertension. Circ Res 2003; 92:984–991.

14. Grover RF, Wagner WW, McMurtry IF, et al. Pulmonary circulation. In: Shepard JT, Aboud FM, eds. Handbook of Physiology. The Cardiovascular System. Peripheral Circulation and Organ Blood Flow. Bethesda MD; Am Physiol Soc, 1983, sect 2, Vol 3, part 1, pp. 103–136.

15. Weir EK, Archer SL. The mechanism of acute hypoxic pulmonary vasoconstriction: the tale of two channels. FASEB J 1995; 9:183–189.

16. Dorrington KL, Clar C, Young JD, et al. Time course of the human pulmonary vascular response to 8 hours of isocapnic hypoxia. Am J Physiol 1997; 273:H1126–H1134.

17. Maggiorini M, Melot C, Pierre S, et al. High-altitude pulmonary edema is initially caused by an increase in capillary pressure. Circulation 2001; 103:2078–2083.

18. Groves BM, Reeves JT, Sutton JR, et al. Operation Everest II: elevated high-altitude pulmonary resistance unresponsive to oxygen. J Appl Physiol 1987; 63:521–530.

19. Minamino T, Christou H, Hsieh CM, et al. Targeted expression of heme oxygenase-1 prevents the pulmonary inflammatory and vascular responses to hypoxia. Proc Natl Acad Sci U S A 2001; 98:8798–8803.

20. Madjdpour C, Jewell UR, Kneller S, et al. Decreased alveolar oxygen induces lung inflammation. Am J Physiol Lung Cell Mol Physiol 2003; 284:L360–L367.

21. Maggiorini M, Brunner-La Rocca HP, Peth S, et al. Both tadalafil and dexamethasone may reduce the incidence of high-altitude pulmonary edema: a randomized trial. Ann Intern Med 2006; 145:497–506.

22. Chen SJ, Chen YF, Meng QC, et al. Endothelin-receptor antagonist bosentan prevents and reverses hypoxic pulmonary hypertension in rats. J Appl Physiol 1995; 79:2122–2131.

23. Stenmark KR, Fasules J, Hyde DM, et al. Severe pulmonary hypertension and arterial adventitial changes in newborn calves at 4,300 m. J Appl Physiol 1987; 62:821–830.

24. Tucker A, Greenlees KJ, Wright ML, et al. Altered vascular responsiveness in isolated perfused lungs from aging rats. Exp Lung Res 1982; 3:29–35.

25. Sugita T, Stenmark KR, Wagner WW Jr., et al. Abnormal alveolar cells in monocrotaline induced pulmonary hypertension. Exp Lung Res 1983; 5:201–215.

26. Tucker A, Anderson KK, Babyak SD, et al. Pulmonary hypertension and increased pulmonary vascular reactivity in rats at 10000 ft since birth. Chest 1988; 93:185S.

27. Peacock AJ, Pickett C, Morris K, et al. The relationship between rapid growth and pulmonary hemodynamics in the fast-growing broiler chicken. Am Rev Respir Dis 1989; 139:1524–1530.

28. Julian RJ, Friars GW, French H, et al. The relationship of right ventricular hypertrophy, right ventricular failure, and ascites to weight gain in broiler and roaster chickens. Avian Dis 1987; 31:130–135.

29. Li H, Chen SJ, Chen YF, et al. Enhanced endothelin-1 and endothelin receptor gene expression in chronic hypoxia. J Appl Physiol 1994; 77:1451–1459.

30. Soma S, Takahashi H, Muramatsu M, et al. Localization and distribution of endothelin receptor subtypes in pulmonary vasculature of normal and hypoxia-exposed rats. Am J Respir Cell Mol Biol 1999; 20:620–630.

31. Tyler RC, Muramatsu M, Abman SH, et al. Variable expression of endothelial NO synthase in three forms of rat pulmonary hypertension. Am J Physiol 1999; 276:L297–L303.

32. Blumberg FC, Lorenz C, Wolf K, et al. Increased pulmonary prostacyclin synthesis in rats with chronic hypoxic pulmonary hypertension. Cardiovasc Res 2002; 55:171–177.
33. Eddahibi S, Fabre V, Boni C, et al. Induction of serotonin transporter by hypoxia in pulmonary vascular smooth muscle cells. Relationship with the mitogenic action of serotonin. Circ Res 1999; 84:329–336.
34. Sebkhi A, Strange JW, Phillips SC, et al. Phosphodiesterase type 5 as a target for the treatment of hypoxia-induced pulmonary hypertension. Circulation 2003; 107:3230–3235.
35. Weir EK, Olschewski A. Role of ion channels in acute and chronic responses of the pulmonary vasculature to hypoxia. Cardiovasc Res 2006; 71:630–641.
36. Frid MG, Brunetti JA, Burke DL, et al. Hypoxia-induced pulmonary vascular remodeling requires recruitment of circulating mesenchymal precursors of a monocyte/macrophage lineage. Am J Pathol 2006; 168:659–669.
37. Takahashi H, Goto N, Kojima Y, et al. Down-regulation of type II bone morphogenetic protein receptor in hypoxic pulmonary hypertension. Am J Physiol Lung Cell Mol Physiol 2006; 290:L450–L458.
38. Kouyoumdjian C, Adnot S, Levame M, et al. Continuous inhalation of nitric oxide protects against development of pulmonary hypertension in chronically hypoxic rats. J Clin Invest 1994; 94:578–584.
39. Dumitrascu R, Weissmann N, Ghofrani HA, et al. Activation of soluble guanylate cyclase reverses experimental pulmonary hypertension and vascular remodeling. Circulation 2006; 113:286–295.
40. Eddahibi S, Raffestin B, Le Monnier de Gouville AC, et al. Effect of DMPPO, a phosphodiesterase type 5 inhibitor, on hypoxic pulmonary hypertension in rats. Br J Pharmacol 1998; 125:681–688.
41. Zhao L, Mason NA, Morrell NW, et al. Sildenafil inhibits hypoxia-induced pulmonary hypertension. Circulation 2001; 104:424–428.
42. Abe Y, Tatsumi K, Sugito K, et al. Effects of inhaled prostacyclin analogue on chronic hypoxic pulmonary hypertension. J Cardiovasc Pharmacol 2001; 37:239–251.
43. Geraci MW, Gao B, Shepherd DC, et al. Pulmonary prostacyclin synthase overexpression in transgenic mice protects against development of hypoxic pulmonary hypertension. J Clin Invest 1999; 103:1509–1515.
44. Marcos E, Adnot S, Pham MH, et al. Serotonin transporter inhibitors protect against hypoxic pulmonary hypertension. Am J Respir Crit Care Med 2003; 168:487–493.
45. Xie W, Wang H, Wang H, et al. Effects of iptakalim hydrochloride, a novel KATP channel opener, on pulmonary vascular remodeling in hypoxic rats. Life Sci 2004; 75:2065–2076.
46. DiCarlo VS, Chen SJ, Meng QC, et al. ETA-receptor antagonist prevents and reverses chronic hypoxia-induced pulmonary hypertension in rat. Am J Physiol 1995; 269: L690–L697.
47. Zaidi SH, You XM, Ciura S, et al. Overexpression of the serine elastase inhibitor elafin protects transgenic mice from hypoxic pulmonary hypertension. Circulation 2002; 105:516–521.
48. Schermuly RT, Dony E, Ghofrani HA, et al. Reversal of experimental pulmonary hypertension by PDGF inhibition. J Clin Invest 2005; 115:2811–2821.
49. Vieillard-Baron A, Frisdal E, Eddahibi S, et al. Inhibition of matrix metalloproteinases by lung TIMP-1 gene transfer or doxycycline aggravates pulmonary hypertension in rats. Circ Res 2000; 87:418–425.
50. Kay JM, Smith P, Heath D. Electron microscopy of Crotalaria pulmonary hypertension. Thorax 1969; 24:511–526.
51. Kay JM, Heath D. Observations on the pulmonary arteries and heart weight of rats fed on Crotalaria spectabilis seeds. J Pathol Bacteriol 1966; 92:385–394.
52. Plestina R, Stoner HB. Pulmonary oedema in rats given monocrotaline pyrrole. J Pathol 1972; 106:235–249.

53. Sugita T, Hyers TM, Dauber IM, et al. Lung vessel leak precedes right ventricular hypertrophy in monocrotaline-treated rats. J Appl Physiol 1983; 54:371–374.

54. Hilliker KS, Roth RA. Alteration of monocrotaline pyrrole-induced cardiopulmonary effects in rats by hydrallazine, dexamethasone or sulphinpyrazone. Br J Pharmacol 1984; 82:375–380.

55. Langleben D, Reid LM. Effect of methylprednisolone on monocrotaline-induced pulmonary vascular disease and right ventricular hypertrophy. Lab Invest 1985; 52:298–303.

56. Miyauchi T, Yorikane R, Sakai S, et al. Contribution of endogenous endothelin-1 to the progression of cardiopulmonary alterations in rats with monocrotaline-induced pulmonary hypertension. Circ Res 1993; 73:887–897.

57. Ono M, Sawa Y, Mizuno S, et al. Hepatocyte growth factor suppresses vascular medial hyperplasia and matrix accumulation in advanced pulmonary hypertension of rats. Circulation 2004; 110:2896–2902.

58. Frasch HF, Marshall C, Marshall BE. Endothelin-1 is elevated in monocrotaline pulmonary hypertension. Am J Physiol 1999; 276:L304–L310.

59. Mathew R, Zeballos GA, Tun H, et al. Role of nitric oxide and endothelin-1 in monocrotaline-induced pulmonary hypertension in rats. Cardiovasc Res 1995; 30:739–746.

60. Yorikane R, Miyauchi T, Sakai S, et al. Altered expression of ETB-receptor mRNA in the lung of rats with pulmonary hypertension. J Cardiovasc Pharmacol 1993; 22(suppl 8): S336–S338.

61. Guignabert C, Raffestin B, Benferhat R, et al. Serotonin transporter inhibition prevents and reverses monocrotaline-induced pulmonary hypertension in rats. Circulation 2005; 111: 2812–2819.

62. McMurtry MS, Archer SL, Altieri DC, et al. Gene therapy targeting survivin selectively induces pulmonary vascular apoptosis and reverses pulmonary arterial hypertension. J Clin Invest 2005; 115:1479–1491.

63. McMurtry MS, Bonnet S, Wu X, et al. Dichloroacetate prevents and reverses pulmonary hypertension by inducing pulmonary artery smooth muscle cell apoptosis. Circ Res 2004; 95:830–840.

64. Voelkel NF, Tuder RM, Bridges J, et al. Interleukin-1 receptor antagonist treatment reduces pulmonary hypertension generated in rats by monocrotaline. Am J Respir Cell Mol Biol 1994; 11:664–675.

65. Jones PL, Rabinovitch M. Tenascin-C is induced with progressive pulmonary vascular disease in rats and is functionally related to increased smooth muscle cell proliferation. Circ Res 1996; 79:1131–1142.

66. Merklinger SL, Jones PL, Martinez EC, et al. Epidermal growth factor receptor blockade mediates smooth muscle cell apoptosis and improves survival in rats with pulmonary hypertension. Circulation 2005; 112:423–431.

67. Roberts JD Jr., Chiche JD, Weimann J, et al. Nitric oxide inhalation decreases pulmonary artery remodeling in the injured lungs of rat pups. Circ Res 2000; 87:140–145.

68. McMurtry MS, Moudgil R, Hashimoto K, et al. Overexpression of human bone morphogenetic protein receptor II does not ameliorate monocrotaline pulmonary arterial hypertension. Am J Physiol Lung Cell Mol Physiol 2006; 292:L872–L878.

69. Inoue M, Harada Y, Watanabe K, et al. The effect of nifedipine on monocrotaline-induced pulmonary hypertension in rats. Acta Paediatr Jpn 1993; 35:273–277.

70. Schermuly RT, Yilmaz H, Ghofrani HA, et al. Inhaled iloprost reverses vascular remodeling in chronic experimental pulmonary hypertension. Am J Respir Crit Care Med 2005; 172:358–363.

71. Ueno M, Miyauchi T, Sakai S, et al. Endothelin-A-receptor antagonist and oral prostacyclin analog are comparably effective in ameliorating pulmonary hypertension and right ventricular hypertrophy in rats. J Cardiovasc Pharmacol 2000; 36:S305–S310.

72. Schermuly RT, Kreisselmeier KP, Ghofrani HA, et al. Chronic sildenafil treatment inhibits monocrotaline-induced pulmonary hypertension in rats. Am J Respir Crit Care Med 2004; 169:39–45.

73. Jasmin JF, Lucas M, Cernacek P, et al. Effectiveness of a nonselective ET(A/B) and a selective ET(A) antagonist in rats with monocrotaline-induced pulmonary hypertension. Circulation 2001; 103:314–318.

74. Nishii Y, Gabazza EC, Fujimoto H, et al. Protective role of protein C inhibitor in monocrotaline-induced pulmonary hypertension. J Thromb Haemost 2006; 4:2331–2339.

75. Ikeda Y, Yonemitsu Y, Kataoka C, et al. Anti-monocyte chemoattractant protein-1 gene therapy attenuates pulmonary hypertension in rats. Am J Physiol Heart Circ Physiol 2002; 283:H2021–H2028.

76. Cowan KN, Heilbut A, Humpl T, et al. Complete reversal of fatal pulmonary hypertension in rats by a serine elastase inhibitor. Nat Med 2000; 6:698–702.

77. Baber SR, Deng W, Master RG, et al. Intratracheal mesenchymal stem cell administration attenuates monocrotaline-induced pulmonary hypertension and endothelial dysfunction. Am J Physiol Heart Circ Physiol 2007; 292:H1120–H1128.

78. Zhao YD, Courtman DW, Deng Y, et al. Rescue of monocrotaline-induced pulmonary arterial hypertension using bone marrow-derived endothelial-like progenitor cells: efficacy of combined cell and eNOS gene therapy in established disease. Circ Res 2005; 96:442–450.

79. Nishida M, Eshiro K, Okada Y, et al. Roles of endothelin ETA and ETB receptors in the pathogenesis of monocrotaline-induced pulmonary hypertension. J Cardiovasc Pharmacol 2004; 44:187–191.

80. Hoffman JI, Rudolph AM, Heymann MA. Pulmonary vascular disease with congenital heart lesions: pathologic features and causes. Circulation 1981; 64:873–877.

81. Eisenmenger V. Die angeborenens Defect der Kammerscheidewand des Herzen, 1897.

82. Wood P. The Eisenmenger syndrome or pulmonary hypertension with reversed central shunt. Br Med J 1958; 2:755–762.

83. Rendas A, Lennox S, Reid L. Aorta-pulmonary shunts in growing pigs. Functional and structural assessment of the changes in the pulmonary circulation. J Thorac Cardiovasc Surg 1979; 77:109–118.

84. De Canniere D, Stefanidis C, Brimioulle S, et al. Effects of a chronic aortopulmonary shunt on pulmonary hemodynamics in piglets. J Appl Physiol 1994; 77:1591–1596.

85. Wauthy P, Abdel Kafi S, Mooi WJ, et al. Inhaled nitric oxide versus prostacyclin in chronic shunt-induced pulmonary hypertension. J Thorac Cardiovasc Surg 2003; 126:1434–1441.

86. Rondelet B, Kerbaul F, Motte S, et al. Bosentan for the prevention of overcirculation-induced experimental pulmonary arterial hypertension. Circulation 2003; 107:1329–1335.

87. Rosenkrantz JG, Carlisle JH, Lynch FP, et al. Ligation of a single pulmonary artery in the pig: a model of chronic pulmonary hypertension. J Surg Res 1973; 15:67–73.

88. Garcia R, Diebold S. Simple, rapid, and effective method of producing aortocaval shunts in the rat. Cardiovasc Res 1990; 24:430–432.

89. Reddy VM, Meyrick B, Wong J, et al. In utero placement of aortopulmonary shunts. A model of postnatal pulmonary hypertension with increased pulmonary blood flow in lambs. Circulation 1995; 92:606–613.

90. van Albada ME, van Veghel R, Cromme-Dijkhuis AH, et al. Treprostinil in advanced experimental pulmonary hypertension: beneficial outcome without reversed pulmonary vascular remodeling. J Cardiovasc Pharmacol 2006; 48:249–254.

91. Silove ED, Tavernor WD, Berry CL. Reactive pulmonary arterial hypertension after pulmonary venous constriction in the calf. Cardiovasc Res 1972; 6:36–44.

92. Esterly JA, Glagov S, Ferguson DJ. Morphogenesis of intimal obliterative hyperplasia of small arteries in experimental pulmonary hypertension. An ultrastructural study of the role of smooth-muscle cells. Am J Pathol 1968; 52:325–347.

93. Heath D, Donald DE, Edwards JE. Pulmonary vascular changes in a dog after aorto-pulmonary anastomosis for four years. Br Heart J 1959; 21:187–196.
94. Rondelet B, Kerbaul F, Van Beneden R, et al. Prevention of pulmonary vascular remodeling and of decreased BMPR-2 expression by losartan therapy in shunt-induced pulmonary hypertension. Am J Physiol Heart Circ Physiol 2005; 289:H2319–H2324.
95. Rondelet B, Kerbaul F, Van Beneden R, et al. Signaling molecules in overcirculation-induced pulmonary hypertension in piglets: effects of sildenafil therapy. Circulation 2004; 110:2220–2225.
96. Rondelet B, Kerbaul F, Vivian GF, et al. Sitaxsentan for the prevention of experimental shunt-induced pulmonary hypertension. Pediatr Res 2007; 61:284–288.
97. Rondelet B, Van Beneden R, Kerbaul F, et al. Expression of the serotonin 1b receptor in experimental pulmonary hypertension. Eur Respir J 2003; 22:408–412.
98. Ovadia B, Reinhartz O, Fitzgerald R, et al. Alterations in ET-1, not nitric oxide, in 1-week-old lambs with increased pulmonary blood flow. Am J Physiol Heart Circ Physiol 2003; 284:H480–H490.
99. Black SM, Bekker JM, Johengen MJ, et al. Altered regulation of the ET-1 cascade in lambs with increased pulmonary blood flow and pulmonary hypertension. Pediatr Res 2000; 47:97–106.
100. Black SM, Mata-Greenwood E, Dettman RW, et al. Emergence of smooth muscle cell endothelin B-mediated vasoconstriction in lambs with experimental congenital heart disease and increased pulmonary blood flow. Circulation 2003; 108:1646–1654.
101. Mata-Greenwood E, Meyrick B, Soifer SJ, et al. Expression of VEGF and its receptors Flt-1 and Flk-1/KDR is altered in lambs with increased pulmonary blood flow and pulmonary hypertension. Am J Physiol Lung Cell Mol Physiol 2003; 285:L222–L231.
102. Mata-Greenwood E, Meyrick B, Steinhorn RH, et al. Alterations in TGF-beta1 expression in lambs with increased pulmonary blood flow and pulmonary hypertension. Am J Physiol Lung Cell Mol Physiol 2003; 285:L209–L221.
103. Black SM, Sanchez LS, Mata-Greenwood E, et al. sGC and PDE5 are elevated in lambs with increased pulmonary blood flow and pulmonary hypertension. Am J Physiol Lung Cell Mol Physiol 2001; 281:L1051–L1057.
104. Cornfield DN, Resnik ER, Herron JM, et al. Pulmonary vascular K+ channel expression and vasoreactivity in a model of congenital heart disease. Am J Physiol Lung Cell Mol Physiol 2002; 283:L1210–L1219.
105. Everett AD, Le Cras TD, Xue C, et al. eNOS expression is not altered in pulmonary vascular remodeling due to increased pulmonary blood flow. Am J Physiol 1998; 274:L1058–L1065.
106. Fratz S, Meyrick B, Ovadia B, et al. Chronic endothelin A receptor blockade in lambs with increased pulmonary blood flow and pressure. Am J Physiol Lung Cell Mol Physiol 2004; 287:L592–L597.
107. Fitzgerald RK, Oishi P, Ovadia B, et al. Tezosentan, a combined parenteral endothelin receptor antagonist, produces pulmonary vasodilation in lambs with acute and chronic pulmonary hypertension. Pediatr Crit Care Med 2004; 5:571–577.
108. Morin FC III. Ligating the ductus arteriosus before birth causes persistent pulmonary hypertension in the newborn lamb. Pediatr Res 1989; 25:245–250.
109. McQueston JA, Kinsella JP, Ivy DD, et al. Chronic pulmonary hypertension in utero impairs endothelium-dependent vasodilation. Am J Physiol 1995; 268:H288–H294.
110. Villamor E, Le Cras TD, Horan MP, et al. Chronic intrauterine pulmonary hypertension impairs endothelial nitric oxide synthase in the ovine fetus. Am J Physiol 1997; 272:L1013–L1020.
111. Steinhorn RH, Russell JA, Morin FC III. Disruption of cGMP production in pulmonary arteries isolated from fetal lambs with pulmonary hypertension. Am J Physiol 1995; 268:H1483–H1489.

112. Hanson KA, Ziegler JW, Rybalkin SD, et al. Chronic pulmonary hypertension increases fetal lung cGMP phosphodiesterase activity. Am J Physiol 1998; 275:L931–L941.

113. Ivy DD, Le Cras TD, Horan MP, et al. Increased lung preproET-1 and decreased ETB-receptor gene expression in fetal pulmonary hypertension. Am J Physiol 1998; 274: L535–L541.

114. Resnik E, Herron J, Keck M, et al. Chronic intrauterine pulmonary hypertension selectively modifies pulmonary artery smooth muscle cell gene expression. Am J Physiol Lung Cell Mol Physiol 2006; 290:L426–L433.

115. Grover TR, Parker TA, Zenge JP, et al. Intrauterine hypertension decreases lung VEGF expression and VEGF inhibition causes pulmonary hypertension in the ovine fetus. Am J Physiol Lung Cell Mol Physiol 2003; 284:L508–L517.

116. Olschewski A, Hong Z, Linden BC, et al. Contribution of the K(Ca) channel to membrane potential and O2 sensitivity is decreased in an ovine PPHN model. Am J Physiol Lung Cell Mol Physiol 2002; 283:L1103–L1109.

117. Thebaud B, Petit T, De Lagausie P, et al. Altered guanylyl-cyclase activity in vitro of pulmonary arteries from fetal lambs with congenital diaphragmatic hernia. Am J Respir Cell Mol Biol 2002; 27:42–47.

118. Deruelle P, Grover TR, Abman SH. Pulmonary vascular effects of nitric oxide-cGMP augmentation in a model of chronic pulmonary hypertension in fetal and neonatal sheep. Am J Physiol Lung Cell Mol Physiol 2005; 289:L798–L806.

119. Thebaud B, de Lagausie P, Forgues D, et al. ET(A)-receptor blockade and ET(B)-receptor stimulation in experimental congenital diaphragmatic hernia. Am J Physiol Lung Cell Mol Physiol 2000; 278:L923–L932.

120. de Buys Roessingh AS, de Lagausie P, Barbet JP, et al. Role of ATP-dependent potassium channels in pulmonary vascular tone of fetal lambs with congenital diaphragmatic hernia. Pediatr Res 2006; 60:537–542.

121. Chu D, Sullivan CC, Du L, et al. A new animal model for pulmonary hypertension based on the overexpression of a single gene, angiopoietin-1. Ann Thorac Surg 2004; 77:449–456; discussion 456–447.

122. Kido M, Du L, Sullivan CC, et al. Gene transfer of a TIE2 receptor antagonist prevents pulmonary hypertension in rodents. J Thorac Cardiovasc Surg 2005; 129:268–276.

123. Eddahibi S, Hanoun N, Lanfumey L, et al. Attenuated hypoxic pulmonary hypertension in mice lacking the 5-hydroxytryptamine transporter gene. J Clin Invest 2000; 105:1555–1562.

124. Guignabert C, Izikki M, Tu LI, et al. Transgenic mice overexpressing the 5-hydroxy-tryptamine transporter gene in smooth muscle develop pulmonary hypertension. Circ Res 2006; 98:1323–1330.

125. Beppu H, Kawabata M, Hamamoto T, et al. BMP type II receptor is required for gastrulation and early development of mouse embryos. Dev Biol 2000; 221:249–258.

126. Beppu H, Ichinose F, Kawai N, et al. BMPR-II heterozygous mice have mild pulmonary hypertension and an impaired pulmonary vascular remodeling response to prolonged hypoxia. Am J Physiol Lung Cell Mol Physiol 2004; 287:L1241–L1247.

127. Long L, MacLean MR, Jeffery TK, et al. Serotonin increases susceptibility to pulmonary hypertension in BMPR2-deficient mice. Circ Res 2006; 98:818–827.

128. Song Y, Jones JE, Beppu H, et al. Increased susceptibility to pulmonary hypertension in heterozygous BMPR2-mutant mice. Circulation 2005; 112:553–562.

129. Song Y, Coleman L, Shi J, et al. Inflammation, endothelial injury, and persistent pulmonary hypertension in heterozygous BMPR2-mutant mice. Am J Physiol Heart Circ Physiol 2008; 295:H677–H690.

130. Mishina Y, Suzuki A, Ueno N, et al. Bmpr encodes a type I bone morphogenetic protein receptor that is essential for gastrulation during mouse embryogenesis. Genes Dev 1995; 9:3027–3037.

131. El-Bizri N, Wang L, Merklinger SL, et al. Smooth muscle protein 22alpha-mediated patchy deletion of Bmpr1a impairs cardiac contractility but protects against pulmonary vascular remodeling. Circ Res 2008; 102:380–388.

132. Winnier G, Blessing M, Labosky PA, et al. Bone morphogenetic protein-4 is required for mesoderm formation and patterning in the mouse. Genes Dev 1995; 9:2105–2116.

133. Sirard C, de la Pompa JL, Elia A, et al. The tumor suppressor gene Smad4/Dpc4 is required for gastrulation and later for anterior development of the mouse embryo. Genes Dev 1998; 12:107–119.

134. Hansmann G, Wagner RA, Schellong S, et al. Pulmonary arterial hypertension is linked to insulin resistance and reversed by peroxisome proliferator-activated receptor-gamma activation. Circulation 2007; 115:1275–1284.

135. Fredenburgh LE, Liang OD, Macias AA, et al. Absence of cyclooxygenase-2 exacerbates hypoxia-induced pulmonary hypertension and enhances contractility of vascular smooth muscle cells. Circulation 2008; 117:2114–2122.

136. Said SI, Hamidi SA, Dickman KG, et al. Moderate pulmonary arterial hypertension in male mice lacking the vasoactive intestinal peptide gene. Circulation 2007; 115:1260–1268.

137. Petkov V, Mosgoeller W, Ziesche R, et al. Vasoactive intestinal peptide as a new drug for treatment of primary pulmonary hypertension. J Clin Invest 2003; 111:1339–1346.

138. Fagan KA, Fouty BW, Tyler RC, et al. The pulmonary circulation of homozygous or heterozygous eNOS-null mice is hyperresponsive to mild hypoxia. J Clin Invest 1999; 103:291–299.

139. Matsui H, Shimosawa T, Itakura K, et al. Adrenomedullin can protect against pulmonary vascular remodeling induced by hypoxia. Circulation 2004; 109:2246–2251.

140. Hoshikawa Y, Voelkel NF, Gesell TL, et al. Prostacyclin receptor-dependent modulation of pulmonary vascular remodeling. Am J Respir Crit Care Med 2001; 164:314–318.

141. Chen YF, Feng JA, Li P, et al. Dominant negative mutation of the TGF-beta receptor blocks hypoxia-induced pulmonary vascular remodeling. J Appl Physiol 2006; 100:564–571.

142. Keegan A, Morecroft I, Smillie D, et al. Contribution of the 5-HT(1B) receptor to hypoxia-induced pulmonary hypertension: converging evidence using 5-HT(1B)-receptor knockout mice and the 5-HT(1B/1D)-receptor antagonist GR127935. Circ Res 2001; 89:1231–1239.

143. Izikki M, Hanoun N, Marcos E, et al. Tryptophan hydroxylase 1 knockout and tryptophan hydroxylase 2 polymorphism: effects on hypoxic pulmonary hypertension in mice. Am J Physiol Lung Cell Mol Physiol 2007; 293:L1045–L1052.

144. Morecroft I, Dempsie Y, Bader M, et al. Effect of tryptophan hydroxylase 1 deficiency on the development of hypoxia-induced pulmonary hypertension. Hypertension 2007; 49:232–236.

145. Wanstall JC, Gambino A, Jeffery TK, et al. Vascular endothelial growth factor-B-deficient mice show impaired development of hypoxic pulmonary hypertension. Cardiovasc Res 2002; 55:361–368.

146. Budts W, Pokreisz P, Nong Z, et al. Aerosol gene transfer with inducible nitric oxide synthase reduces hypoxic pulmonary hypertension and pulmonary vascular remodeling in rats. Circulation 2000; 102:2880–2885.

147. Nagaya N, Yokoyama C, Kyotani S, et al. Gene transfer of human prostacyclin synthase ameliorates monocrotaline-induced pulmonary hypertension in rats. Circulation 2000; 102:2005–2010.

148. Clapp LH, Finney P, Turcato S, et al. Differential effects of stable prostacyclin analogs on smooth muscle proliferation and cyclic AMP generation in human pulmonary artery. Am J Respir Cell Mol Biol 2002; 26:194–201.

149. Wharton J, Strange JW, Moller GM, et al. Antiproliferative effects of phosphodiesterase type 5 inhibition in human pulmonary artery cells. Am J Respir Crit Care Med 2005; 172:105–113.

150. Morrell NW, Yang X, Upton PD, et al. Altered growth responses of pulmonary artery smooth muscle cells from patients with primary pulmonary hypertension to transforming growth factor-beta(1) and bone morphogenetic proteins. Circulation 2001; 104:790–795.

151. Yang X, Long L, Southwood M, et al. Dysfunctional Smad signaling contributes to abnormal smooth muscle cell proliferation in familial pulmonary arterial hypertension. Circ Res 2005; 96:1053–1063.
152. Eddahibi S, Guignabert C, Barlier-Mur AM, et al. Cross talk between endothelial and smooth muscle cells in pulmonary hypertension: critical role for serotonin-induced smooth muscle hyperplasia. Circulation 2006; 113:1857–1864.
153. Welsh DJ, Peacock AJ, MacLean M, et al. Chronic hypoxia induces constitutive p38 mitogen-activated protein kinase activity that correlates with enhanced cellular proliferation in fibroblasts from rat pulmonary but not systemic arteries. Am J Respir Crit Care Med 2001; 164:282–289.
154. Welsh DJ, Harnett M, MacLean M, et al. Proliferation and signaling in fibroblasts: role of 5-hydroxytryptamine2A receptor and transporter. Am J Respir Crit Care Med 2004; 170:252–259.

6
Genetics of PAH

ERIC D. AUSTIN, JAMES E. LOYD, and JOHN A. PHILLIPS III
Vanderbilt University School of Medicine, Nashville, Tennessee, U.S.A.

I. Introduction

Originally known as primary pulmonary hypertension (PPH), idiopathic pulmonary arterial hypertension (IPAH) was first described by Dresdale et al. in 1951 (1). Three years later, the same authors described the occurrence of pulmonary hypertension among several members of the same family, providing the first report of what until recently has been known as familial pulmonary arterial hypertension (FPAH) (2). It is now recognized that PAH comes in many forms, including idiopathic (IPAH), heritable (HPAH), and associated with drug exposures (such as anorectic fenfluramine compounds) or other medical conditions (3).

PAH was reported as a heritable disease for 13 different families in the United States following Dresdale's initial description. In 1984, a follow-up analysis of these 13 families was published; this included a 14th family. There were eight new cases in those initial 13 families, while the additional family contained the largest number of affected family members described to that time, with six deaths due to PAH over two generations (4). Loyd et al. concluded that the inheritance patterns were suggestive of an autosomal dominant mode of inheritance indicative of a single gene defect. They also speculated that cases of PAH, which appeared to occur in isolation, could in fact have a familial basis, but were difficult to recognize as such, due in part to skipped generations, which resulted from reduced penetrance (5).

A research registry of PAH in the 1980s provided the foundation for the clinical definition of PAH, and facilitated interaction of participating investigators to collect and organize sufficient numbers of families to provide robust statistical power for a genome wide search for HPAH loci (6). Meanwhile, the genetic defect underlying the majority of cases of HPAH was mapped to chromosome 2q31–32 in 1997 (7,8). Subsequently, mutations in the gene encoding bone morphogenetic protein receptor type 2 (*BMPR2*), a member of the transforming growth factor β (TGF-β) superfamily of receptors, were found to be responsible for the majority of cases of the autosomal dominant familial disease now known as HPAH (9,10). It is currently believed that the majority of individuals with HPAH have an identifiable germline mutation in *BMPR2* (~80%). It is suspected that mutations in one or more other genes related to the BMPR2 pathway are responsible for the majority of the remaining HPAH cases. HPAH associated with hereditary hemorrhagic telangiectasia (HHT), which can be caused by mutations in activin-like kinase type 1 (*ALK1*) or endoglin (*ENG*), supports this assumption (11,12).

II. Clinical Expression of PAH is Variable

BMPR2 mutations have reduced penetrance, which can make establishing familial transmission difficult since generations of mutation-carrying individuals may not express disease (4,13). Penetrance refers to the frequency with which a specific trait (phenotype) is expressed by individuals with a genotype known to be able to cause that trait. Disorders with reduced penetrance may not be recognized as familial in a highly mobile society such as ours, because full family genealogical history is often impaired (14). Because of reduced penetrance, only about 20% of individuals with an HPAH-causing genetic mutation in *BMPR2* will develop detectable PAH during their lifetime. In addition, HPAH is a disease with variable expressivity (extent to which a genetic defect is expressed), such that patients with the same mutation may express disease at different ages, respond in different manners to the same mutations, and have variable durations of survival. Several other interesting findings characterize HPAH, including female pre-dominance ($\sim 2{:}1$ female:male ratio) and genetic anticipation. Most but not all families demonstrate these interesting characteristics to some degree, as demonstrated in the pedigree of one of the most heavily affected families followed by our research group at Vanderbilt University (Fig. 1). This family has a mutation in exon 9, which presumably causes haploinsufficiency (HI) due to the activation of the nonsense-mediated decay

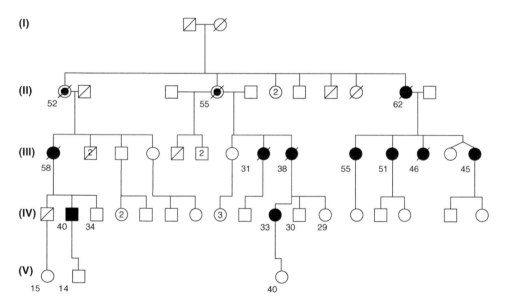

Figure 1 Pedigree of an extended kindred with HPAH due to a *BMPR2* mutation with reduced penetrance. This pedigree contains 10 total patients (9 females, 1 male) with HPAH, as well as 2 known carriers for the family's *BMPR2* mutation. Solid symbols represent individuals with disease. Circles represent women; squares represent men. Line through symbol represents death. Dot inside symbol represents carrier of the *BMPR2* mutation. Numbers below symbols represent age at death or current living age. Numbers inside symbols represent numbers of unaffected siblings of each gender. *Abbreviation*: HPAH, heritable pulmonary arterial hypertension.

(NMD) pathway of RNA surveillance, which destroys mutant mRNAs. This family's pedigree demonstrates pronounced female predominance of the disease (9 females and 1 male with HPAH), as well as reduced disease penetrance with variable ages at disease onset, and appears to support the concept of genetic anticipation.

A. Reduced Penetrance

This characteristic of mutant *BMPR2* alleles suggests that possession of one mutant allele that is sufficient to cause HPAH (heterozygosity) is required but not sufficient to precipitate clinical expression of disease in most cases (15). To date, the mechanisms of reduced penetrance are unknown and suggest a role for additional genetic and/or environmental modifiers of disease expression (16).

At Vanderbilt University, we follow a research cohort of 120 families with HPAH, each with reduced *BMPR2* penetrance. Of 64 families with comprehensive genetic testing for germline *BMPR2* mutations completed, 52 have a detectable mutation, while 12 do not. Of the 351 individuals formally diagnosed with HPAH, 253 are females and 98 are males (ratio $\sim 2.6{:}1$). The age at death spans the entire age spectrum, although a greater percentage of male deaths occur in childhood compared with percentage of female deaths in childhood. There are another 4085 bloodline family members at risk to develop HPAH. In total, 18% of bloodline family members have been diagnosed with PAH to date. Of note, among the six most heavily affected families, 26% of first-degree relatives of patients with PAH have also been diagnosed with the disease. Figure 1 shows the family with the second-largest number of affected subjects in our research registry (9 affected subjects). Not surprisingly, this family's pedigree demonstrates female predominance of the disease, as well as reduced disease penetrance and variable ages at disease onset.

B. Variable Expressivity

It is believed that the variable age of onset of HPAH reflects the variable expressivity of disease in *BMPR2* carriers (17). Efforts to correlate genotype with phenotype to date have not stratified by the type of *BMPR2* mutation, although some studies suggest that patients with HPAH due to any type of *BMPR2* mutation may have more severe disease than those with IPAH (no detectable mutation). Sztrymf et al. reported more severe disease among patients with a *BMPR2* mutation, and noted a younger age at diagnosis and death. In addition, *BMPR2* mutation carriers had more severe hemodynamic compromise at diagnosis, including higher mean pulmonary artery pressure, lower cardiac index, and higher pulmonary vascular resistance. However, *BMPR2* mutation status did not substantially influence survival (18).

Elliott et al. sought to compare the results of vasoreactivity testing according to *BMPR2* mutation type, under the presumption that patients with improvement during cardiac catheterization testing are more likely to respond to chronic therapy with calcium channel blockers (19,20). Interestingly, those with *BMPR2* mutations were nine times less likely to demonstrate vasoreactivity by standard testing [vasoreactivity in 3.7% of 27 patients with nonsynonymous *BMPR2* variations vs. 35% of 40 patients without it ($p = 0.003$)] (21). Similarly, Rosenzweig et al. also found diminished vasoreactivity in patients with a *BMPR2* mutation, as well as worse hemodynamic parameters consistent with the report of Sztrymf et al. mentioned earlier (22).

C. Female Predominance

After the documentation of a *BMPR2* mutation, gender is the most reliable determinant of HPAH. While it has been speculated that the gender discrepancy results from increased male fetal losses, this has not been substantiated (13). Alternatively, it may be that females possess a detrimental risk factor or males possess a protective factor. A hormonal effect has been suggested because of the reported association of HPAH and IPAH with exogenous hormone therapy and pregnancy, but the role of hormones remains unproven (23–26). Interestingly, using genome expression arrays confirmed by real-time polymerase chain reaction (PCR), West et al. recently found significantly decreased transcript levels of cytochrome P450 1B1 (*CYP1B1*) (a cytochrome p450 family enzyme critical to estrogen metabolism) in affected female compared with unaffected female *BMPR2* mutation carriers (27). The significance of this finding is yet to be determined.

D. Genetic Anticipation

Several reports have demonstrated genetic anticipation, which is the increased severity or an earlier age of onset in subsequent generations in HPAH. In many families, the age at death in successive generations decreases serially by about a decade in each generation (4). While controversial as some argue that genetic anticipation is an artifact of ascertainment bias, progressively earlier ages of death have been demonstrated by several investigators, most recently those studying a large registry of patients with PAH in France (28).

The molecular mechanism of genetic anticipation in HPAH remains unknown. It is seen in several neurological diseases, including fragile X syndrome and Huntington disease, both of which exhibit genetic anticipation as well as reduced penetrance and variable age of onset in association with specific trinucleotide repeat expansions (TREs). To date, TREs have not been identified in *BMPR2* genes, nor has an alternative cause of anticipation (progressive telomere shortening) been found (29).

III. *BMPR2* Mutations Cause the Majority of HPAH Cases

The discovery of the genetic basis of HPAH has made possible advances in molecular genetics and the availability of information from the human genome project, as well as the cooperation of several families heavily affected by HPAH (30). Two separate groups utilized microsatellite markers and linkage analysis to focus the search to chromosome 2q33. Nichols et al. used a microsatellite marker search to analyze DNA collected from 19 affected and 58 unaffected family members from 6 families with HPAH, and established linkage to a 30 million base pair (30 Mb) region on chromosome 2q33 (7). Simultaneously, Morse et al. identified the locus of the causative gene using similar techniques (31).

Since at that time 30 Mb of DNA was a challenge to sequence rapidly, a positional candidate gene approach was employed to test genes in this region with products of potential relevance (14). In 2000, two separate teams of investigators identified multiple mutations in the gene that encodes BMPR2, a member of the TGF-β superfamily of receptors, as the cause of disease in several affected kindreds (9,10). A large gene, *BMPR2*, resides on chromosome 2q33 and has 13 exons.

While the discovery that *BMPR2* mutations provide the genetic basis of the majority of cases of HPAH, many unanswered genetic and molecular questions remain (30). Among these is the question that since 2q33 is not the only locus at which a detectable mutation results in phenotypic expression of HPAH, abnormalities at how many other loci can cause disease?

At least two additional loci have subsequently been identified as causing a PAH phenotype, with both found in conjunction with a larger heritable disease known as HHT. HHT is a vascular dysplasia characterized by mucocutaneous telangiectasias, recurrent epistaxis, and gastrointestinal bleeding, as well as arteriovenous malformations of the pulmonary, hepatic, and cerebral circulations. While not uniformly seen, PAH that is clinically and histologically identical to HPAH and IPAH has recently been described in multiple unique kindreds with HTT. Mutations in *ALK1* located on chromosome 12 and *ENG* on chromosome 9 cause HHT (32,33). Interestingly, both genes encode proteins of the TGF-β superfamily of receptors, and like *BMPR2* signal intracellularly via the Smad family of coactivators (34,35).

IV.   Prevalence of *BMPR2* Mutations in Heritable PAH

Since its discovery in 2000, investigators have worked to identify *BMPR2* mutations in other families, as well as in those with apparently "sporadic" PAH (IPAH). While the precise rate of *BMPR2* mutations in the general population is unknown, it is extremely low (14). *BMPR2* is highly conserved, and mutations have been identified in many different ethnic groups (36–38). By 2005, approximately 65% of known HPAH families had *BMPR2* mutations identifiable by gene sequencing. A summary report described 144 distinct mutations among 210 subjects, and the majority of these coded frameshift, nonsense, or splice site donor/acceptance site mutations (39).

Because direct sequencing of genomic DNA does not detect other types of heterozygous mutations such as exonic deletions or duplications, Cogan et al. expanded the mutation screening methods in 2005 using multiplex ligation-dependent probe amplification (MLPA) analysis of genomic DNA with confirmation by real-time PCR. Using MLPA, they demonstrated that 48% of the 21 mutations discovered in 30 unrelated affected families were deletions or duplications of exons. They concluded that such techniques would improve the identification of genetic abnormalities in *BMPR2* in FPAH, such that 70% or more of such families have identifiable *BMPR2* mutations (40). A separate group used MLPA analysis of genomic DNA to identify mutations in 28% of families previously reported to lack *BMPR2* mutations when tested by direct sequencing of genomic DNA (41). These reports further support the primary role of *BMPR2* in the central pathogenesis of disease in HPAH. Interestingly, with few exceptions, each family with HPAH has a different *BMPR2* mutation regardless of ethnicity, such that there is no dominant mutation as seen in other genetic diseases such as cystic fibrosis.

V.   *BMPR2* Mutations in Idiopathic PAH

A small but significant proportion of IPAH patients harbor mutations in the *BMPR2* gene. These mutations may occur in the setting of low-penetrance germline mutations, in which other family members transmit the mutation without disease expression, or the

mutations may develop de novo (42). This is not surprising, given that reduced penetrance and genetic anticipation are both hallmarks of HPAH. While the detection rates
vary in part due to the availability of detailed family histories, mutations are typically
detected in about 10% to 20% of patients (41–44).

VI. *BMPR2* Mutations and Disease Expression

HI describes the condition in which heterozygosity for a gene mutation leads to insufficient protein product, or products with decreased function that is insufficient to reach
the threshold level of activity needed to prevent phenotypic expression of disease. HI is
believed to be the predominant molecular mechanism by which a *BMPR2* mutation
predisposes to PAH (36,45). Consistent with this, various deletions within exons 2 to 13,
which lead to nonfunctional peptides, have been reported (40,41). In addition, approximately 60% of the reported pathogenic mutations should result in a premature truncation codon, which in most cases activate the NMD pathway (36). NMD activation
destroys the mutant transcripts causing HI. In total, these studies suggest that HI contributes to the molecular mechanisms underlying PAH. However, it is unclear what
percentage of *BMPR2* mutations results in disease due to an overtly detrimental

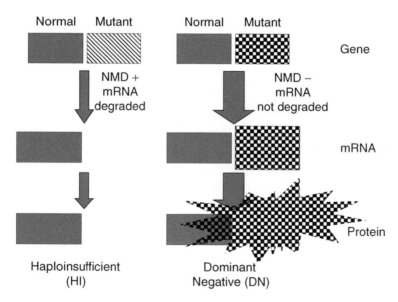

Figure 2 (*See color insert*) Comparison of a heterozygous mutation that results in a haploinsufficient effect versus one that results in a potentially DN effect in the context of NMD. In the
case of HI, the heterozygous state results in one normal (wild-type) allele and one mutant allele.
The mutant allele is degraded by activation of the NMD pathway, such that the only protein
product that results is from the wild-type allele. In contrast, a potentially DN effect occurs when
products of a mutant allele interact with and reduce the expression of normal (wild-type) allele
products. The potential result is even less normal protein is available to function than in the
HI situation. *Abbreviations*: DN, dominant negative; NMD, nonsense-mediated decay; HI,
haploinsufficiency.

(dominant negative, DN) effect on BMP signaling. A DN effect occurs when products of a mutant allele interact and reduce the expression of normal allele products (46,47).

Complete disruption of BMP signaling can lead to absence of critical mechanisms in the antiproliferative and differentiation mechanisms in the pulmonary vasculature (39). In vitro functional studies have demonstrated DN effects on BMP signaling due to mutations or truncations in the kinase domain of *BMPR2* (48). While it is unclear whether reproducible phenotypic differences will emerge in comparing HI and DN mutations, some data suggests that DN mutations are more detrimental (Fig. 2) (49).

In the setting of an HI effect due to a *BMPR2* mutation, the production of *BMPR2* by the remaining wild-type allele may be a critical modifier of disease expression. Studying lymphoblastoid cell lines derived from *BMPR2* mutation carriers with four different HI mutations, Hamid et al. used real-time PCR assays to determine wild-type and mutated *BMPR2* transcript levels. As expected, HI mutant alleles contribute very little to the total *BMPR2* transcript levels (0–2.5%), such that the wild-type *BMPR2* allele is the major determinant of total transcript. Interestingly, they found that HPAH patients had significantly lower wild-type *BMPR2* transcript levels compared with unaffected mutation carriers with the same HI mutation. The authors concluded that the extent of transcript production by the wild-type *BMPR2* allele may be a critical modifier of disease penetrance (50).

VII. *BMPR2* Mutations and Genetic Modifiers

As noted above, HPAH has reduced penetrance and variable expressivity, suggesting that genetic and environmental modifiers may influence the clinical expression of a *BMPR2* mutation. A number of biologically relevant candidate genes have been investigated and implicated, but the studies are limited by the large number of research subjects needed for confirmation (49,51–56).

Data suggests that *BMPR2* mutations can alter a delicate signaling balance among the various members of the TGF-β superfamily of receptors, which may facilitate the development of PAH (11,57). In support of this finding, Phillips et al. investigated a cohort of individuals with varying types of *BMPR2* mutations and found that subjects with *BMPR2* mutations and polymorphic *TGF-β1* alleles predicted to increase pathway activity were more likely to be penetrant than those without these polymorphic alleles (49). Meanwhile, Zaiman et al. demonstrated reduced markers of pulmonary vascular remodeling and prevention of pulmonary hypertension by inhibition of the TGF-β type 1 receptor in an animal model of pulmonary hypertension (58).

Vasoactive intestinal peptide (VIP) is an endogenous modulator of pulmonary vascular remodeling and inflammation, which may modify disease expression in PAH. In animal studies, VIP gene deletions promote a PAH phenotype (59). However, efforts to identify polymorphic variations in VIP, which might modify disease expression in HPAH and IPAH, have not been successful (60).

Serotonin (5-hydroxytryptamine, 5-HT) is a cellular mitogen, and stimulates pulmonary artery smooth muscle cell (PASMC) proliferation through a signaling pathway mediated via the serotonin transporter (*SERT*) (61). Internalization of 5-HT by *SERT* leads to downstream activation of the MAPK cascade, in part via the production of reactive oxygen species, which ultimately acts to stimulate transcription of genes to drive cellular proliferation, including within PASMCs (62,63). Several studies have suggested that genetic polymorphisms in the *SERT* gene, or polymorphisms in the serotonin (5-HT) pathway, may play a role in the development of HPAH.

In support of this, Eddahibi et al. found increased growth of PASMCs in culture from patients with PAH compared with controls when stimulated by serotonin or serum, and attributed these mitogenic effects to increased expression of the *SERT* (64,65). To determine the role of *SERT* overexpression, they studied a common polymorphism in the *SERT* gene promoter in 89 PAH patients and 84 control subjects and found that it modified PAH susceptibility (65). However, work by Machado et al. (in a population consisting of 133 patients with a *BMPR2* mutation, 259 IPAH patients, and 353 control subjects) concluded that this *SERT* polymorphism was unlikely to contribute to phenotypic expression of PAH in subjects with or without *BMPR2* mutation. Likewise, genetic variation of the *SERT* promoter gene locus did not correlate with differences in the age at diagnosis (54). Finally, Willers and colleagues studied the role of *SERT* polymorphisms in a separate cohort of 127 patients with a *BMPR2* mutation. While no *SERT* genotype had a significant association with disease penetrance, subset analysis did show an earlier age at diagnosis according to *SERT* genotype (55). The variable results of these studies emphasize the challenges of associating common genetic polymorphisms with disease expression in a rare disease with small numbers of subjects available for study. Both positive and negative findings are potentially false in this setting, and neither type of finding definitively implicates nor eliminates a gene as a modifier of phenotype without independent validation.

VIII. Genetic Implications for Clinical Evaluation and Therapy

The impact of *BMPR2* genotype on clinical outcomes and therapeutic response in PAH is an area of intense study, but much work is still needed for complete understanding. As noted above, there is growing evidence that patients with a *BMPR2* mutation will have more severe disease as dictated by earlier age at diagnosis and death as well as worse hemodynamic parameters than PAH patients without a detectable mutation (18,21,22). However, the implications for treatment and survival remain to be determined (18,66).

Studies such as these correlating genotype and phenotype are critical to define the molecular variations that are predictive of PAH variability (66). In addition, they may provide clinical evidence that not all *BMPR2* mutations result in equal effects. Furthermore, kindred individuals with the same *BMPR2* mutation may have differences, such as gender or environmental exposures, which modify the severity of their shared *BMPR2* mutations. There may come a day when physicians and *BMPR2* mutation carriers will be able to implement a prevention and/or management strategy based in part on one's genotype and environmental exposures (66).

IX. Genetic Testing and Screening

Genetic testing for known *BMPR2* mutations is currently available from several laboratories in North America and Europe. At present, its use is best reserved for unaffected individuals with a known family history of PAH, or PAH patients. Given the vast number of potential mutations in the large *BMPR2* gene (~300 are currently known), screening for mutations best starts with the patient, so that, if present, the specific mutation in the family can be identified (3). Genetic testing should only be provided in concert with professional genetic counseling by experienced counselors (14,67). It is important to consider that for presumably sporadic cases of PAH (IPAH), the discovery of a *BMPR2* mutation reveals a heritable family disease, which can be emotionally devastating to families (68). For asymptomatic family members of patients with HPAH, current screening recommendations include a surveillance echocardiogram at three to five year intervals (67).

X. Summary

Great strides have been made in identifying some of the genetic underpinnings of this devastating disease. The discovery that mutations in the *BMPR2* gene contribute to the majority of cases of familial PAH, and of a subset of cases of IPAH, has energized the field and prompted significant progress in understanding the molecular basis of PAH. In addition, progress has been made in correlating genotype with phenotypic expression of disease. However, work is still needed to elucidate the causes of reduced penetrance, variable expressivity, and gender discrepancy in HPAH, including the identity and role of various modifiers of disease expression. Ultimately, a greater understanding of the genetic and molecular mechanisms of PAH should lead to earlier diagnosis, advanced pharmacogenomics, and, perhaps one day in the future, disease prevention.

XI. Acknowledgments

The authors thank the many patients and families who graciously contributed to this work, and Mrs. Lisa Wheeler, whose service is invaluable as coordinator of the Vanderbilt Familial Primary Pulmonary Hypertension study.

XII. Support

This work was supported by NIH PO1 HL072058, NIH K12 RR1 7697, and GCRC RR000095.

References

1. Dresdale DT, Schultz M, Michtom RJ. Primary pulmonary hypertension. I. Clinical and hemodynamic study. Am J Med 1951; 11:686–705.
2. Dresdale DT, Michtom RJ, Schultz M. Recent studies in primary pulmonary hypertension, including pharmacodynamic observations on pulmonary vascular resistance. Bull N Y Acad Med 1954; 30:195–207.
3. Machado R, Chung W, Eickelberg O, et al. Genetics and genomics of pulmonary arterial hypertension. J Am Coll Cardiol 2009.
4. Loyd JE, Primm RK, Newman JH. Familial primary pulmonary hypertension: clinical patterns. Am Rev Respir Dis 1984; 129:194–197.

5. Thomas AQ, Gaddipati R, Newman JH, et al. Genetics of primary pulmonary hypertension. Clin Chest Med 2001; 22:477–491, ix.
6. Rich S, Dantzker DR, Ayres SM, et al. Primary pulmonary hypertension. A national prospective study. Ann Intern Med 1987; 107:216–223.
7. Nichols WC, Koller DL, Slovis B, et al. Localization of the gene for familial primary pulmonary hypertension to chromosome 2q31–32. Nat Genet 1997; 15:277–280.
8. Morse JH, Barst RJ. Detection of familial primary pulmonary hypertension by genetic testing. N Engl J Med 1997; 337:202–203.
9. Lane KB, Machado RD, Pauciulo MW, et al. Heterozygous germline mutations in BMPR2, encoding a TGF-beta receptor, cause familial primary pulmonary hypertension. The International PPH Consortium. Nat Genet 2000; 26:81–84.
10. Deng Z, Morse JH, Slager SL, et al. Familial primary pulmonary hypertension (gene PPH1) is caused by mutations in the bone morphogenetic protein receptor-II gene. Am J Hum Genet 2000; 67:737–744.
11. Newman JH, Phillips JA III, Loyd JE. Narrative review: the enigma of pulmonary arterial hypertension: new insights from genetic studies. Ann Intern Med 2008; 148:278–283.
12. Sztrymf B, Yaici A, Girerd B, et al. Genes and pulmonary arterial hypertension. Respiration 2007; 74:123–132.
13. Loyd JE, Butler MG, Foroud TM, et al. Genetic anticipation and abnormal gender ratio at birth in familial primary pulmonary hypertension. Am J Respir Crit Care Med 1995; 152:93–97.
14. Newman JH, Trembath RC, Morse JA, et al. Genetic basis of pulmonary arterial hypertension: current understanding and future directions. J Am Coll Cardiol 2004; 43:33S–39S.
15. Gaine SP, Rubin LJ. Primary pulmonary hypertension. Lancet 1998; 352:719–725.
16. Machado RD, James V, Southwood M, et al. Investigation of second genetic hits at the BMPR2 locus as a modulator of disease progression in familial pulmonary arterial hypertension. Circulation 2005; 111:607–613.
17. Runo JR, Loyd JE. Primary pulmonary hypertension. Lancet 2003; 361:1533–1544.
18. Sztrymf B, Coulet F, Girerd B, et al. Clinical outcomes of pulmonary arterial hypertension in carriers of BMPR2 mutation. Am J Respir Crit Care Med 2008.
19. Montani D, Marcelin AG, Sitbon O, et al. Human herpes virus 8 in HIV and non-HIV infected patients with pulmonary arterial hypertension in France. AIDS 2005; 19:1239–1240.
20. Archer SL, Michelakis ED. An evidence-based approach to the management of pulmonary arterial hypertension. Curr Opin Cardiol 2006; 21:385–392.
21. Elliott CG, Glissmeyer EW, Havlena GT, et al. Relationship of BMPR2 mutations to vasoreactivity in pulmonary arterial hypertension. Circulation 2006; 113:2509–2515.
22. Rosenzweig EB, Morse JH, Knowles JA, et al. Clinical implications of determining BMPR2 mutation status in a large cohort of children and adults with pulmonary arterial hypertension. J Heart Lung Transplant 2008; 27:668–674.
23. Irey NS, Manion WC, Taylor HB. Vascular lesions in women taking oral contraceptives. Arch Pathol 1970; 89:1–8.
24. Irey NS, Norris HJ. Intimal vascular lesions associated with female reproductive steroids. Arch Pathol 1973; 96:227–234.
25. Kleiger RE, Boxer M, Ingham RE, et al. Pulmonary hypertension in patients using oral contraceptives. A report of six cases. Chest 1976; 69:143–147.
26. Morse JH, Horn EM, Barst RJ. Hormone replacement therapy: a possible risk factor in carriers of familial primary pulmonary hypertension. Chest 1999; 116:847.
27. West J, Cogan J, Geraci M, et al. Gene expression in BMPR2 mutation carriers with and without evidence of pulmonary arterial hypertension suggests pathways relevant to disease penetrance. BMC Med Genomics 2008; 1:45.
28. Sztrymf B, Yaici A, Jais X, et al. Idiopathic pulmonary hypertension: what did we learn from genes? Sarcoidosis Vasc Diffuse Lung Dis 2005; 22(suppl 1):S91–S100.

29. Armanios M, Chen JL, Chang YP, et al. Haploinsufficiency of telomerase reverse transcriptase leads to anticipation in autosomal dominant dyskeratosis congenita. Proc Natl Acad Sci U S A 2005; 102:15960–15964.

30. Newman JH. Pulmonary hypertension. Am J Respir Crit Care Med 2005; 172:1072–1077.

31. Morse JH, Jones AC, Barst RJ, et al. Mapping of familial primary pulmonary hypertension locus (PPH1) to chromosome 2q31–q32. Circulation 1997; 95:2603–2606.

32. Johnson DW, Berg JN, Baldwin MA, et al. Mutations in the activin receptor-like kinase 1 gene in hereditary haemorrhagic telangiectasia type 2. Nat Genet 1996; 13:189–195.

33. McAllister KA, Grogg KM, Johnson DW, et al. Endoglin, a TGF-beta binding protein of endothelial cells, is the gene for hereditary haemorrhagic telangiectasia type 1. Nat Genet 1994; 8:345–351.

34. Shi Y, Massague J. Mechanisms of TGF-beta signaling from cell membrane to the nucleus. Cell 2003; 113:685–700.

35. Fernandez LA, Sanz-Rodriguez F, Blanco FJ, et al. Hereditary hemorrhagic telangiectasia, a vascular dysplasia affecting the TGF-beta signaling pathway. Clin Med Res 2006; 4:66–78.

36. Machado RD, Pauciulo MW, Thomson JR, et al. BMPR2 haploinsufficiency as the inherited molecular mechanism for primary pulmonary hypertension. Am J Hum Genet 2001; 68: 92–102.

37. Koehler R, Grunig E, Pauciulo MW, et al. Low frequency of BMPR2 mutations in a German cohort of patients with sporadic idiopathic pulmonary arterial hypertension. J Med Genet 2004; 41:e127.

38. Morisaki H, Nakanishi N, Kyotani S, et al. BMPR2 mutations found in Japanese patients with familial and sporadic primary pulmonary hypertension. Hum Mutat 2004; 23:632.

39. Elliott CG. Genetics of pulmonary arterial hypertension: current and future implications. Semin Respir Crit Care Med 2005; 26:365–371.

40. Cogan JD, Pauciulo MW, Batchman AP, et al. High Frequency of BMPR2 Exonic Deletions/duplications in familial pulmonary arterial hypertension. Am J Respir Crit Care Med 2006.

41. Aldred MA, Vijayakrishnan J, James V, et al. BMPR2 gene rearrangements account for a significant proportion of mutations in familial and idiopathic pulmonary arterial hypertension. Hum Mutat 2006; 27:212–213.

42. Machado RD, Aldred MA, James V, et al. Mutations of the TGF-beta type II receptor BMPR2 in pulmonary arterial hypertension. Hum Mutat 2006; 27:121–132.

43. Thomson JR, Machado RD, Pauciulo MW, et al. Sporadic primary pulmonary hypertension is associated with germline mutations of the gene encoding BMPR-II, a receptor member of the TGF-beta family. J Med Genet 2000; 37:741–745.

44. Fujiwara M, Yagi H, Matsuoka R, et al. Implications of mutations of activin receptor-like kinase 1 gene (ALK1) in addition to bone morphogenetic protein receptor II gene (BMPR2) in children with pulmonary arterial hypertension. Circ J 2008; 72:127–133.

45. Humbert M, Deng Z, Simonneau G, et al. BMPR2 germline mutations in pulmonary hypertension associated with fenfluramine derivatives. Eur Respir J 2002; 20:518–523.

46. Rudarakanchana N, Flanagan JA, Chen H, et al. Functional analysis of bone morphogenetic protein type II receptor mutations underlying primary pulmonary hypertension. Hum Mol Genet 2002; 11:1517–1525.

47. Khajavi M, Inoue K, Lupski JR. Nonsense-mediated mRNA decay modulates clinical outcome of genetic disease. Eur J Hum Genet 2006; 14:1074–1081.

48. Yang X, Long L, Southwood M, et al. Dysfunctional Smad signaling contributes to abnormal smooth muscle cell proliferation in familial pulmonary arterial hypertension. Circ Res 2005; 96:1053–1063.

49. Phillips JA III, Poling JS, Phillips CA, et al. Synergistic heterozygosity for TGFbeta1 SNPs and BMPR2 mutations modulates the age at diagnosis and penetrance of familial pulmonary arterial hypertension. Genet Med 2008; 10:359–365.

50. Hamid R. Penetrance of Pulmonary Arterial Hypertension is modulated by the Expression of Normal BMPR2 allele. Hum Mutat 2008 (in press).
51. Abraham WT, Raynolds MV, Badesch DB, et al. Angiotensin-converting enzyme DD genotype in patients with primary pulmonary hypertension: increased frequency and association with preserved haemodynamics. J Renin Angiotensin Aldosterone Syst 2003; 4:27–30.
52. Hoeper MM, Tacacs A, Stellmacher U, et al. Lack of association between angiotensin converting enzyme (ACE) genotype, serum ACE activity, and haemodynamics in patients with primary pulmonary hypertension. Heart 2003; 89:445–446.
53. Koehler R, Olschewski H, Hoeper M, et al. Serotonin transporter gene polymorphism in a cohort of German patients with idiopathic pulmonary arterial hypertension or chronic thromboembolic pulmonary hypertension. Chest 2005; 128:619S.
54. Machado RD, Koehler R, Glissmeyer E, et al. Genetic association of the serotonin transporter in pulmonary arterial hypertension. Am J Respir Crit Care Med 2006; 173:793–797.
55. Willers ED, Newman JH, Loyd JE, et al. Serotonin transporter polymorphisms in familial and idiopathic pulmonary arterial hypertension. Am J Respir Crit Care Med 2006; 173:798–802.
56. Remillard CV, Tigno DD, Platoshyn O, et al. Function of Kv1.5 channels and genetic variations of KCNA5 in patients with idiopathic pulmonary arterial hypertension. Am J Physiol Cell Physiol 2007; 292:C1837–C1853.
57. Morrell NW. Pulmonary hypertension due to BMPR2 mutation: a new paradigm for tissue remodeling? Proc Am Thorac Soc 2006; 3:680–686.
58. Zaiman AL, Podowski M, Medicherla S, et al. Role of TGF-{beta}/ALK5 kinase in Monocrotaline-Induced Pulmonary Hypertension. Am J Respir Crit Care Med 2008.
59. Said SI. The vasoactive intestinal peptide gene is a key modulator of pulmonary vascular remodeling and inflammation. Ann N Y Acad Sci 2008; 1144:148–153.
60. Haberl I, Frei K, Ramsebner R, et al. Vasoactive intestinal peptide gene alterations in patients with idiopathic pulmonary arterial hypertension. Eur J Hum Genet 2007; 15:18–22.
61. Lee SL, Wang WW, Moore BJ, et al. Dual effect of serotonin on growth of bovine pulmonary artery smooth muscle cells in culture. Circ Res 1991; 68:1362–1368.
62. Liu Y, Suzuki YJ, Day RM, et al. Rho kinase-induced nuclear translocation of ERK1/ERK2 in smooth muscle cell mitogenesis caused by serotonin. Circ Res 2004; 95:579–586.
63. Lee SL, Wang WW, Finlay GA, et al. Serotonin stimulates mitogen-activated protein kinase activity through the formation of superoxide anion. Am J Physiol 1999; 277:L282–L291.
64. Eddahibi S, Hanoun N, Lanfumey L, et al. Attenuated hypoxic pulmonary hypertension in mice lacking the 5-hydroxytryptamine transporter gene. J Clin Invest 2000; 105:1555–1562.
65. Eddahibi S, Humbert M, Fadel E, et al. Serotonin transporter overexpression is responsible for pulmonary artery smooth muscle hyperplasia in primary pulmonary hypertension. J Clin Invest 2001; 108:1141–1150.
66. Rubin LJ. BMPR2 mutation and outcome in pulmonary arterial hypertension: clinical relevance to physicians and patients. Am J Respir Crit Care Med 2008; 177:1300–1301.
67. McGoon M, Gutterman D, Steen V, et al. Screening, early detection, and diagnosis of pulmonary arterial hypertension: ACCP evidence-based clinical practice guidelines. Chest 2004; 126:14S–34S.
68. Jones DL, Sandberg JC, Rosenthal MJ, et al. What patients and their relatives think about testing for BMPR2. J Genet Couns 2008; 17:452–458.

7

Imaging of Pulmonary Hypertension

DOMINIQUE MUSSET and SOPHIE MAÎTRE
Université Paris-Sud 11, UPRES EA 2705, Centre National de Référence de l'Hypertension
Artérielle Pulmonaire, Service de Radiologie, Hôpital Antoine Béclère, Assistance Publique
Hôpitaux de Paris, Clamart, France

I. Introduction

Pulmonary hypertension (PH) comprises a spectrum of diseases characterized by elevated pulmonary artery pressure leading to right-heart failure and death (1,2). A recent clinical classification (2) distinguishes pulmonary arterial hypertension (PAH), PH due to left-heart diseases, chronic respiratory diseases, and chronic thromboembolic disease (obstructive PH). PAH includes various forms of PH of different etiologies but similar clinical presentation, and in many cases similar response to medical treatment: idiopathic PAH (IPAH), familial PAH, PAH associated with other conditions (connective tissue disease, congenital heart diseases with systemic to pulmonary shunts, portal hypertension, human immunodeficiency virus infection, and exposure to drugs and/or toxins), and PAH associated with significant venous (pulmonary veno-occlusive disease, PVOD) or capillary involvement (pulmonary capillary hemangiomatosis, PCH). Among these various causes of PAH, it is very important to distinguish PVOD because the classic treatment of PAH can induce life-threatening pulmonary edema. The diagnosis of chronic thromboembolic pulmonary hypertension (CTEPH) is also critical as this disease may be potentially curable by pulmonary thromboendarterectomy (PTE).

Initial evaluation of all patients in whom PH is suspected is based on electrocardiogram, chest radiography, and echocardiography. The latter is the initial investigation of choice for noninvasive detection of PH, but measurement of pulmonary pressures during right-heart catheterization is required to confirm the diagnosis of PH.

According to the 2004 guidelines on diagnosis of PH (3,4), the next step after the confirmation of PH is the identification of the cause of PH on the basis of the clinical classification.

Screening includes several diagnostic imaging procedures: ventilation and perfusion (V/Q) lung scan, chest high-resolution computed tomography (HRCT), multidetector computed tomography (MDCT), and if required pulmonary angiography, selective digital substraction angiography (DSA), and, more recently, magnetic resonance angiography (MRA) (5,6). However, there is no benefit in performing all tests on every patient.

This chapter describes noninvasive tools that are appropriate for the detection of PH, techniques of MDCT and pulmonary angiography, as well as how these techniques are used in the diagnosis of CTEPH, used to assess operability when CTEPH is present, and used for the diagnosis of non-CTEPH causes. The role of MR imaging in diagnosis of CTEPH is also reviewed.

II. Diagnostic Tools

A. Chest Radiography

In 90% of IPAH patients, the chest radiograph is abnormal at the time of diagnosis (7). However, a normal chest radiograph may also be seen. Chest radiographic findings of PH (7–9) include main and hilar pulmonary arterial dilatation with attenuation of peripheral pulmonary vascular markings (pruning or loss). On the posteroanterior chest radiograph, a transverse diameter of the right descending pulmonary artery of 17 mm or greater is a reliable indicator of PH. Enlargement of the main pulmonary artery causes a left second arc protrusion (Fig. 1). Cardiomegaly (cardiothoracic ratio greater than 0.5) with predominant right ventricular (RV) enlargement may be present. A lateral radiograph may also demonstrate enlargement of both the right and left pulmonary arteries and RV enlargement by anterior displacement of the right ventricle into the retrosternal space. The chest radiograph is also useful in evaluating underlying pulmonary parenchymal disease (chronic obstructive pulmonary disease, interstitial lung disease) or pulmonary venous congestion, due to left-heart abnormalities. The presence of Kerley B lines, pleural effusion, and patchy irregularities on a standard chest X ray may provide important clues to suggest pulmonary venous congestion. No correlation appears to exist between the extent of the radiographic parenchymal abnormalities and the degree of PH (4).

The following two investigations provide directions to help establish the diagnosis.

B. Transthoracic Doppler Echocardiography

Transthoracic Doppler echocardiography (TTE) is the initial noninvasive test that may suggest or screen for the diagnosis of PH (10,11). TTE also provides important information on cardiac causes of PH, with evaluation of the RV and left ventricular (LV) dimensions and function. TTE identifies left-heart valvular abnormalities, left atrial enlargement, and myocardial problems responsible for pulmonary venous hypertension. Congenital heart diseases with systemic to pulmonary shunts, patent foramen ovale, or small sinus venosus–type atrial septal defects can be easily identified with contrast intravenous injection of agitated saline microbubbles while performing TTE. TTE can evaluate complications due to CTEPH such as atrial and ventricular enlargement, RV and LV impairment, tricuspid regurgitation, flattening and displacement of the interventricular septum, and pericardial effusion, which is a poor prognostic sign in patients with PH (12). Other imaging tests are required if no cardiac etiology of PH is found.

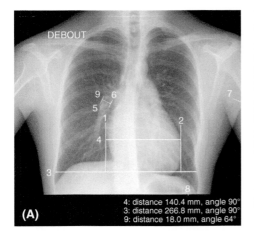
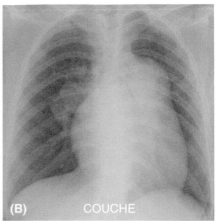

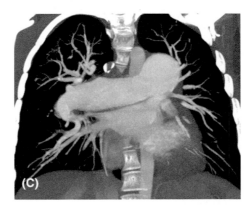

Figure 1 Pulmonary arterial hypertension. (**A**) Posteroanterior chest X ray in a young patient with PH: The dilatation of the main pulmonary artery results in an increased convexity of the second left mediastinal contour. The presence of a cardiomegaly is considered if the cardiothoracic ratio is greater than 0.5. The transverse diameter of the right descending pulmonary artery measures 18 mm (normal size of this artery is 9 to 16 mm). (**B**) Posteroanterior X ray in a 24-year-old woman with primary pulmonary arterial hypertension shows cardiomegaly and major enlargement of the main pulmonary and hilar arteries. (**C**) Corresponding frontal MPR from MDCT angiography shows central arterial dilatation with tortuous distal pulmonary vessels. *Abbreviations*: MPR, multiplanar reconstruction; MDCT, multidetector computed tomography.

C. Ventilation and Perfusion Lung Scan

The V/Q lung scan plays a central role in the diagnostic approach to the patient with PH and distinguishes CTEPH from other causes of PH (Fig. 2). In CTEPH, multiple large segmental perfusion defects are usually found bilaterally, which are typically mismatched to normally ventilated regions or where the perfusion abnormalities are out of proportion to the ventilation abnormalities (13,14).

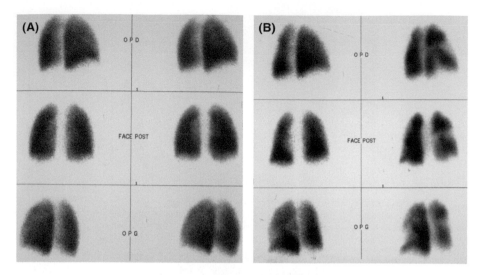

Figure 2   Pulmonary arterial hypertension: V/Q lung scan. (**A**) Patient with idiopathic pulmonary hypertension: the V/Q lung scan is near normal. (**B**) Patient with chronic thromboembolic disease: the V/Q lung scan shows multiple segmental mismatched perfusion defects.

In PAH, the lung V/Q scans may be normal or show patchy nonsegmental defects best seen as a mottled appearance (15). In patients with parenchymal lung disease, the perfusion defects are typically matched by ventilation defects. V/Q scanning has a sensitivity of 90% to 100% and a specificity of 94% to 100% for the distinction between IPAH and CTEPH (13).

Lung perfusion scanning does not, however, establish the severity of CTEPH, suggest the prognosis, or predict the response to various types of therapy (16).

Although a normal V/Q scintigraphy practically rules out the presence of CTEPH, mismatched perfusion defects may also be seen in veno-occlusive disease, pulmonary arterial sarcoma, large-vessel pulmonary arteritis, or extrinsic vascular compression, which can be confused with CTEPH. Such patients require careful additional imaging tests.

D. MDCT Angiography of the Pulmonary Arteries

The CT technique using multidetectors (4 to 320 detectors) is known as MDCT and is widely available and easy to perform. High-quality CT imaging is essential to distinguish CTEPH from other forms of PH and to identify potential candidates for surgery. Accurate evaluation of the patient with suspected PH and with an abnormal perfusion lung scan requires meticulous scanning technique.

Technique

MDCT with contrast media administration (MDCT angiography) is necessary to evaluate the pulmonary arteries as well as the heart and the vessels of the chest. The choice of iodinated contrast media concentration in the range of 300 to 400 mg I/mL has an effect on the diagnostic image quality. The detection rate of fifth- and sixth-order arteries appears significantly higher when using a contrast media concentration of 400 mg I/mL than with a concentration of 300 mg I/mL (16).

Typically, 90 to 100 mL of a nonionic contrast medium is administrated in an antecubital vein via an 18-gauge peripheral venous catheter with a flow rate of 4 to 5 mL/sec using a power injector. The delay between the contrast agent administration and the start of the scan acquisition is the single, most critical element in optimizing scan quality, determined by bolus tracking or test injection of 20 mL. The average time of acquisition is 8 to 10 seconds with MDCT angiography.

The key to optimizing scan quality is the acquisition of the thinnest possible sections during the short period of peak opacification of the pulmonary arterial vasculature (17). Several studies (18–22) showed that a narrow collimation of 1.25 mm or less significantly improved visualization of segmental and subsegmental pulmonary arteries. MDCT technique allows acquisition of contiguous sections with a section thickness of 1 mm or less throughout the entire chest with a reduced acquisition time in a single breath-hold (8–10 seconds). This short time yields optimal contrast enhancement and high spatial resolution (i.e., $0.6 \times 0.6 \times 0.6$ mm in the x, y, and z extensions) of the MDCT data, which permit evaluation of pulmonary vessels down to sixth-order branches. MDCT angiography images allow for characterization of the pulmonary vasculature, heart, mediastinum, and lung parenchyma.

Because the entire lung is scanned with a section thickness of 1 mm or less, the MDCT technique can also provide thin-section images of the lung parenchyma. For this specific analysis, MDCT angiography should systematically include an initial reconstruction with a combination of thin-section and high-frequency reconstruction algorithms known as HRCT.

CT Image Postprocessing

MDCT angiography allows the high-resolution multiplanar reconstruction (MPR) of images. Because of quasi-isotropic voxel size, MPR images taken in the coronal, sagittal, and axial planes allow for the distinction of intra-arterial from extra-arterial anomalies. Maximum intensity projection (MIP) images are useful to obtain a complete road map of the pulmonary arteries (Fig. 3). These postprocessing images also include minimum intensity projections (mIP). mIP reconstructions (23) can identify different patterns of pulmonary parenchyma attenuation (subtle emphysema, mosaic pattern).

CT Signs of PH and RV Dysfunction

In PH patients, increased vascular resistance leads to dilatation of the central pulmonary arteries, resulting in dilatation of the right cardiac chambers. An enlargement of the main pulmonary artery greater than 29 mm (24) may be seen on the CT scan (Fig. 4). This finding has a sensitivity of 87% and a specificity of 89% for the diagnosis of PH.

When the ratio of the diameter of the main pulmonary artery to the diameter of the aorta is greater than 1:1, a strong correlation with elevated pulmonary artery pressure also has been described, especially in patients younger than 50 years (25). A more specific feature of chronic right cardiac strain is dilatation of the right-sided cardiac

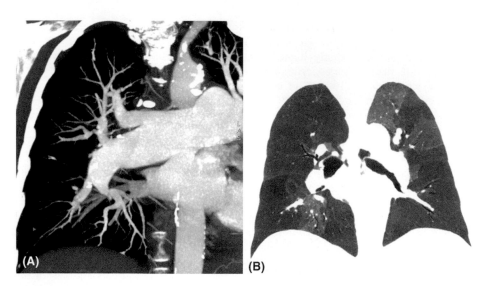

Figure 3 Chronic thromboembolic pulmonary hypertension. (**A**) Thick MIP–MPR image supplies a road map of pulmonary arterial tree. A simplified global view of vessels is helpful to demonstrate the number of obstructed segmental or subsegmental arteries and the major abnormalities. In contrast, the arterial detail is studied on thin MIP–MPR reconstructions. (**B**) mIP: coronal mIP (4-mm-thick slab) reformatted CT image with a lung window demonstrates mosaic lung perfusion. *Abbreviations*: MIP, maximum intensity projection; MPR, multiplanar reconstruction; mIP, minimum intensity projection.

chambers when compared with the left-heart chambers. Dilatation of the right ventricle is considered present when the ratio of the RV diameter to LV diameter is greater than 1:1 and there is bowing of the interventricular septum toward the left ventricle (26).

It has been demonstrated that ventricular measurements could be based on axial views using MDCT scanners (27). The RV myocardial thickness (less than 4 mm in normal subjects) is often associated with PH.

The presence of elevated right-heart pressure or tricuspid valve regurgitation should be suspected when there is dilatation of the coronary sinus or reflux of contrast material into the inferior vena cava and hepatic veins (28). Patients with PH often have mild pericardial thickening or a small pericardial effusion, which is a poor prognosis factor.

A recent study (29) shows that the measurement of right pulmonary artery (RPA) distensibility is possible from ECG-gated CT and is calculated from highest and lowest cross-sectional area measurements between diastole and systole. RPA distensibility is more strongly correlated with mean pulmonary arterial pressure (mPAP) than with right ventricular outflow tract (RVOT) systolic dimensions and diastolic wall thickness. This functional approach could overcome the limitations of PH diagnosis based on CT measurement of pulmonary trunk diameter and could identify patients with PH.

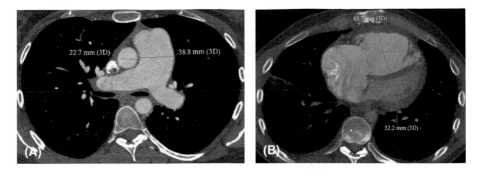

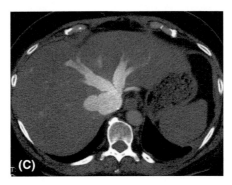

Figure 4 Pulmonary hypertension: cardiac evaluations on MDCT. (**A**) Axial contrast-enhanced MDCT section shows an enlargement of the main pulmonary artery with a maximum diameter of 38 mm. The CT diameter of the main pulmonary artery is measured in the scanning plane of its bifurcation, at a right angle to its long axis just lateral to the ascending aorta. Note the ratio of the diameter of the main pulmonary artery to the diameter of the aorta greater than 1:1, which suggests an eventual pulmonary hypertension. (**B**) Axial CT image shows an enlargement of the right ventricle with a ratio of the diameter of the right ventricle to that of the left ventricle greater than 1:1. The bowing of the interventricular septum toward the left ventricles is also visible. (**C**) Axial CT section obtained through the liver in a different patient than **A** and **B**. There is a reflux of contrast material into the dilated IVC and hepatic veins. The reflux suggests right-heart strain and/ or tricuspid value regurgitation. *Abbreviation*: MDCT, multidetector computed tomography.

E. Digital Subtraction Angiography

Pulmonary artery DSA is considered as an invasive method. However, right-sided cardiac catheterization is ultimately required to confirm the presence of PH, definitively establish its cause, assess severity, and guide therapy. Pulmonary DSA can be performed at the same time as right cardiac catheterization.

Pulmonary DSA is performed by the antecubital or jugular venous approach. The main pulmonary artery (pulmonary trunk) and the right and the left pulmonary arteries are selectively catheterized by using a 5.0-Fr pigtail catheter. Five injection series are performed by administering 40 mL of iodinated contrast material at a flow rate of 20 mL/sec. Arteriograms are acquired at 10 frames/sec. Two view projections of each lung are taken: anterior and lateral views for the right pulmonary arterial tree, while the left anterior oblique 30° and lateral views for the left pulmonary arterial tree. Lateral views are used to discriminate the segmental arteries of the middle lobe on the right and that of the ligula on the left from the basilar segmental arteries.

Angiographic data must include serial pictures, from the time of dye injection into the pulmonary artery until its venous return into the pulmonary veins, including parenchymography to show the nonperfused areas (6).

The data of these different imaging modalities allow for the identification of CTEPH, PVOD, and other causes of PH according to the Venice clinical classification.

III. Etiological Diagnosis of PH

The accurate diagnosis of the cause of PH influences the management and prognosis of patients with PH. Once the diagnosis of left-heart disease is excluded, the first step is CT evaluation to distinguish CTEPH from other forms of PH. Indeed, chronic thromboembolic PH is potentially curable and should be sought in all patients with PH.

A. Chronic Thromboembolic PH

CTEPH is caused by obstruction of the large pulmonary arteries by acute and recurrent pulmonary emboli, and organization of these blood clots (6). Incomplete resolution of thrombi has been noted in approximately 4% of patients with acute pulmonary emboli (30). The remaining embolic material is transformed into fibrous tissue with disappearance of the intima and infiltration of the pulmonary arterial media (6). The fibrous material is incorporated into the intima resulting in a thrombotic wall thickening, a decrease of the pulmonary arterial lumen, and finally obstruction of the pulmonary arterial vessel (6,31). These lesions can be partially recanalized resulting in intravascular webs, bands, and abnormal proximal to distal tapering of vessel diameter. Pseudo-intimal fibrous thickening usually starts at the level of the intrapericardial segment of the pulmonary artery and becomes progressively thicker downstream in lobar and segmental arteries that eventually become occluded (6). In addition to pulmonary arterial occlusion, vascular changes also are due to lesions of distal arteriolar vasculopathy in non-obstructed and obstructed regions (6,32,33). Both vascular remodeling and occluding lesions contribute to the increased pulmonary vascular resistance (PVR). These various anatomic findings explain mixed imaging pictures.

The aim of imaging tools (MDCT angiography, angiography DSA, MRI) is to diagnose CTEPH, to evaluate the extent of proximal disease, and to assess operability when CTEPH is present.

MDCT Angiography

Direct Signs

Only vascular signs (34–40) represent direct signs of CTEPH and include the following:

1. Complete endovascular filling defects (pouching or occlusion) (Fig. 5): this result from an abrupt cutoff of the vessel with or without opacification of the vessel segment distal to the pouching (39). This sharp cutoff is not

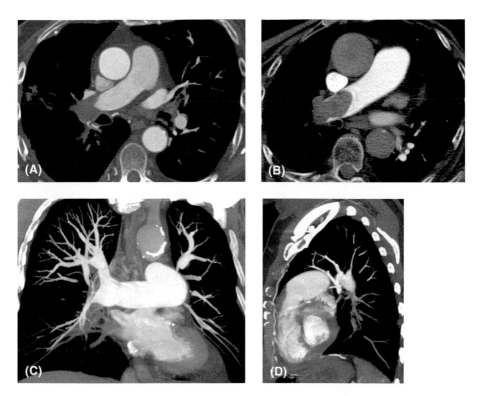

Figure 5 Chronic thromboembolic pulmonary hypertension. (**A, B**) Axial MDCT angiogram shows complete obstruction with an aspect of pouching defect of the right interlobar pulmonary artery. The material contrast column stops on intravascular filling defect with a convex margin. This characteristic allows for differing from a complete obstruction caused by acute pulmonary embolism where the column of contrast material has a concave margin with the filling defect as shown in (**B**). (**C, D**) Coronal and sagittal MIP reformated CT angiogram shows a pouching defect of the right pulmonary artery with (**C**) or without opacification (**D**) of vessels beyond the level of obstruction. *Abbreviations*: MDCT, multidetector computed tomography; MIP, maximum intensity projection.

cupuliform, contrary to the presentation of occlusion in cases of acute pulmonary embolism. Recanalization of thromboembolic material is possible and can also cause abrupt vessel narrowing. Calcification within thromboembolic material may be seen.

2. Partial filling defects (Fig. 6): eccentric endovascular filling defects named as thrombotic wall thickening are characterized by the formation of broad-based oblique margins with adjacent arterial walls. This organized mural thromboembolic material lines the arterial wall.

These defects result in a reduction in the diameter of the arterial lumen when compared with the external diameter of the pulmonary artery (6) and also result in

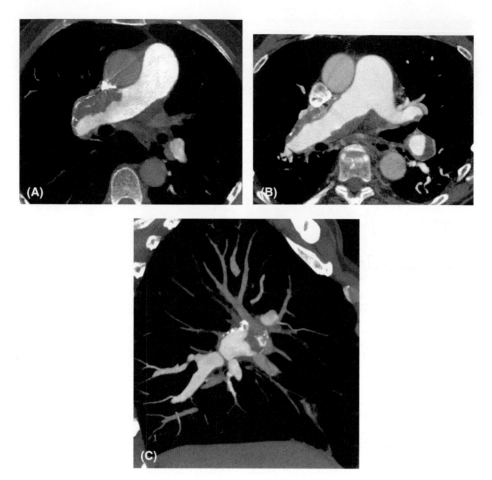

Figure 6 Chronic thromboembolic pulmonary hypertension. (**A**) Axial MDCT angiogram shows a partially calcified, eccentric, thrombus with a broad base forming obtuse angles with the vessel wall. This filling defect entails intimal irregularities of the right pulmonary artery. Note the calcification of the wall of the pulmonary artery. (**B**) Axial-oblique MIP MDCT angiogram shows a chronic thrombus of the right interlobar pulmonary artery as a cause of intimal irregularities. Note an eccentric filling defect that lines the wall of the left lower lobe pulmonary artery. (**C**) Sagittal MIP reformated MDCT angiogram shows a web or band crossing the lumen of the right posterobasal pulmonary artery, which result from of chronic thrombus. Note an eccentric filling defect of the right pulmonary artery. *Abbreviations*: MDCT, multidetector computed tomography; MIP, maximum intensity projection.

arterial narrowing and an abnormal proximal to distal tapering of the vessel diameter. These also cause intimal irregularities. Intraluminal webs or bands result from synechiae and appear as a decreased linear attenuation that transversally or longitudinally crosses the arterial lumen.

Indirect Signs

Pulmonary Vessels and Mediastinum. Irregular and tortuous vessel walls are indirect signs of PH.

CT scans also delineate atheromatous calcifications of the pulmonary artery in long-standing disease, which increase the technical difficulty of the endarterectomy.

Other findings include enlarged mediastinal lymph nodes due to vascular transformation of the lymph node sinus (41).

Collateral Systemic Circulation. An increase in bronchial arterial flow may appear when the pulmonary arterial flow is diminished. Under normal conditions, the bronchial arteries follow the large bronchi down to the alveoli, form an anastomotic network with pulmonary arterioles, and drain via the pulmonary veins into the left atrium (42). Under pathological conditions, these anastomoses, normally closed, open resulting in their appearance. Thereafter, the bronchial arteries take part in pulmonary oxygenation. In patients with CTEPH, bronchial flow may represent almost 30% of the systemic blood flow as compared with 1% to 2% of the cardiac output in healthy adults (42).

Bronchial arteries (Fig. 7) with a diameter of more than 1.5 mm are considered to be enlarged (43). Transpleural systemic collateral vessels (intercostals, internal mammary, inferior phrenic arteries) may develop (44). Systemic to pulmonary arterial anastomoses may also develop beyond the level of obstruction.

MIP reconstructions may depict the development of the bronchial or nonbronchial systemic circulation, which is indicative of an obstructive cause of PH, more often seen in thromboembolic PH than in patients with IPAH (44). Moreover, development of this circulation is a good predictor of surgical success (45). The presence of a significant collateral circulation may identify patients who have a potential for more technically difficult surgical endarterectomy (6).

Parenchymal Involvement. Parenchymal signs are nonspecific and include scars from prior lung infarctions and features of mosaic attenuation (28,34,39) (Fig. 8).

The presence of mosaic attenuation of the lung parenchyma, defined as sharply demarcated areas of increased and decreased attenuation (Fig. 8A), is seen in up to 75% of patients with CTEPH but in only 5% to 10% of patients with PH due to other causes, including patients with IPAH (46–48). Increased attenuation is explained by a redistribution of blood flow to the nonoccluded vascular areas. These regions include enlarged segmental arteries. Decreased attenuation is due either to hypoperfusion in areas distal to occluded vessels or to distal vasculopathy in nonoccluded regions (39,49). Pseudodilatation of the segmental and/or subsegmental bronchi may be observed in areas of decreased attenuation with occluded pulmonary arteries (50).

The association of mosaic attenuation and the disparity in the size of segmental arteries is highly specific for CTEPH (39).

However, Bergin et al. noted that segmental vessels were not always diminished in size in areas of decreased attenuation in patients with CTEPH (45). This feature named "the small-vessel factor" may help to define the contribution of distal arteriopathy to the total PVR (45).

Pulmonary Angiography

Pulmonary angiography (51,52) is the definitive test to confirm the diagnosis of CTEPH and determine the operability according to the location of disease: proximal versus distal (53–55).

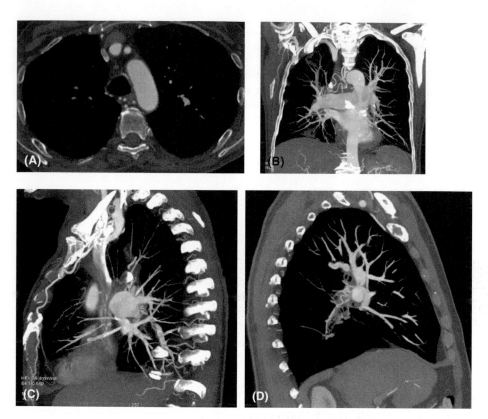

Figure 7 Chronic thromboembolic pulmonary hypertension: (**A**) Axial MDCT angiogram shows enlargement of bronchial arteries in the mediastinum at the level of the esophagus and the trachea. (**B, C**) Coronal (**B**) and sagittal (**C**) reformatted CT angiograms show bronchial and nonbronchial collateral circulation. Note intercostal arteries filling the posterobasal lower artery downstream, beyond the stenosis of the left pulmonary artery (**C**). (**D**) Sagittal reformatted CT angiogram shows enlargement of bronchial arteries beyond the level of pouching defect of the right inferior pulmonary artery with an opacification of a thin posterobasal inferior pulmonary artery. *Abbreviation*: MDCT, multidetector computed tomography.

Interpretation of angiography in cases of CTEPH is more difficult than in acute pulmonary emboli. Five angiographic features are characteristic of chronic thromboembolic disease (51) (Fig. 9): (*i*) a sacciform stop (pouching defect) of the pulmonary artery with a similar presentation of that described in MDCT angiography, (*ii*) transverse bands or webs resembling chordae tethering the arterial lumen, (*iii*) irregularities of the arterial wall, (*iv*) abrupt change in the caliber of the artery, and (*v*) absence of segmental or lobar arterial branches with parenchymal defects in these territories.

Because of the patient risk and the level of expertise necessary to its realization and interpretation, pulmonary angiography must be performed in the reference centers of PH.

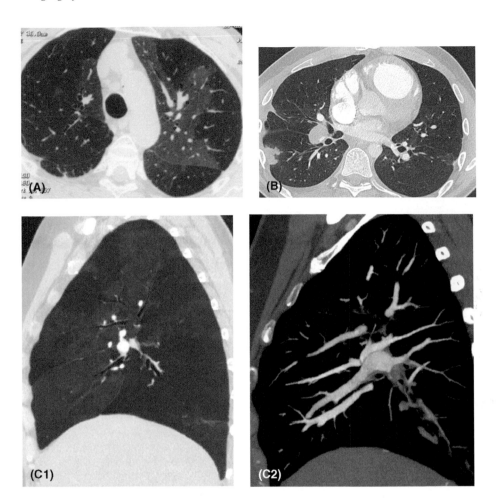

Figure 8 Chronic thromboembolic pulmonary hypertension: MDCT pulmonary parenchymal evaluation. (**A**) Axial CT image with lung windows shows the characteristic appearance of mosaic attenuation. Note that enlarged arteries are in areas of higher lung attenuation and smaller arteries in areas of lower attenuation. (**B**) Axial CT image with lung windows shows subpleural wedge-shaped area of consolidation in the right lower lobe from prior infarction. (**C1**) Sagittal mIP reformatted image demonstrates heterogeneous attenuation patterns with areas of low attenuation into the right inferior lobe. (**C2**) Corresponding sagittal multiplanar CT image with mediastinal windows demonstrates occlusive arterial changes producing mosaic attenuation founded in **C**: no opacification of vessels distal to the pouching defect of lower pulmonary artery in areas of lower attenuation. *Abbreviation*: MDCT, multidetector computed tomography.

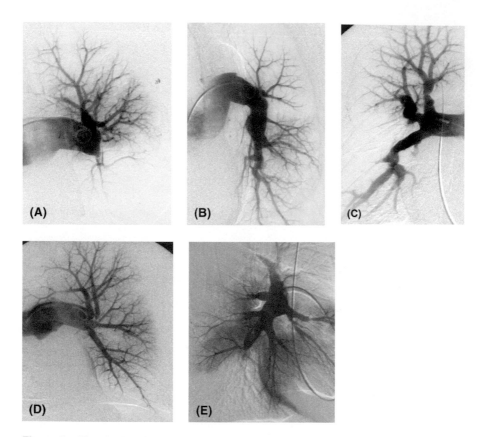

Figure 9 Chronic thromboembolic pulmonary hypertension: pulmonary angiography evaluation. (**A**) Selective pulmonary angiogram of the left pulmonary artery with left anterior oblique view shows a pouching defect of the left pulmonary artery with parenchymal defect in the territory. (**B**) Selective left pulmonary angiogram shows intimal irregularities beginning at the origin of the left pulmonary artery. Mediastinal arteries are also occluded. (**C**) Selective right pulmonary angiography on frontal view shows an abrupt change in the caliber between the right main pulmonary artery and the interlobar pulmonary artery. Note webs, bands, and obstruction of segmental lower arteries. (**D**) Selective left angiogram shows a pouching defect of the left lower lobe artery. Among segmental arteries of the lower lobe, only the posterobasal lower pulmonary artery is opacified. Note also stenoses of the superior mediastinal and Fowler segmental arteries. (**E**) Right pulmonary angiography lateral view shows multiple stenoses of segmental arteries and a pouching defect of posterobasal artery with parenchymal defects.

Magnetic Resonance Imaging

Magnetic resonance (MR) imaging of the chest is a rapidly evolving tool. Techniques include contrast-enhanced MR angiography (ce-MRA), with retrospective MPR, MR perfusion imaging, phase-contrast imaging of the great vessels, cine imaging of the heart, and combined perfusion-ventilation MR imaging with hyperpolarized noble gases. These techniques seem to be promising for the characterization of patients with CTPEH.

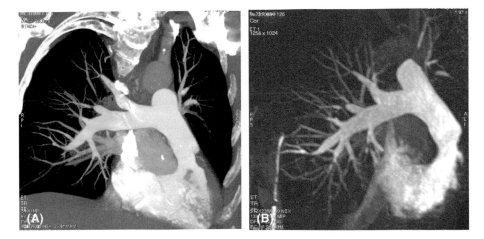

Figure 10 Patient with CTEPH: Coronal reformation performed after MDCT angiogram (**A**) and MPR reconstruction from a magnetic resonance (**B**) give comparative informations on the pulmonary arterial tree. Note especially the stenosis of the hilar artery and the pouching of the left inferior pulmonary artery. *Abbreviations*: CTEPH, chronic thromboembolic pulmonary hypertension; MDCT, multidetector computed tomography.

Ce-MRA describes morphological vascular features in patients with CPETH as well as MDCT angiography down to segmental pulmonary arteries (56–59) (Fig. 10).

The combination of MR perfusion and MRA is useful for the knowledge of regional pulmonary microcirculation (59).

Cine imaging and phase-contrast MR imaging of the heart provide information related to the extent of the right-heart impairment with measurement of several hemodynamic parameters. Kreitner et al. (57) studied a series of 34 patients with CTEPH who were examined with MR imaging techniques before and after PTE and showed a significant increase of RV ejection fractions and pulmonary peak velocities after PTE, a good correlation of RV ejection fraction with PVR and mPAP, a postoperative decrease in mPAP correlated well with the increase in RV ejection fraction, and a postoperatively complete reduction of a preoperatively existing bronchosystemic shunt volume.

MR has also been proposed for evaluating pulmonary artery distensibility (60), which seems to be an accurate noninvasive marker of PH.

Both techniques noted above, as well as ventilation imaging with helium, have potential value for the future and will play a role in the diagnosis and follow-up of patients with CTEPH.

Preoperative Imaging Evaluation

The goal of pulmonary surgery is to decrease the extent of pulmonary vascular obstruction, thereby reducing PAP and the total PVR. However, in some cases, elevated PVR persists after surgery due to the inaccessibility of lesions of small-vessel arteriopathy to surgical treatment (53–55,61,62).

Currently, the preoperative assessment of CTEPH includes the systematic evaluation of proximal disease and microvascular disease (distal organized thrombi and/or small-vessel arteriopathy) and its contribution to overall PVR (62). Evaluations of both proximal and distal pathology are considered equally important in decision making for PTE (62).

- Imaging techniques play a primary role in the evaluation of the surgical accessibility of these vascular lesions.
- Patients with CTEPH and thromboembolic defects at the main, lobar, or proximal segmental levels are characterized as having proximal disease and represent the main cases for operability, while patients with significant PH but with little or no visible evidence of thromboembolic pathology are considered poor candidates for surgery (62).

Presently, MDCT angiography in combination with pulmonary angiography represents the standard for imaging obstructive changes (6). However, only the comparison between the absolute elevation of PVR and the extent and location of obstructive changes by imaging techniques (pulmonary angiography and MDCT angiography) may allow an estimate of the "proximal" versus "distal" disease, which can give an estimate of the existing small-vessel vasculopathy in areas distal to open arteries (32).

Differential Diagnosis of Chronic Thromboembolic PH

MDCT also is essential to exclude rare conditions that may present with similar symptoms as chronic pulmonary thromboembolic disease. Other causes of pulmonary arterial obstruction include endovascular lesions, extrinsic compression, and parietal lesions of the pulmonary arteries.

B.   In Situ Pulmonary Artery Thrombosis

Although the diagnosis of chronic thromboembolic disease relies on precise vascular features, the distinction of CTEPH from in situ pulmonary artery thrombosis in patients with IPAH (Fig. 11) or PH associated with Eisenmenger syndrome is necessary (63,64).

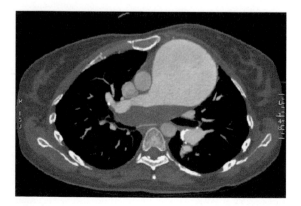

Figure 11   In situ thrombosis in patients with severe pulmonary hypertension. Axial contrast-enhanced CT shows large defect in the right pulmonary artery in a patient with idiopathic pulmonary hypertension. The distal lobar and segmental pulmonary arteries (not shown) are normal.

Eisenmenger syndrome is defined as a congenital heart defect that initially causes large left to right shunt that subsequently induces severe pulmonary vascular disease and PAH.

These intravascular filling defects may mimic pulmonary arterial occlusions caused by thrombotic material of embolic origin. In situ thrombosis is depicted on CT as an intravascular filling defect seen in the proximal pulmonary arteries. However on CT, the distal pulmonary arteries are normal and the diagnosis is suggested on the basis of absence of other findings of CTEPH (abrupt narrowing, variation in size of segmental vessels, webs, mosaic attenuation, pulmonary infarcts). These large central thrombi are not hemodynamically significant. The V/Q lung scan is near normal, without segmental or large defects. It is critical to identify patients with in situ thrombi as they are not candidates for surgical extraction.

C. Angiosarcoma of the Pulmonary Artery

Primary and metastatic tumors may be seen as intravascular filling defects on MTDC angiography mimicking acute or chronic pulmonary embolism, but treatment with anti-coagulants provides no improvement of clinical signs. On MDCT angiography (Fig. 12), the inhomogeneous pattern and especially the delayed contrast enhancement of the

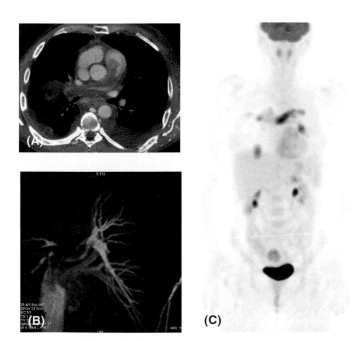

Figure 12 Pulmonary artery sarcoma. (**A**) Axial MDCT angiogram shows an inhomogeneous filling defect of the pulmonary artery trunk with a contrast enhancement of the proximal part of the defect. (**B**) MR imaging shows irregular filling defect of the main pulmonary artery extending into the right pulmonary artery. (**C**) Positron-emission tomography scan shows a strong contrast enhancement of the "thrombus." *Abbreviation*: MDCT, multidetector computed tomography.

intravascular filling defects (65) strongly suggest the diagnosis. Extravascular extension into the mediastinum or lung is another finding that may be helpful to distinguish a pulmonary artery sarcoma from thromboembolic material.

Once the diagnosis is suspected, positive positron-emission tomography (PET) scan (66) activity along the pulmonary artery and MR imaging using gadolinium injection showing a contrast enhancement of the thrombus support the diagnosis of angiosarcoma, but it must be confirmed at the time of surgery, on pathological analysis.

Undifferentiated sarcoma and leiomyosarcoma are the most frequent types of sarcoma of the pulmonary arteries. Other malignancies can induce emboli of the pulmonary arteries: renal, thyroid, testicular, and uterine cancers. Benign tumors such as uterine leiomyomatosis or hydatid cysts of the liver can also migrate spontaneously into the inferior vena cava and the pulmonary arteries.

Tumors arising within the lung or bronchi, hilum mediastinum, heart or extrathoracic metastases may also invade both pulmonary veins and arteries.

D. Fibrous Mediastinitis

Mediastinal fibrosis (67) is an uncommon chronic inflammatory condition characterized by progressive proliferation of dense fibrous tissue within the mediastinum. Fibrous mediastinitis can cause severe PH and can closely mimic chronic thromboembolic disease on angiography.

There are two types of mediastinal fibrosis: focal and diffuse. The focal type is probably caused by a fibroinflammatory reaction to a previous histoplasmosis or tuberculosis infection. The diffuse type often occurs in association with autoimmune disorders, retroperitoneal fibrosis, sclerosing thyroiditis, and certain drugs; while occasionally it is idiopathic.

On MDCT angiography, the focal type appears as a localized calcified mass or as mediastinal hypodense tissue infiltration in the pulmonary hila that encases and compresses the pulmonary arteries (Fig. 13). The paratracheal or subcarinal regions of the mediastinum can be involved. The diffuse type manifests on CT scanning as a diffusely infiltrative noncalcified mass that affects multiple mediastinal compartments. This diffuse type may encase other structures, such as the superior vena cava, esophagus, phrenic and recurrent nerves, pulmonary veins with possible postcapillary hypertension, and the bronchi (6).

On pulmonary angiography, involvement of the pulmonary arteries may be unilateral or bilateral, but is most commonly limited to the RPA. Asymmetric narrowing or obstruction of a pulmonary artery may also be seen.

E. Pulmonary Arteritis

Takayasu arteritis is a chronic nonspecific inflammatory disease that mainly affects the wall of the elastic arteries of the aorta and its major branches (65); pulmonary artery involvement can reveal the disease (68) or be a late manifestation of the disease. The most characteristic findings are stenosis, occlusion, or false aneurysm formation mainly of the segmental and subsegmental arteries, and less commonly of the lobar or main pulmonary arteries.

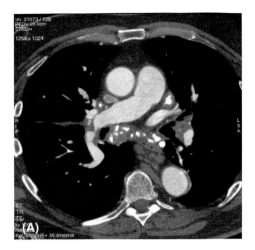 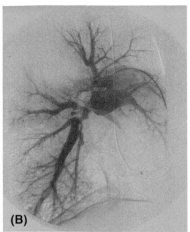

Figure 13 Mediastinal fibrosis in a 50-year-old patient with pulmonary hypertension and sarcoidosis. (**A**) Axial and sagittal reformatted CT images show a mediastinal subcarinal partial calcified mass extending to the right and left hila, narrowing the right interlobar pulmonary artery. (**B**) Corresponding lateral pulmonary angiogram shows the involvement of the right interlobar pulmonary artery.

CT angiography (Fig. 14) depicts circumferential or noncircumferential wall thickening and enhancement in early phases, and mural calcium deposition and luminal stenosis or occlusions in chronic phases. The presence of mural enhancement is suggestive of active disease. The diagnosis is easy in cases of typical lesions with false aneurysm of the pulmonary artery associated with in situ thrombosis on angiography and on MDCT. Collateral systemic vessels also develop in response to decreased arterial pulmonary circulation.

F. Non-CTEPH Forms of PH

Once the diagnosis of left-heart disease is excluded, and in the absence of CTEPH vascular changes or other diseases that directly affect the proximal pulmonary arteries, imaging methods may be useful in discriminating between other PAH conditions. Following the establishment of the Venice classification of PH, imaging techniques, particularly MDCT, are essential tools in the evaluation of PH associated with connective tissue disorders and the differentiation of PVOD from plexogenic PH.

PAH Complicating Connective Tissue Diseases

PAH may be observed in all of the connective tissue diseases (69), but it is most common in systemic sclerosis disease (SSD). Two forms of SSD are described: a limited variant form defined as CREST syndrome and an associated form with pulmonary fibrosis. PH is a risk factor for mortality (69) and can be observed in the two forms of the

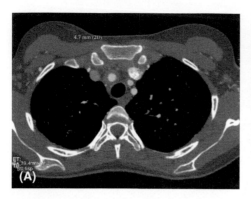 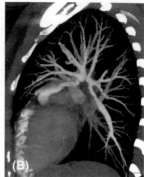

Figure 14 Takayasu arteritis. (**A**) Axial MDCT image shows mural thickening of the brachiocephalic artery. (**B**) Sagittal reformatted MIP CT images shows a decreased diameter of the entire left pulmonary vasculature with a mild, smooth stenosis of the lower pulmonary artery. The mural thickening of the pulmonary artery is not visible. *Abbreviations*: MDCT, multidetector computed tomography; MIP, maximum intensity projection.

SSD. The mechanism of PH is different: If PH is a purely vascular disease (characterized by vascular lesions similar to those of IPAH) in the limited form of SSD, PH can be secondary to hypoxia (which is induced by pulmonary fibrosis). Therefore, the therapeutic management of these patients is not similar.

HRCT is useful mainly to exclude significant fibrosis. On HRCT, signs of fibrosis (ground-glass opacities, fine reticular pattern superimposed, traction bronchiectasis, architectural distortion) usually have a basal, posterior, and peripheral predominance (Fig. 15). Honeycombing may involve 10% of the lungs. Other findings include enlarged mediastinal nodes and a dilated esophagus. These findings may be helpful in the differential diagnosis between idiopathic fibrosis and fibrosis in SSD.

Interestingly, the measurement of pulmonary arterial diameter is not a reliable criterion of PH in cases of pulmonary fibrosis regardless of causality. Indeed pulmonary arterial diameter may be increased even in the absence of PH. However, the ratio of the diameter of the main pulmonary artery to the diameter of the aorta remains reliable (70).

In patients with PH and systemic sclerosis but no evidence of interstitial lung disease, a recent study has demonstrated a uniform pattern of perfusion throughout the lung sections. The vertical gradient of perfusion on CT observed in healthy subjects disappeared. The perfusion values are reduced. Both findings reflect the diffuse pattern of disease and possibly a loss of compliance of the small pulmonary vessels (71).

Pulmonary Veno-Occlusive Disease/Pulmonary Capillary Hemangiomatosis

PVOD (72) is a rare cause of PH characterized by obstructions of the pulmonary septal veins and venules by intimal fibrosis, cellular proliferation, and muscularization.

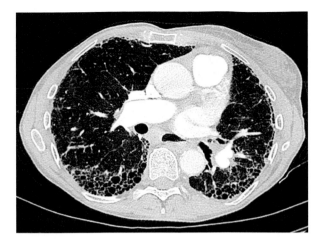

Figure 15 Systemic sclerosis disease in patients with severe pulmonary hypertension. Axial high-resolution CT shows extensive bilateral ground-glass opacities with honeycombing and reticulation. The dilatation of the esophagus is also visible.

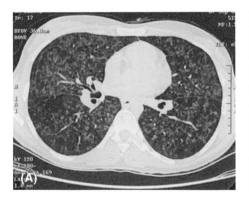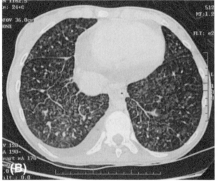

Figure 16 PVOD in patient with severe pulmonary hypertension. (**A**) HRCT CT scan shows ground-glass opacity with centrilobular pattern and poorly defined nodular opacities with diameters ranging from only a few millimeters to 1 cm. Nodules have a random distribution. (**B**) Pretherapeutic HRCT scan in a different patient shows centrilobular ground-glass opacities, with poorly defined nodular opacities and septal thickening. *Abbreviations*: PVOD, pulmonary veno-occlusive disease; HRCT, high-resolution multidetector.

Pulmonary capillary hemangiomatosis (PCH) is characterized by proliferation of small blood vessels that result in infiltration and compression of pulmonary veins with secondary PVOD. These vasculopathies are rare entities that have many pathological similarities and may in fact overlap (72). Imaging tools are useful allowing

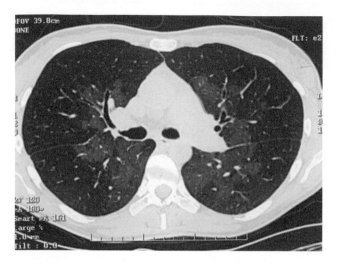

Figure 17 Primary pulmonary hypertension. Pretherapeutic transverse HRCT scan shows central panlobular of ground-glass opacities with relatively well-defined borders and with a predominantly central distribution. Primary pulmonary hypertension was confirmed at postmortem examination. *Abbreviation*: HRCT, high-resolution multidetector.

for avoidance prostacyclin therapy, which may result in life-threatening pulmonary edema (73).

On pretherapeutic HRCT (Fig. 16), poorly defined centrilobular ground-glass opacities (diameter from a few millimeters to 1 cm), smooth thickened interlobular septa (septal lines), and mediastinal lymph node enlargement are depicted with significantly higher frequency in patients with PVOD and PCH compared with patients with IPAH (74–76). In patients with PAH, centrilobular ground-grass opacities (Fig. 17) have been described as isolated, without septal lines or adenopathy, and can represent cholesterol granulomas (77). In contrast, the absence or presence of only one of these radiological abnormalities could not rule out PVOD. Neither pleural effusion nor any other abnormal parenchymal findings correlated with the presence of PVOD.

Panlobular ground-glass opacities (geographic regions of lung attenuation with relatively well-defined borders) are seen in both diseases and are not predictive. In both diseases, the size of the primary pulmonary veins is normal.

IV. Conclusion

In summary, the initial evaluation of PH is based on chest X ray and echocardiography. Imaging techniques (V/Q lung scan scintigraphy, MDCT, MRI, pulmonary angiography) represent the essential tools for the diagnosis, combined with the clinical presentation and the hemodynamic data.

V/Q lung scan is indicated to differentiate patients with CTEPH from those with IPAH.

Since the introduction of MDCT machines with high spatial and temporal resolution, MDCT angiography has become the noninvasive method of choice to study the pulmonary vasculature, especially to differentiate CTEPH from the other causes of vascular obstructive diseases. MDCT can define the thickness of the proximal pulmonary arterial walls and detects arterial obstruction down to subsegmental level. MDCT allows identification of other alternative diagnoses. Among them, MDCT often shows features suggesting IPAH or veno-occlusive disease.

Pulmonary angiography remains necessary for the diagnosis of CTEPH as it allows an assessment of the proximal-distal extent and surgical accessibility. At present, the association of MDCT and pulmonary angiography is considered the reference standard to establish the diagnosis and determine the operability of patients with CTEPH.

At this time, MRI is not systematically included among the screening techniques for patients with PH. However, improvements in MRI spatial and temporal resolution due to the development of multiple sequences have led to a noninvasive assessment of cardiopulmonary vascular structures. MRI provides hemodynamical parameters that correlate with the data of right-sided cardiac catheterization. Because MRI does not emit any radiation, it should be reassessed in the future to determine its place among the imaging methods of PH, especially for the prognosis and follow-up of patients with CPEPH.

References

1. Rubin L. Primary pulmonary hypertension. N Engl J Med 1997; 336:111–117.
2. Simonneau G, Galie N, Rubin LJ, et al. Clinical classification of pulmonary hypertension. J Am Coll Cardiol 2004; 43:5S–12S.
3. Galie N, Torbicki A, Barst R. Guidelines on diagnosis and treatment of pulmonary arterial hypertension The Task Force on Diagnosis and Treatment of Pulmonary Arterial Hypertension of the European Society of Cardiology. Eur Heart J 2004; 25:2243–2278.
4. McGoon M, Gutterman D, Steen V, et al. Screening, early detection, and diagnosis of pulmonary arterial hypertension. Chest 2004; 126:14S–34S.
5. Hoeper MM, Mayer E, Simonneau G, et al. Chronic thromboembolic pulmonary hypertension. Circulation 2006; 113:2011–2020.
6. Dartevelle P, Fadel E, Mussot S, et al. Chronic thromboembolic pulmonary hypertension. Eur Respir J 2004; 23:637–648.
7. Rich S, Dantzker DR, Ayres SM, et al. Primary pulmonary hypertension. A national prospective study. Ann Intern Med 1987; 107:216–223.
8. Rubin L, Badesch DB. Evaluation and management of the patient with pulmonary arterial hypertension. Ann Intern Med 2005; 143:282–292.
9. Satoh T, Kyotani S, Okano Y, et al. Descriptive patterns of severe chronic pulmonary hypertension by chest radiography. Respir Med 2005; 99:329–336.
10. Bossone E, Rubenfire M, Bach DS, et al. Range of tricuspid regurgitation velocity at rest and during exercise in normal adult men: implications for the diagnosis of pulmonary hypertension. J Am Coll Cardiol 1999; 33:1662–1666.

11. Ommen SR, Nishimura RA, Hurrell DG, et al. Assessment of right atrial pressure with two-dimensional and Doppler echocardiography: a simultaneous catheterization and echocardiographic study. Mayo Clin Proc 2000; 75:24–29.
12. Raymond RJ, Hinderliter AL, Willis PW, et al. Echocardiographic predictors of adverse outcomes in primary pulmonary hypertension. J Am Coll Cardiol 2002; 39:1214–1219.
13. Fedullo PF, Auger WR, Kerr KM, et al. Chronic thromboembolic pulmonary hypertension. N Engl J Med. 2001; 345:1465–1472.
14. Azarian R, Wartski M, Collignon MA, et al. Lung perfusion scans and hemodynamics in acute and chronic pulmonary embolism. J Nucl Med 1997; 38(6):980–983.
15. Ryan KL, Fedullo PF, Davis GB, et al. Perfusion scan findings understate the severity of angiographic and hemodynamic compromise in chronic thromboembolic pulmonary hypertension. Chest 1988; 93:1180–1185.
16. Schoellnast H, Deutschmann HA, Fritz GA, et al. MDCT angiography of the pulmonary arteries: influence of iodine flow concentration on vessel attenuation and visualization. AJR Am J Roentgenol 2005; 184:1935–1939.
17. Remy-Jardin M, Remy J, Artaud, D, et al. Peripheral pulmonary arteries: optimization of the spiral CT acquisition protocol. Radiology 1997; 204:157–163.
18. Schoepf U, Holzknecht N, Helmberger TK, et al. Subsegmental pulmonary emboli: improved detection with thin-collimation multidetector-row spiral CT. Radiology 2002; 222:483–490.
19. Qanadli SD, Hajjam ME, Mesurolle B, et al. Pulmonary embolism detection: prospective evaluation of dual-section helical CT versus selective pulmonary arteriography in 157 patients. Radiology 2000; 217:447–455.
20. Patel S, Kazerooni EA, Cascade PN. Pulmonary embolism: optimization of small pulmonary artery visualization at multi-detector row CT. Radiology 2003; 227:455–460.
21. Remy-Jardin M, Mastora I, Remy J. Pulmonary embolus imaging with multislice CT. Radiol Clin North Am 2003; 41:507–519.
22. Revel MP, Petrover D, Hernigou A, et al. Diagnosing pulmonary embolism with four–detector row helical CT: prospective evaluation of 216 outpatients and inpatients. Radiology 2005; 234:265–273.
23. Beigelman-Aubry C, Hill C, Guibal A, et al. Multi-detector row CT and postprocessing techniques in the assessment of diffuse lung disease. Radiographics 2005; 25:1639–1652.
24. Frazier AA, Galvin JR, Franks TJ, et al. From the archives of the AFIP: pulmonary vasculature—hypertension and infarction. Radiographics 2000; 20:491–524.
25. Ng CS, Wells AU, Padley SP. A CT sign of chronic pulmonary arterial hypertension: the ratio of main pulmonary artery to aortic diameter. J Thorac Imaging 1999; 14:270–278.
26. Oliver TB, Reid JH, Murchison JT. Interventricular septal shift due to massive pulmonary embolism shown by CT pulmonary angiography: an old sign revisited. Thorax 1998; 53:1092–1094.
27. Kamel EM, Schmidt S, Doenz F, et al. Computed tomographic angiographic in acute pulmonary embolism: do we need multiplanar reconstruction to evaluate the right ventricular dysfunction? J Comput Assist Tomogr 2008; 32:438–443.
28. Groves AM, Win T, Charman SC, et al. Semi-quantitative assessment of tricuspid regurgitation on contrast-enhanced multidetector CT. Clin Radiol 2004; 59:715.
29. Revel MP, Faivre JB, Remy-Jardin M, et al. Pulmonary Hypertension: ECG gated 64-Section CT angiographic evaluation of new functional parameters as diagnostic criteria. Radiology 2009; 250:558–566.
30. Tapson VF, Humbert M. Incidence and prevalence of chronic thromboembolic pulmonary hypertension: from acute to chronic pulmonary embolism. Proc Am Thorac Soc 2006; 3:564–567.

31. Jamieson SW, Kapelanski DP. Pulmonary endarterectomy. Curr Probl Surg 2000; 37:165–252.
32. Galiè N, Kim NH. Pulmonary microvascular disease in chronic thromboembolic pulmonary hypertension. Proc Am Thorac Soc 2006; 3:571–576.
33. Moser KM, Bloor CM. Pulmonary vascular lesions occurring in patients with chronic major vessel thromboembolic pulmonary hypertension. Chest 1993; 103:685–692.
34. King MA, Ysrael M, Bergin CJ. Chronic thromboembolic pulmonary hypertension: CT findings. AJR Am J Roentgenol 1998; 170:955–960.
35. Wittram C, Kalra MK, Maher MM, et al. Acute and chronic pulmonary emboli: angiography-CT correlation. AJR Am J Roentgenol 2006; 186(6 suppl 2):S421–S429.
36. Paul JF, Khallil A, Sigal-Cinqualbre A, et al. Findings on submillimeter MDCT are predictive of operability in chronic thromboembolic pulmonary hypertension. AJR Am J Roentgenol 2007; 188:1059–1062.
37. Oikonomou A, Dennie CJ, Müller NL, et al. Chronic thromboembolic pulmonary arterial hypertension: correlation of postoperative results of thromboendarterectomy with preoperative helical contrast-enhanced computed tomography. J Thorac Imaging 2004; 19:67–73.
38. Heinrich M, Uder M, Tscholl D, et al. CT scan findings in chronic thromboembolic pulmonary hypertension: predictors of hemodynamic improvement after pulmonary thromboendarterectomy. Chest 2005; 127:1606–1613.
39. Bergin CJ, Rios G, King MA, et al. Accuracy of high-resolution CT in identifying chronic pulmonary thromboembolic disease. AJR Am J Roentgenol 1996; 166:1371–1377.
40. Tardivon AA, Musset D, Maitre S, et al. Role of CT in chronic pulmonary embolism: comparison with pulmonary angiography. J Comput Assist Tomogr 1993; 17:345–351.
41. Meysman M, Diltoer M, Raeve HD, et al. Chronic thromboembolic pulmonary hypertension and vascular transformation of the lymph node sinuses. Eur Respir J 1997; 10:1191–1193.
42. Ley S, Kreitner KF, Morgenstern I, et al. Bronchopulmonary shunts in patients with chronic thromboembolic pulmonary hypertension: evaluation with helical CT and MR imaging. AJR Am J Roentgenol 2002; 179:1209–1215.
43. Kauczor HU, Schwickert HC, Mayer E, et al. Spiral CT of bronchial arteries in chronic thromboembolism. J Comput Assist Tomogr 1994; 18:855–861.
44. Remy-Jardin M, Duhamel A, Deken V, et al. Systemic collateral supply in patients with chronic thromboembolic and primary pulmonary hypertension: assessment with multidetector row helical CT angiography. Radiology 2005; 235:274–281.
45. Bergin CJ, Sirlin C, Deutsch R, et al. Predictors of patient response to pulmonary thromboendarterectomy. AJR Am J Roentgenol 2000; 174:509–515.
46. King MA, Bergin CJ, Yeung DWC, et al. Chronic pulmonary thromboembolism: detection of regional hyperperfusion with CT. Radiology 1994; 191:359–363.
47. Schwickert HC, Schweden F, Schildt HH, et al. Pulmonary arteries and lung parenchyma in chronic pulmonary embolism: preoperative and postoperative CT findings. Radiology 1994; 191:351–357.
48. Sherrick AD, Swensen SJ, Hartman TE. Mosaic pattern of lung attenuation on CT scans: frequency among patients with pulmonary artery hypertension of different causes. AJR Am J Roentgenol 1997; 169:79–82.
49. Moser KM, Auger WR, Fedullo PF, et al. Chronic thromboembolic pulmonary hypertension: clinical picture and surgical treatment. Eur Respir J 1992; 5:334–342.
50. Remy-Jardin M, Remy J, Louvegny S, et al. Airway changes in chronic pulmonary embolism: CT findings in 33 patients. Radiology 1997; 203:355–360.
51. Auger WR, Fedullo PF, Moser KM, et al. Chronic major-vessel thromboembolic pulmonary artery obstruction: appearance at angiography. Radiology 1992; 182:393–398.
52. Nicod P, Peterson K, Levine M, et al. Pulmonary angiography in severe chronic pulmonary hypertension. Ann Intern Med 1987; 107:565–568.

53. Kim NHS. Assessment of operability in chronic thromboembolic pulmonary hypertension. Proc Am Thorac Soc 2006; 3:584–588.
54. Peacock A, Simonneau G, Rubin L. Controversies, uncertainties and future research on the treatment of chronic thromboembolic pulmonary hypertension. Proc Am Thorac Soc 2006; 3:608–614.
55. Coulden R. State-of-the-art imaging techniques in chronic thromboembolic pulmonary hypertension. Proc Am Thorac Soc 2006; 3:577–583.
56. Ley S, Kauczor HU, Heussel CP, et al. Value of contrast-enhanced MR angiography and helical CT angiography in chronic thromboembolic pulmonary hypertension. Eur Radiol 2003; 13:2365–2371.
57. Kreitner KF, Ley S, Kauczor HU, et al. Chronic thromboembolic pulmonary hypertension: pre and postoperative assessment with breath-hold MR imaging techniques. Radiology 2004; 232:535–543.
58. Kreitner KF, Kunz RP, Ley S, et al. Chronic thromboembolic pulmonary hypertension—assessment by magnetic resonance imaging. Eur Radiol 2007; 17:11–21.
59. Nikolaou K, Schoenberg SO, Attenberg U, et al. Pulmonary arterial hypertension: diagnosis with fast perfusion MR imaging and high-spatial-resolution MR angiography-preliminary experience. Radiology 2005; 236:694–703.
60. Paz R, Mohiaddin RH, Longmore DB. Magnetic resonance assessment of the pulmonary arterial trunk anatomy, flow, pulsatility and distensibility. Eur Heart J 1993; 14(11):1524–1530.
61. Jamieson SW, Kapelanski DP, Sakakibara N, et al. Pulmonary endarterectomy: experience and lessons learned in 1,500 cases. Ann Thorac Surg 2003; 76:1457–1462.
62. Rubin LJ, Hoeper MM, Klepetko W, et al. Current and future management of chronic thromboembolic pulmonary hypertension from diagnosis to treatment responses. Proc Am Thorac Soc 2006; 3:601–607.
63. Caramuru LH, Maeda NY, Bydlowski SP, et al. Age-dependent likelihood of in situ thrombosis in secondary pulmonary hypertension. Clin Appl Thromb Hemost 2004; 10(3):217–223.
64. Moser KM, Fedullo PF, Finkbeiner WE, et al. Do patients with primary pulmonary hypertension develop extensive central thrombi? Circulation 1995; 91:741–745.
65. Castaner E, Gallardo X, Rimola J, et al. Congenital and acquired pulmonary artery anomalies in the adult: radiologic overview. Radiographics 2006; 26:349–371.
66. Chong S, Kim BS, Kim BT, et al. Pulmonary artery sarcoma mimicking pulmonary thromboembolism: integrated FDG PET/CT. AJR Am J Roentgenol 2007; 188:1691–1693.
67. Rossi SE, McAdams HP, Rosado-de-Christenson ML, et al. Fibrosing mediastinitis. Radiographics 2001; 21:737–757.
68. Hayashi K, Nagasaki M, Matsunaga N, et al. Initial pulmonary artery involvement in Takayasu arteritis. Radiology 1986; 159:401–403.
69. Behr J, Ryu JH. Pulmonary hypertension in interstitial lung disease. Eur Respir J 2008; 31:1357–1367.
70. Devaraj A, Wells A, Meister M, et al. The effect of diffuse pulmonary fibrosis on the reliability of CT signs of pulmonary hypertension. Radiology 2008:249:1042–1049.
71. Jones AT, Hansell DM, Evans TW. Quantifiying pulmonary perfusion in primary pulmonary hypertension using electron-beam computed tomography. Eur Respir J 2004; 23:202–207.
72. Montani D, Price LC, Dorfmuller P, et al. Pulmonary veno-occlusive disease. Eur Respir J 2009; 33:189–200.
73. Humbert M, Maıtre S, Capron F, et al. Pulmonary edema complicating continuous intravenous prostacyclin in pulmonary capillary hemangiomatosis. Am J Respir Crit Care Med 1998; 157:1681–1685.
74. Dufour B, Maitre S, Humbert M, et al. High-resolution CT of the chest in four patients with pulmonary capillary hemangiomatosis or pulmonary venoocclusive disease. AJR Am J Roentgenol 1998; 171:1321–1324.

75. Resten A, Maitre S, Humbert M, et al. Pulmonary arterial hypertension: thin-section CT predictors of epoprostenol therapy failure. Radiology 2002; 222:782–788.
76. Resten A, Maitre S, Humbert M, et al. Pulmonary hypertension: CT of the chest in pulmonary veno-occlusive disease. AJR Am J Roentgenol 2004; 183:65–70.
77. Nolan RL, McAdams HP, Sporn TA, et al. Pulmonary cholesterol granulomas in patients with pulmonary artery hypertension. AJR Am J Roentgenol 1999; 172:1317–1319.

8
Echocardiography of Pulmonary Arterial Hypertension

ADAM TORBICKI and ANNA FIJAŁKOWSKA
Institute of Tuberculosis and Lung Diseases, Warsaw, Poland

I. Introduction

This chapter will discuss the current role and future perspectives of echocardiography in

- noninvasive estimation of pulmonary arterial pressure (PAP),
- diagnosis of pulmonary arterial hypertension (PAH),
- staging of PAH, and
- follow-up of PAH.

II. Noninvasive Estimation of Pulmonary Arterial Pressure

The search for a noninvasive method of estimation of PAP went on for decades. It was only after the simplified Bernoulli equation was applied to assess right-heart hemodynamics that clinically useful estimation of systolic pulmonary arterial pressure (sPAP) based on Doppler measurement of tricuspid insufficiency (TI) peak jet velocity ("tricuspid jet method") became possible.

Several early papers reported excellent correlations between Doppler-derived sPAP assessment and direct catheter measurements. Other echo-Doppler variables based either on pulmonary regurgitation velocity or right ventricular (RV) systolic and diastolic time intervals had been suggested as useful for noninvasive estimation of PAP. However, when compared with tricuspid jet method, some were found less reliable (1, 2), others more difficult to assess, and none gained much popularity in clinical practice.

The main drawback of the tricuspid jet method is that it provides an estimate of sPAP, while both diagnosis and assessment of pulmonary hypertension (PH) are based on mean pulmonary arterial pressure (mPAP) values.

A recent review of data available from high-fidelity direct pressure measurements showed strong correlation of sPAP and mPAP across a wide range of pressure levels. According to the equation suggested by Chemla et al., mPAP = 0.61 sPAP + 2 mmHg (3, 4). This seems true not only for idiopathic pulmonary arterial hypertension (IPAH) but also for patients with left-heart disease, lung disease, or chronic thromboembolic PH. These data may renew the clinical interest in noninvasive estimation of sPAP.

However, the applicability of the Chemla equation derived from high-fidelity catheter measurements to clinical Doppler measurements has not been tested and remains questionable. This is due to intrinsic and operator-dependent limitations of Doppler echocardiography. Main problems are related to

- inaccuracies of tricuspid jet method for individual noninvasive measurements of peak systolic gradient between the contracting right ventricle and right atrium (5, 6) and
- error introduced by assumption of right atrial pressure required for calculation of sPAP (7).

It remained unclear to what extent the discrepancies in Doppler-derived and catheter-measured systolic pulmonary pressures were due to nonsimultaneous acquisition of data (8). A recent trial compared tricuspid jet method results with direct sPAP measurements obtained in patients with PH within one hour from each other in clinically stable conditions (9). The majority of the 65 patients had PAH, while PH due to interstitial lung disease, pulmonary venous hypertension, and obstructive sleep apnea was represented by 11 patients. For the whole studied group, there was no systematic over- or underestimation of sPAP with the tricuspid jet method. However, 95% limits of agreement ranged from +38.8 to −40.0 mmHg. Doppler echocardiography over- or underestimated sPAP by >10 mmHg when compared with right-heart catheterization (RHC) in 31 out of 68 persons (48%). The magnitude of pressure underestimation was greater than overestimation and would more often result in misclassification of the severity of the PH. In 12 out of 15 (80%) patients, pressure underestimates were >20 mmHg. Pressure overestimates were >20 mmHg in 6 out of 16 patients (38%). Half of all the cases of pulmonary arterial (PA) systolic pressure overestimation were related solely to right atrial pressure overestimation by echocardiography.

However, problems with right atrial pressure estimation did not account for most of the observed inaccuracies of Doppler-derived assessment of sPAP. Indeed 95% limits of (dis)agreement between systolic right ventricular–right atrial gradient by the two methods remained high (+33.6 and −37.2 mmHg, respectively).

While discrepancies were large, the studied group was characterized by significant PH and therefore by high velocities of tricuspid regurgitation. Bernoulli equation requires this velocity to be raised to second power and multiplied by 4. This amplifies any initial error in Doppler measurement, particularly performed in higher-velocity range. Therefore, the cited results do not necessarily imply that tricuspid jet method is useless for the early detection of PH.

III. Echocardiographic Diagnosis of Pulmonary Hypertension/Pulmonary Arterial Hypertension

Two main approaches were used to provide echo-Doppler criteria of PH: defining upper limits of normal for Doppler-derived sPAP estimates and attempting to find a Doppler sPAP cutoff value corresponding to catheter definition of PH.

A. Upper Limits of Normal Doppler-Derived Systolic Pulmonary Arterial Pressure

Most of the trials that attempted to define the upper normal limits of tricuspid jet velocity at rest were small. As an example, Aessopos et al. studied 53 healthy nonsmokers aged 14 to 55 years. Tricuspid gradient ranged from 12.6 to 29.3 mmHg (mean 19.3 ± 4.0) (10); Even relatively small studies, such as that by Dib et al. who selected 134 echocardiographic Doppler examinations considered as normal, reported a significant correlation between sPAP and the age of the studied person ($r = 0.47$, $p = 0.0001$). SPAP increased progressively with age from 13 ± 5 mmHg between 20 and 29 years of age to 22 ± 6 mmHg for 80 years of age or more (11). The largest data set came from Massachusetts General Hospital, where echograms of 3212 patients with otherwise normal transthoracic examination and no clinically suspected diseases potentially leading to elevated PAP were analyzed for tricuspid jet velocities (12). Mean peak tricuspid jet velocity was 2.61 m/sec, and RV to right atrial peak systolic gradient [tricuspid insufficiency *pressure gradient* (TIPG)] 18.0 ± 4.7 mmHg, with 95% confidence interval (CI) 8.8 − 27.2 mmHg. Multiple linear regression revealed that age, body mass index (BMI), sex, left ventricular (LV) ejection fraction, and clinical referral category independently influenced tricuspid velocity. In patients aged over 60 years and/or presenting with BMI > 30 kg/m^2, the 95% confidence intervals for pressure gradient derived from tricuspid jet velocity measurement exceeded 30 mmHg (Table 1).

Thus, on the basis of existing evidence, it appeared justified to consider TI jet velocities exceeding 2.8 m/sec at rest and corresponding to TIPG > 30.56 mmHg, as elevated, except for patients >60 years of age and/or very obese subjects. Arbitrarily set cutoff criteria for noninvasive diagnosis of PH in the presence of TIPG ≥ 30 mmHg were used by some authors (13,14). During the World Health Organization (WHO) meeting in Evian (1998), mild PH was defined, arbitrarily, as tricuspid jet velocity between 2.8 and 3.4 m/sec, which corresponds to TIPG between 31 and 46 mmHg and to sPAP between 36 and 51 mmHg, if fixed right atrial pressure of 5 mmHg was used for its calculation (15).

However, very few data were collected regarding prospective specificity and sensitivity of these criteria. Also, there are no published data regarding the clinical outcome of patients with diagnosis of PH made according to this criterion.

Table 1　Upper Ranges for TIPG and sPAP: the Influence of Age and Sex

Age (yr)	N	Upper 95% CI for TIPG (sPAP) (mmHg)	
		Women ($N = 2065$)	Men ($N = 1147$)
<20	856	24.2 (29.2)	26.2 (31.2)
20–29	669	24.4 (29.4)	26.3 (31.3)
30–39	650	25.7 (30.7)	27.5 (32.5)
40–49	494	27.5 (32.5)	28.3 (33.3)
50–59	344	29.4 (34.4)	30.6 (35.6)
>60	199	32.1 (37.1)	33.6 (38.6)

TIPG: Doppler-estimated RV to RA peak systolic gradient. SPAP: Doppler-estimated systolic pulmonary pressure, fixed value for right atrial pressure (5 mmHg) was used in calculations.
Abbreviations: RV, right ventricular; RA, right atrial; TIPG, tricuspid instantaneous peak gradient; sPAP, systolic pulmonary arterial pressure.
Source: From Ref. 12.

B. Doppler Vs. Catheter Definition of Pulmonary Hypertension

Two large programs aimed at prospective verification of abnormal echographic results were undertaken in France and referred to scleroderma- and human immunodeficiency virus (HIV)-infected patients, respectively. ItinerAIR study enrolled 599 patients with scleroderma. RHC was performed either if TI peak velocity was >3.0 m/sec regardless of symptoms or in patients with dyspnea and TI peak velocity of 2.5 to 3.0 m/sec. Among 33 patients without previous diagnosis of PAH who met these criteria, 14 had mild to moderate PH at RHC at rest and an additional 4 patients developed PAP > 30 mmHg at exercise (16). These data were compatible with 45% false-positive results of echo-Doppler "screening."

Another trial assessed the prevalence of PAH in 7646 patients with HIV infection (17). In that cohort, 10% of HIV patients presented with dyspnea and 247 without a previous diagnosis of PAH were included in the screening program and were eligible for echo. Among 18 patients with TI peak velocity >2.5 m/sec, only 5 were found to have PAH at RHC. A retrospective resetting of the cutoff value to TI peak velocity >2.8 m/sec (which would correspond to the mPAP of 24 mmHg according to Chemla equation) reduced the number of false-positive echo results from 18 to 7 (72% to 29%). In summary, these two programs aimed at early detection of PAH in populations at risk were disappointing not only because of many false-positive results but also because of high number of patients needed to test (NNT) with echo to detect a PAH patient.

More stringent criteria based on tricuspid jet gradient >45 mmHg, after adding 5 mmHg for right atrial pressure corresponding to sPAP > 50 mmHg, were suggested earlier by Mukerjee et al. (18), and recently similar approach (tricuspid jet >40 mmHg + 10 mmHg for right atrial pressure) was applied by Launay et al. (19) in scleroderma patients. In the latter trial, Doppler diagnosis was confirmed in all 32 (out of 38) patients who were submitted to RHC. However, while reducing the number of patients unnecessarily referred to RHC, such approach inevitably leads to increased prevalence of false-negative results, as evident from the scatter plot showing individual Doppler and catheter measurements based on data by Mukerjee et al. (Fig. 1).

Therefore, additional echocardiographic and clinical variables should be considered to improve accuracy of noninvasive assessment in future programs aimed at early PAH detection in at-risk populations. Echocardiography could be used to define the likelihood of PH, and this information could be incorporated into a score defining pretest probability of PAH as low, intermediate, or high. Such a score could take into account not only symptoms and risk factors for PAH but also data supporting alternative causes of PH. After appropriate validation of the score, decisions whether to continue with noninvasive follow-up or to consider RHC could be based on pretest PAH probability.

C. Echocardiographic Tests for Latent Pulmonary Hypertension

Similar to catheter evaluation, Doppler echocardiography may be used to assess PAP at exercise. Though technically difficult, tricuspid jets were recorded and their velocity could be measured during supine exercise, especially after tilting the patient to the left during pedaling or after enhancing the jet signal with peripheral saline contrast injection. The correlation with simultaneously performed catheter measurements of pulmonary

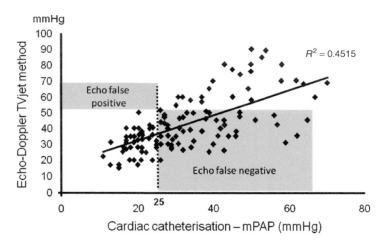

Figure 1 Attempts at improving specificity of echo-Doppler diagnosis of pulmonary arterial hypertension based on tricuspid jet method will lead to increase in prevalence of false-negative echocardiographic results. *Source*: From Ref. 18.

artery systolic pressure was reported as excellent ($r = 0.98$) (20). Exercise echo was used to assess sPAP in several specific groups of patients: with chronic lung diseases, after heart transplantation (21), with atrial septal defect (ASD) (22) as well as high-altitude lung edema (23), and in asymptomatic carriers of a primary pulmonary hypertension (PPH) gene mutation (24). In all these studied groups, sPAP significantly increased on exercise when compared with controls. Prolonged hypoxia (FiO_2 12.5%) was also used as a stress test to induce PH, which could be quantified with Doppler echocardiography.

In healthy controls sPAP, as assessed with the Doppler tricuspid jet method, remained low despite exercise and averaged to 31 ± 7 mmHg, 20.5 ± 3.8 mmHg, 19 ± 8 mmHg, 36 ± 3 mmHg, and 37 ± 3 mmHg for the five studies listed above, respectively. One of the groups arbitrarily defined sPAP < 40 mmHg, calculated after assuming fixed right atrial pressure of 5 mmHg, as a normal hemodynamic reaction during stress echocardiography. Interestingly, athletes were reported to generate higher PAP when exercising under the same workload as nonathletes when assessed with tricuspid jet method (25).

Results of a multicenter trial assessing by exercise echo the genetic predisposition to PAH among family members of index patients with IPAH are awaited soon. They might shed more light on the normal values observed during exercise with echo in the control group. However, it should be emphasized that the current definition of PH no longer refers to exercise. The exercise mPAP > 30 mmHg criterion was removed at the recent Dana Point Consensus Conference because of lack of standardized methodology of exercise tests that could be currently recommended. A review of the existing literature revealed significant differences in response to exercise due to the age of the patient and intensity and type of the exercise.

Another approach to latent PH was attempted with the pulsed-wave Doppler method assessing flow velocity curve in the RV outflow tract during various interventions. Acceleration time showed divergent trends during RV preload challenge induced by passive legs raising or inspiration in patients with normal and abnormal pulmonary circulation

(26–28). In summary, various echocardiographic stress tests are promising but not validated as far as sensitivity and specificity of cutoff criteria for PH are considered.

D. Differential Diagnosis of Pulmonary Arterial Hypertension

Echocardiography is a mainstay of noninvasive diagnosis in general cardiology. Consequently, it is most useful for detecting many of the potential causes of PH. The detailed echocardiographic diagnostic criteria for left-heart valvular disease, systolic and diastolic dysfunctions, cardiomyopathies, congenital heart disease, and hyperkinetic states are beyond the scope of this chapter. However, a few issues should be particularly considered when using echocardiography for differential diagnosis of PH.

- Mild to moderate signs of RV pressure overload found concomitantly with a well-established diagnosis of left-heart dysfunction might not require immediate confirmation by RHC. However, severe or progressive echocardiographic signs compatible with PH, particularly when considered out of proportion to the severity of presumed cause of PH, should prompt direct assessment of hemodynamics.
- Diastolic LV dysfunction might be suggested by typical pulmonary venous and mitral flow patterns as well as concentric LV hypertrophy and dilated left atrium. Diastolic position and shape of interatrial and interventricular septae might be of additional help. However, echocardiography cannot exclude LV diastolic dysfunction as a cause of PH, and therefore, RHC is recommended to avoid false diagnosis of PAH.
- Congenital shuts leading to potentially reversible RV pressure and volume overload might sometimes be missed at contrast transthoracic echocardiography. Therefore, particularly in cases with dilatation of the right ventricle and/ or proximal pulmonary arteries, out-of-proportion to mild to moderate RV pressure overload additional tests should be performed. They may consist of contrast transesophageal echo, cardiac magnetic resonance (cMR), or comprehensive heart catheterization with oximetry and contrast examination.

IV. Echocardiographic Staging of Pulmonary Arterial Hypertension

Theoretically, echocardiography may provide noninvasive estimates of recognized hemodynamic markers of prognosis in PAH, such as right atrial pressure, cardiac index, and even pulmonary vascular resistance. Interestingly, echocardiographic variables that were reported as useful for baseline prognostic staging of patients with PAH were different. Baseline echocardiographic prognostic markers reflected either morphological or functional consequences of RV overload:

A. Morphological Consequences of RV Overload

Leftward shifting of the interventricular septum resulting in increased LV eccentricity index, supramedian right atrial area, and the presence and quantitative score of pericardial effusion were all found to be related to the risk of death among 81 IPAH patients followed up for a mean of 36.9 ± 15.4 months (29). Particularly, the presence of pericardial effusion on echocardiography was consistently reported to indicate poor prognosis in patients with idiopathic (primary) PAH (30,31). All these markers can be considered as relatively late consequences of chronically increased RV filling pressure.

B. Functional Consequences of RV Overload

RV failure is the main cause of death in patients with PAH. Echocardiography may provide noninvasive insight into RV function. However, echocardiographic estimation of RV ejection fraction is difficult because of the complex shape of this chamber. RV area change or tricuspid annular plane systolic excursion (TAPSE) can be considered its surrogate. TAPSE is of particular interest: it is easy to measure with apical approach by 2D guided M-mode echocardiography and is therefore quite reproducible.

Forfia et al. reported on prognostic significance of TAPSE in PAH. Patients with TAPSE below a cutoff value of 18 mm, as defined by receiver-operator curve analysis, had significantly worse prognosis, with survival estimates at two years of 50% compared with 88% in subjects with a TAPSE above 18 mm (32).

Assessment of RV *dP/dt* from the rate of rise of tricuspid jet velocity is feasible with Doppler, but this index of contractility is influenced by PAP (33). Tissue Doppler allows for measurement of isovolumetric acceleration (IVA) of the tricuspid annulus. IVA is considered as directly related to RV elastance, reflecting RV contractility. However, prognostic implications of Doppler-derived IVA measurements have not been adequately validated (34).

Doppler index of global RV dysfunction was suggested by Tei et al. It is calculated by subtracting RV ejection time (ET) from total RV systolic time (the latter measured as the interval between cessation and reappearance of tricuspid diastolic flow) (35). In such a way, total duration of systolic and diastolic isovolumetric time intervals of RV can be assessed. In a retrospective study involving 53 IPAH patients, this index of myocardial dysfunction was independent of heart rate, RV systolic pressure, dilation, or tricuspid regurgitation but correlated with symptoms and survival (36).

Acute vasoreactivity test with inhaled nitric oxide (NO) can identify patients with PH, in whom vigorous pulmonary vasodilatation can still be pharmacologically induced. In PAH, such a result is usually related to excellent long-term prognosis. Continuous imaging with echocardiography can be attempted during NO inhalation. In some patients, it reveals immediate reverse remodeling, and regression of signs of RV over-load, suggestive of significant acute pulmonary vasodilatation. However, the sensitivity of such indirect echocardiographic detection of vasoreactivity is unknown and probably not clinically satisfactory. Moreover, non-PAH patients with PH due to hypoxia or LV dysfunction and even patients with pulmonary veno-occlusive disease (PVOD) might respond acutely to vasodilators, with equivocal prognostic and therapeutic implications.

V. Echocardiographic Follow-up of Pulmonary Arterial Hypertension

Doppler echocardiography offers a plethora of noninvasive variables potentially useful for follow-up of patients with PAH. A landmark blinded trial compared baseline and 16-week echocardiograms between patients randomized to placebo or to bosentan (37). All twenty assessed morphological and functional echo-Doppler variables showed positive trends in actively treated group compared with placebo-treated group. However, significant changes were restricted to 11 variables, 10 of which could be assessed in >80% of recorded tracings. Importantly, many of those variables carried pathophysiologically relevant message (LV systolic and diastolic area and filling pattern, inspiratory diameter of the inferior vena cava, RV ejection time, LV stroke volume), and some had previously recognized baseline prognostic significance when assessed with echocardiography (LV eccentricity index) or at RHC (cardiac index)

Altogether, echocardiography was found useful to document differences in the trends between two studied groups despite a relatively short interval of four months between the baseline and follow-up evaluations. Whether the observed echocardiographic changes reflected the treatment-induced modification in prognosis remains speculative.

In addition, follow-up of individual PAH patients with echocardiography is difficult in view of well-known problems with inter- and intraobserver reproducibility of echocardiographic measurements. The optimal balance between a strategy maximizing the number of monitored variables versus a strategy focusing on few most relevant ones remains a challenge. Some recently suggested variables, such as TAPSE, might simplify echocardiographic follow-up, while others—such as monitoring regional RV strain rate changes (38)—seem rather of pathophysiological interest.

Suggestions for echocardiographic monitoring may also emerge from recent trials implementing cMR (known also as "rich men's echo") to follow up patients with PAH (39). Van Volferen et al. used this technique to identify variables, which changes at one year were related to subsequent three-year survival (40). Several of those cMR variables can also be evaluated by echocardiography and were earlier found to respond to targeted treatment (37). Consequently, focusing on monitoring the changes in stroke volume and RV and LV area might improve the efficiency of echocardiographic follow-up assessment in PAH.

References

1. Chan KL, Currie PJ, Seward JB, et al. Comparison of three Doppler ultrasound methods in the prediction of pulmonary artery pressure. J Am Coll Cardiol 1987; 9(3):549–554.
2. Torbicki A, Skwarski K, Hawrylkiewicz I, et al. Attempts at measuring pulmonary arterial pressure by means of Doppler echocardiography in patients with chronic lung disease. Eur Respir J 1989; 2(9):856–860.
3. Chemla D, Castelain V, Humbert M, et al. New formula for predicting mean pulmonary artery pressure using systolic pulmonary artery pressure. Chest 2004; 126(4):1313–1317.
4. Chemla D, Castelain V, Provencher S, et al. Evaluation of various empirical formulas for estimating mean pulmonary artery pressure by using systolic pulmonary artery pressure in adults. Chest 2009; 135(3):760–768.
5. Brecker SJ, Gibbs JS, Fox KM, et al. Comparison of Doppler derived haemodynamic variables and simultaneous high fidelity pressure measurements in severe pulmonary hypertension. Br Heart J 1994; 72(4):384–389.
6. Vachiery JL, Brimioulle S, Crasset V, et al. False-positive diagnosis of pulmonary hypertension by Doppler echocardiography. Eur Respir J 1998; 12(6):1476–1478.
7. Pepi M, Tamborini G, Galli C, et al. A new formula for echo-Doppler estimation of right ventricular systolic pressure. J Am Soc Echocardiogr 1994; 7(1):20–26.

8. Currie PJ, Seward JB, Chan KL, et al. Continuous wave Doppler determination of right ventricular pressure: a simultaneous Doppler-catheterization study in 127 patients. J Am Coll Cardiol 1985; 6(4):750–756.

9. Fisher MR, Forfia PR, Chamera E, et al. Accuracy of Doppler Echocardiography in the hemodynamic assessment of pulmonary hypertension. Am J Respir Crit Care Med 2009; 179(7):615–621.

10. Aessopos A, Farmakis D, Taktikou H, et al. Doppler-determined peak systolic tricuspid pressure gradient in persons with normal pulmonary function and tricuspid regurgitation. J Am Soc Echocardiogr 2000; 13(7):645–649.

11. Dib JC, Abergel E, Rovani C, et al. The age of the patient should be taken into account when interpreting Doppler assessed pulmonary artery pressures. J Am Soc Echocardiogr 1997; 10 (1):72–73.

12. McQuillan BM, Picard MH, Leavitt M, et al. Clinical correlates and reference intervals for pulmonary artery systolic pressure among echocardiographically normal subjects. Circulation 2001; 104(23):2797–2802.

13. Murata I, Takenaka K, Yoshinoya S, et al. Clinical evaluation of pulmonary hypertension in systemic sclerosis and related disorders. A Doppler echocardiographic study of 135 Japanese patients. Chest 1997; 111(1):36–43.

14. Elstein D, Klutstein MW, Lahad A, et al. Echocardiographic assessment of pulmonary hypertension in Gaucher's disease [see comments]. Lancet 1998; 351(9115):1544–1546.

15. McGoon MD. The assessment of pulmonary hypertension. Clin Chest Med 2001; 22(3):493–508, ix.

16. Hachulla E, Gressin V, Guillevin L, et al. Early detection of pulmonary arterial hypertension in systemic sclerosis: a French nationwide prospective multicenter study. Arthritis Rheum 2005; 52(12):3792–3800.

17. Sitbon O, Lascoux-Combe C, Delfraissy JF, et al. Prevalence of HIV-related pulmonary arterial hypertension in the current antiretroviral therapy era. Am J Respir Crit Care Med 2008; 177(1):108–113.

18. Mukerjee D, St GD, Knight C, et al. Echocardiography and pulmonary function as screening tests for pulmonary arterial hypertension in systemic sclerosis. Rheumatology (Oxford) 2004; 43(4):461–466.

19. Launay D, Mouthon L, Hachulla E, et al. Prevalence and characteristics of moderate to severe pulmonary hypertension in systemic sclerosis with and without interstitial lung disease. J Rheumatol 2007; 34(5):1005–1011.

20. Himelman RB, Stulbarg M, Kircher B, et al. Noninvasive evaluation of pulmonary artery pressure during exercise by saline-enhanced Doppler echocardiography in chronic pulmonary disease. Circulation 1989; 79(4):863–871.

21. Barbant SD, Redberg RF, Tucker KJ, et al. Abnormal pulmonary artery pressure profile after cardiac transplantation: an exercise Doppler echocardiographic study. Am Heart J 1995; 129 (6):1185–1192.

22. Oelberg DA, Marcotte F, Kreisman H, et al. Evaluation of right ventricular systolic pressure during incremental exercise by Doppler echocardiography in adults with atrial septal defect. Chest 1998; 113(6):1459–1465.

23. Grunig E, Mereles D, Hildebrandt W, et al. Stress Doppler echocardiography for identification of susceptibility to high altitude pulmonary edema. J Am Coll Cardiol 2000; 35(4):980–987.

24. Grunig E, Janssen B, Mereles D, et al. Abnormal pulmonary artery pressure response in asymptomatic carriers of primary pulmonary hypertension gene. Circulation 2000; 102 (10):1145–1150.

25. Bossone E, Rubenfire M, Bach DS, et al. Range of tricuspid regurgitation velocity at rest and during exercise in normal adult men: implications for the diagnosis of pulmonary hypertension. J Am Coll Cardiol 1999; 33(6):1662–1666.

26. Torbicki A, Tramarin R, Fracchia F, et al. Effect of increased right ventricular preload on pulmonary artery flow velocity in patients with normal or increased pulmonary artery pressure. Am J Noninvasive Cardiol 1994; 8:151–155.
27. Ohashi M, Sato K, Suzuki S, et al. Doppler echocardiographic evaluation of latent pulmonary hypertension by passive leg raising. Coron Artery Dis 1997; 8(10):651–655.
28. Bossone E, Avelar E, Bach DS, et al. Diagnostic value of resting tricuspid regurgitation velocity and right ventricular ejection flow parameters for the detection of exercise induced pulmonary arterial hypertension. Int J Card Imaging 2000; 16(6):429–436.
29. Raymond RJ, Hinderliter AL, Willis PW, et al. Echocardiographic predictors of adverse outcomes in primary pulmonary hypertension. J Am Coll Cardiol 2002; 39(7):1214–1219.
30. Hinderliter AL, Willis PW, Long W, et al. Frequency and prognostic significance of pericardial effusion in primary pulmonary hypertension. PPH study group. Primary pulmonary hypertension. Am J Cardiol 1999; 84(4):481–4, A10.
31. Eysmann SB, Palevsky HI, Reichek N, et al. Two-dimensional and Doppler-echocardiographic and cardiac catheterization correlates of survival in primary pulmonary hypertension. Circulation 1989; 80(2):353–360.
32. Forfia PR, Fisher MR, Mathai SC, et al. Tricuspid annular displacement predicts survival in pulmonary hypertension. Am J Respir Crit Care Med 2006; 174(9):1034–1041.
33. Pai RG, Bansal RC, Shah PM. Determinants of the rate of right ventricular pressure rise by Doppler echocardiography: potential value in the assessment of right ventricular function. J Heart Valve Dis 1994; 3(2):179–184.
34. Vogel M, Schmidt MR, Kristiansen SB, et al. Validation of myocardial acceleration during isovolumic contraction as a novel noninvasive index of right ventricular contractility: comparison with ventricular pressure-volume relations in an animal model. Circulation 2002; 105(14):1693–1699.
35. Tei C, Dujardin KS, Hodge DO, et al. Doppler echocardiographic index for assessment of global right ventricular function. J Am Soc Echocardiogr 1996; 9(6):838–847.
36. Yeo TC, Dujardin KS, Tei C, et al. Value of a Doppler-derived index combining systolic and diastolic time intervals in predicting outcome in primary pulmonary hypertension. Am J Cardiol 1998; 81(9):1157–1161.
37. Galie N, Hinderliter AL, Torbicki A, et al. Effects of the oral endothelin-receptor antagonist bosentan on echocardiographic and doppler measures in patients with pulmonary arterial hypertension. J Am Coll Cardiol 2003; 41(8):1380–1386.
38. Borges AC, Knebel F, Eddicks S, et al. Right ventricular function assessed by two-dimensional strain and tissue Doppler echocardiography in patients with pulmonary arterial hypertension and effect of vasodilator therapy. Am J Cardiol 2006; 98(4):530–534.
39. Torbicki A. Cardiac magnetic resonance in pulmonary arterial hypertension: a step in the right direction. Eur Heart J 2007; 28(10):1187–1189.
40. van Wolferen SA, Marcus JT, Boonstra A, et al. Prognostic value of right ventricular mass, volume, and function in idiopathic pulmonary arterial hypertension. Eur Heart J 2007; 28(10):1250–1257.

9

Diagnosis and Hemodynamic Assessment of Pulmonary Arterial Hypertension

RAJAN SAGGAR, RAJEEV SAGGAR, JOHN A. BELPERIO, DAVID A. ZISMAN,
JOSEPH P. LYNCH III, and JAMIL ABOULHOSN
David Geffen School of Medicine at UCLA, Los Angeles, California, U.S.A.

I. Introduction

Pulmonary hypertension (PH) can occur as either a primary or secondary process and, in general, its presence increases overall morbidity and mortality. Importantly, the majority of prior study has been in the setting of idiopathic pulmonary arterial hypertension (IPAH), and as such, the following discussion will focus on IPAH. As most available diagnostic strategies lack sensitivity and specificity, the physician must maintain a high index of suspicion in considering PAH. This chapter will provide an overview of the available diagnostic studies for PAH with a particular focus on hemodynamic assessment. Novel approaches to the often-delayed diagnosis of PAH are being studied and will also be discussed.

Pulmonary arterial hypertension (PAH) was first described by Romberg (1) in 1891 as "sclerosis of the pulmonary arteries". Since PAH is often diagnosed years after symptom onset (2) and hemodynamic severity correlates with subsequent mortality (3), early diagnostic strategies are essential. Importantly, the extensive vascular reserve inherent to the pulmonary circulation (4,5) and the paucity of diagnostic findings by current standard testing early in the course of disease can further delay the diagnosis. Right-heart catheterization (RHC) is the gold standard to diagnose PAH. However, noninvasive parameters (particularly echocardiography) and ancillary studies may suggest the diagnosis and, in some cases, provide an assessment of severity of PAH.

II. Symptomatology and Physical Exam

The symptoms of idiopathic PAH are often nonspecific. The most common presenting symptom is dyspnea (60%) (2), while other symptoms increase during the course of the disease and include fatigue (73%), chest pain (47%), syncope (36%), Raynaud's phenomena (10%), and edema (37%). The likelihood of PAH is increased when the physical exam suggests signs of right-heart strain or failure such as an increased pulmonic component of the second heart sound (P2), prominent jugular venous pulsation +/− hepatojugular reflux, right-sided S3 and/or S4, holosystolic murmur of tricuspid regurgitation, and ascites/edema (6). Interestingly, a more contemporary registry approach is currently being completed and plans to report on 3500 PAH patients from World Health Organization (WHO) group 1 (not just IPAH) (7).

III. Chest Radiograph

A chest radiograph is necessary in the diagnostic evaluation of PAH, but lacks sensitivity as a screening test for PAH (8). The chest radiograph in the setting of PAH can show enlarged main pulmonary and hilar artery shadows, peripheral "pruning" of vessels, loss of the retrosternal airspace (lateral radiograph) suggesting right ventricular (RV) enlargement, increased radiological index of PAH (9), and increased right (>16 mm) and/or left (>18 mm) descending pulmonary artery caliber (10,11). In general, the degree of PAH is not reflected by any specific radiographic abnormality (9,12,13). Finally, most studies evaluating chest radiography and PH were performed in individuals with chronic obstructive pulmonary disease (COPD) and mitral stenosis, not WHO group 1 PAH.

IV. Other Radiological Modalities

A. High-Resolution Chest Tomography

Chest tomography (CT) imaging can be very helpful in the diagnostic algorithm of PH, apart from its obvious utility in the assessment of chronic thromboembolic disease. In IPAH, there are mural calcific deposits in the proximal pulmonary arteries (23%), mosaic attenuation (14), and bronchial/systemic arterial collaterals (15). Right ventricular hypertrophy (RVH), dilation of the proximal pulmonary arteries (or the diameter ratio of the pulmonary artery to aorta) (16–18), and pericardial thickening or effusion (19) can be present. IPAH has also been reported to present with diffuse micronodules on CT (20), possibly representing cholesterol granulomas formed after repeated pulmonary hemorrhage (21), or in the setting of pulmonary capillary hemangiomatosis and/ or pulmonary veno-occlusive disease (22,23). CT also serves to evaluate other clues for disorders associated with PAH [e.g., parenchymal lung disease, mediastinal abnormalities (fibrosis or lymphadenopathy with extrinsic compression of the pulmonary artery), pulmonary artery sarcoma, patulous esophagus (in systemic sclerosis), and intrinsic left-sided heart disease]. Extrinsic compression of the left main artery has also been visualized by CT in an IPAH patient (24).

B. Magnetic Resonance Imaging

Magnetic resonance imaging (MRI) is an emerging modality for assessing pulmonary vascular disease and concurrent cardiac evaluation (25). The complex RV geometry, which is difficult to assess by Doppler echocardiography (DE), is well visualized by MRI and allows precise noninvasive measurements of cardiac volumes and function. In addition, cine phase contrast allows for vascular flow measurements. Normal ranges of cardiac parameters have been established (26,27), and reproducibility between studies regarding right and left ventricular functions is strong (28,29). A recent report found MRI-determined pulmonary artery stiffness to predict mortality in a cohort of WHO group 1 patients (30). Several completed and ongoing studies (31,32) are evaluating MRI parameter(s) as an endpoint in drug intervention trials. Finally, MRI angiography can visualize differential pulmonary perfusion, which may allow for a better under-standing of the types of blood vessels involved and the physiology in a given patient with PH.

V. Electrocardiogram

The electrocardiogram (ECG) findings of PAH reflect right-heart chamber adaptations to increased pulmonary vascular resistance (PVR). Right-axis deviation (79%) and RVH (87%) are common in severe IPAH (2). In one study, significant predictors of decreased survival in an IPAH cohort included ECG evidence for right atrial enlargement (2.8-fold) and RVH (4.3-fold) (33). Furthermore, recent data suggest that ECG changes in the P-wave amplitude in lead II (right atrial enlargement), QRS axis, and T axis can predict the hemodynamic response to therapy as assessed by RHC (34). Nevertheless, as a single test, ECG is inadequate as a screening tool to rule out clinically relevant PAH (8,35).

A. Pulmonary Function Testing

Several studies have shown that up to 50% of IPAH individuals have mild spirometric restriction with moderate reduction in diffusing capacity for carbon monoxide (D_LCO) (3,36). While obstructive lung disease is uncommon, peripheral airway obstruction has been reported and is more pronounced with severe IPAH (37). A component of inspiratory and expiratory respiratory muscle weakness has also been described in IPAH (38,39). Contrary to IPAH, scleroderma represents a unique patient population that is routinely screened for PAH, given its strong association with subsequent mortality (40). In scleroderma, a decreased or decreasing D_LCO (41,42) and/or increased forced vital capacity (FVC)/D_LCO ratio (43,44) can predict the development or progression of PAH.

B. Cardiopulmonary Exercise Testing and Gas Exchange

Most patients with PAH first experience symptoms during exertion or exercise, thus making cardiopulmonary exercise testing (CPET) a potential diagnostic modality (45). In a recent study of 406 patients who underwent concurrent CPET and RHC testing, 75% were referred for dyspnea of unknown etiology, and the two most common CPET diagnoses included PAH (23%) and pulmonary venous hypertension (48%) (46). Importantly, the impairment of gas exchange due to altered ventilation-perfusion rela-tionships (47) and cardiac output limitation (48) in PAH drives the CPET findings. Exercise capacity is severely reduced and peak oxygen uptake (VO_{2peak}) is about 40% of normal (49). Other CPET findings for PAH include a decreased lactic acidosis threshold (LAT), high LAT/VO_{2peak} ratio (opposite to deconditioning), decreased $\Delta VO_2/\Delta WR$ (above the LAT), decreased mixed venous O_2 saturation at maximum exercise (50), low oxygen pulse [O_2 pulse = VO_2/HR = stroke volume $\times$ C(a$-$v)O_2], increased ventilatory equivalents for O_2 and CO_2, and low $P_{ET}CO_2$ (48,51,52). In addition, CPET might be useful for the assessment of exercise-induced PAH (46,53) and determining response to therapy (54). In fact, the peak systolic blood pressure and VO_{2max} based on CPET are independent predictors of survival in untreated IPAH patients (55). Importantly, the six-minute walk (6MW) test (56) has been shown to reflect CPET findings (57), and the total distance and extent of desaturation (58) from 6MW testing also have prognostic significance. The ease and reproducibility of 6MW testing, as opposed to the expertise and time required for CPET, favors its use as a primary endpoint in most PAH trials. Gas exchange is also affected during sleep without evidence for apneas/hypopneas (59,60), and daytime hypocapnea at rest and during exertion independently predict mortality for IPAH (61).

VI. Serology

No specific blood test(s) is diagnostic of PAH. However, a serological evaluation helps characterize whether the PAH is idiopathic or associated with another WHO group 1 condition (6). In addition, several biomarkers are prognostic predictors once WHO group 1 PAH is established, including uric acid (62,63), brain natriuretic peptide (BNP) (64–66), N-terminus fragment (NT)-proBNP (67,68), anticentromere antibodies (69), and serum creatinine (70). Other biomarkers have an association with WHO group 1 PAH and include thyroid function (71), anticardiolipin antibodies (72,73), and low-titer antinuclear antibodies (74,75). Plasma von Willebrand factor Antigen (vWF:Ag) has been shown to be elevated in patients with IPAH (76). A relatively standard battery of serological testing should also incorporate liver function, viral hepatitis panels (77), and HIV status (78). Recently, several investigators are evaluating other serum markers of inflammation in PAH (79–81), and their association with disease severity (e.g., procoagulant membrane particles) (82).

VII. Transthoracic Doppler Echocardiography

DE is currently considered to be the noninvasive screening test of choice for evaluating PH (6). The sensitivity and specificity of DE is 0.79 to 1.0 and 0.68 to 0.98, respectively for detecting PAH (6). DE estimation of systolic pulmonary artery pressure (PAP) requires a detectable and adequate (83) tricuspid jet velocity and an assessment of right atrial pressure (RAP) either by inferior vena cava collapsibility (84–86), a standardized value (5 or 10 mmHg) (87,88), or a clinical estimation of jugular venous pressure (89). By use of the maximum velocity of the tricuspid regurgitant (TR) jet (v), the systolic pressure gradient between the right ventricle and right atrium is calculated using the modified Bernoulli's equation (4 v^2); the sum of this pressure gradient and the RAP estimates the pulmonary artery systolic pressure (PASP), assuming no obstruction to RV blood flow (89).

A. "Normal" Echocardiographic Pulmonary Artery Pressure

Most prior studies noted a strong statistical correlation ($r = 0.78$ to 0.95) between PASP determined by DE and the gold standard RHC for WHO group 1 PAH (89–94).

Importantly, this correlation is substantially weakened in the setting of parenchymal lung disease (WHO group 3 PAH), especially interstitial lung disease (95). While patients with signs of right-heart failure invariably have a TR signal (90–100%) (89,90), DE in normal populations detects a TR signal only 50% to 70% of the time (88,96). Furthermore, only 24% of normals have both a TR signal and a recordable estimation of the PASP (88), highlighting that a TR signal does not always provide a PASP. This TR signal might be enhanced using contrast to better estimate the PASP (97). The available echocardiographic studies on normal populations have found a mean estimated PASP between 26.6 and 30.2 mmHg (87,88,98,99) with the largest of these studies demonstrating a 95% upper limit of 37.9 mmHg, corresponding to a TR velocity of 2.64 m/sec (88). Importantly, the normal values estimated by DE are dependent on body mass index, gender, age, left ventricular posterior wall thickness and ejection fraction (87,88, 100–102). These factors should be taken into account especially when assessing marginal elevations in DE-estimated PASP.

B. Echocardiography as an Effective Screening Tool

DE evaluates the degree of PH and also evaluates for prognosticating variables [right atrial and/or ventricular enlargement, pericardial effusion (103,104), RV ejection fraction] and other potential causes of PH (left ventricular systolic/diastolic dysfunction, valvular heart disease, intracardiac shunting). DE can be used to determine most hemodynamic variables that are routinely assessed by RHC including mean pulmonary artery pressure (mPAP) (97,105), diastolic PAP (106,107), PVR (108,109), and cardiac output (Q_T) (110,111). With careful study, DE can also document the presence and degree of diastolic dysfunction (112) and might distinguish pulmonary arterial from venous hypertension (113). Currently, however, DE is not an acceptable replacement for RHC especially since nonsimultaneous assessments have been shown to be statistically inaccurate in a high-PH prevalence population (114). The role of echocardiography in PAH is discussed in depth by Dr Torbicki and coworkers in chapter 8.

VIII. Cardiac Catheterization

The confirmatory test for PH is RHC (6), and appropriate guidelines and risks have been published for this invasive procedure (3, 115–117). The RHC technique and application was described by Swan et al. in 1970 (118) and is standardly conducted at rest, in the supine position, and via the internal jugular, femoral, or subclavian vein approach. RHC allows for the precise establishment of the diagnosis and type of PH, the severity of disease, prognosticating hemodynamic data (3), and pulmonary vascular reserve. Importantly, an individual's hemodynamic profile has an inherent variability of 8% in PAP and 13% in PVR over a given six-hour period (119).

A. Hemodynamic Definition of PH and PAH

The current definition of PH by the NIH registry is a mean PAP >25 mmHg at rest; PAH is defined as PH combined with a pulmonary artery occlusion pressure (PAOP) of

<15 mmHg and a calculated pulmonary vascular resistance (PVR) >3 Wood units (2). When a PVR is unable to be calculated given an unobtainable PAOP, one can calculate the total pulmonary resistance (mPAP/Q_T). In addition, the RHC provides the following measured hemodynamic data: RAP, right ventricular pressure (RVP), mixed venous oxygenation (mvO$_2$) ± oxygenation of superior vena cava/inferior vena cava (SVC/IVC), transpulmonary gradient (mean PAP − downstream pressure), and cardiac output [either by thermodilution (120) or using the Fick's principle (121)]. The interpretation of hemodynamic tracings should be performed by experienced clinicians, and all measurements should be made during end-expiration (122). The hemodynamic definition of resting PH has varied in the literature with the upper limit of normal as low as 19 mmHg (123). In fact, a new definition scheme for PH was proposed at the recent Fourth World Symposium on Pulmonary Hypertension (Dana Point, California, February 2008) suggesting that mean PAP <21 mmHg (corresponding TR jet velocity of <2.5 m/sec) was more suitable for normalcy (124). Appropriately, some investigators have questioned the current practice of using fluid-filled catheters to measure instantaneous pressures and PVR (125), pointing out the inherent pulsatility of the pulmonary circulation (126). In this context, there are ongoing efforts to better understand pulmonary hemodynamics including the study of pulmonary resistance partitioning, closing pressure (pressure axis intercept of the mPAP/flow relationship), pulmonary vascular impedance, and pulmonary pressure pulsatility (125,127).

B. Vasodilator Testing

An RHC also allows for acute vasodilator testing to assess for vasoreactivity, which is present when a short-acting vasodilator [usually inhaled nitric oxide, intravenous epoprostenol, or intravenous adenosine (128)] causes a decrease of >10 mmHg in mean PAP to an absolute value of <40 mmHg, without a concurrent decrease in cardiac output (129) (Fig. 1). Approximately 7% of IPAH patients qualify as "vasoreactive," which independently portends an excellent five-year survival (95%) with calcium channel blocker therapy (130). Vasodilator testing might also help to unmask pulmonary veno-occlusive disease (23).

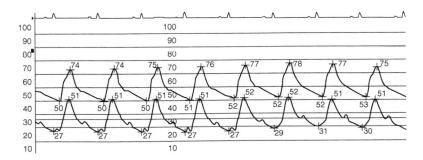

Figure 1 Hemodynamic tracings of pulmonary artery pressure demonstrating a positive response to inhaled nitric oxide (*bottom tracing*) during acute vasoreactivity testing in a 28-year-old male with IPAH. The cardiac output improved with nitric oxide administration.

C. Evaluation of Intracardiac Shunt and Pulmonary Venous Hypertension

While contrast can be used with DE to reliably detect right to left shunting, RHC [usually in concert with left-heart catheterization (LHC)] or transesophageal echocardiography are superior modalities for detecting potential shunts, often in the setting of congenital abnormalities. Concurrent LHC also allows for shunt quantification and accurate calculation of the pulmonary to systemic blood flow ratio (Q_p/Q_s). In cases of intracardiac shunt (including patent foramen ovale), blood flow must be calculated using the Fick's method since the thermodilution technique is inadequate in this setting. Furthermore, an LHC is often necessary to adequately determine left-sided filling pressures (LVEDP, left ventricular end-diastolic pressure) when an accurate PAOP is unable to be obtained (131), especially given the poor interobserver variability of PAOP interpretation (132). The LVEDP is affected by the status of the mitral valve and left atrial and ventricular compliance (133). One can also consider volume loading, exercise provocation, or pharmacological manipulation (i.e., nitroprusside) to further evaluate for pulmonary venous hypertension (134) during cardiac catheterization. In normoxic, healthy subjects, the difference between mPAP and PAOP (transpulmonary gradient) is 5 to 9 mmHg (135), and a widening of this gradient suggests a component of "fixed" pulmonary vascular disease.

D. Hemodynamic Assessment of Left-Heart Disease

The contour of the left ventricular filling pressure is of importance in identifying patients with restrictive diastolic filling, usually consisting of a sharp dip and plateau appearance (Fig. 2). Simultaneous right and left ventricular pressure measurement throughout the respiratory cycle is the gold standard method for differentiating restrictive from constrictive physiology (136). Simultaneous PAOP and left ventricular pressure measurement is still the gold standard method for identifying and quantifying the severity of obstruction to left atrial emptying (Fig. 3) (most often from mitral valve stenosis but rarely from supravalvar stenosis or cor triatriatum). Elevation of left atrial, pulmonary venous, pulmonary capillary, and pulmonary arterial pressure results from the pressure gradient across the obstruction, while the magnitude of the pressure elevation is related to the severity of stenosis and rate of flow across the segment of stenosis. The formulae of Gorlin and Gorlin define the relationship of flow and pressure in mitral stenosis (137–140):

$$\text{Mitral valve flow (mL/sec)} = \frac{\text{Cardiac output (mL/min)}}{\text{Diastolic filling time (sec/min)}}$$

$$\text{Mitral valve area(cm}^2) = \frac{\text{Mitral valve flow(ml/sec)}}{31 \times \sqrt{\text{pressure gradient}}}$$

The rate of mitral valve flow increases if there is an increase in cardiac output or a decrease in diastolic filling time with increased heart rate. The pressure gradient increases logarithmically with any increase in flow; once the left atrial pressure is above 25 mmHg, the oncotic pressure in the pulmonary capillaries is exceeded and pulmonary edema occurs. The rise in left atrial pressure results in an obligate increase in pulmonary arterial and RV pressure to maintain forward flow, resulting in "passive" PH. In patients with long-standing mitral stenosis, there is pronounced pulmonary vasoconstriction that further

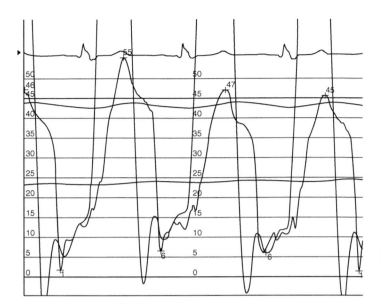

Figure 2 Simultaneous left ventricular (LV) and right ventricular (RV) pressure recordings (50 mmHg scale) in a 35-year-old patient with repaired tetralogy of Fallot and pulmonary hypertension. Note the "dip and plateau" appearance of the left ventricular pressure waveform in early and mid-diastole, consistent with a restrictive filling pattern. Both the RVEDP and LVEDP are elevated ($\sim$ 15 mmHg). RV systolic pressure is moderately elevated (45–55 mmHg) and RV contractility is reduced (RV dp/dt = 384 mmHg/sec). LV contractility is normal (dp/dt = 1250 mmHg/sec).

elevates PVR and pressures in the right ventricle and pulmonary artery. This elevation in PVR is "protective" in that it limits the flow rate into the pulmonary venous system, thereby lowering the oncotic pressure and shifting the hemodynamic burden to the right heart. With relief of the obstruction to left atrial emptying, the passive component of PH may be alleviated immediately; however, the protective component, consisting of increased resistance within the pulmonary arteries and arterioles, may not normalize in older patients with long-standing severe mitral stenosis, concomitant mitral regurgitation, and those with chronic atrial fibrillation (141). Isolated mitral valve regurgitation (MR) may result in severe PH if it is acute (e.g., papillary muscle rupture or ischemic dysfunction), despite the fact that the left atrium and left ventricle are subjected to a lesser volume overload compared to chronic regurgitation. Chronic MR is usually well tolerated because the left heart can compensate for the volume overload by increasing compliance and ventricular stroke volume. In acute, poorly tolerated MR, the left ventricular diastolic pressure and left atrial pressure (or PAOP) rises precipitously (specifically the V wave), and forward cardiac output may be compromised by the inability of the left ventricle to accommodate the increased volume load and generate an adequate forward stroke volume, a situation that is often made worse if coronary ischemia is present. Reflex systemic and pulmonary arterial vasoconstriction further decreases cardiac output, increases left ventricular filling pressure, and augments the regurgitation fraction. This vasoconstriction can be ameliorated by the use of vasodilators such as nitroglycerin. LVEDP and PAOP in

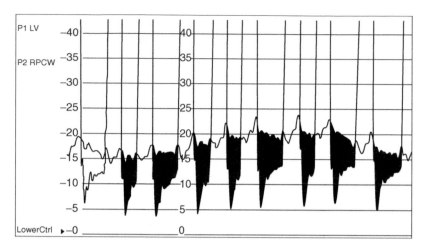

Figure 3 Simultaneous right–pulmonary capillary wedge pressure (RPCW) and left ventricular (LV) pressure tracings in a 47-year-old male with atrial fibrillation and cor triatriatum (the presence of a partially obstructive membrane within the left atrium). The mean pressure gradient over eight cardiac cycles is 7 mmHg, consistent with a moderate degree of obstruction to left atrial emptying. This lesion imposes the same hemodynamic burden as valvular mitral stenosis. It is important to measure the gradient over at least five cycles if atrial fibrillation is present given the random variability in diastolic filling periods.

patients without obstruction to left atrial emptying (e.g., mitral stenosis) are inversely related to ventricular compliance. The left ventricle becomes less compliant with age, hypertrophy, and ischemia. An elevation in LVEDP and PAOP (>12 mmHg) reflects abnormal compliance and can be unmasked with volume loading during the catheterization procedure. Left ventricular contractility can be assessed by the rate of rise of ventricular pressure (*dp/dt*) during systole ($\geq$1200 mmHg/sec). Contractility refers to a reflection of the force-velocity relationship of the myocardium and is independent of volume.

E. RHC and Exercise

The definition of PH also incorporates exercise; a mean PAP >30 mmHg during exercise is consistent with PH (2). Tolle and colleagues recently defined exercise PAH as a mean PAP $\geq$ 30 mmHg, PVR $\geq$ 1 Wood unit, and a PAWP <20 mmHg (46). However, normal PAWP measurements during supine exercise appear age dependent and can exceed 30 mmHg in older, healthy individuals (61–83 years old); PAWP during exercise in older normals increases by 1.93 $\pm$ 0.94 mmHg for each liter of cardiac output, compared with 0.30 $\pm$ 0.35 for normal young individuals (142). In addition, the potential swings in pleural pressure during heavy exercise might affect the accurate determination of PAWP. Unlike PAWP, there is no significant difference in the transpulmonary gradient (mPAP $-$ PAWP) during exercise between older and younger normals (0.64 $\pm$ 0.57 vs. 0.53 $\pm$ 0.44 for each liter of cardiac output, respectively) (142). Importantly, the PVR in normals during exercise either stays unchanged or decreases; in a group of young athletes, the PVR at peak exercise was 0.5 ± 0.1 Wood units with cardiac output elevations of 20 to 30 L/min (143). During higher levels of exercise, the alveolar-arterial O_2 actually widens and is most related to diffusion limitation and, less so, to ventilation-perfusion mismatch (144). There are currently no standards or practice guidelines related to exercise provocation during RHC. The physiology during exercise is potentially complicated by patient position (upright vs. supine), type of exercise (upper vs. lower extremity), blood oxygenation, and acid-base balance (145). The mPAP/cardiac output slope in normal man has been calculated as 1.5 mmHg/L/min/m^2 and 1.6 mmHg/L/min/m^2 using exercise-derived data (146) and unilateral pulmonary artery occlusion (147), respectively. Recent studies are incorporating exercise hemo-dynamics as an endpoint in IPAH (148,149) and systemic sclerosis (150) and lending supportive evidence to the concept that PAH may be a spectrum, originating as an exercise-related phenomenon before eventually manifesting at rest (46). In support, a study in COPD-associated PH found exercise-induced PH to be a significant predictor of developing resting PH based on sequential cardiac catheterization (151). Whether exercise echocardiography will prove to be a noninvasive screening test for exercise cardiac catheterization clearly requires further study.

IX. Lung Biopsy

There is a paucity of literature around the diagnostic utility of either thoracoscopic or open lung biopsy in a patient with PAH. The original NIH registry reported on 23 open lung biopsies; one patient clearly died as a result of the surgery; information was unavailable in 18 of those 23 patients (152). Indeed, there are no distinctive histological findings that would alter a planned trial of therapy in this group of patients [with the possible exception of pulmonary veno-occlusive disease (23)]. Given its possible mor-bidity and mortality, surgical lung biopsy has little diagnostic utility for PAH (153).

X. Summary

PAH has several potential diagnostic modalities; however, several of these have limited sensitivity and specificity, especially early in the disease process. Currently, there is uniform agreement that DE is the accepted screening tool of choice for PAH; however, cardiac catheterization is essential for the final diagnosis. The importance in evaluating for concurrent left-heart disease cannot be overemphasized. Using exercise to "unmask" PAH in symptomatic individuals (without resting PAH) might allow for earlier diagnosis and perhaps alter the natural history of the disease. Newer diagnostic modalities such as MRI imaging are emerging and will likely augment our noninvasive armamentarium in the diagnosis of PAH.

References

1. Romberg E. Ueber sklerose der lungen arterie. Dtsch Arch Klin Med 1891; 48:197–206.
2. Rich S, Dantzker DR, Ayres SM, et al. Primary pulmonary hypertension. A national pro-spective study. Ann Intern Med 1987; 107:216–223.

3. D'Alonzo GE, Barst RJ, Ayres SM, et al. Survival in patients with primary pulmonary hypertension. Results from a national prospective registry. Ann Intern Med 1991; 115:343–349.
4. Fishman AP. Handbook of physiology. Bethesda, MD: American Physiological Society, 1985.
5. West J. Respiratory Physiology: The Essentials. 8th ed. Lippincott Williams & Wilkins, 2008.
6. McGoon M, Gutterman D, Steen V, et al. Screening, early detection, and diagnosis of pulmonary arterial hypertension: ACCP evidence-based clinical practice guidelines. Chest 2004; 126:14S–34S.
7. McGoon MD, Krichman A, Farber HW, et al. Design of the REVEAL registry for US patients with pulmonary arterial hypertension. Mayo Clin Proc 2008; 83:923–931.
8. Algeo S, Morrison D, Ovitt T, et al. Noninvasive detection of pulmonary hypertension. Clin Cardiol 1984; 7:148–156.
9. Lupi E, Dumont C, Tejada VM, et al. A radiologic index of pulmonary arterial hypertension. Chest 1975; 68:28–31.
10. Teichmann V, Jezek V, Herles F. Relevance of width of right descending branch of pulmonary artery as a radiological sign of pulmonary hypertension. Thorax 1970; 25:91–96.
11. Matthay RA, Schwarz MI, Ellis JH Jr., et al. Pulmonary artery hypertension in chronic obstructive pulmonary disease: determination by chest radiography. Invest Radiol 1981; 16:95–100.
12. Chetty KG, Brown SE, Light RW. Identification of pulmonary hypertension in chronic obstructive pulmonary disease from routine chest radiographs. Am Rev Respir Dis 1982; 126:338–341.
13. Schmidt HC, Kauczor HU, Schild HH, et al. Pulmonary hypertension in patients with chronic pulmonary thromboembolism: chest radiograph and CT evaluation before and after surgery. Eur Radiol 1996; 6:817–825.
14. Sherrick AD, Swensen SJ, Hartman TE. Mosaic pattern of lung attenuation on CT scans: frequency among patients with pulmonary artery hypertension of different causes. AJR Am J Roentgenol 1997; 169:79–82.
15. Perloff JK, Hart EM, Greaves SM, et al. Proximal pulmonary arterial and intrapulmonary radiologic features of Eisenmenger syndrome and primary pulmonary hypertension. Am J Cardiol 2003; 92:182–187.
16. Kuriyama K, Gamsu G, Stern RG, et al. CT-determined pulmonary artery diameters in predicting pulmonary hypertension. Invest Radiol 1984; 19:16–22.
17. Haimovici JB, Trotman-Dickenson B, Halpern EF, et al. Relationship between pulmonary artery diameter at computed tomography and pulmonary artery pressures at right-sided heart catheterization. Massachusetts General Hospital Lung Transplantation Program. Acad Radiol 1997; 4:327–334.
18. Ng CS, Wells AU, Padley SP. A CT sign of chronic pulmonary arterial hypertension: the ratio of main pulmonary artery to aortic diameter. J Thorac Imaging 1999; 14:270–278.
19. Hansell DM. Small-vessel diseases of the lung: CT-pathologic correlates. Radiology 2002; 225:639–653.
20. Horton MR, Tuder RM. Primary pulmonary arterial hypertension presenting as diffuse micronodules on CT. Crit Rev Comput Tomogr 2004; 45:335–341.
21. Nolan RL, McAdams HP, Sporn TA, et al. Pulmonary cholesterol granulomas in patients with pulmonary artery hypertension: chest radiographic and CT findings. AJR Am J Roentgenol 1999; 172:1317–1319.
22. Lippert JL, White CS, Cameron EW, et al. Pulmonary capillary hemangiomatosis: radiographic appearance. J Thorac Imaging 1998; 13:49–51.
23. Mandel J, Mark EJ, Hales CA. Pulmonary veno-occlusive disease. Am J Respir Crit Care Med 2000; 162:1964–1973.
24. Eksinar S, Gedevanishvili A, Koroglu M, et al. Extrinsic compression of the left main coronary artery in pulmonary hypertension. JBR-BTR 2005; 88:190–192.

25. Kovacs G, Reiter G, Reiter U, et al. The emerging role of magnetic resonance imaging in the diagnosis and management of pulmonary hypertension. Respiration 2008; 76:458–470.

26. Maceira AM, Prasad SK, Khan M, et al. Reference right ventricular systolic and diastolic function normalized to age, gender and body surface area from steady-state free precession cardiovascular magnetic resonance. Eur Heart J 2006; 27:2879–2888.

27. Alfakih K, Plein S, Thiele H, et al. Normal human left and right ventricular dimensions for MRI as assessed by turbo gradient echo and steady-state free precession imaging sequences. J Magn Reson Imaging 2003; 17:323–329.

28. Grothues F, Moon JC, Bellenger NG, et al. Interstudy reproducibility of right ventricular volumes, function, and mass with cardiovascular magnetic resonance. Am Heart J 2004; 147:218–223.

29. Chatzimavroudis GP, Oshinski JN, Franch RH, et al. Evaluation of the precision of magnetic resonance phase velocity mapping for blood flow measurements. J Cardiovasc Magn Reson 2001; 3:11–19.

30. Gan CT, Lankhaar JW, Westerhof N, et al. Noninvasively assessed pulmonary artery stiffness predicts mortality in pulmonary arterial hypertension. Chest 2007; 132:1906–1912.

31. Chin KM, Kingman M, de Lemos JA, et al. Changes in right ventricular structure and function assessed using cardiac magnetic resonance imaging in bosentan-treated patients with pulmonary arterial hypertension. Am J Cardiol 2008; 101:1669–1672.

32. Gan CT, Holverda S, Marcus JT, et al. Right ventricular diastolic dysfunction and the acute effects of sildenafil in pulmonary hypertension patients. Chest 2007; 132:11–17.

33. Bossone E, Paciocco G, Iarussi D, et al. The prognostic role of the ECG in primary pulmonary hypertension. Chest 2002; 121:513–518.

34. Henkens IR, Gan CT, van Wolferen SA, et al. ECG monitoring of treatment response in pulmonary arterial hypertension patients. Chest 2008; 134(6):1250–1257 [Epub July 18, 2008].

35. Ahearn GS, Tapson VF, Rebeiz A, et al. Electrocardiography to define clinical status in primary pulmonary hypertension and pulmonary arterial hypertension secondary to collagen vascular disease. Chest 2002; 122:524–527.

36. Sun XG, Hansen JE, Oudiz RJ, et al. Pulmonary function in primary pulmonary hypertension. J Am Coll Cardiol 2003; 41:1028–1035.

37. Meyer FJ, Ewert R, Hoeper MM, et al. Peripheral airway obstruction in primary pulmonary hypertension. Thorax 2002; 57:473–476.

38. Meyer FJ, Lossnitzer D, Kristen AV, et al. Respiratory muscle dysfunction in idiopathic pulmonary arterial hypertension. Eur Respir J 2005; 25:125–130.

39. Kabitz HJ, Schwoerer A, Bremer HC, et al. Impairment of respiratory muscle function in pulmonary hypertension. Clin Sci (Lond) 2008; 114:165–171.

40. Chang B, Schachna L, White B, et al. Natural history of mild-moderate pulmonary hypertension and the risk factors for severe pulmonary hypertension in scleroderma. J Rheumatol 2006; 33:269–274.

41. Steen V, Medsger TA Jr. Predictors of isolated pulmonary hypertension in patients with systemic sclerosis and limited cutaneous involvement. Arthritis Rheum 2003; 48:516–522.

42. Launay D, Mouthon L, Hachulla E, et al. Prevalence and characteristics of moderate to severe pulmonary hypertension in systemic sclerosis with and without interstitial lung disease. J Rheumatol 2007; 34:1005–1011.

43. Steen VD, Graham G, Conte C, et al. Isolated diffusing capacity reduction in systemic sclerosis. Arthritis Rheum 1992; 35:765–770.

44. Hsu VM, Moreyra AE, Wilson AC, et al. Assessment of pulmonary arterial hypertension in patients with systemic sclerosis: comparison of noninvasive tests with results of right-heart catheterization. J Rheumatol 2008; 35:458–465.

45. Oudiz RJ. The role of exercise testing in the management of pulmonary arterial hypertension. Semin Respir Crit Care Med 2005; 26:379–384.
46. Tolle JJ, Waxman AB, Van Horn TL, et al. Exercise-induced pulmonary arterial hypertension. Circulation 2008; 118:2183–2189.
47. Dantzker DR, D'Alonzo GE, Bower JS, et al. Pulmonary gas exchange during exercise in patients with chronic obliterative pulmonary hypertension. Am Rev Respir Dis 1984; 130:412–416.
48. Riley MS, Porszasz J, Engelen MP, et al. Gas exchange responses to continuous incremental cycle ergometry exercise in primary pulmonary hypertension in humans. Eur J Appl Physiol 2000; 83:63–70.
49. D'Alonzo GE, Gianotti LA, Pohil RL, et al. Comparison of progressive exercise performance of normal subjects and patients with primary pulmonary hypertension. Chest 1987; 92:57–62.
50. Dantzker DR, Bower JS. Mechanisms of gas exchange abnormality in patients with chronic obliterative pulmonary vascular disease. J Clin Invest 1979; 64:1050–1055.
51. Hansen JE, Ulubay G, Chow BF, et al. Mixed-expired and end-tidal CO_2 distinguish between ventilation and perfusion defects during exercise testing in patients with lung and heart diseases. Chest 2007; 132:977–983.
52. Sun XG, Hansen JE, Oudiz RJ, et al. Exercise pathophysiology in patients with primary pulmonary hypertension. Circulation 2001; 104:429–435.
53. Markowitz DH, Systrom DM. Diagnosis of pulmonary vascular limit to exercise by cardiopulmonary exercise testing. J Heart Lung Transplant 2004; 23:88–95.
54. Oudiz RJ, Roveran G, Hansen JE, et al. Effect of sildenafil on ventilatory efficiency and exercise tolerance in pulmonary hypertension. Eur J Heart Fail 2007; 9:917–921.
55. Wensel R, Opitz CF, Anker SD, et al. Assessment of survival in patients with primary pulmonary hypertension: importance of cardiopulmonary exercise testing. Circulation 2002; 106:319–324.
56. Guyatt GH, Sullivan MJ, Thompson PJ, et al. The 6-minute walk: a new measure of exercise capacity in patients with chronic heart failure. Can Med Assoc J 1985; 132:919–923.
57. Miyamoto S, Nagaya N, Satoh T, et al. Clinical correlates and prognostic significance of six-minute walk test in patients with primary pulmonary hypertension. Comparison with cardiopulmonary exercise testing. Am J Respir Crit Care Med 2000; 161:487–492.
58. Paciocco G, Martinez FJ, Bossone E, et al. Oxygen desaturation on the six-minute walk test and mortality in untreated primary pulmonary hypertension. Eur Respir J 2001; 17:647–652.
59. Rafanan AL, Golish JA, Dinner DS, et al. Nocturnal hypoxemia is common in primary pulmonary hypertension. Chest 2001; 120:894–899.
60. Minai OA, Pandya CM, Golish JA, et al. Predictors of nocturnal oxygen desaturation in pulmonary arterial hypertension. Chest 2007; 131:109–117.
61. Hoeper MM, Pletz MW, Golpon H, et al. Prognostic value of blood gas analyses in patients with idiopathic pulmonary arterial hypertension. Eur Respir J 2007; 29:944–950.
62. Njaman W, Iesaki T, Iwama Y, et al. Serum uric Acid as a prognostic predictor in pulmonary arterial hypertension with connective tissue disease. Int Heart J 2007; 48:523–532.
63. Nagaya N, Uematsu M, Satoh T, et al. Serum uric acid levels correlate with the severity and the mortality of primary pulmonary hypertension. Am J Respir Crit Care Med 1999; 160:487–492.
64. Nagaya N, Nishikimi T, Uematsu M, et al. Plasma brain natriuretic peptide as a prognostic indicator in patients with primary pulmonary hypertension. Circulation 2000; 102:865–870.
65. Leuchte HH, Holzapfel M, Baumgartner RA, et al. Clinical significance of brain natriuretic peptide in primary pulmonary hypertension. J Am Coll Cardiol 2004; 43:764–770.
66. Hargett CW, Tapson VF. Brain natriuretic peptide: diagnostic and therapeutic implications in pulmonary arterial hypertension. Semin Respir Crit Care Med 2005; 26:385–393.

67. Gan CT, McCann GP, Marcus JT, et al. NT-proBNP reflects right ventricular structure and function in pulmonary hypertension. Eur Respir J 2006; 28:1190–1194.
68. Andreassen AK, Wergeland R, Simonsen S, et al. N-terminal pro-B-type natriuretic peptide as an indicator of disease severity in a heterogeneous group of patients with chronic precapillary pulmonary hypertension. Am J Cardiol 2006; 98:525–529.
69. Kampolis C, Plastiras S, Vlachoyiannopoulos P, et al. The presence of anticentromere antibodies may predict progression of estimated pulmonary arterial systolic pressure in systemic sclerosis. Scand J Rheumatol 2008; 37:278–283.
70. Shah SJ, Thenappan T, Rich S, et al. Association of serum creatinine with abnormal hemodynamics and mortality in pulmonary arterial hypertension. Circulation 2008; 117:2475–2483.
71. Chu JW, Kao PN, Faul JL, et al. High prevalence of autoimmune thyroid disease in pulmonary arterial hypertension. Chest 2002; 122:1668–1673.
72. Falcao CA, Alves IC, Chahade WH, et al. Echocardiographic abnormalities and anti-phospholipid antibodies in patients with systemic lupus erythematosus. Arq Bras Cardiol 2002; 79:285–291.
73. Asherson RA, Higenbottam TW, Dinh Xuan AT, et al. Pulmonary hypertension in a lupus clinic: experience with twenty-four patients. J Rheumatol 1990; 17:1292–1298.
74. Rich S, Kieras K, Hart K, et al. Antinuclear antibodies in primary pulmonary hypertension. J Am Coll Cardiol 1986; 8:1307–1311.
75. Isern RA, Yaneva M, Weiner E, et al. Autoantibodies in patients with primary pulmonary hypertension: association with anti-Ku. Am J Med 1992; 93:307–312.
76. Lopes AA, Maeda NY, Goncalves RC, et al. Endothelial cell dysfunction correlates differentially with survival in primary and secondary pulmonary hypertension. Am Heart J 2000; 139:618–623.
77. Golbin JM, Krowka MJ. Portopulmonary hypertension. Clin Chest Med 2007; 28:203–218, ix.
78. Sitbon O. HIV-related pulmonary arterial hypertension: clinical presentation and management. AIDS 2008; 22(suppl 3):S55–S62.
79. Dorfmuller P, Perros F, Balabanian K, et al. Inflammation in pulmonary arterial hypertension. Eur Respir J 2003; 22:358–363.
80. Sanchez O, Marcos E, Perros F, et al. Role of endothelium-derived CC chemokine ligand 2 in idiopathic pulmonary arterial hypertension. Am J Respir Crit Care Med 2007; 176:1041–1047.
81. Dorfmuller P, Zarka V, Durand-Gasselin I, et al. Chemokine RANTES in severe pulmonary arterial hypertension. Am J Respir Crit Care Med 2002; 165:534–539.
82. Bakouboula B, Morel O, Faure A, et al. Procoagulant membrane microparticles correlate with the severity of pulmonary arterial hypertension. Am J Respir Crit Care Med 2008; 177:536–543.
83. Miyatake K, Okamoto M, Kinoshita N, et al. Evaluation of tricuspid regurgitation by pulsed Doppler and two-dimensional echocardiography. Circulation 1982; 66:777–784.
84. Simonson JS, Schiller NB. Sonospirometry: a new method for noninvasive estimation of mean right atrial pressure based on two-dimensional echographic measurements of the inferior vena cava during measured inspiration. J Am Coll Cardiol 1988; 11:557–564.
85. Ommen SR, Nishimura RA, Hurrell DG, et al. Assessment of right atrial pressure with 2-dimensional and Doppler echocardiography: a simultaneous catheterization and echocardiographic study. Mayo Clin Proc 2000; 75:24–29.
86. Kircher BJ, Himelman RB, Schiller NB. Noninvasive estimation of right atrial pressure from the inspiratory collapse of the inferior vena cava. Am J Cardiol 1990; 66:493–496.
87. Bossone E, Rubenfire M, Bach DS, et al. Range of tricuspid regurgitation velocity at rest and during exercise in normal adult men: implications for the diagnosis of pulmonary hypertension. J Am Coll Cardiol 1999; 33:1662–1666.

88. McQuillan BM, Picard MH, Leavitt M, et al. Clinical correlates and reference intervals for pulmonary artery systolic pressure among echocardiographically normal subjects. Circulation 2001; 104:2797–2802.
89. Yock PG, Popp RL. Noninvasive estimation of right ventricular systolic pressure by Doppler ultrasound in patients with tricuspid regurgitation. Circulation 1984; 70:657–662.
90. Currie PJ, Seward JB, Chan KL, et al. Continuous wave Doppler determination of right ventricular pressure: a simultaneous Doppler-catheterization study in 127 patients. J Am Coll Cardiol 1985; 6:750–756.
91. Berger M, Haimowitz A, Van Tosh A, et al. Quantitative assessment of pulmonary hypertension in patients with tricuspid regurgitation using continuous wave Doppler ultrasound. J Am Coll Cardiol 1985; 6:359–365.
92. Denton CP, Cailes JB, Phillips GD, et al. Comparison of Doppler echocardiography and right heart catheterization to assess pulmonary hypertension in systemic sclerosis. Br J Rheumatol 1997; 36:239–243.
93. Shapiro SM, Oudiz RJ, Cao T, et al. Primary pulmonary hypertension: improved long-term effects and survival with continuous intravenous epoprostenol infusion. J Am Coll Cardiol 1997; 30:343–349.
94. Kim WR, Krowka MJ, Plevak DJ, et al. Accuracy of Doppler echocardiography in the assessment of pulmonary hypertension in liver transplant candidates. Liver Transpl 2000; 6:453–458.
95. Arcasoy SM, Christie JD, Ferrari VA, et al. Echocardiographic assessment of pulmonary hypertension in patients with advanced lung disease. Am J Respir Crit Care Med 2003; 167:735–740.
96. Berger M, Hecht SR, Van Tosh A, et al. Pulsed and continuous wave Doppler echocardiographic assessment of valvular regurgitation in normal subjects. J Am Coll Cardiol 1989; 13:1540–1545.
97. Celermajer DS, Marwick T. Echocardiographic and right heart catheterization techniques in patients with pulmonary arterial hypertension. Int J Cardiol 2008; 125:294–303.
98. Aessopos A, Farmakis D, Taktikou H, et al. Doppler-determined peak systolic tricuspid pressure gradient in persons with normal pulmonary function and tricuspid regurgitation. J Am Soc Echocardiogr 2000; 13:645–649.
99. Dib JC, Abergel E, Rovani C, et al. The age of the patient should be taken into account when interpreting Doppler assessed pulmonary artery pressures. J Am Soc Echocardiogr 1997; 10:72–73.
100. de Divitiis O, Fazio S, Petitto M, et al. Obesity and cardiac function. Circulation 1981; 64:477–482.
101. Davidson WR Jr., Fee EC. Influence of aging on pulmonary hemodynamics in a population free of coronary artery disease. Am J Cardiol 1990; 65:1454–1458.
102. Ekelund LG, Holmgren A. Central hemodynamics during exercise. Circ Res 1967:XX, XXI.
103. Eysmann SB, Palevsky HI, Reichek N, et al. Two-dimensional and Doppler-echocardiographic and cardiac catheterization correlates of survival in primary pulmonary hypertension. Circulation 1989; 80:353–360.
104. Raymond RJ, Hinderliter AL, Willis PW, et al. Echocardiographic predictors of adverse outcomes in primary pulmonary hypertension. J Am Coll Cardiol 2002; 39:1214–1219.
105. Kitabatake A, Inoue M, Asao M, et al. Noninvasive evaluation of pulmonary hypertension by a pulsed Doppler technique. Circulation 1983; 68:302–309.
106. Lanzarini L, Fontana A, Lucca E, et al. Noninvasive estimation of both systolic and diastolic pulmonary artery pressure from Doppler analysis of tricuspid regurgitant velocity spectrum in patients with chronic heart failure. Am Heart J 2002; 144:1087–1094.

107. Stephen B, Dalal P, Berger M, et al. Noninvasive estimation of pulmonary artery diastolic pressure in patients with tricuspid regurgitation by Doppler echocardiography. Chest 1999; 116:73–77.

108. Scapellato F, Temporelli PL, Eleuteri E, et al. Accurate noninvasive estimation of pulmonary vascular resistance by Doppler echocardiography in patients with chronic failure heart failure. J Am Coll Cardiol 2001; 37:1813–1819.

109. Abbas AE, Fortuin FD, Schiller NB, et al. A simple method for noninvasive estimation of pulmonary vascular resistance. J Am Coll Cardiol 2003; 41:1021–1027.

110. Ihlen H, Amlie JP, Dale J, et al. Determination of cardiac output by Doppler echocardiography. Br Heart J 1984; 51:54–60.

111. Lewis JF, Kuo LC, Nelson JG, et al. Pulsed Doppler echocardiographic determination of stroke volume and cardiac output: clinical validation of two new methods using the apical window. Circulation 1984; 70:425–431.

112. Rakowski H, Appleton C, Chan KL, et al. Canadian consensus recommendations for the measurement and reporting of diastolic dysfunction by echocardiography: from the Investigators of Consensus on Diastolic Dysfunction by Echocardiography. J Am Soc Echocardiogr 1996; 9:736–760.

113. Willens HJ, Chirinos JA, Gomez-Marin O, et al. Noninvasive differentiation of pulmonary arterial and venous hypertension using conventional and Doppler tissue imaging echocardiography. J Am Soc Echocardiogr 2008; 21:715–719.

114. Selimovic N, Rundqvist B, Bergh CH, et al. Assessment of pulmonary vascular resistance by Doppler echocardiography in patients with pulmonary arterial hypertension. J Heart Lung Transplant 2007; 26:927–934.

115. Oudiz RJ, Langleben, D. Cardiac catheterization in pulmonary arterial hypertension: an updated guide to proper use. Adv Pulm Hypertens 2005; 4:15–25.

116. Guillinta P, Peterson KL, Ben-Yehuda O. Cardiac catheterization techniques in pulmonary hypertension. Cardiol Clin 2004; 22:401–15, vi.

117. Grossman W. Cardiac Catheterization and Angiography. Philadelphia: Lea & Febiger, 1980.

118. Swan HJ, Ganz W, Forrester J, et al. Catheterization of the heart in man with use of a flow-directed balloon-tipped catheter. N Engl J Med 1970; 283:447–451.

119. Rich S, D'Alonzo GE, Dantzker DR, et al. Magnitude and implications of spontaneous hemodynamic variability in primary pulmonary hypertension. Am J Cardiol 1985; 55:159–163.

120. Khalil HH. Determination of cardiac output in man by a new method based on thermodilution. Lancet 1963; 1:1352–1354.

121. Yung GL, Fedullo PF, Kinninger K, et al. Comparison of impedance cardiography to direct Fick and thermodilution cardiac output determination in pulmonary arterial hypertension. Congest Heart Fail 2004; 10:7–10.

122. Kaluski E, Shah M, Kobrin I, et al. Right heart catheterization: indications, technique, safety, measurements, and alternatives. Heart Drug 2003; 3:225–235.

123. Fowler NO, Westcott RN, Scott RC. Normal pressure in the right heart and pulmonary artery. Am Heart J 1953; 46:264–267.

124. Olschewski H. [Dana Point: what is new in the diagnosis of pulmonary hypertension?]. Dtsch Med Wochenschr 2008; 133(suppl 6):S180–S182.

125. McGregor M, Sniderman A. On pulmonary vascular resistance: the need for more precise definition. Am J Cardiol 1985; 55:217–221.

126. Naeije R, Torbicki A. More on the noninvasive diagnosis of pulmonary hypertension: Doppler echocardiography revisited. Eur Respir J 1995; 8:1445–1449.

127. Chemla D, Castelain V, Herve P, et al. Haemodynamic evaluation of pulmonary hypertension. Eur Respir J 2002; 20:1314–1331.

128. McLaughlin VV, Shillington A, Rich S. Survival in primary pulmonary hypertension: the impact of epoprostenol therapy. Circulation 2002; 106:1477–1482.
129. Sitbon O, Humbert M, Jais X, et al. Long-term response to calcium channel blockers in idiopathic pulmonary arterial hypertension. Circulation 2005; 111:3105–3111.
130. Rich S, Kaufmann E, Levy PS. The effect of high doses of calcium-channel blockers on survival in primary pulmonary hypertension. N Engl J Med 1992; 327:76–81.
131. Ghofrani HA, Wilkins MW, Rich S. Uncertainties in the diagnosis and treatment of pulmonary arterial hypertension. Circulation 2008; 118:1195–1201.
132. Komadina KH, Schenk DA, LaVeau P, et al. Interobserver variability in the interpretation of pulmonary artery catheter pressure tracings. Chest 1991; 100:1647–1654.
133. Braunwald E, Ross J Jr. The ventricular end-diastolic pressure. Appraisal of its value in the recognition of ventricular failure in man. Am J Med 1963; 34:147–150.
134. Nootens M, Wolfkiel CJ, Chomka EV, et al. Understanding right and left ventricular systolic function and interactions at rest and with exercise in primary pulmonary hypertension. Am J Cardiol 1995; 75:374–377.
135. Reeves J, Groves, BM. Approach to patient with pulmonary hypertension. Mount Kisco, NY: Futura, 1984.
136. Hurrell DG, Nishimura RA, Higano ST, et al. Value of dynamic respiratory changes in left and right ventricular pressures for the diagnosis of constrictive pericarditis. Circulation 1996; 93:2007–2013.
137. Gorlin R, Gorlin SG. Hydraulic formula for calculation of the area of the stenotic mitral valve, other cardiac valves, and central circulatory shunts. I. Am Heart J 1951; 41:1–29.
138. Gorlin R, Haynes FW, Goodale WT, et al. Studies of the circulatory dynamics in mitral stenosis. II. Altered dynamics at rest. Am Heart J 1951; 41:30–45.
139. Gorlin R, Lewis BM, Haynes FW, et al. Factors regulating pulmonary capillary pressure in mitral stenosis. IV. Am Heart J 1951; 41:834–854.
140. Gorlin R, Sawyer CG, Haynes FW, et al. Effects of exercise on circulatory dynamics in mitral stenosis. III. Am Heart J 1951; 41:192–203.
141. Gamra H, Zhang HP, Allen JW, et al. Factors determining normalization of pulmonary vascular resistance following successful balloon mitral valvotomy. Am J Cardiol 1999; 83:392–395.
142. Reeves JT, Dempsey JA, Grover RF. Pulmonary circulation during exercise. New York: Marcel Dekker, 1989.
143. Groves BM, Reeves JT, Sutton JR, et al. Operation everest II: elevated high-altitude pulmonary resistance unresponsive to oxygen. J Appl Physiol 1987; 63:521–530.
144. Wagner PD, Gale GE, Moon RE, et al. Pulmonary gas exchange in humans exercising at sea level and simulated altitude. J Appl Physiol 1986; 61:260–270.
145. Fowler NO. The normal pulmonary arterial pressure-flow relationships during exercise. Am J Med 1969; 47:1–6.
146. Bevegard S, Holmgren A, Jonsson B. The effect of body position on the circulation at rest and during exercise, with special reference to the influence on the stroke volume. Acta Physiol Scand 1960; 49:279–298.
147. Brofman BL, Charms BL, Kohn PM, et al. Unilateral pulmonary artery occlusion in man; control studies. J Thorac Surg 1957; 34:206–227.
148. Provencher S, Herve P, Sitbon O, et al. Changes in exercise haemodynamics during treatment in pulmonary arterial hypertension. Eur Respir J 2008; 32:393–398.
149. Castelain V, Chemla D, Humbert M, et al. Pulmonary artery pressure-flow relations after prostacyclin in primary pulmonary hypertension. Am J Respir Crit Care Med 2002; 165:338–340.
150. Steen V, Chou M, Shanmugam V, et al. Exercise-induced pulmonary arterial hypertension in patients with systemic sclerosis. Chest 2008; 134:146–151.

151. Kessler R, Faller M, Weitzenblum E, et al. "Natural history" of pulmonary hypertension in a series of 131 patients with chronic obstructive lung disease. Am J Respir Crit Care Med 2001; 164:219–224.

152. Pietra GG, Edwards WD, Kay JM, et al. Histopathology of primary pulmonary hypertension. A qualitative and quantitative study of pulmonary blood vessels from 58 patients in the National Heart, Lung, and Blood Institute, Primary Pulmonary Hypertension Registry. Circulation 1989; 80:1198–1206.

153. Nicod P, Moser KM. Primary pulmonary hypertension. The risk and benefit of lung biopsy. Circulation 1989; 80:1486–1488.

10

Idiopathic, Familial, and Anorexigen-Associated Pulmonary Arterial Hypertension

JEROME LE PAVEC and MARC HUMBERT
Université Paris Sud 11, Service de Pneumologie et Réanimation Respiratoire, Hôpital Antoine Béclère, Assistance Publique Hôpitaux de Paris, Clamart, France

I. Introduction

Pulmonary arterial hypertension (PAH) is defined by right-heart catheterization (RHC) showing a mean pulmonary artery pressure >25 mmHg at rest and a normal pulmonary artery wedge pressure <15 mmHg (1,2). PAH is a disease of the small pulmonary arteries, characterized by vascular proliferation and remodeling resulting in a progressive increase in pulmonary vascular resistance and, ultimately, right ventricular failure and death (1–5). Multiple risk factors and associated conditions that trigger and/or worsen the progression of the disease have been recognized, including anorexigen exposure, connective tissue diseases, portal hypertension, human immunodeficiency virus (HIV) infection, and congenital heart diseases (5). A diagnosis of idiopathic PAH (IPAH) is made when no known risk factor is identified (5). When PAH occurs in a familial context, germline mutations in the bone morphogenetic protein receptor 2 (*BMPR2*) gene are detected in at least 70% of cases (6). Recent studies have shown that BMPR2 mutations can also be found in 10% to 40% of apparently sporadic or anorexigen-associated cases (6–10).

PAH in patients with idiopathic, familial, or anorexigen-associated disease has similar clinical, functional, and hemodynamic characteristics, and overall survival (6–11). These similarities contrast with PAH occurring in the setting of comorbidities, which influence patients' clinical characteristics and survival, such as connective tissue diseases (12–14), portal hypertension (15), HIV infection (16,17), and congenital heart diseases (5,13). For instance, survival of PAH in patients with systemic sclerosis is significantly worse than that of IPAH (12–14).

PAH is a severe condition for which the trend is for management in designated centers with multidisciplinary teams working in a shared-care approach (18,19). Information relative to the natural history of IPAH was mostly derived from a national registry conducted in the United States in the early 1980s (20,21). This study confirmed that primary pulmonary hypertension (corresponding to idiopathic and familial PAH in the recent classification) bears a very poor prognosis, with a median survival of 2.8 years after diagnosis (21). Significant medical advances have occurred in the last 20 years, which include a more systematic assessment of patients with objective parameters [such as six-minute walk test (6MWT) and acute vasodilator challenge] and availability of new treatments (such as prostacyclin derivatives, endothelin receptor antagonists, and phosphodiesterase type 5 inhibitors) (22,23). Prompted by the rapid evolution of knowledge in the field of PAH and the absence of large multicenter registry since the 1980s, several epidemiological studies have been initiated with the goal to describe the disease characteristics, risk factors, and outcomes in the modern management era (19,24,25). In the present chapter, we will discuss the current knowledge of IPAH, as well as closely linked variants such as familial PAH and anorexigen-associated PAH.

II. Epidemiology

IPAH is a rare disease, with an estimated incidence of two cases per million in industrialized countries (19,24,25). To overcome the limitations of sporadic reports, the National Institute of Health (NIH) established the prospective National Registry for the Characterization of Primary Pulmonary Hypertension (20). One hundred and eighty-seven patients from 32 centers were enrolled between 1981 and 1985 (20,21). The disease affected patients of all ages, both men and women, and all ethnic groups. The mean age of patients in the registry was 36.4 years, similar for men and women. Women were affected more frequently, with a female to male ratio of 1.7:1. Nine percent of patients were older than 60. Race and ethnicity were similar to those of the general population. Similar demographic trends have been reported in series from other countries (19,24,25).

In the French Registry, IPAH was the leading cause of PAH, representing 39.2% of the cases. Anorexigen-associated PAH represented 9.5% of the patients, and 3.9% were familial cases. Thus, half of the cases from the French Registry corresponded to idiopathic, familial, and anorexigen-associated PAH, and the remaining patients suffered from PAH associated with known comorbid conditions (19). As in prior studies, IPAH was seen more commonly in women, with a ratio to men of 1.6:1 (19). The mean age at IPAH diagnosis was 52 years, older than that in prior series (19,20) (Table 1). Eighty percent of IPAH presented with New York Heart Association (NYHA) functional class III or IV at diagnosis. Interestingly, familial PAH had a similar female predominance (female to male ratio of 2.2:1), while familial cases occurred earlier than IPAH (mean age at diagnosis was 37 years). Nearly 70% of familial PAH cases presented with NYHA functional class III or IV at diagnosis (Table 1). Anorexigen-associated PAH mostly occurred in females, with a female to male ratio of 14:9, a mean age of 57 years, and NYHA functional class III or IV in 81% of cases (19) (Table 1). On the basis of the 674 PAH cases in the French Registry, the low estimates of PAH prevalence and PAH yearly incidence in France in 2002 to 2003 were 15.0 cases per million adult inhabitants

Table 1 Clinical Data Obtained at Diagnosis for Each Subgroup of PAH

Subgroup of PAH	Males (%)	Females (%)	Age (yr)	New York Heart Association III–IV (%)	6-Min walk distance (m)
Idiopathic ($N = 259$)	37.9	62.1	52 ± 15	80.5	328 ± 112
Familial ($N = 26$)	30.8	69.2	37 ± 11	69.2	368 ± 103
Anorexigens ($N = 63$)	6.3	93.7	57 ± 11	78.1	289 ± 120

Data expressed as mean ± SD. *Abbreviation*: PAH, pulmonary arterial hypertension.

and 2.4 cases per million adult inhabitants, respectively (19). Half corresponded to idiopathic, familial, and anorexigen-associated PAH (19).

Since the 1960s, anorexigen-associated PAH has been a difficult and recurrent problem in pulmonary vascular medicine (10,24,26–29). In the late 1960s, an increased incidence of severe PAH cases was described in Austria, Germany, and Switzerland (26). More than 60% of newly diagnosed patients had a history of intake of the ano-rexigen aminorex fumarate. The fact that epidemic started two years after commercial availability of aminorex fumarate and disappeared two years after drug withdrawal allowed the recognition of temporal and geographic relationship between the use of the drug and PAH outbreak (26). Although this clearly indicated a role as a risk factor, the clinical course of aminorex-associated PAH was not conclusively different from that of the so-called primary pulmonary hypertension (26). In the early 1980s, the first descriptions of a possible relationship between the use of fenfluramine derivatives and PAH were published (27,28). Following this, the results of the International Primary Pulmonary Hypertension Study (24) definitely demonstrated a strong association between PAH and the use of anorexigens (mainly fenfluramine derivatives). The relation of fenfluramine derivatives use and PAH was further confirmed in a subsequent study (29). In a recent series, Souza et al. retrospectively studied the records of all patients with the diagnosis of fenfluramine-associated PAH evaluated at the French Reference Center for Pulmonary Hypertension from 1986 to 2004 (10). Median duration of exposure was of six months, with 4.5 years between fenfluramine exposure and beginning of symptoms. Median survival was of 6.4 years, without significant difference between anorexigen-associated PAH patients and a control group of idiopathic and familial PAH patients referred over the same time frame and treated identically. Duration of fenfluramine exposure presented no relation to survival, while cardiac index was the only independent predictor in multivariate analysis. This study confirmed that anorexigen-associated PAH shares clinical, functional, hemodynamic, and genetic fea-tures with IPAH, as well as the same overall survival. It was therefore concluded that fenfluramine exposure characterizes a potent trigger for PAH without influencing its clinical course.

III. Genetics

The first description of familial PAH in 1954 included a description of three related subjects displaying severe PAH with hemodynamic confirmation (30). Since the first report, a large number of familial cases have been described (19,20,31,32). Genealogies provided the first characteristics of familial PAH, which segregates as an autosomal dominant trait according to genetic anticipation phenomenon (31). Recognition of a genetic basis enabled chromosomal localization of the locus designated PPH1 on chro-mosome 2q33 using linkage analysis (33,34). At this location, in a familial context of PAH (2,12–14), germline mutations in the *BMPR2* gene have been detected in at least 70% of cases (35–39). In apparently sporadic IPAH cases and in anorexigen-associated PAH, BMPR2 mutations have also been identified in 11% to 40% of cases (8,35,40–42). However, the penetrance of BMPR2 mutations is about 20% (31,32), and neither the factors involved in the initiation of the disease in affected subjects nor the precise molecular mechanisms underlying the responsibility of BMPR2 haploinsufficiency in the disease are identified (11). Interestingly, Sztrymf et al. have shown that BMPR2 status may be associated with distinct disease phenotypes (6). Indeed, compared with non-carriers, BMPR2 mutation carriers present with a more severe hemodynamic compromise at diagnosis and approximately 10 years earlier, with fatal events occurring at earlier age (6). A better understanding of the mechanisms by which BMPR2 mutations define a subclass of patients with a more severe disease would be critical for improving our knowledge of PAH.

Several lines of evidence point to the potential requirement of additional factors, either environmental or genetic, in the pathogenesis of the disease. In addition, a proportion of so-called IPAH as well as anorexigen-associated PAH turn out to have an inherited basis, as demonstrated by detection of germline BMPR2 mutations (7,39,42). The distinction between idiopathic and familial BMPR2 mutation carriers may, in fact, be artificial as these subjects have an inherited condition and may all correspond to a potential familial disease. Recent expert discussion pleads in favor of the term "hereditable" PAH to describe these genetic forms of the disease. BMPR2 mutation represents the major identified genetic predisposing factor for idiopathic, familial, and anorexigen-associated PAH. In patients with fenfluramine-associated PAH, the duration of exposure to fenfluramine derivatives in patients with BMPR2 mutation was significantly shorter than that in patients without the mutation (10). This is in agreement with the "multiple-hit" concept, fenfluramine exposure being a trigger/risk factor in genetically predisposed individuals (10).

Analysis of other genes encoding transforming growth factor (TGF)-β receptor proteins led to the demonstration that PAH, in association with hereditary hemorrhagic telangiectasia, an autosomal dominant vascular dysplasia, can involve activin-like kinase type 1 (ALK-1) mutations (a gene encoding a type I TGF-β receptor) (43,44). The relevance of the TGF-β superfamily in the etiology of PAH is further emphasized by a report of endoglin germline mutation in a patient who had hereditary hemorrhagic telangiectasia and anorexigen-associated PAH (45). These observations support the hypothesis that mutations in the TGF-β superfamily may be a trigger for pulmonary vascular remodeling.

IV. Clinical Presentation

The symptoms of IPAH are nonspecific and include breathlessness, fatigue, weakness, angina, syncope, and abdominal distention (46). These nonspecific symptoms explain why many patients with severe IPAH are diagnosed late in the course of the disease, after months or years of symptoms (19). Symptoms at rest are reported only in very advanced cases. The physical signs of PAH include left parasternal lift, an accentuated pulmonary component of S_2, a pansystolic murmur of tricuspid regurgitation, and a diastolic murmur of pulmonary insufficiency. Jugular vein distension, hepatomegaly, peripheral edema, ascites, and cool extremities characterize patients in a more advanced state (46). Lung sounds are usually normal. Clinical examination may also provide clues as to the cause (or the absence of cause) of pulmonary hypertension. If digital clubbing is encountered in PAH, an alternative diagnosis such as congenital heart disease, liver cirrhosis, pulmonary veno-occlusive disease, or comorbid respiratory conditions disease should be sought.

V.   Diagnostic Methods

Since IPAH is a diagnosis of exclusion, the diagnostic process of PAH requires a series of investigations that are intended to establish the diagnosis, to clarify the clinical class of PAH and the type of PAH and to evaluate the functional and hemodynamic impairment (47).

A.   Electrocardiography

Electrocardiography may provide suggestive or supportive evidence of PAH by demonstrating right ventricular and atrial hypertrophy (47). Right ventricular hypertrophy on electrocardiogram is present in 87% and right axis deviation in 79% of patients with IPAH (20). The absence of these findings does not exclude the presence of PAH, nor does it exclude severe hemodynamic abnormalities. The electrocardiogram has inadequate sensitivity (55%) and specificity (70%) to be a screening tool for PAH.

B.   Chest X Ray

In 90% of IPAH patients, the chest X ray is abnormal at the time of diagnosis (20,47). Findings include central pulmonary arterial dilatation, which contrasts with "pruning" (loss) of the peripheral pulmonary vessels. Right atrial and ventricular enlargement may be seen in more advanced cases. Pleural effusion, more often right sided, may be observed in advanced cases, either isolated or in the context of significant right-heart failure with ascites. Overall, the degree of pulmonary hypertension in any given patient does not correlate with the extent of radiographic abnormalities.

C.   Pulmonary Function Tests

Patients with IPAH usually have decreased lung diffusion capacity for carbon monoxide (DLCO) (it is typically in the range of 40–80% predicted) and mild to moderate reduction of lung volumes (20, 47). Arterial oxygen tension (PaO_2) is normal or only slightly lower than normal, and arterial carbon dioxide tension ($PaCO_2$) is decreased as a result of alveolar hyperventilation.

D.   Echocardiography

Transthoracic echocardiography (TTE) is an excellent noninvasive screening test for the patient with suspected pulmonary hypertension (47–49). TTE estimates pulmonary artery systolic pressure and can provide additional information about the cause and consequences of pulmonary hypertension (see chap. 8).

Besides identification of pulmonary hypertension, TTE also allows a differential diagnosis of the possible causes of pulmonary hypertension. TTE can recognize valvular and myocardial diseases responsible for postcapillary pulmonary hypertension, as well as congenital heart diseases with systemic to pulmonary shunts, which may lead to PAH. The venous injection of agitated saline as contrast medium can help the identification of a patent foramen ovale or small sinus venosus–type atrial septal defects that can be overlooked on the standard TTE examination. Transesophageal echocardiography is rarely required.

Table 2 Hemodynamic Data Obtained by Right-Heart Catheterization at Diagnosis for Each Subtype of PAH.

Subgroup of PAH	RAP (mmHg)	mPAP (mmHg)	PAWP (mmHg)	CI (L/min/m^2)	S$_V$O$_2$ (%)	PVRI (mmHg/L/ min/m^2)	Acute vasodilator responders (%)
Idiopathic (N = 259)	9 ± 5	56 ± 14	8 ± 3	2.3 ± 0.7	61 ± 10	22.8 ± 10	10.3
Familial (N = 26)	7 ± 4	61 ± 12	8 ± 3	2.3 ± 0.7	63 ± 9	24.7 ± 8.5	0
Anorexigens (N = 63)	9 ± 5	56 ± 12	8 ± 4	2.5 ± 0.7	63 ± 9	20.0 ± 8.3	6.8

Data expressed as mean ± SD. *Abbreviations*: HIV, human immunodeficiency virus; mPAP, mean pulmonary arterial pressure; NYHA, New York Heart Association; PAWP, pulmonary arterial wedge pressure; PVRI, pulmonary vascular resistance index; RAP, right atrial pressure; S$_V$O$_2$, venous oxygen saturation; PAH, pulmonary arterial hypertension. *Source*: Adapted from Ref. 19.

E. Right-Heart Catheterization

RHC is mandatory to confirm the diagnosis of PAH, to assess the severity of the hemodynamic impairment, and to test the vasoreactivity of the pulmonary circulation (47,50,51) (Table 2). Adequate recording of pulmonary artery wedge pressure is required for the differential diagnosis of pulmonary hypertension due to left-heart disease. In rare cases, left-heart catheterization may be necessary for direct assessment of left ventricular end diastolic pressure (LVEDP). Some hemodynamic variables have important prognostic relevance, including elevated mean right atrial pressure and pulmonary vascular resistance, as well as reduced cardiac output and mixed venous oxygen saturation (21).

In PAH, acute vasoreactivity testing should be performed at the time of diagnosis to identify patients who may benefit from long-term therapy with calcium channel blockers (47,50–52). Acute vasodilator challenge should only be performed with short-acting, safe, and easy-to-administer drugs with no or limited systemic effects. Currently, the agent most used in acute testing is nitric oxide (51). On the basis of previous experience, intravenous epoprostenol or intravenous adenosine may also be used as an alternative (47,50–52). Because of the risk of potentially life-threatening complications, the use of calcium channel blockers (given orally or intravenously as acute test) should be discouraged (51). A positive acute response is defined as a reduction of mean PAP ≥ 10 mmHg to reach an absolute value of mean PAP ≤ 40 mmHg with an increase or unchanged cardiac output (22,52). Only about 10% of patients with IPAH or anorexigen-associated PAH and only a few with familial PAH will meet these criteria (6,19,52) (Table 2). Positive acute responders are most likely to show a sustained response to long-term treatment with high doses of calcium channel blockers and are the only patients who can safely be treated with this type of therapy (19,52).

F.   Exercise Capacity

For objective assessment of exercise capacity, the 6MWT and cardiopulmonary exercise testing are commonly used in patients with PAH. The 6MWT is technically simple, inexpensive, reproducible, and well standardized (53). Besides, distance walked, dyspnea on exertion (Borg scale), heart rate, and percutaneous oxygen saturation are recorded. Lack of standardization and insufficient expertise in performing cardiopulmonary exercise testing have led to a poor correlation between cardiopulmonary exercise testing and 6MWT in randomized controlled trials (54,55). The 6MWT remains the only accepted exercise end point for studies evaluating treatment effects in PAH for the Food and Drug Administration and the European Agency for the Evaluation of Medicinal Products.

G.   Ventilation/Perfusion Lung Scan

The ventilation/perfusion lung scan should be performed in patients with pulmonary hypertension to look for multiple segmental perfusion defects characteristic of chronic thromboembolic pulmonary hypertension (56). In IPAH the ventilation/perfusion lung scan may be normal or it may show mild to moderate peripheral unmatched and non-segmental perfusion defects (20).

H.   High-Resolution Computed Tomography of the Chest

High-resolution computed tomography of the chest provides detailed views of the lung parenchyma and facilitates the diagnosis of alternative forms of pulmonary hypertension (47). High-resolution computed tomography of the chest may be very helpful where there is a clinical suspicion of pulmonary veno-occlusive disease and/or pulmonary capillary hemangiomatosis (57). Helical computed tomography of the chest may be used as a complementary investigation for the diagnosis of surgically accessible chronic thromboembolic pulmonary hypertension (56).

I.   Pulmonary Angiography

Conventional pulmonary angiography is still mandatory in most centers for the workup of chronic thromboembolic pulmonary hypertension to select patients who are good candidates for pulmonary endarterectomy (56). Angiography can be performed safely by experienced staff in patients with severe pulmonary hypertension using modern contrast media and with selective injections (56). Pulmonary angiography may also be useful in the evaluation of pulmonary vasculitis, such as Takayasu's disease, and pulmonary arteriovenous malformations, such as hereditary hemorrhagic telangiectasia. Nevertheless, helical computed tomography often provides valuable information in such cases.

J.   Other Tests

Liver cirrhosis and/or portal hypertension can be reliably excluded by the use of abdominal ultrasound. When suspected, the diagnosis of portal hypertension is based on hemodynamic measurement of a hepatic venous pressure gradient of >5 mmHg or the presence of esophageal varices at endoscopy (15). Routine biochemistry, hematology, and thyroid function tests, as well as a number of other mandatory blood tests, including identification of antinuclear antibodies and HIV serology, are performed in all patients. Brain natriuretic peptide (BNP) is released from myocardium in response to wall stress. The level of BNP or N-terminus (NT) fragment pro-BNP strongly correlate with right-heart function and prognosis in IPAH, and this test is now commonly performed in PAH patients (58,59).

VI. Survival, Prognosis Factors, and Impact of Therapy

PAH therapies will be discussed in detail in other chapters. PAH basic treatment is based on lifestyle modification and nonspecific treatment (warfarin, diuretics, oxygen) (22). As discussed above, calcium channel blockers are vasodilators that have been shown to be of great efficacy in a very specific PAH subpopulation of acute-testing responders (22,53). Of note, acute vasodilator responders represent around 10% of IPAH or anorexigen-associated PAH, but acute vasodilator response is uncommon in case of familial/hereditable disease (6,10,22,53) (Table 2). For the vast majority of IPAH patients, targeted medical therapy will include one or a combination of the following agents: prostacyclin derivatives, endothelin receptor antagonists, and phosphodiesterase type 5 inhibitors (22). Nonpharmacological treatments include atrioseptostomy and surgical procedures such as lung transplantation, which can be valuable strategies in well-characterized patients. American and European therapeutic guidelines are now available and regularly updated (23,60,61). Despite these important advances, there is still no cure for PAH, and further improvements are needed to treat this dismal condition.

The prognosis of IPAH is very poor in the absence of effective treatment (21). The median survival is 2.8 years, with estimated survival rates of 68%, 48%, and 34% at one, three, and five years, respectively (21). Both clinical and hemodynamic assessments yield important prognostic information, which may guide clinical management. Predictors of outcome will be discussed in other chapters. Briefly, NYHA functional class, 6MWD, pulmonary hemodynamics, and biomarkers such as BNP, measured at baseline and after three-month therapy, are important predictors of outcome in IPAH (61–63). Recent data from the French Registry indicate that idiopathic, familial, and anorexigen-associated PAH remains a progressive fatal disease in the modern management era, with a 12-month survival of 89% versus an expected survival, based on the NIH registry, of 72% (19,20).

VII. Conclusion

IPAH is a rare disease with a mean survival from diagnosis of <3 years in the absence of treatment. Nevertheless, remarkable advances have been achieved in elucidating the pathogenesis and management of IPAH over the past decades, leading to the development of disease-targeted therapies for this condition. Despite these achievements, the response to therapy is often incomplete in many patients and survival remains unsatisfactory. Accordingly, novel therapeutic targets and strategies need to be developed for IPAH to improve survival.

References

1. Rubin LJ. Primary pulmonary hypertension. N Engl J Med 1997; 336:111–117.
2. Runo JR, Loyd JE. Primary pulmonary hypertension. Lancet 2003; 361:1533–1544.
3. Humbert M, Morrell NW, Archer SL, et al. Cellular and molecular pathobiology of pulmonary arterial hypertension. J Am Coll Cardiol 2004; 43:13S–24S.
4. Farber HW, Loscalzo J. Pulmonary arterial hypertension. N Engl J Med 2004; 351:1655–1665.
5. Simonneau G, Galie N, Rubin LJ, et al. Clinical classification of pulmonary hypertension. J Am Coll Cardiol 2004; 43:5S–12S.
6. Sztrymf B, Coulet F, Girerd B, et al. Clinical outcomes of pulmonary arterial hypertension in carriers of BMPR2 mutation. Am J Respir Crit Care Med 2008; 177:1377–1383.
7. Thomson JR, Machado RD, Pauciulo MW, et al. Sporadic primary pulmonary hypertension is associated with germline mutations of the gene encoding BMPR-II, a receptor member of the TGF-beta family. J Med Genet 2000; 37:741–745.
8. Humbert M, Deng Z, Simonneau G, et al. BMPR2 germline mutations in pulmonary hypertension associated with fenfluramine derivatives. Eur Respir J 2002; 20:518–523.
9. Simonneau G, Fartoukh M, Sitbon O, et al. Primary pulmonary hypertension associated with the use of fenfluramine derivatives. Chest 1998; 114:195S–199S.
10. Souza R, Humbert M, Sztrymf B, et al. Pulmonary arterial hypertension associated with fenfluramine exposure: report of 109 cases. Eur Respir J 2008; 31:343–348.
11. Sztrymf B, Yaïci A, Girerd B, et al. Genes and pulmonary arterial hypertension. Respiration 2007; 74:123–132.
12. Kawut SM, Taichman DB, Archer-Chicko CL, et al. Hemodynamics and survival in patients with pulmonary arterial hypertension related to systemic sclerosis. Chest 2003; 123:344–350.
13. Kuhn KP, Byrne DW, Arbogast PG, et al. Outcome in 91 consecutive patients with pulmonary arterial hypertension receiving epoprostenol. Am J Respir Crit Care Med 2003; 167:580–586.
14. Fisher MR, Mathai SC, Champion HC, et al. Clinical differences between idiopathic and scleroderma-related pulmonary hypertension. Arthritis Rheum 2006; 54:3043–3050.
15. Le Pavec J, Souza R, Herve P, et al. Portopulmonary hypertension: survival and prognostic factors. Am J Respir Crit Care Med 2008; 178:637–643.
16. Opravil M, Pechère M, Speich R, et al. HIV-associated primary pulmonary hypertension. A case control study. Swiss HIV Cohort Study. Am J Respir Crit Care Med 1997; 155:990–995.
17. Nunes H, Humbert M, Sitbon O, et al. Prognostic factors for survival in human immunodeficiency virus-associated pulmonary arterial hypertension. Am J Respir Crit Care Med 2003; 167:1433–1439.
18. Galie N, Rubin LJ. New insights into a challenging disease: a review of the third world symposium on pulmonary arterial hypertension. J Am Coll Cardiol 2004; 43:1S.
19. Humbert M, Sitbon O, Chaouat A, et al. Pulmonary arterial hypertension in France: results from a national registry. Am J Respir Crit Care Med 2006; 173:1023–1030.
20. Rich S, Danzker DR, Ayres SM, et al. Primary pulmonary hypertension: a national prospective study. Ann Intern Med 1987; 107:216–223.
21. D'Alonzo GE, Barst RJ, Ayres SM, et al. Survival in patients with primary pulmonary hypertension. Ann Intern Med 1991; 115:343–349.
22. Humbert M, Sitbon O, Simonneau G. Treatment of pulmonary arterial hypertension. N Engl J Med 2004; 351:1425–1436.
23. Badesch DB, Abman SH, Ahearn GS, et al. Medical therapy for pulmonary arterial hypertension: ACCP evidence-based clinical practice guidelines. Chest 2004; 35S–62S.
24. Abenhaim L, Moride Y, Brenot F, et al. Appetite-suppressant drugs and the risk of primary pulmonary hypertension. N Engl J Med 1996; 335:609–616.

25. Peacock A, Murphy NF, McMurray JJV, et al. An epidemiological study of pulmonary arterial hypertension in Scotland. Eur Respir J 2007; 30:104–109.

26. Gurtner HP. Aminorex and pulmonary hypertension. A review. Cor Vasa 1985; 27:160–171.

27. Douglas JG, Munro JF, Kitchin AH, et al. Pulmonary hypertension and fenfluramine. Br Med J 1981; 283:881–883.

28. Brenot F, Herve P, Petitpretz P, et al. Primary pulmonary hypertension and fenfluramine use. Br Heart J 1993; 70:537–5341.

29. Rich S, Rubin L, Walker AM, et al. Anorexigens and pulmonary hypertension in the United States: results from the surveillance of North American pulmonary hypertension. Chest 2000; 117:870–874.

30. Dresdale DT, Michtom RJ, Schultz M. Recent studies in primary pulmonary hypertension, including pharmacodynamic observations on pulmonary vascular resistance. Bull N Y Acad Med 1954; 30:195–207.

31. Loyd JE, Butler MG, Foroud TM, et al. Genetic anticipation and abnormal gender ratio at birth in familial primary pulmonary hypertension. Am J Respir Crit Care Med 1995; 152:93–97.

32. Loyd JE, Primm RK, Newman JH. Familial primary pulmonary hypertension: Clinical patterns. Am Rev Resp Dis 1984; 129:194–197.

33. Morse JH, Jones AC, Barst RJ, et al. Mapping of familial primary pulmonary hypertension locus (PPH1) to chromosome 2q31-q32. Circulation 1997; 95:2603–2606.

34. Nichols WC, Koller DL. Localization of the gene for familial primary pulmonary hypertension to chromosome 2q31-32. Nat Genet 1997; 15:277–280.

35. Aldred MA, Vijayakrishnan J, James V, et al. BMPR2 gene rearrangements account for a significant proportion of mutations in familial and idiopathic pulmonary arterial hypertension. Hum Mutat 2006; 27:212–213.

36. Cogan JD, Pauciulo MW, Batchman AP, et al. High frequency of BMPR2 exonic deletions/duplications in familial pulmonary arterial hypertension. Am J Respir Crit Care Med 2006; 174:590–598.

37. Deng Z, Morse JH, Slager SL, et al. Familial primary pulmonary hypertension (gene PPH1) is caused by mutations in the bone morphogenetic protein receptor-ii gene. Am J Hum Genet 2000; 67:737–744.

38. Lane KB, Machado RD, Pauciulo MW, et al. Heterozygous germline mutations in BMPR2, encoding a tgf-beta receptor, cause familial primary pulmonary hypertension. Nat Genet 2000; 26:81–84.

39. Newman JH, Wheeler L, Lane KB, et al. Mutation in the gene for bone morphogenetic protein receptor II as a cause of primary pulmonary hypertension in a large kindred. N Engl J Med 2001; 345:319–324.

40. Koehler R, Grunig E, Pauciulo MW, et al. Low frequency of BMPR2 mutations in a German cohort of patients with sporadic idiopathic pulmonary arterial hypertension. J Med Genet 2004; 41:e127.

41. Machado RD, Pauciulo MW, Thomson JR, et al. BMPR2 haploinsufficiency as the inherited molecular mechanism for primary pulmonary hypertension. Am J Hum Genet 2001; 68:92–102.

42. Morisaki H, Nakanishi N, Kyotani S, et al. BMPR2 mutations found in Japanese patients with familial and sporadic primary pulmonary hypertension. Hum Mutat 2004; 23:632.

43. Abdalla SA, Gallione CJ, Barst RJ, et al. Primary pulmonary hypertension in families with hereditary haemorrhagic telangiectasia. Eur Respir J 2004; 23:373–377.

44. Trembath RC, Thomson JR, Machado RD, et al. Clinical and molecular genetic features of pulmonary hypertension in patients with hereditary hemorrhagic telangiectasia. N Engl J Med 2001; 345:325–334.

45. Chaouat A, Coulet F, Favre C, et al. Endoglin germline mutation in a patient with hereditary haemorrhagic telangiectasia and dexfenfluramine associated pulmonary arterial hypertension. Thorax 2004; 59:446–448.

46. Gaine SP, Rubin LJ. Primary pulmonary hypertension. Lancet 1998; 352:719–725.
47. Barst RJ, McGoon M, Torbicki A, et al. Diagnosis and differential assessment of pulmonary arterial hypertension. J Am Coll Cardiol 2004; 43:40S–47S.
48. Hachulla E, Gressin V, Guillevin L, et al. Early detection of pulmonary arterial hypertension in systemic sclerosis: a French nationwide prospective multicenter study. Arthritis Rheum 2005; 52:3792–3800.
49. Sitbon O, Lascoux-Combe C, Delfraissy JF, et al. Prevalence of HIV-related pulmonary arterial hypertension in the current antiretroviral therapy era. Am J Respir Crit Care Med 2008; 177:108–113.
50. Rich S, Kaufmann E, Levy PS. The effect of high doses of calcium-channel blockers on survival in primary pulmonary hypertension. N Engl J Med 1992; 327:76–81.
51. Sitbon O, Humbert M, Jagot JL, et al. Inhaled nitric oxide as a screening agent for safely identifying responders to oral calcium-channel blockers in primary pulmonary hypertension. Eur Respir J 1998; 12:265–270.
52. Sitbon O, Humbert M, Jais X, et al. Long-term response to calcium channel blockers in idiopathic pulmonary arterial hypertension. Circulation 2005; 111:3105–3111.
53. ATS Committee on Proficiency Standards for Clinical Pulmonary Function Laboratories. ATS statement: guidelines for the six-minute walk test. Am J Respir Crit Care Med 2002; 166:111–117.
54. Barst RJ, Langleben D, Frost A, et al. Sitaxsentan therapy for pulmonary arterial hypertension. Am J Respir Crit Care Med 2004; 169:441–447.
55. Barst RJ, McGoon M, McLaughlin V, et al. Beraprost therapy for pulmonary arterial hypertension. J Am Coll Cardiol 2003; 41:2119–2125.
56. Dartevelle P, Fadel E, Mussot S, et al. Chronic thromboembolic pulmonary hypertension. Eur Respir J 2004; 23:637–648.
57. Montani D, Price LC, Dorfmüller P, et al. Pulmonary veno-occlusive disease. Eur Respir J 2009; 33:189–200.
58. Fijalkowska A, Kurzyna M, Torbicki A, et al. Serum N-terminal brain natriuretic peptide as a prognostic parameter in patients with pulmonary hypertension. Chest 2006; 129:1313–1321.
59. Nagaya N, Nishikimi T, Uematsu M, et al. Plasma brain natriuretic peptide as a prognostic indicator in patients with primary pulmonary hypertension. Circulation 2000; 102:865–870.
60. Badesch DB, Abman SH, Simonneau G, et al. Medical therapy for pulmonary arterial hypertension: updated ACCP evidence-based clinical practice guidelines. Chest 2007; 131:1917–1928.
61. Galie N, Torbicki A, Barst R, et al. Task force. Guidelines on diagnosis and treatment of pulmonary arterial hypertension. The task force on diagnosis and treatment of pulmonary arterial hypertension of the European Society of Cardiology. Eur Heart J 2004; 25:2243–2278.
62. Miyamoto S, Nagaya N, Satoh T, et al. Clinical correlates and prognostic significance of six-minute walk test in patients with primary pulmonary hypertension. Comparison with cardiopulmonary exercise testing. Am J Respir Crit Care Med 2000; 161:487–492.
63. Sitbon O, Humbert M, Nunes H, et al. Long-term intravenous epoprostenol infusion in primary pulmonary hypertension. Prognostic factors and survival. J Am Coll Cardiol 2002; 40:780–788.

11

Pulmonary Arterial Hypertension Complicating Connective Tissue Diseases

PAUL M. HASSOUN
Johns Hopkins University, Baltimore, Maryland, U.S.A.

I. Introduction

Pulmonary arterial hypertension (PAH), defined as a mean pulmonary arterial pressure of greater than 25 mmHg in the absence of elevation of the pulmonary capillary wedge pressure, is a cause of significant morbidity and mortality (1). PAH is characterized by increased pulmonary vascular resistance due to remodeling and occlusion of the small pulmonary arterioles. Left untreated it leads irremediably to right ventricular (RV) hypertrophy, pressure overload, and dilation resulting in death within two to three years (1). PAH that encompasses a heterogeneous group of clinical entities sharing similar pathological changes can be associated with various connective tissue diseases (CTDs) such as systemic sclerosis (SSc), systemic lupus erythematosus (SLE), rheumatoid arthritis (RA), and mixed CTD (MCTD).

Although the mechanisms involved in the pathogenesis of PAH are unknown, the association of PAH with autoimmune diseases (such as CTD) suggests an underlying inflammatory component in the pathogenesis of this syndrome. From a histological standpoint, the pulmonary vascular lesions in PAH complicating CTD are fairly indistinguishable from those present in idiopathic PAH (IPAH). Although serological and pathological features suggestive of inflammation are found in both IPAH and CTD-associated PAH such as SSc-PAH, it is likely that more pronounced inflammatory pathways in the latter may explain survival discrepancies between the two syndromes and a differential response to therapy (2,3). As such, SSc-PAH may be considered an ideal prototypic example to study inflammatory processes potentially operative in the pathogenesis of PAH. Other CTDs such as SLE, MCTD, and to a lesser extent RA, dermatomyositis, and Sjögren syndrome can also be complicated by PAH and will be discussed separately in this chapter.

II. PAH Associated with Systemic Sclerosis

SSc is a heterogeneous disorder characterized by dysfunction of the endothelium, dysregulation of fibroblasts resulting in excessive production of collagen, and abnormalities of the immune system (4). These processes lead to progressive fibrosis of the skin and internal organs resulting in organ failure and death. Although the etiology of SSc is unknown, genetic and environmental factors are thought to contribute to host susceptibility (5) in the context of autoimmune dysregulation. SSc, whether presenting in the limited or diffuse form, is a systemic disease with the potential for multiple organ system involvement including the gastrointestinal, cardiac, renal, and pulmonary systems (6). Pulmonary manifestations include PAH, interstitial fibrosis, and increased susceptibility to lung neoplasms.

Estimates of incidence and prevalence of SSc have varied widely by the period of observation, disease definition, and population studied (7). Although the incidence seemed to be increasing over the period from 1940 to 1970, the rate of occurrence has stabilized since the widespread use of a standard classification system (8). However, there continues to be a marked geographic variation in the occurrence of the disease, supporting a role for environmental factors in disease pathogenesis. Prevalence of SSc ranges from 30 to 70 cases per million in Europe and Japan (9,10) to approximately 240 cases per million in the United States (8). Incidence varies similarly by geographic area, with the highest rates found in the United States (~ 19 persons per million per year) (7).

Estimates of the prevalence of PAH in patients with SSc have varied widely based on the definition of pulmonary hypertension and the method of diagnosis. In patients with limited SSc (formerly called CREST syndrome for *C*alcinosis cutis, *R*aynaud phenomenon, *E*sophageal dysfunction, *S*clerodactyly, and *T*elangiectasias), the prevalence of elevated RV systolic pressure may be as high as 60% (11–14) when based on echocardiographic criteria. Using strict cardiac catheterization criteria for diagnosis, the prevalence of pulmonary hypertension is closer to 8% to 12% (15,16). However, it is likely that SSc-PAH remains underdiagnosed as suggested by the lower than predicted prevalence of the disease in the few registries available (17,18).

A. Evidence for Autoimmunity as a Central Component of Pulmonary Vascular Remodeling

Vascular changes occur at an early state in SSc (19), and include endothelial cell apoptosis (20) and activation with expression of cell adhesion molecules, inflammatory cell recruitment, procoagulant state (21), and intimal proliferation and adventitial fibrosis leading to vessel obliteration. Prognosis and outcome of patients with SSc depend on the extent and severity of the vascular lesions (22). Endothelial injury is reflected by increased levels of soluble vascular cell adhesion molecule 1 (sVCAM-1) (23), disturbances in angiogenesis as reflected by increased levels of circulating vascular endothelial growth factor (VEGF) (24,25), and presence of angiostatic factors (24,26). Increased VEGF, a glycoprotein with potent angiogenic and vascular permeability-enhancing properties, may be a consequence of increased angiogenesis or profound disturbances in signaling in SSc. Thus, the role of dysregulated angiogenesis in SSc-PAH, whether driven by the inflammatory process or other mechanisms, appears to be a predominant feature of the disease and should be the focus of future studies.

B. Autoantibodies in Scleroderma-Related PAH

Antifibrillarin antibodies (anti-U3 RNP) are frequently found in SSc-PAH patients (27), and the poorly characterized antiendothelial antibodies (aECA) correlate with digital infarcts (28). IgG antibodies directed against endothelial cells and obtained from patients with IPAH and SSc-PAH display distinct reactivity profiles against antigens from the micro- and macrovascular beds (29). Antibodies to fibrin-bound tissue plasminogen activator in CREST patients (30) and antitopoisomerase II-α antibodies, particularly in association with HLA-B35 antigen (31), have been reported in SSc-PAH. Nicolls et al. suggested that aECA, which can activate endothelial cells and induce the expression of adhesion molecules, as well as trigger apoptosis, can potentially play a role in the pathogenesis of APAH (32). In vitro, autoantibodies from patients with CTD (anti-U1-RNP and anti-dsDNA) can upregulate adhesion molecules (e.g., endothelial leukocyte adhesion molecule-1) and histocompatibility complex class II molecules in human pulmonary arterial endothelial cells (33), suggesting that such an inflammatory process could lead to proliferative and inflammatory pulmonary vasculopathy.

Fibroblasts are essential components of the pulmonary vascular wall remodeling in PAH and can be found in the remodeled neointimal layer in both SSc-PAH and IPAH. The detection of antifibroblast antibodies in the serum of SSc and IPAH patients (29,34) has significant pathogenic importance since these antibodies can activate fibroblasts and induce collagen synthesis, thus contributing potentially directly to the remodeling process. Antibodies from sera of patients with SSc can induce a proadhesive and proinflammatory response in normal fibroblasts (34). IgG antifibroblast antibodies are present in sera of patients with IPAH and SSc-PAH and have distinct reactivity profiles (35). Several fibroblast antigens recognized by serum IgG from IPAH and SSc-PAH patients that have been identified include proteins involved in regulation of cytoskeletal function, cell contraction, cell and oxidative stress, and other key cellular pathways (36). It is thought that these fibroblast autoantibodies mediate the release of cytokines and growth factors that in turn contribute to the pathogenesis of vascular remodeling in PAH (35).

Taken together, particularly in light of the positive response to immunosuppressive therapy for some patients with PAH associated with SLE and MCTD (37), these studies suggest that inflammation and autoimmunity could play a major role in the pathogenesis of PAH.

C.   Genetic Factors in SSc and Scleroderma-Related PAH

A genetic contribution to the development of PAH has been recognized in idiopathic and familial PAH. Polymorphisms involving the bone morphogenetic protein receptor 2 *BMPR2* are present in about 80% of familial IPAH and up to 20% of sporadic cases of IPAH (38). Additional candidate genes have been proposed to influence the pathogenesis of PAH (39). Polymorphisms of the activin receptor–like kinase 1 (*ALK1*) gene, which encodes the TGF-β receptor, have been reported in patients with hereditary hemorrhagic telangiectasia (HHT) and PAH (40).

Although case studies to date suffer from limited statistical power, an increasing number of candidate genes have been reported to be associated with SSc in different populations. However, despite these recent advances in genetics, little is known about genetic involvement in SSc-PAH. *BMPR2* mutations have not been identified in two small cohorts of SSc-PAH patients (41,42). Recently, an association between an endoglin gene (*ENG*) polymorphism and SSc-related PAH was identified. Wipff and colleagues demonstrated a significant lower frequency of the 6bINS allele in SSc-PAH patients compared with controls or patients with SSc but no PAH (43). Endoglin, a homodimeric membrane glycoprotein primarily present on human vascular endothelium,

Table 1 Risk Factors for Development of Pulmonary
Arterial Hypertension in Systemic Sclerosis

Risk factors	Reference
Limited systemic sclerosis	46
Late age of onset	44
Raynaud phenomenon	46
↓ $D_L CO$	45
$FVC/D_L CO < 1.6$	46
↑ NT-pro-BNP serum level	47,52
Antibodies (e.g., anti-U3 RNP)	27

is part of the TGF-β receptor complex. The functional significance of the *ENG* polymorphism in SSc patients remains to be determined.

D. Clinical Features

Risk factors for the development of PAH in SSc patients include late-onset disease (44),
an isolated reduction in diffusing capacity for carbon monoxide ($D_L CO$), a forced vital
capacity $(FVC)/D_L CO$ ratio of less than 1.6 (45,46), or a combined decreased $D_L CO/$
alveolar volume with elevation of serum N-terminal pro-brain natriuretic peptide (NT-
pro-BNP) levels (47) (Table 1). Typically, patients with SSc-PAH are predominantly
women, have limited SSc, are older and have seemingly less severe hemodynamic
impairment compared with IPAH patients (3). Like in IPAH, clinical symptoms are
nonspecific, including dyspnea, and functional limitation that may be more severe than
in IPAH not only due to older age but also frequent involvement of the musculoskeletal
system in these patients. SSc-PAH patients also tend to have other organ involvement
such as renal dysfunction and intrinsic heart disease. Indeed patients with SSc (even in
the absence of PAH) tend to have depressed RV function (48,49) and left ventricular
(LV) systolic as well as diastolic dysfunction (50). Like IPAH patients, SSc-PAH
patients have severe RV dysfunction at time of presentation but have more severely
depressed RV contractility compared to IPAH patients (51). In addition, SSc-PAH
patients tend to have more commonly LV diastolic dysfunction and a high prevalence of
pericardial effusion (34% compared with 13% for IPAH) (3). In both groups, pericardial
effusion portends a particularly poor prognosis (3). SSc-PAH patients also tend to have
more severe hormonal and metabolic dysfunction such as high levels of NT-pro-BNP
(52) and hyponatremia (53). Both NT-pro-BNP and hyponatremia have been shown at
baseline (52,53), and with serial changes [for NT-pro-BNP (52)] to correlate with survival in PAH.

E. Detection of the Disease

An algorithm for detection of PAH in patients with SSc may be helpful if based on a
combination of symptoms and screening echocardiography (Fig. 1). In a large French
study, patients with SSc with tricuspid regurgitation velocity (TRV) jet by transthoracic
echocardiography greater than 3 m/sec or between 2.5 and 3 m/sec if accompanied by
unexplained dyspnea were systematically referred for right-heart catheterization (15).

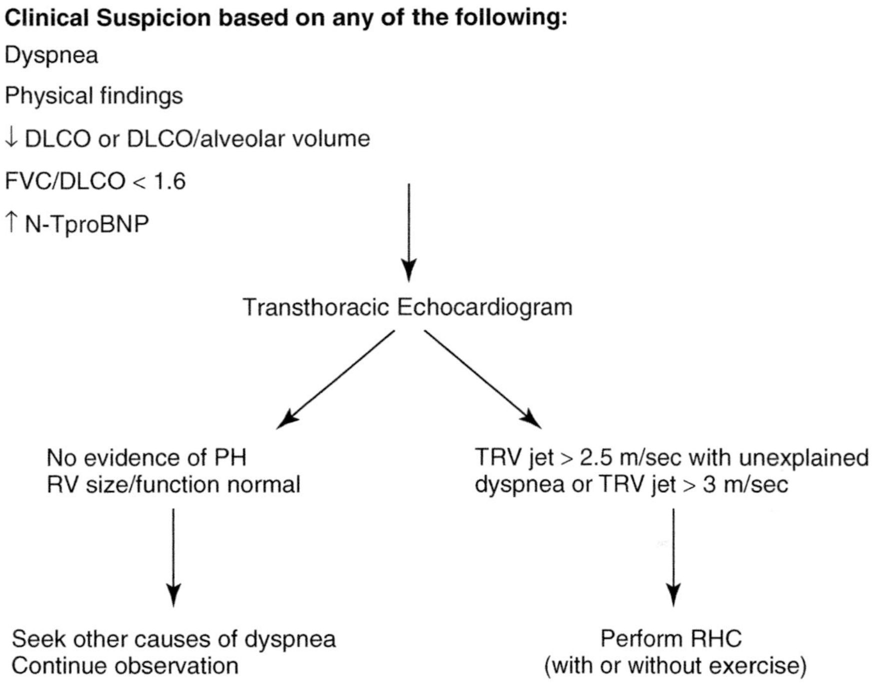

Clinical Suspicion based on any of the following:

Dyspnea

Physical findings

↓ DLCO or DLCO/alveolar volume

FVC/DLCO < 1.6

↑ N-TproBNP

Transthoracic Echocardiogram

No evidence of PH
RV size/function normal

TRV jet > 2.5 m/sec with unexplained
dyspnea or TRV jet > 3 m/sec

Seek other causes of dyspnea
Continue observation

Perform RHC
(with or without exercise)

Figure 1 Algorithm for detection of PAH in patients with systemic sclerosis. Proposed algorithm for performance of routine clinical tests in patients with systemic sclerosis that may allow early detection of pulmonary arterial hypertension or other causes of cardiac dysfunction (e.g., LV dysfunction). *Abbreviations*: PFTs, pulmonary function tests; $D_L CO$, single breath diffusing capacity to carbon momoxide; FVC, forced vital capacity; RV, right ventricle; TRV, tricuspid regurgitation jet; RHC, right-heart catheterization.

This approach allowed detection of incident cases of SSc-PAH with less severe disease (as judged by hemodynamic data) compared with patients with known disease. Therefore, unexplained dyspnea should prompt a search for PAH in these patients, in particular in the setting of a low single-breath $D_L CO$ or declining $D_L CO$ over time (46), echocardiographic findings suggestive of the disease (elevated TRV jet or dilated RV or atrium), or elevated levels of NT-pro-BNP, which can reflect cardiac dysfunction and have been found to predict the presence of SSc-PAH (52). Systematic screening should allow for detection of early disease and prompt therapy, which may theoretically be beneficial from a prognostic standpoint (54).

F. Prognosis

In general, patients with SSc-PAH tend to have a worse prognosis compared with patients with other forms of PAH such as IPAH. Indeed, one-year survival rates for SSc-PAH patients range from 50% to 81% (2,3,14,16), considerably lower than the estimated 88% one-year survival for IPAH patients (55). In all patients with SSc, PAH significantly worsens survival and is one of the leading causes of mortality in these patients (56).

III. PAH Associated with Other Connective Tissue Diseases

A. Systemic Lupus Erythematosus

There are many reasons for a pulmonary vascular involvement in SLE. Like in SSc, there is evidence of endothelial dysfunction in SLE with a potential consequent imbalance between vasodilators and vasoconstrictors. Endothelin levels are high in patients with SLE and particularly in those patients with pulmonary hypertension. Other causes of pulmonary vascular disease that may lead to pulmonary hypertension in SLE include recurrent thromboembolic disease, in particular in patients with a hypercoagulable state from antiphospholipid antibodies (such as anticardiolipin antibody present in up to 10% of patients with SLE) (57), pulmonary vasculitis, and parenchymal disease (including interstitial lung disease), and the shrinking lung syndrome from myositis of the diaphragm. Combined vasculitis and chronic hypoxia are frequent contributing offenders in these syndromes. In addition, pulmonary venous hypertension can be a consequence of LV dysfunction, myocarditis, or Libman Sachs endocarditis.

The prevalence of PAH is unclear but likely to be about 0.5% to 14% in patients with SLE in a large review of the literature (58). These patients are predominantly female (90%), young (average age of 33 at the time of diagnosis), and often suffer from Raynaud syndrome. The pathological lesions are often indistinguishable from IPAH or SSc-PAH lesions, with intimal hyperplasia, smooth muscle cell hypertrophy, and medial thickening. Survival, which was thought to be quite poor (25–50% at 2 years) even compared with SSc-PAH in studies antedating specific pulmonary hypertension treatment, is now estimated at 75% (18).

B. Mixed Connective Tissue Disease

Patients with MCTD have clinical features that overlap between those of SSc, SLE, RA, and polymyositis. The exact prevalence of PAH in MCTD is unknown and has been reported as high as 50% (59). PAH in these patients may occasionally respond to immunosuppressive drugs (37).

C. Rheumatoid Arthritis

Both the prevalence and impact of pulmonary hypertension in patients with RA is not well known. PAH is however a rather rare complication of RA.

D. Primary Sjögren Syndrome

Although primary Sjögren syndrome (pSS) is a relatively common autoimmune disease with glandular and extraglandular manifestations, it is very rarely complicated by PAH. In a recent review by Launay et al., the mean age at diagnosis of PAH of these almost exclusively female patients (27/28) with pSS and PAH was 50 years (60). Patients had severe functional class (FC III and IV) and hemodynamic impairment. Standard pulmonary hypertension therapy was ineffective, although some patients were reported to respond to immunosuppressive treatment. However, conclusion regarding treatment is limited by the small size of this case report. Survival rate was low (66% at 3 years).

IV. Therapy

Evidence of chronically impaired endothelial function (61), affecting vascular tone and remodeling, has been the basis for current therapy of PAH. Vasodilator therapy using high-dose calcium channel blockers is an effective long-term therapy, but only for a minority of patients (less than 7% of IPAH patients) who demonstrate acute vasodilation (e.g., to NO or adenosine) during hemodynamic testing (62), and an even smaller number of patients with PAH related to CTD who typically fail to show a vasodilator response to acute testing [only about 2.6% responders in one large study (63)]. Therefore, high-dose calcium channel therapy is usually not indicated for patients with PAH associated with CTD such as SSc-PAH, although most patients often receive these drugs at low dosage, typically for Raynaud syndrome.

A. Anti-inflammatory Drugs

As discussed earlier, inflammation may play a significant role in PAH, particularly CTD. Interestingly, some patients with severe PAH associated with some forms of CTD (such as SLE, primary Sjögren syndrome, and MCTD) have had dramatic improvement of their pulmonary vascular disease with corticosteroids and/or immunosuppressive therapy (37), emphasizing the relevance of inflammation in these subsets of patients. However, patients with SSc-PAH are usually refractory to these drugs (37).

B. Prostaglandins

In SSc-PAH, continuous intravenous epoprostenol marginally improves exercise capacity and hemodynamics (64), compared with conventional therapy, and there has been no demonstrable effect on survival.

Treprostinil, an analogue of epoprostenol suitable for continuous subcutaneous administration, has been shown to have modest effects on symptoms and hemodynamics in PAH (65). In a small study of 16 patients (among whom 6 had CTD-related PAH), recently FDA-approved intravenous treprostinil was shown to improve hemodynamics, six-minute walk distance (6MWD), functional class, and hemodynamics after 12 weeks of therapy (66). Although the safety profile of this drug is similar to IV epoprostenol, required maintenance doses are usually twice as much as for epoprostenol. However, for patients with SSc-PAH, the lack of requirement of ice packing and less frequent mixing of the drug offer significant advantages.

Several reports of pulmonary edema in SSc-PAH patients treated with prostaglandin derivatives, both in acute and chronic settings, have raised the suspicion of increased prevalence of veno-occlusive disease in these patients (67,68), and concern about usefulness of these drugs for this entity. Nevertheless, intravenous prostaglandin therapy remains a viable option for patients with SSc-PAH with NYHA functional class IV. Considering the frequent digital problems and disabilities that these patients often experience, this form of therapy can be quite challenging and may increase the already heavy burden of disease in these patients.

C. Endothelin Receptor Antagonists

Bosentan therapy improves functional class, six-minute walk distance, time to clinical worsening, and hemodynamics in PAH (69,70). In these studies, roughly one-fifth of the population consisted of SSc-PAH patients, while a large majority had a diagnosis of IPAH. A subgroup analysis, performed by Rubin et al., reported a nonsignificant trend toward a positive treatment effect on six-minute walk distance among the SSc-PAH patients treated with bosentan compared with placebo (70). At most, bosentan therapy prevented deterioration in these patients (as assessed by an increase of 3 m in the 6MWD in the treated group compared with a decrease of 40 m in the placebo group). This less than optimal effect of therapy in patients with SSc-PAH is unclear but may be related to the severity of PAH at time of presentation, as well as other factors such as, hypothetically, more severe RV and pulmonary vascular dysfunction, compared with patients with other forms of PAH (e.g., IPAH) (Fig. 2).

In a recent analysis of patients with associated PAH related to CTD (e.g., patients with SLE, overlap syndrome, and other rheumatological disorders) included in randomized clinical trials of bosentan, there was a trend toward improvement in 6MWD

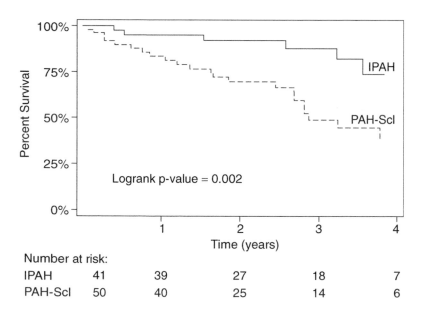

Figure 2 Survival differences between SSc-PAH and IPAH patients treated with modern therapy: a single center experience. One- and three-year survival rates are around 87% and 48%, respectively in patients with SSc-PAH and 95% and 83%, respectively in IPAH patients. SSc-PAH patients are three times more likely to die than IPAH patients despite similar treatment (endothelin receptor antoagonists, prostaglandins, or phosphodiesterase inhibitors). *Source*: From Ref. 3.

and improved survival compared with historical cohorts (71). Our experience suggests that long-term outcome of first-line bosentan monotherapy is inferior in SSc-PAH compared with IPAH patients, with no change in functional class and worse survival in the former group (72). Since ET-1 appears to play an important pathogenic role in the development of SSc-PAH, contributing to vascular damage and fibrosis, inhibiting ET-1 remains a rational and viable therapeutic strategy in these patients. In fact, in a small study of 35 patients with SSc (10 of whom had SSc-PAH), bosentan treatment appeared to reduce endothelial cell (as determined by endothelial soluble serum factors such as ICAM-1, VCAM-1, P-selection, and PECAM-1) and T cell subset (assessed by expression of lymphocyte function–associated antigen-1, very late antigen-4, and L-selectin on CD3 T cells) activation (73). Aside from improving pulmonary hypertension, ET-1 receptor antagonists (specifically bosentan) cause significant reductions in the occurrence of new digital ulcerations without, however, healing preexisting ulcers (74).

D. Phosphodiesterase Inhibitors

Sildenafil, a phosphodiesterase type 5 inhibitor that reduces the catabolism of cGMP, thereby enhancing the cellular effects mediated by nitric oxide, has become a widely used and highly efficacious therapy for PAH. A recent clinical trial showed that sildenafil therapy led to an improvement in the 6MWD in patients with IPAH and PAH related to CTD or repaired congenital heart disease (patients were predominantly FC II or III) at all three doses tested (20, 40, and 80 mg, given three times daily) (75). In a post hoc subgroup analysis of 84 patients with PAH related to CTD (45% of whom had SSc-PAH), sildenafil at a dose of 20 mg improved exercise capacity (6MWD), hemodynamic measures, and functional class after 12 weeks of therapy (76). However, for reasons that remain unclear (but in part related to the limitations of that study such as post hoc subgroup analysis), there was no effect for the dose of 80 mg three times a day on hemodynamics in this subgroup of patients with CTD-related PAH (76). For this reason and because of the potential of increased side effects (such as bleeding from arteriovenous malformations) at high doses, a sildenafil dosage of 20 mg three times a day is recommended for SSc-PAH patients (and perhaps patients with PAH associated with other forms of CTD) as standard therapy. The impact of long-term sildenafil therapy on survival in these patients remains to be determined.

E. Combination Therapy

It is now common practice to add drugs when patients fail to improve on monotherapy. Combining drugs with different targets is mechanistically appealing because of potential synergy. The Pulmonary Arterial Hypertension Combination Study of Epoprostenol and Sildenafil (PACES) trial demonstrates that adding sildenafil (at a dose of 80 mg three times a day) to intravenous epoprostenol improves exercise capacity, hemodynamic measurements, time to clinical worsening, and quality of life (77). About 21% of these patients had CTD, including 11% with SSc-PAH. Although no specific subgroup analysis is provided, improvement was apparently mainly in patients with IPAH. In a smaller one-center clinical trial, adding sildenafil to patients with IPAH or SSc-PAH after they failed initial monotherapy with bosentan demonstrates that combination therapy improved the 6MWD and FC in IPAH patients. The outcome in patients with

SSc-PAH was less favorable, and there were more side effects reported in the SSc-PAH compared with the IPAH patients, including hepatotoxicity that developed after addition of sildenafil to bosentan monotherapy (78).

F. Anticoagulation

Anticoagulation is generally recommended in the treatment of IPAH patients. However, the role of anticoagulation in other forms of PAH, in particular CTD, is much less clear. Theoretically, there is potential for increased bleeding in patients with CTD, particularly with SSc where intestinal telangiectasias may be common. In our experience, less than 50% of patients with CTD who are prescribed anticoagulation for PAH remain on therapy. The reason for discontinuing anticoagulation in these patients is often related to occult bleeding in the gastrointestinal tract, but the exact source of bleeding is often difficult to diagnose.

G. Tyrosine Kinase Inhibitors

The finding that there is pathologically aberrant proliferation of endothelial and smooth muscle cells in PAH, as well increased expression of secreted growth factors such as VEGF and bFGF, has caused a shift in paradigm in treatment strategies for this disease, as some investigators have likened this condition to a neoplastic process reminiscent of advanced solid tumors (79). As a result, antineoplastic drugs have been tested in experimental models (80) and some patients (81,82). Whether drugs with antityrosine kinase activity will have a role in PAH associated with CTD such as SSc-PAH (where there is evidence for both dysregulated proliferation and increased expression of growth factors such as VEGF) remains to be determined.

H. Lung Transplantation

Lung transplantation (LT) is typically offered as a last resort to patients with PAH who fail medical therapy. Although CTD is not an absolute contraindication to LT, patients with CTD often have associated morbidity and organ dysfunction other than the lung that place them at a specifically high risk for LT. The involvement of the esophagus with severe motility disorder and gastroesophageal reflux in patients with SSc can be problematic as it enhances postoperative potential of aspiration and damage to the recipient lung. However, if properly screened and approved for LT, patients with SSc experience similar rates of survival two years after the procedure compared with patients who receive LT for pulmonary fibrosis or IPAH (83).

V. Conclusion

Pulmonary hypertension is a common complication of CTD, particularly SSc where it has a significantly worse outcome compared with other diseases (such as IPAH) within group 1 of the WHO classification. In addition, modern therapy for PAH appears to be of limited value in SSc-PAH. Similarly, currently available markers of disease severity or response to therapy in SSc-PAH and other CTDs are either limited or lacking.

Therefore, there is an urgent need to identify potential genetic causes and novel physiological, molecular, and imaging biomarkers that will allow a better understanding of the underlying pathogenesis and serve as reliable tools to monitor therapy in this devastating syndrome.

References

1. D'Alonzo GE, Barst RJ, Ayres SM, et al. Survival in patients with primary pulmonary hypertension. Results from a national prospective registry. Ann Intern Med 1991; 115(5): 343–349.
2. Kawut SM, Taichman DB, Archer-Chicko CL, et al. Hemodynamics and survival in patients with pulmonary arterial hypertension related to systemic sclerosis. Chest 2003; 123(2): 344–350.
3. Fisher MR, Mathai SC, Champion HC, et al. Clinical differences between idiopathic and scleroderma-related pulmonary hypertension. Arthritis Rheum 2006; 54(9):3043–3050.
4. Jimenez SA, Derk CT. Following the molecular pathways toward an understanding of the pathogenesis of systemic sclerosis. Ann Intern Med 2004; 140(1):37–50.
5. Tan FK. Systemic sclerosis: the susceptible host (genetics and environment). Rheum Dis Clin North Am 2003; 29(2):211–237.
6. LeRoy EC, Black C, Fleischmajer R, et al. Scleroderma (systemic sclerosis): classification, subsets and pathogenesis. J Rheumatol 1988; 15(2):202–205.
7. Mayes MD, Lacey JV Jr., Beebe-Dimmer J, et al. Prevalence, incidence, survival, and disease characteristics of systemic sclerosis in a large US population. Arthritis Rheum 2003; 48(8):2246–2255.
8. Mayes MD. Scleroderma epidemiology. Rheum Dis Clin North Am 2003; 29(2):239–254.
9. Tamaki T, Mori S, Takehara K. Epidemiological study of patients with systemic sclerosis in Tokyo. Arch Dermatol Res 1991; 283(6):366–371.
10. Allcock RJ, Forrest I, Corris PA, et al. A study of the prevalence of systemic sclerosis in northeast England. Rheumatology (Oxford) 2004; 43(5):596–602.
11. Battle RW, Davitt MA, Cooper SM, et al. Prevalence of pulmonary hypertension in limited and diffuse scleroderma. Chest 1996; 110(6):1515–1519.
12. Stupi AM, Steen VD, Owens GR, et al. Pulmonary hypertension in the CREST syndrome variant of systemic sclerosis. Arthritis Rheum 1986; 29(4):515–524.
13. Sacks DG, Okano Y, Steen VD, et al. Isolated pulmonary hypertension in systemic sclerosis with diffuse cutaneous involvement: association with serum anti-U3RNP antibody. J Rheumatol 1996; 23(4):639–642.
14. MacGregor AJ, Canavan R, Knight C, et al. Pulmonary hypertension in systemic sclerosis: risk factors for progression and consequences for survival. Rheumatology (Oxford) 2001; 40(4): 453–459.
15. Hachulla E, Gressin V, Guillevin L, et al. Early detection of pulmonary arterial hypertension in systemic sclerosis: a French nationwide prospective multicenter study. Arthritis Rheum 2005; 52(12):3792–3800.
16. Mukerjee D, St George D, Coleiro B, et al. Prevalence and outcome in systemic sclerosis associated pulmonary arterial hypertension: application of a registry approach. Ann Rheum Dis 2003; 62(11):1088–1093.
17. Peacock AJ, Murphy NF, McMurray JJ, et al. An epidemiological study of pulmonary arterial hypertension. Eur Respir J 2007; 30(1):104–109.
18. Condliffe R, Kiely DG, Peacock AJ, et al. Connective tissue disease associated pulmonary arterial hypertension in the modern treatment era. Am J Respir Crit Care Med 2009; 179(2): 151–157.

19. LeRoy EC. Systemic sclerosis. A vascular perspective. Rheum Dis Clin North Am 1996; 22(4): 675–694.
20. Sgonc R, Gruschwitz MS, Boeck G, et al. Endothelial cell apoptosis in systemic sclerosis is induced by antibody-dependent cell-mediated cytotoxicity via CD95. Arthritis Rheum 2000; 43(11):2550–2562.
21. Cerinic MM, Valentini G, Sorano GG, et al. Blood coagulation, fibrinolysis, and markers of endothelial dysfunction in systemic sclerosis. Semin Arthritis Rheum 2003; 32(5):285–295.
22. Altman RD, Medsger TA Jr., Bloch DA, et al. Predictors of survival in systemic sclerosis (scleroderma). Arthritis Rheum 1991; 34(4):403–413.
23. Denton CP, Bickerstaff MC, Shiwen X, et al. Serial circulating adhesion molecule levels reflect disease severity in systemic sclerosis. Br J Rheumatol 1995; 34(11):1048–1054.
24. Distler O, Del Rosso A, Giacomelli R, et al. Angiogenic and angiostatic factors in systemic sclerosis: increased levels of vascular endothelial growth factor are a feature of the earliest disease stages and are associated with the absence of fingertip ulcers. Arthritis Res 2002; 4(6):R11.
25. Choi JJ, Min DJ, Cho ML, et al. Elevated vascular endothelial growth factor in systemic sclerosis. J Rheumatol 2003; 30(7):1529–1533.
26. Hebbar M, Peyrat JP, Hornez L, et al. Increased concentrations of the circulating angiogenesis inhibitor endostatin in patients with systemic sclerosis. Arthritis Rheum 2000; 43(4): 889–893.
27. Okano Y, Steen VD, Medsger TA Jr. Autoantibody to U3 nucleolar ribonucleoprotein (fibrillarin) in patients with systemic sclerosis. Arthritis Rheum 1992; 35(1):95–100.
28. Negi VS, Tripathy NK, Misra R, et al. Antiendothelial cell antibodies in scleroderma correlate with severe digital ischemia and pulmonary arterial hypertension. J Rheumatol 1998; 25(3):462–466.
29. Tamby MC, Chanseaud Y, Humbert M, et al. Anti-endothelial cell antibodies in idiopathic and systemic sclerosis associated pulmonary arterial hypertension. Thorax 2005; 60(9):765–772.
30. Fritzler MJ, Hart DA, Wilson D, et al. Antibodies to fibrin bound tissue type plasminogen activator in systemic sclerosis. J Rheumatol 1995; 22(9):1688–1693.
31. Grigolo B, Mazzetti I, Meliconi R, et al. Anti-topoisomerase II alpha autoantibodies in systemic sclerosis-association with pulmonary hypertension and HLA-B35. Clin Exp Immunol 2000; 121(3):539–543.
32. Nicolls MR, Taraseviciene-Stewart L, Rai PR, et al. Autoimmunity and pulmonary hypertension: a perspective. Eur Respir J 2005; 26(6):1110–1118.
33. Okawa-Takatsuji M, Aotsuka S, Fujinami M, et al. Up-regulation of intercellular adhesion molecule-1 (ICAM-1), endothelial leucocyte adhesion molecule-1 (ELAM-1) and class II MHC molecules on pulmonary artery endothelial cells by antibodies against U1-ribonucleoprotein. Clin Exp Immunol 1999; 116(1):174–180.
34. Chizzolini C, Raschi E, Rezzonico R, et al. Autoantibodies to fibroblasts induce a proadhesive and proinflammatory fibroblast phenotype in patients with systemic sclerosis. Arthritis Rheum 2002; 46(6):1602–1613.
35. Tamby MC, Humbert M, Guilpain P, et al. Antibodies to fibroblasts in idiopathic and scleroderma-associated pulmonary hypertension. Eur Respir J 2006; 28(4):799–807.
36. Terrier B, Tamby MC, Camoin L, et al. Identification of target antigens of antifibroblast antibodies in pulmonary arterial hypertension. Am J Respir Crit Care Med 2008; 177(10): 1128–1134.
37. Sanchez O, Sitbon O, Jais X, et al. Immunosuppressive therapy in connective tissue diseases-associated pulmonary arterial hypertension. Chest 2006; 130(1):182–189.
38. Austin ED, Loyd JE. Genetics and mediators in pulmonary arterial hypertension. Clin Chest Med 2007; 28(1):43–57, vii–viii.

39. Morse JH, Deng Z, Knowles JA. Genetic aspects of pulmonary arterial hypertension. Ann Med 2001; 33(9):596–603.
40. Trembath RC, Thomson JR, Machado RD, et al. Clinical and molecular genetic features of pulmonary hypertension in patients with hereditary hemorrhagic telangiectasia. N Engl J Med 2001; 345(5):325–334.
41. Morse J, Barst R, Horn E, et al. Pulmonary hypertension in scleroderma spectrum of disease: lack of bone morphogenetic protein receptor 2 mutations. J Rheumatol 2002; 29(11):2379–2381.
42. Tew MB, Arnett FC, Reveille JD, et al. Mutations of bone morphogenetic protein receptor type II are not found in patients with pulmonary hypertension and underlying connective tissue diseases. Arthritis Rheum 2002; 46(10):2829–2830.
43. Wipff J, Kahan A, Hachulla E, et al. Association between an endoglin gene polymorphism and systemic sclerosis-related pulmonary arterial hypertension. Rheumatology (Oxford) 2007; 46(4):622–625.
44. Schachna L, Wigley FM, Chang B, et al. Age and risk of pulmonary arterial hypertension in scleroderma. Chest 2003; 124(6):2098–2104.
45. Chang B, Schachna L, White B, et al. Natural history of mild-moderate pulmonary hypertension and the risk factors for severe pulmonary hypertension in scleroderma. J Rheumatol 2006; 33(2):269–274.
46. Steen V, Medsger TA Jr. Predictors of isolated pulmonary hypertension in patients with systemic sclerosis and limited cutaneous involvement. Arthritis Rheum 2003; 48(2):516–522.
47. Allanore Y, Borderie D, Avouac J, et al. High N-terminal pro-brain natriuretic peptide levels and low diffusing capacity for carbon monoxide as independent predictors of the occurrence of precapillary pulmonary arterial hypertension in patients with systemic sclerosis. Arthritis Rheum 2008; 58(1):284–291.
48. Hsiao SH, Lee CY, Chang SM, et al. Right heart function in scleroderma: insights from myocardial Doppler tissue imaging. J Am Soc Echocardiogr 2006; 19(5):507–514.
49. Lee CY, Chang SM, Hsiao SH, et al. Right heart function and scleroderma: insights from tricuspid annular plane systolic excursion. Echocardiography 2007; 24(2):118–125.
50. Meune C, Avouac J, Wahbi K, et al. Cardiac involvement in systemic sclerosis assessed by tissue-Doppler echocardiography during routine care: a controlled study of 100 consecutive patients. Arthritis Rheum 2008; 58(6):1803–1809.
51. Overbeek MJ, Lankhaar JW, Westerhof N, et al. Right ventricular contractility in systemic sclerosis-associated and idiopathic pulmonary arterial hypertension. Eur Respir J 2008; 31(6): 1160–1166.
52. Williams MH, Handler CE, Akram R, et al. Role of N-terminal brain natriuretic peptide (N-TproBNP) in scleroderma-associated pulmonary arterial hypertension. Eur Heart J 2006; 27(12):1485–1494.
53. Forfia PR, Mathai SC, Fisher MR, et al. Hyponatremia predicts right heart failure and poor survival in pulmonary arterial hypertension. Am J Respir Crit Care Med 2008; 177(12): 1364–1369.
54. Williams MH, Das C, Handler CE, et al. Systemic sclerosis associated pulmonary hypertension: improved survival in the current era. Heart 2006; 92(7):926–932.
55. McLaughlin VV, Shillington A, Rich S. Survival in primary pulmonary hypertension: the impact of epoprostenol therapy. Circulation 2002; 106(12):1477–1482.
56. Steen VD, Medsger TA. Changes in causes of death in systemic sclerosis, 1972–2002. Ann Rheum Dis 2007; 66(7):940–944.
57. Pope J. An update in pulmonary hypertension in systemic lupus erythematosus—do we need to know about it? Lupus 2008; 17(4):274–277.
58. Haas C. Pulmonary hypertension associated with systemic lupus erythematosus. Bull Acad Natl Med 2004; 188(6):985–997; discussion 97.

59. Sullivan WD, Hurst DJ, Harmon CE, et al. A prospective evaluation emphasizing pulmonary involvement in patients with mixed connective tissue disease. Medicine (Baltimore) 1984; 63(2): 92–107.
60. Launay D, Hachulla E, Hatron PY, et al. Pulmonary arterial hypertension: a rare complication of primary Sjogren syndrome: report of 9 new cases and review of the literature. Medicine (Baltimore) 2007; 86(5):299–315.
61. Budhiraja R, Tuder RM, Hassoun PM. Endothelial dysfunction in pulmonary hypertension. Circulation 2004; 109(2):159–165.
62. Sitbon O, Humbert M, Jais X, et al. Long-term response to calcium channel blockers in idiopathic pulmonary arterial hypertension. Circulation 2005; 111(23):3105–3111.
63. Humbert M, Sitbon O, Chaouat A, et al. Pulmonary arterial hypertension in France: results from a national registry. Am J Respir Crit Care Med 2006; 173(9):1023–1030.
64. Badesch DB, Tapson VF, McGoon MD, et al. Continuous intravenous epoprostenol for pulmonary hypertension due to the scleroderma spectrum of disease. A randomized, controlled trial. Ann Intern Med 2000; 132(6):425–434.
65. Simonneau G, Barst RJ, Galie N, et al. Continuous subcutaneous infusion of treprostinil, a prostacyclin analogue, in patients with pulmonary arterial hypertension: a double-blind, randomized, placebo-controlled trial. Am J Respir Crit Care Med 2002; 165(6):800–804.
66. Tapson VF, Gomberg-Maitland M, McLaughlin VV, et al. Safety and efficacy of IV treprostinil for pulmonary arterial hypertension: a prospective, multicenter, open-label, 12-week trial. Chest 2006; 129(3):683–688.
67. Farber HW, Graven KK, Kokolski G, et al. Pulmonary edema during acute infusion of epoprostenol in a patient with pulmonary hypertension and limited scleroderma. J Rheumatol 1999; 26(5):1195–1196.
68. Palmer SM, Robinson LJ, Wang A, et al. Massive pulmonary edema and death after prostacyclin infusion in a patient with pulmonary veno-occlusive disease. Chest 1998; 113(1): 237–240.
69. Channick RN, Simonneau G, Sitbon O, et al. Effects of the dual endothelin-receptor antagonist bosentan in patients with pulmonary hypertension: a randomised placebo-controlled study. Lancet 2001; 358(9288):1119–1123.
70. Rubin LJ, Badesch DB, Barst RJ, et al. Bosentan therapy for pulmonary arterial hypertension. N Engl J Med 2002; 346(12):896–903.
71. Denton CP, Humbert M, Rubin L, et al. Bosentan treatment for pulmonary arterial hypertension related to connective tissue disease: a subgroup analysis of the pivotal clinical trials and their open-label extensions. Ann Rheum Dis 2006; 65(10):1336–1340.
72. Mathai SC, Hummers LK, Champion HC, et al. Survival in pulmonary hypertension associated with the scleroderma spectrum of diseases: impact of interstitial lung disease. Arthritis Rheum 2009; 60(2):569–577.
73. Iannone F, Riccardi MT, Guiducci S, et al. Bosentan regulates the expression of adhesion molecules on circulating T cells and serum soluble adhesion molecules in systemic sclerosis-associated pulmonary arterial hypertension. Ann Rheum Dis 2008; 67(8):1121–1126.
74. Jain M, Varga J. Bosentan for the treatment of systemic sclerosis-associated pulmonary arterial hypertension, pulmonary fibrosis and digital ulcers. Expert Opin Pharmacother 2006; 7(11):1487–1501.
75. Galie N, Ghofrani HA, Torbicki A, et al. Sildenafil citrate therapy for pulmonary arterial hypertension. N Engl J Med 2005; 353(20):2148–2157.
76. Badesch DB, Hill NS, Burgess G, et al. Sildenafil for pulmonary arterial hypertension associated with connective tissue disease. J Rheumatol 2007; 34(12):2417–2422.
77. Simonneau G, Rubin LJ, Galie N, et al. Addition of sildenafil to long-term intravenous epoprostenol therapy in patients with pulmonary arterial hypertension: a randomized trial. Ann Intern Med 2008; 149(8):521–530.

78. Mathai SC, Girgis RE, Fisher MR, et al. Addition of sildenafil to bosentan monotherapy in pulmonary arterial hypertension. Eur Respir J 2007; 29(3):469–475.
79. Adnot S. Lessons learned from cancer may help in the treatment of pulmonary hypertension. J Clin Invest 2005; 115(6):1461–1463.
80. Schermuly RT, Dony E, Ghofrani HA, et al. Reversal of experimental pulmonary hypertension by PDGF inhibition. J Clin Invest 2005; 115(10):2811–2821.
81. Ghofrani HA, Seeger W, Grimminger F. Imatinib for the treatment of pulmonary arterial hypertension. N Engl J Med 2005; 353(13):1412–1413.
82. Patterson KC, Weissmann A, Ahmadi T, et al. Imatinib mesylate in the treatment of refractory idiopathic pulmonary arterial hypertension. Ann Intern Med 2006; 145(2): 152–153.
83. Schachna L, Medsger TA Jr., Dauber JH, et al. Lung transplantation in scleroderma compared with idiopathic pulmonary fibrosis and idiopathic pulmonary arterial hypertension. Arthritis Rheum 2006; 54(12):3954–3961.

12

Pulmonary Arterial Hypertension in Congenital Heart Disease

DANIEL S. LEVI
Mattel Children's Hospital at UCLA, Los Angeles, California, U.S.A.

VICTORIA SCOTT, and JAMIL ABOULHOSN
David Geffen School of Medicine at UCLA, Los Angeles, California, U.S.A.

I. Introduction

Increasingly effective surgical therapies for congenital heart disease (CHD) over the past four decades have caused a rapid increase in the number of adults who have some form of CHD (1). Many of the adult patients managed in congenital heart centers continue to have pulmonary hypertension caused by unrepaired systemic to pulmonary shunts. Pulmonary hypertension also continues to be a significant problem in pediatric patients with repaired, palliated, and unrepaired CHD. While CHD patients are predisposed to have high pulmonary vascular resistance because of excessive pulmonary blood flow and/or high left atrial pressures, patients with "single ventricle" CHD physiology require especially low pulmonary vascular resistance so that they can benefit from cavopulmonary shunts (the Glenn and Fontan operations).

This chapter reviews the relationship between pulmonary arterial hypertension (PAH) and various forms of CHD, as well as possible pathophysiological mechanisms driving the development of PAH in the context of CHD. The specific structural heart lesions that cause PAH are considered and both the diagnostic and treatment choices for patients with CHD-associated PAH are reviewed.

II. Epidemiology of Congenital Heart Disease

CHD encompasses a large number of defects that vary across a wide range of severities and can often go undiagnosed or even self-correct. Because many arterial ducts and some atrial and ventricular septal defects (VSDs) can close without intervention, the incidence and prevalence of CHD has been difficult to characterize. The most recent studies suggest incidence rates of 5 to 10/1000 live births for CHD (1–4). Despite a wide variance in quoted incidence rates, there is no evidence of global geographical differences. (1) While high altitude and genetic predispositions (such as Down syndrome) can contribute to the development of pulmonary hypertension, the incidence of pulmonary hypertension with CHD is most closely correlated with the ability of the health care system to recognize and treat large systemic to pulmonary shunts, such as atrial septal defects (ASDs), VSDs, and the patent ductus arteriosus (PDA). For

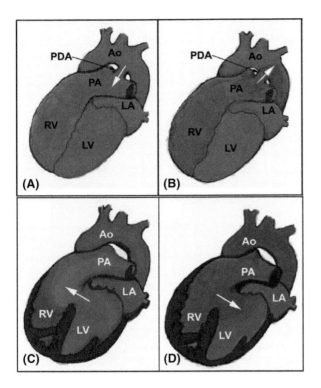

Figure 1 (*See color insert*) (**A**) PDA with left to right shunt (*white arrow*) of oxygenated blood from the Ao to the PA. The RV, LA, and LV are also labeled. (**B**) PDA with Eisenmenger syndrome. Pulmonary vascular resistance is now suprasystemic and the shunt has reversed, deoxygenated blood from the PA is shunted to the Ao via the PDA. Most of this deoxygenated blood flows to the lower extremities given the typical location of a PDA at the distal aortic arch, resulting in differential cyanosis where the upper extremity digits are typically not cyanotic while the lower extremity digits are cyanotic. (**C**) Nonrestrictive ventricular septal defect during infancy, prior to the development of elevated pulmonary vascular resistance. The shunt is left to right (*arrow*) with highly oxygenated pulmonary venous blood entering the LA, to the LV, and thereafter to the Ao as well as shunting to the PA. This leads to LA and LV volume overload and pulmonary edema. (**D**) Gradually over the first few years of life the pulmonary vascular resistance rises to approximate or exceed systemic vascular resistance and the VSD shunt reverses (*arrow*). Now, deoxygenated blood from the RV is shunted leftward to the LV and Ao, resulting in systemic cyanosis and the Eisenmenger complex. Note that the RV is now enlarged and severely hypertrophied. *Abbreviations*: PDA, patent ductus arteriosus; Ao, aorta; PA, pulmonary artery; LV, right ventricle; LA, left atrium; LV, left ventricle; VSD, ventricular septal defect; RV, right ventricle.

example, cases of children with large PDAs and pulmonary hypertension are not common in the United States, but have high incidence in high altitude towns in South America (5).

The prevalence of adolescents and adults with CHD has risen rapidly since the 1940s because of improved recognition, diagnosis, devices, drugs for treating pulmonary hypertension, and surgical techniques (6,7). Survival has also been affected by improved access to prenatal care in some parts of the world. For complex lesions, survival to one year improved from 20% during the 1940s and 1950s to 85% during the 1980s. For moderate lesions, one-year survival improved from 60% to 90% during the same period. The most recent U.S. estimates suggest prevalence figures of 100,000 to 150,000 adults with complex CHD, roughly 300,000 with moderate CHD, and 400,000 with persistent simple lesions (6,7).

PAH is a relatively uncommon syndrome that may arise idiopathically or as a complication of CHD, connective tissue disease (CTD), portal hypertension, HIV, or other medical conditions (8,9). While most PAH in the context of CHD is generally a consequence of congenital systemic to pulmonary shunts (left to right shunts) (9), the physiology of structural heart disease such as transposition of the great arteries with a large VSD can be much more complex with respect to its effects on the pulmonary vasculature.

The final common pathway of CHD-PAH is Eisenmenger syndrome, in which elevated pulmonary vascular resistance leads to the reversal of an intracardiac or systemic to pulmonary shunt (Fig. 1). Over the past decade, significant improvements have been achieved in the management of PAH, including new pharmacological agents and treatment targets. As the prevalence of idiopathic PAH (IPAH) is three- to fourfold greater than CHD-associated PAH, most clinical studies have involved a preponderance of patients with IPAH. While the prognosis for Eisenmenger syndrome patients has historically been extremely poor (8,10), early subgroup analyses from older studies with small numbers of patients suggest potential benefit of treating select Eisenmenger patients with pulmonary vasodilators and surgical intervention. To date, only one randomized, double-blind, clinical trial, BREATHE-5, has been conducted exclusively in patients with CHD—with the endothelin blocker bosentan (11). Results of this study will be discussed in detail later in this chapter.

III. Classification of CHD That Causes Pulmonary Hypertension

It is helpful to classify the types of CHD that cause pulmonary hypertension into several categories. Table 1 provides a summary of the following classification:

1. Heart lesions that produce left to right shunts and cause pulmonary hypertension by volume and pressure loading of the pulmonary vasculature. This category includes some of the most common types of CHDs including large ASDs, VSDs, atrioventricular canals (AV canals), the PDA, and aortopulmonary windows. The rate at which these defects cause pulmonary hypertension and the severity of PAH depends on the size of the shunt, the location of the shunt (i.e., atrial vs. ventricular vs. great arterial level), and the patient. For example,

Table 1 Classification of Congenital Heart Anomalies Associated with PAH

Left to right shunts
  Atrial septal defects
  Ventricular septal defects
  Atrioventricular canal
  Patent ductus arteriosis
  Aortopulmonary window
  Surgically placed aortopulmonary shunt
  Arteriovenous fistula
Left-sided obstruction
  Obstructed pulmonary venous return (often TAPVR)
  Cor triatriatum
  Mitral stenosis
  Pulmonary vein stenosis or hypoplasia
  Coarctation of the aorta
  Aortic stenosis
  Restrictive cardiomyopathy
Cyanotic congenital heart disease (with increased pulmonary blood flow)
  Truncus arteriosus
  Transposition of the great vessels
  Single ventricles with increased pulmonary blood flow
    Double outlet right ventricle (some variants)
    Tricuspid atresia with transposed great vessels
    Double inlet left ventricle (some variants)
Anomalies of the pulmonary arteries or veins
  Scimitar syndrome
  Tetralogy of Fallot with pulmonary atresia with MAPCAs
  Absence of a pulmonary artery
  TAPVR
  Hemitruncus

Abbreviations: TAPVR, total anomalous venous return; MAPCA, major aortopulmonary collateral artery.

patients with Down syndrome, patients who live at high altitude, and patients with other forms of chronic lung disease have a known predisposition for developing PAH in the setting of large left to right shunts. While small ASDs and even small VSDs rarely cause PAH, even if left unrepaired for many years, a large VSD or PDA results in PAH from birth. Conversely, patients with large ASDs can go many decades without congestive heart failure or severe PAH (less than 20% of ASD patients have PAH by the third decade of life) (12–14). The combination of high flow and high pressure as found in the AV canal can produce an especially rapid onset of PAH. Importantly, surgical aortopulmonary shunts such as the Blalock-Taussig, Waterson, or Potts shunt can also mediate an excessive left to right shunt and lead to elevation in pulmonary vascular resistance. This is most common with the Potts and Waterston anastomoses and has led to direct anastomoses between the aorta and pulmonary artery (essentially a surgically created aortopulmonary window) falling out of favor. Figure 1 graphically represents the progression of a PDA and VSD to Eisenmenger's physiology.

2. Any congenital heart lesion that causes left-sided inflow obstruction will cause PAH not only by increasing pulmonary venous pressures but also by causing a reactive increase in pulmonary vascular resistance. Types of CHDs in this category include pulmonary vein stenosis, total anomalous venous return (TAPVR), Shone's complex, cor triatriatum, mitral stenosis (valvar or supravalvar), and even aortic stenosis and coarctations, which are severe enough to increase the left ventricular end-diastolic pressure (LVEDP). Although they are not usually considered congenital heart lesions, restrictive cardiomyopathies fall in this category. In the rare setting of left ventricular (LV) dysfunction and PAH in a newborn, it is especially important to determine the contribution of elevation of LVEDP to PAH. Many of these infants can become candidates for heart transplant if their heart is decompressed, as with an assist device [left ventricular assist device (LVAD) or extracorporeal membrane oxygenator (ECMO)]. Patients with hypoplastic left-heart syndrome and an intact or highly restrictive ASD also fall into this category; however, these patients require immediate intervention, which quickly changes their physiology.

3. A subset of cyanotic heart lesions can also cause PAH. These forms of CHD include lesions in which patients are cyanotic in the setting of high pulmonary blood flow. These include truncus arteriosus, transposition of the great vessels, and some forms of double outlet right ventricle and tricuspid atresia (i.e., the Taussig-Bing malformation) but not lesions such as Tetralogy of Fallot (TOF) in which there is an obstruction to pulmonary blood flow which "protects" the pulmonary arteries from overcirculation (with the notable exception of TOF with pulmonary atresia and multiple unobstructed arteriopulmonary collaterals, described later). All patients with single ventricle physiology and high pulmonary flow fall into this category. Patients with truncus arteriosus and transposition of the great arteries with nonrestrictive VSD typically have systemic levels of pulmonary hypertension from birth and rapidly develop suprasystemic pulmonary vascular resistance of uncorrected early in infancy. The circulation of highly oxygenated blood in the setting of very high pulmonary blood flow and often high pressures is an especially profound stimulus for PAH (15).

4. The final group of patients with structural heart disease predisposed to PAH are patients in whom there are congenital anomalies of the pulmonary arteries or veins. Many of the lesions in this group such as TAPVR (which can cause an obstruction to left-sided inflow) or a single pulmonary artery arising from the aorta (which clearly mediates a left to right shunt and is often classified as a hemitruncus) could easily be also classified in one of the above groups. However, we believe that it is important for this category to stand alone as a reminder to clinicians of the consequences of pulmonary arterial and vein anomalies. Perhaps the best-known example of this physiology is Scimitar syndrome in which there is partial anomalous venous drainage of the right lung to the inferior vena cava, hypoplasia of the right pulmonary artery, and a lung sequestration that often receives its arterial supply from the descending aorta. Unilateral absence of a pulmonary artery can in and of itself cause PAH in the contralateral lung from a relative increase in flow to this lung—absence of one pulmonary artery by definition doubles the flow to the other lung.

Finally, patients with TOF and complete pulmonary atresia often form large aortopulmonary collaterals that supply pulmonary blood flow. If free of stenoses and left untreated, the lung segments supplied by this collateral flow are hypertensive and develop elevated pulmonary vascular resistance.

IV. Pathophysiology of CHD-Associated PAH

Despite the range of congenital defects that can lead to PAH, they appear to share common pathophysiological mechanisms linking increased blood flow, pressure, and shear stress to endothelial cell damage and dysfunction. There is both activation and shifts in the signaling and response pathways that favor vasoconstriction and inhibit vasodilation (16–18). Although it is clear that PAH involves multiple biochemical pathways and cell types, the precise processes that initiate the pathological changes in PAH are still unknown.

The simplistic view of PAH associated with CHD simply links high pressure and high flow to endothelial dysfunction and a resultant chronic deficiency of vasodilators with antiproliferative and antimigratory properties such as nitric oxide (NO) and prostacyclin. Overexpression of vasoconstrictors such as thromboxane A_2 (TxA_2) and endothelin-1 (ET-1) is known to play a large role in pulmonary hypertension associated with CHD and is the basis for treatment of these patients with bosentan (9).

Endothelial dysfunction leads initially to an elevation of vascular tone and eventually triggers vascular remodeling. Abnormal flow promotes production of elastases, which release biologically active mitogens such as basic fibroblast growth factor (bFGF) and transforming growth factor β (TGF-β) (19). An increase in the glycoproteins tenascin and fibronectin is also observed, amplifying the proliferative responses and smooth muscle cell migration and contributing to hypertrophy of the media of the arterial wall (20).

Recently it has been shown that circulating endothelial progenitor cells (EPCs) are reduced in Eisenmenger syndrome (21). EPCs from bone marrow are significant for postnatal vasculogenesis and vascular homeostasis. Studies on monocrotaline-treated rats showed a reversal of PAH after bolus administration of EPCs, suggesting that bone marrow–derived EPCs can integrate into the pulmonary vasculature (22). It has been hypothesized that a deficiency of such an endogenous repair mechanism could predispose to Eisenmenger syndrome in the presence of a left to right shunt from CHD by impairing maintenance of endothelial function (21).

All layers of the vessel wall are involved in subsequent pulmonary vascular remodeling. This remodeling is characterized by proliferative and obstructive changes that involve several cell types, including endothelial cells, smooth muscle cells, and fibroblasts (8). The first change observed in vessel walls in PAH is extension of muscle into the peripheral nonmuscular arteries. Medial hypertrophy can be found in normally muscular arteries as a result of hypertrophy and hyperplasia of existing smooth muscle cells. Additionally, there is also an increase in extracellular matrix. Increases in the growth factors bFGF and TGF-β induce differentiation of precursor cells to mature smooth muscle cells in normally small nonmuscular peripheral arteries and the hypertrophy and proliferation of smooth muscle in muscular arteries (20). Impaired growth and loss of arterioles causes a loss of arterial density over time. Ultimately, dilation complexes with plexiform lesions and fibroid necrosis form. Blood flow changes from laminar to turbulent as the PAH progresses (18). While inflammatory cells, platelets, and prothrombotic abnormalities have also been shown to have important roles in IPAH, there is no evidence for their significance in CHD-associated PAH (23).

Clinically, there is a large variation in the rate at which patients develop pulmonary hypertension. For example, given two patients with a similar sized ASD and shunt or Q_p:Q_s (ratio of systemic flow to pulmonary flow), one patient may live her entire life without pulmonary hypertension while the other progresses to Eisenmenger syndrome. Although a single mechanism for this difference has not been definitely identified, there is clearly more to pulmonary hypertension than simply increased pulmonary flow, pressure, or left atrial hypertension.

V. Pathophysiology: Persistent Pulmonary Hypertension of the Newborn

The establishment of a normal postnatal cardiopulmonary circulation depends on a series of relatively rapid changes at birth that remodel the pulmonary arteries and arterioles into thin-walled vessels characteristic of the low-pressure pulmonary circulation (24). Failure of these adaptive pathways leads to the pathological condition called persistent pulmonary hypertension of the newborn (PPHN). Although the use of NO has made a significant improvement in the outcomes of newborns with PPHN, this condition continues to be associated with high morbidity and mortality. Although PPHN is not a form of pulmonary hypertension caused by CHD, it is a form of PAH managed by neonatologists and pediatric cardiologists and pulmonologists.

Although most often associated with congenital and acquired hypoxic lung disease and congenital heart defects, PPHN can be related to other causes or can be idiopathic (23). Regardless of its origin, PPHN results from a disruption of the rapid reduction in pulmonary arterial wall thickness that occurs immediately after birth in the normal lung. An increase in medial thickness will eventually cause the onset of pulmonary vascular obstructive disease (PVOD) if the pressure remains elevated. The normal process of remodeling allows cells to elongate and thin as they extend around an enlarging lumen. This process occurs through transient disassembly of the actin cytoskeleton of smooth muscle cells.

In addition to the structural abnormality, PPHN also appears to occur as a result of failure of endothelial dependent and independent relaxation (there is an excess of vasoconstrictor activity) (19). A disturbance of the NO pathway, occasionally a deficiency of L-arginine, increased concentrations of endogenous inhibitor asymmetric dimethylarginine, and high levels of endothelin concentrations have been shown to contribute to PPHN (23). In patients with PPHN, the low nitric oxide synthetase (NOS) activity and poor endothelial dependent relaxation normally overcome at birth remain intact. ET_A receptors (with vasoconstrictor properties) increase while endothelial vasodilation receptor ET_B decreases. (It should be noted that diaphragmatic hernias are also a very large cause of PAH in children. However, as this entity is clearly distinct from CHD, it is considered to be beyond the scope of this chapter.)

Many pathways exist to mediate pulmonary vascular relaxation (prostaglandin, endothelium-derived hyperpolarizing factor, NO), and all of these pathways mature at different rates and times and are susceptible to insult. Multiple signaling pathways have been implicated in the processes of endothelial dysfunction and vascular remodeling. These include impaired NO synthesis and response, increased serum elastases, increased vascular endothelial growth factor (VEGF), elevated serotonin, elevated thromboxane, reduced prostacyclin, and alterations in pathways mediated by TGF-β (16–18,25).

Endothelin-1 (ET-1) appears to be a central component in several of the pathways thought to mediate PPHN (17,25). Beyond its well-characterized, potent activity as a vasoconstrictor, ET-1 may also mediate several other pathways leading to structural and functional derangements in CHD-associated PAH. These including inflammation, cardiac and vascular hypertrophy, proliferation of smooth muscle and fibroblasts, and fibrosis (17). ET-1 levels are elevated in both IPAH and CHD-associated PAH (26). Animal studies using a sheep model of CHD (with an artificial shunt) demonstrate increased ET-1 levels, which may be the result of increased expression of endothelin-converting enzyme (ECE), and temporal and spatial shifts in expression of ET_A and ET_B receptor subtypes. Both of these findings appear to be important in the development of early CHD-associated vasoconstriction and vascular remodeling (17,27–29). ET-1 also appears to be a critical component of acute postsurgical vascular damage (in the coronary, pulmonary, and systemic circulation) associated with ischemia-reperfusion injury following CHD repair (17,30–32).

VI. Diagnosis and Assessment of Pulmonary Hypertension in CHD

The assessment of pulmonary hypertension in the setting of CHD requires an anatomic assessment of the structural heart disease, an understanding of the intracardiac shunting and pulmonary blood flow, and an accurate assessment of the pulmonary vascular resistance and reactivity. The assessement of resistance in the pulmonary vasculature is very complex and often cannot be done using conventional methods such as right-heart catheterization because of intracardiac shunting.

In many patients with PAH and CHD, the PAH develops because of a delay in diagnosis or management of CHD. Upon diagnosis of any patient with a left to right shunt, with cyanotic heart disease, or with left-sided obstructive lesions, arterial pressure and resistance must be evaluated before surgical or transcatheter interventions are performed. Transthoracic echocardiography with Doppler is a very useful, cost-effective, and nearly universal method to evaluate patients with CHD for presence of PAH. In patients in whom there is an increased suspicion of PAH by history, physical examination, X ray, or echocardiography (i.e., a Down syndrome patient with the delayed diagnosis of a large VSD), it is absolutely necessary to assess both the degree of pulmonary vascular resistance elevation and reactivity of the pulmonary vascular bed before considering any interventions aimed at eliminating a shunt.

The physical cardiovascular examination is often revealing and should be approached in a methodical manner. Physical examination signs suggestive of pulmonary hypertension include the following:

- Accentuated jugular venous A wave
- Right ventricular (RV) S4 gallop
- Loud pulmonic closure sound
- Absence of or minimal inspiratory splitting of the second heart sound
- RV heave (parasternal and subxiphoid)
- High-pitched early diastolic murmur of high-pressure pulmonary regurgitation

The Graham Steell murmur of pulmonary regurgitation is best heard at the left upper, mid, and lower sternal borders in patients with normal cardiac situs and great arterial anatomy. Careful examination of the upper and lower extremities should be performed to rule out differential cyanosis (blue toes, pink fingers) in patients with PDA and suprasystemic pulmonary vascular resistance with right to left shunting of deoxygenated blood via the ductus to the lower extremities.

The chest X ray (CXR) and electrocardiogram (ECG) provide additional information on the type of CHD, the degree of shunting, and the degree of pulmonary hypertension. As in non-CHD patients, the CXR of patients with CHD will show the typical pulmonary changes of large main and branch pulmonary arteries that taper (or "prune") quickly. The peripheral lung fields are dark from the paucity of distal pulmonary vessels and there is often RV enlargement. In contrast, patients with increased left to right shunts (increased pulmonary blood flow) may have elevated pulmonary artery pressure, but subsystemic pulmonary vascular resistance and a CXR with a dilated main and branch pulmonary arteries but with absence of peripheral pruning and increased pulmonary vascular markings.

Because the presence of CHD can complicate the evaluation of a CXR for PAH, the approach to the CXR should be systematic without any assumptions, given the heterogeneity of CHD subtypes. Available clinical texts and electronic media should be used as references (33). While patients with pulmonary stenosis have very large PAs but almost never have PAH, other patients such as those with truncus arteriosus or TOF with pulmonary atresia may have no main PA. Patients with congenitally corrected transposition have ventricular inversion with the pulmonary artery arising posteriorly from the dextraposed left ventricle with subsequent absence of the main pulmonary artery "mogul" usually seen in a patient with normal anatomy of frontal CXR. Patients with single ventricle physiology can have very minor findings of increased PVR that can have a devastating effect on a cavopulmonary (Glenn or Fontan) repair.

With advances in imaging techniques such as ECHO, CT, and MRI, the ECG has diminished in importance as a diagnostic tool for structural heart disease. It can, however, give many important clues as to the presence and degree of pulmonary hypertension and CHD. With or without CHD, PAH patients manifest signs of right atrial enlargement (RAE), signs of RV hypertrophy, right axis deviation, and even RV conduction delay. While the ECG has a high sensitivity for the detection of PAH, it is not specific. This is especially true for patients with CHD who have RV hypertrophy, RAE, and a rightward axis from structural heart diseases such has valvar pulmonary stenosis, double-chambered RV, and supravalvar or branch pulmonary artery stenosis.

ECG signs of RV strain are always important indicators that the right ventricle is beginning to fail.

Because ECHO can both define most types of intracardiac CHD and assess the degree of PAH and RV function, it is in the current era, arguably the most important diagnostic tool in the setting of PAH in CHD. ECHO is a cost-effective, time efficient, and nearly universally available diagnostic test for the wide variety of CHD types that cause PAH: ASDs, VSDs, AV canals, PDAs, cyanotic CHD, and all left-sided obstructive lesions. ECHO can be used to assess both LV and RV systolic functions and to provide clues to the presence of restrictive cardiomyopathy and diastolic dysfunction. Because elevation of left atrial pressure from diastolic dysfunction causes a functional obstruction to left-heart filling, it can cause PAH. It is imperative to distinguish intrinsic pulmonary hypertension from pulmonary hypertension caused by left atrial hypertension, specifically because the pulmonary vasodilator therapies that are so effective in treating intrinsic pulmonary hypertension may worsen symptoms in those with left atrial hypertension as the cause of PH. Atrial enlargement and abnormal mitral valve (MV) in flow signals on ECHO must be examined carefully in all patients with PAH.

Figure 2 represents three different techniques that can be used to quantitatively and qualitatively assess PAH by ECHO in a patient with CHD. Bernoulli's equation allows us to estimate pressure gradients from velocities of blood flow acquired using Doppler (e.g., the velocity of tricuspid or pulmonary regurgitation or of valvar pulmonary stenosis or a VSD) (34). Thus, ECHO can be used in many ways to assess the degree of pulmonary hypertension. (Bernoulli's equation states that the total pressure is equal to static pressure plus dynamic pressure. With several assumptions, this concept can be mathematically simplified to: pressure gradient $= 4v^2$, where v is the velocity at the region of interest.) The maximum instantaneous pressure gradient of a left to right PDA or VSD shunt is an extremely useful variable in the assessment of PAH in CHD. For example, a VSD or PDA with a high-velocity shunt (pressure gradients of >50–80 mmHg) is likely to have mild or no PAH. The PA pressures can be estimated in this setting by subtracting the maximum instantaneous pressure gradient from the systolic blood pressure. For example, a child with a blood pressure of 90/50 and a maximum

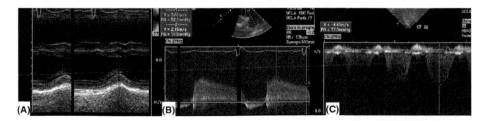

Figure 2   (*See color insert*) (**A**) ECHO M-mode of a patient with a large ASD and PAH. Note the large RV and flattened interventricular septum. (**B**) Pulse-wave Doppler signal form the pulmonary valve of the same patient. There is high-velocity pulmonary insufficiency with a gradient of 52 mmHg in early diastole. (**C**) Estimation of RV pressures by tricuspid regurgitation jet velocity. By the Bernouli's equation, this patient's RV and PA systolic pressure is 79 mmHg plus the central venous pressure. In this case it was suprasystemic. *Abbreviations*: ASD, atrial septal defect; PAH, pulmonary arterial hypertension; PA, pulmonary artery; RV, right ventricle.

instantaneous peak gradient (MIG) across a PDA of 70 mmHg is likely to have normal PA pressures (about 20 mmHg in systole). On the other hand, a VSD or a PDA (or an AP window) with a very low velocity shunt is likely to have systemic of near systemic PA pressures. Large PDAs often have low-velocity bidirectional shunting that is primarily left to right in the first decade of life. As the pulmonary vascular resistance rises to systemic levels, the shunt will reverse direction. Patients with moderate or severe degrees of obstruction to pulmonary blood flow (i.e., TOF patients or patients with pulmonary stenosis, subpulmonary stenosis, or even branch PA stenoses) always have high RV pressures but rarely have true PAH. The pulmonary vascular bed of these patients is "protected" from insult by RV outflow obstruction.

MRI and CT scans are increasingly being used to compliment ECHO and heart catheterization for the assessment of PAH patients with CHD. CT scans can give structural information about cardiovascular structures, can assess lung pathology, and are becoming the gold standard for the diagnosis of thromboembolism. MRI scans can give very accurate assessment of structural heart disease without radiation exposure. MRI scans can estimate pulmonary pressures from jets of tricuspid regurgitation and pulmonary insufficiency just as done with ECHO. The anatomy of the proximal pulmonary vasculature is very well seen by both MRI and CT, but the peripheral pulmonary artery windows by MRI are more limited. Although both CT and MR remain as auxillary tests for PAH in CHD, both technologies are rapidly evolving tools in both the field of pulmonary hypertension and in the field of CHD.

It is very important to distinguish between an elevation in PA pressures and an elevation in PVR (34). Many patients with CHD have elevated PA pressures from increased flow. "An increase in PA pressures in the presence of CHD does not necessarily mean that the PVR is increased or that patients will benefit from pulmonary vasodilator therapy. Many patients with large left to right shunts can have high pulmonary flow (increased Q_p:Q_s), high PA pressures, and a relatively low PVR." Although many publications have attempted to define pulmonary hypertension by an elevation in PA pressures, these definitions are not acceptable for patients with CHD. PAH in CHD patients must be defined in terms of PVR rather than PA pressures. While left to right shunt patients can have high flow and lower PVR, cyanotic CHD patients may have very low pulmonary blood flow but an elevation of the PVR that often benefits from treatment. Furthermore, patients with elevated pulmonary venous pressures as from mitral valve stenosis or pulmonary vein stenosis always have elevated PA pressures, but do not necessarily have an elevation in PVR or transpulmonary gradient and do not derive benefit from pulmonary vasodilators.

Because it is the most accurate way to assess PVR, cardiac catheterization is the gold standard for quantifying the severity of PAH in CHD. While heart catheterization allows for a direct and accurate measurement of transpulmonary gradient (the mean pressure in the PA minus the LA or pulmonary wedge pressure), an estimation of pulmonary blood flow can be more complex if a left to right shunt is present. Thermodilution estimates of cardiac output and pulmonary blood flow as made by the Swan Ganz catheter should "only be used if a left to right shunt is *not* present." Unless the operator knows how to account for a left to right shunt, any large shunt will introduce huge errors into the thermodilution methodology. Thus, the preferred method for estimation of flow in patients with CHD and PAH is the Fick's method. Simplified, the Fick's equation states that flow through a vessel (such as the pulmonary vascular bed) is proportional to the rate of extraction of an indicator (such as oxygen) divided by the difference of the content of this indicator before entering and after leaving a given vessel. To calculate pulmonary blood flow, it is necessary to measure or accurately estimate both pulmonary arterial and venous PA oxygen saturations (SATs), oxygen extraction across the pulmonary bed (VO_2 can be measured or estimated) and hemoglobin. The following equation is used by congenital cardiologists to estimate pulmonary blood flow:

$$PBF \, (L/min/m^2) = \frac{VO_2 \, (oxygen \, extraction \, in \, cc/min)^\alpha}{\begin{array}{c} 10 \, (dL/L) \times hemoglobin \, (g \, HGB/dL) \\ \times 1.34 \, (ccO_2/g \, HGB) \times (PA \, O_2 \, SAT - PV \, O_2 \, SAT)^\dagger \end{array}}$$

When using the Fick's equation, it is vital that close attention is paid to units. This can help any operator avoid costly errors. It also helps to both understand and to remember this important formula, resistance is easily calculated as:

$$PVR \, (WU \, indexed) = \frac{transpulmonary \, gradient \, (mmHg)}{pulmonary \, blood \, flow \, (L/min/m^2)}$$

Heart catheterization is not only used to assess absolute PVR, but it is used to assess "reactivity" to pulmonary vasodilator therapies (usually inhaled NO and oxygen). Baseline pressure and saturation measurements are taken on room air, on 100% oxygen, and on oxygen with 20 ppm (and 40 ppm) of NO. PVR, SVR, and pulmonary and systemic blood flows are then estimated for each condition. Reactivity to NO and oxygen in the cath lab likely correlate with response to vasodilator therapies.

Heart catheterization is often necessary to assess surgical candidacy for closure of a left to right shunt, to assess candidacy for vasodilator therapy, and to monitor the effects of therapy. However, it is certainly not without pitfalls. In the setting of severe PAH, the procedural risks approach and exceed even the riskier transcatheter interventions for CHD patients. Both anesthesia and cardiac catheterizations can induce a pulmonary hypertensive crisis that can often be life-threatening. A large injection of contrast in the PAs or even simply the presence of a catheter in the PA can cause a life-threatening pulmonary hypertensive crisis. The operator should consult with his or her anesthesiologist (if the patient needs to be placed under deep sedation or general anesthesia, usually necessary in children and infants) prior to the procedure so that anesthesia-induced pulmonary hypertensive spells can be minimized. A consideration of the risks and benefits must also be considered. Although noninvasive tests such has ECHO can be used to avoid catheterization on the very mild and very severe patients; advances in pulmonary vasodilator therapies have made it difficult to forgo an assessment of PVR, and reactivity in even the most severe cases of PAH are associated with a left to right shunt. At our institution, very high risk CHD-PAH patients are sometimes pretreated with pulmonary vasodilators to minimize risks of PAH crises.

[α]Oxygen extraction ideally should be measured using a metabolic rate meter in the catheterization laboratory. However, VO_2 can also be approximated based on body surface area.

[†]O_2 SATs must be used as decimals (e.g., an O_2 SAT of 99% should be 0.99 when used in the calculation of PBF).

VII. Eisenmenger Syndrome

The Eisenmenger complex refers to the reversal of a left to right shunt through a nonrestrictive VSD. Eisenmenger syndrome refers to a variety of CHD lesions that can cause pulmonary vascular disease and a reverse left to right shunt through a VSD, ASD, AV canal, etc. Figure 1 illustrates the progression of PAH in a patient with VSD and PDA.

During the first few years of life, the small muscular pulmonary artery branches are capable of relaxing, and a VSD or AV canal can be closed with a subsequent gradual fall in pulmonary vascular resistance. After two to three years, reactive intimal fibrosis begins to obliterate the lumen of the muscular arteries. By this time, these arteries have minimal if any response to vasodilating agents. Atrial level shunts have a very different natural history; they often go undetected for decades, may not present with pulmonary hypertension, and only rarely result in cyanosis. Patients with trisomy 21 are especially susceptible to developing pulmonary vascular disease (35). Cyanosis with pulmonary vascular disease and shunt reversal results in severely decreased exercise capacity that is multifactorial, but is mainly driven by worsening of right to left shunting during exercise (as a result of decreased systemic vascular resistance) and resultant CO_2 elevation in the systemic circulation, leading to hyperpnea and reduced ventilatory efficiency (36,37).

Death from Eisenmenger syndrome is usual by the fourth decade though some patients can survive into the seventh decade. Patients with unrepaired truncus arteriosus and those with single ventricle morphology have a poorer prognosis than patients with a nonrestrictive VSD (38). Causes of death include pulmonary hemorrhage, pulmonary arterial thrombosis, pulmonary artery dissection, ventricular arrhythmias, and RV failure. All cyanotic patients are at risk for infective endocarditis and should receive antibiotic prophylaxis prior to any bacteremic procedures (39). Patients with cyanotic CHD demonstrate an antiatherogenic substrate and are less susceptible to atherosclerotic heart disease than noncyanotic controls (40–42).

The coronary arterial tree in Eisenmenger's patients is markedly dilated with tortuous extramural coronary arteries and a well-developed microcirculation within the myocardium (43). The antiatherogenic state of these patients is characterized by low lipid levels, elevated bilirubin levels, increased NO production by vascular endothelial cells, and low platelet levels incurring less thrombotic risk. Patients with chronic cyanosis also develop defective hemostasis from abnormalities in platelet function and in the coagulation and fibrinolytic systems (44,45). Interestingly, although the systemic arterial circulation is seemingly devoid of atherosclerosis, the pulmonary arterial circulation is not spared from atherosclerosis and thrombosis (46). While pulmonary arterial in situ thrombosis is common, chronic anticoagulation increases the risk of pulmonary hemorrhage, particularly with thrombocytopenia, and should be avoided unless the patient has other definitive indications (e.g., atrial fibrillation or deep venous thrombosis) (38,47).

Chronic cyanosis leads to secondary erythrocytosis and increased blood viscosity. The absolute risk of symptomatic hyperviscosity is low with a hemoglobin level <20 g/dL. Symptoms include headache, dizziness, fatigue, bony pain, and blurry vision. Phlebotomy may improve symptoms but should be reserved for patients who do not improve with hydration (48). Phlebotomies on a regular basis result in iron deficiency and microcytic less deformable red blood cells that may not traverse the microcirculation, increasing the risk of stroke (49). While hyperuricemia is common due to increased red blood cell turnover and decreased renal excretion of uric acid, gouty flares and urate nephropathy are rare, as are tophaceous deposits within the soft tissue of the elbows or digits. Patients with right to left shunts are at risk for paradoxical emboli, leading to cerebrovascular accidents, renal impairment, or myocardial infarction. Septic emboli can cause cerebral abscesses and should be considered in the cyanotic patient with fever and neurological symptoms. Particle filters should be utilized with intravenous lines, and chronic indwelling venous catheters should be avoided. Anticoagulation may be considered in patients who must have chronic indwelling lines. However, unlike in patients with IPAH, those with Eisenmenger syndrome are generally not placed on chronic anticoagulation, because they have a higher risk of developing hemoptysis and are at increased risk of bleeding because of chronic thrombocytopenia (see preceding text).

VIII. Therapies for PAH in CHD

Over the past decade, a number of therapeutic options have become available for patients with PAH. Most clinical studies on the various pharmacological agents have involved a preponderance of patients with idiopathic pulmonary hypertension and are discussed elsewhere. Only one randomized, double-blind and placebo-controlled clinical trial was conducted exclusively in patients with CHD. The BREATHE-5 trial randomized 54 patients with atrial and/or VSDs, pulmonary hypertension, and cyanosis, to treatment with the dual selective endothelin blocker bosentan or placebo for 16 weeks (11). Patients on bosentan had significant improvement in six-minute walk distance (+53 m) without deterioration in pulse oximetry, the primary safety endpoint of the study. Patients also had a significant reduction in pulmonary vascular resistance. An open-label extension of this study for an additional 24 weeks did not demonstrate any decrement in 6-minute walk distance or World Health Association functional class (50). A smaller nonrandomized study demonstrated clinical stability with bosentan over two years but a slow return to baseline of VO_2 max and six-minute walk distance (51). The ET_A selective endothelin blocker ambrisentan is now commercially available and is increasingly being used in clinical practice; however, no trials in patients with Eisenmenger syndrome have been performed.

Phosphodiesterase 5 (PDE-5) inhibitors potentiate the vasodilatory and anti-proliferative effects of endogenous NO by increasing cyclic GMP levels. Sildenafil has been evaluated in small nonrandomized case series of patients with congenital heart defects and appears effective in reducing pulmonary vascular resistance and improving functional capacity (52,53). The once daily oral PDE-5 inhibitor tadalafil resulted in improved hemodynamics and functional capacity in an elegant prospective non-randomized study and may eventually be a viable alternative to the short-acting sildenafil (54). There are limited available clinical data on the combination of endothelin blockade and PDE-5 inhibition in patients with CHD, the available data suggests that combination therapy is well tolerated and additional improvement in functional capacity may occur; however, more extensive evaluation of combination therapies is warranted (55). Intravenous prostanoids are effective in reducing pulmonary vascular resistance in patients with congenital cardiac shunts, but there continues to be concerns about infection and thromboembolic complications related to chronic indwelling venous catheters in patients with right to left cardiac shunts. These issues have certainly limited the use of intravenous pulmonary vasodilators. Inhaled prostacyclin is well tolerated and has demonstrated efficacy in children with pulmonary hypertension related to CHD, but has not been specifically tested in adults with Eisenmenger syndrome (56).

The effects of therapy must be carefully monitored. Patients with mitral stenosis, LV restrictive physiology, or pulmonary venous stenosis can have flash pulmonary venous congestion with initiation of pulmonary vasodilator therapy. Similarly, if pulmonary vasodilators have a dramatic effect on a patient with a left to right shunt, the shunt volume can increase significantly and cause congestive heart failure and pulmonary edema. As above, these patients will have an increase in the Q_p:Q_s but may have relatively constant PA pressures. This effect is seen with VSDs, AV canals, and PDAs but not as much with ASD patients as atrial level shunt is primarily a function of relative ventricular compliance rather than systolic pressures.

Prostacyclin and prostacyclin analogue therapy is based on vasodilatory and antiplatelet properties, as well as implication of prostacyclin/thromboxane imbalance in PAH pathogenesis. A small study of 20 patients with CHD-associated PAH demonstrated significant reduction in PAP and PVR, with intravenous epoprostenol and improvements in cardiac index, exercise capacity, and functional class (57). These advantages do come at a substantial inconvenience and cost, as well as serious risks from the indwelling central venous catheter. Continuous subcutaneous (SC) treprostanil, a prostacyclin analogue, has demonstrated some efficacy in a large ($n = 469$) double-blind, placebo-controlled randomized study of PAH with mixed etiologies (58); however, only 10% of the enrolled patients had CHD-associated PAH, and no subgroup analysis was provided.

Two other prostacyclin analogues have shown some potential promise in treating CHD-associated PAH, but have only been evaluated in studies of mixed populations, in studies of short-term response, or in case reports. Short-term administration of the inhaled analogue iloprost reduced the ratio of PVR to systemic resistance in children with CHD to a degree comparable to NO. Combined iloprost plus NO had no additional effect (59). The oral analogue beraprost demonstrated some positive effects on disease progression and exercise capacity in a mixed PAH population (mostly IPAH), but significant improvement over placebo was only noted for the six-month time point (60).

NO remains an effective, inhaled continuous therapy for patients with PAH and CHD. While its use is often in intubated patients or those undergoing provocative testing in the catheterization laboratory (see preceding text), it can also be effective when administered by facemask as its therapeutic effects can be detected at doses less than five parts per million (61–63). The availability of NO in the postoperative cardiothoracic ICU has allowed both surgeons and interventionalists to be much more aggressive in closing lesions mediating left to right shunts in patients shown to be reactive to NO (64). Not only has NO become the gold standard for the treatment of PPHN, but it has also been shown to decrease intraventricular hemorrhage and death in newborns with respiratory distress syndrome (65–67). It is also used very commonly in patients both before an after CHD in the ICU setting, especially for patients with single ventricle physiology after a cavopulmonary shunt, and has well-defined uses in ARDS and for patients with V/Q mismatching (68).

The side effects of NO must be carefully monitored and long-term use of NO can lead to rebound pulmonary hypertension, which is ameliorated by use of other pulmonary vasodilators such as sildenafil (65,69,70). Methemaglobin levels should also be carefully monitored (70). Ironically, PPHN is the only disease for which NO use is FDA approved. All other applications of NO are off-label.

Transcatheter and surgical creation of an interatrial shunt may be life saving and can delay transplant in patients with RV failure and severely elevated right-sided filling pressures (71,72). Atrial septostomy provides hemodynamic and symptomatic improvement in patients with PAH and repaired CHD (73). The ASD serves as a "pop-off" for a volume-overloaded right atrium and right ventricle and results in a reduction in the RV volume. The failing right ventricle in patients with PAH is noncompliant and demonstrates restrictive physiology; therefore, a reduction in the filling volume often results in significant hemodynamic improvements. Right to left shunting across the interatrial septum with resultant cyanosis is expected. Creation of an ASD can ameliorate pulmonary hypertension by both decompression of the right or left atrium. While the Rashkind septostomy, blade septostomies, and static balloon septostomy can be temporary, transcatheter stenting of the atrial septum can produce more permanent atrial communication (74). Figure 3 demonstrates the use of transseptal puncture and stenting of an atrial septum in the setting of severe PAH in a newborn associated with single ventricle physiology and severe left-heart hypoplasia and left atrial hypertension.

Conversely, controlled and gradual closure of atrial level communications that are thought to be contributing to increased pulmonary artery pressures and causing RV volume overload may be achieved with fenestration of transcatheter devices (75,76). However, these fenestrations often will close slowly over time; in a study of

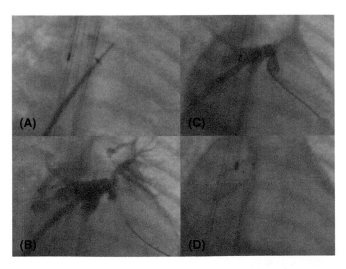

Figure 3 These series of angiograms demonstrate transcatheter stent decompression of the left atrial in a newborn with severe PAH secondary to left-heart hypoplasia and severe left atrial hypertension. (**A**) Use of a transseptal needle to cross the thick intra-atrial septum. (**B, C**) Positioning of a sheath and stent across the atrial septum. (**D**) Stent shown well positioned and fully inflated in the interatrial septum. *Abbreviation*: PAH, pulmonary arterial hypertension.

10 fenestrated devices implanted in children with PAH, 5 remained patent on echocardiography at 26 months of follow-up (75).

Lung transplant continues to be a final option therapy for pediatric patients with PAH. When PAH is caused by CHD, lung transplantation is of especially limited usefulness as there is always associated pathology of the heart and/or pulmonary veins or ateries (77). Heart and lung transplantation is sometimes the only viable transplantation option. Given the poor results of both lung and combined heart-lung transplantation in children, these therapies continue to an absolute last resort (78). The early diagnosis and treatment of CHD and associated PAH is of paramount importance in avoiding these much less desirable last resort therapies.

References

1. Hoffman JI, Kaplan S. The incidence of congenital heart disease. J Am Coll Cardiol 2002; 39:1890–1900.
2. Schulze-Neick I, Gilbert N, Ewert R, et al. Adult patients with congenital heart disease and pulmonary arterial hypertension: first open prospective multicenter study of bosentan therapy. Am Heart J 2005; 150:716.
3. Wren C, O'Sullivan JJ. Survival with congenital heart disease and need for follow up in adult life. Heart 2001; 85:438–443.
4. Hoffman JI, Christianson R. Congenital heart disease in a cohort of 19,502 births with long-term follow-up. Am J Cardiol 1978; 42:641–647.
5. Bialkowski J, Szkutnik M. Percutaneous closure of patent ductus arteriosus at high altitude. Congenit Cardiol Today 2007; 5:1–2.
6. Warnes CA, Liberthson R, Danielson GK, et al. Task force 1: the changing profile of congenital heart disease in adult life. J Am Coll Cardiol 2001; 37:1170–1175.
7. Hoffman JI, Kaplan S, Liberthson RR. Prevalence of congenital heart disease. Am Heart J 2004; 147:425–439.
8. Humbert M, Sitbon O, Simonneau G. Treatment of pulmonary arterial hypertension. N Engl J Med 2004; 351:1425–1436.
9. Galie N, Torbicki A, Barst R, et al. Guidelines on diagnosis and treatment of pulmonary arterial hypertension. The Task Force on Diagnosis and Treatment of Pulmonary Arterial Hypertension of the European Society of Cardiology. Eur Heart J 2004; 25:2243–2278.
10. Humbert M, Sitbon O, Chaouat A, et al. Pulmonary arterial hypertension in France: results from a national registry. Am J Respir Crit Care Med 2006; 173:1023–1030.
11. Galie N, Beghetti M, Gatzoulis MA, et al. Bosentan therapy in patients with Eisenmenger syndrome: a multicenter, double-blind, randomized, placebo-controlled study. Circulation 2006; 114:48–54.
12. Engelfriet P, Meijboom F, Boersma E, et al. Repaired and open atrial septal defects type II in adulthood: an epidemiological study of a large European cohort. Int J Cardiol 2008; 126:379–385.
13. Kidd L, Driscoll DJ, Gersony WM, et al. Second natural history study of congenital heart defects. Results of treatment of patients with ventricular septal defects. Circulation 1993; 87:138–151.
14. Horvath KA, Burke RP, Collins JJ Jr, et al. Surgical treatment of adult atrial septal defect: early and long-term results. J Am Coll Cardiol 1992; 20:1156–1159.
15. Newfeld EA, Paul MM, Muster AJ, et al. Pulmonary vascular disease in complete transposition of the great arteries: a study of 200 patients. Am J Cardiol 1974; 34:75–82.
16. Tullow R. Congenital heart disease in relation to pulmonary hypertension in paediatric practice. Paediatr Respir Rev 2005; 6:174–180.

17. Beghetti M, Black SM, Fineman JR. Endothelin-1 in congenital heart disease. Pediatr Res 2005; 57:16R–20R.
18. Haworth SG. Pulmonary hypertension in the young. Heart 2002; 88:658–664.
19. Tulloh RM. Congenital heart disease in relation to pulmonary hypertension in paediatric practice. Paediatr Respir Rev 2005; 6:174–180.
20. Rabinovitch M. Elastase and the pathobiology of unexplained pulmonary hypertension. Chest 1998; 114:213S–224S.
21. Diller GP, van Eijl S, Okonko DO, et al. Circulating endothelial progenitor cells in patients with Eisenmenger syndrome and idiopathic pulmonary arterial hypertension. Circulation 2008; 117:3020–3030.
22. Zhao YD, Courtman DW, Deng Y, et al. Rescue of monocrotaline-induced pulmonary arterial hypertension using bone marrow-derived endothelial-like progenitor cells: efficacy of combined cell and eNOS gene therapy in established disease. Circ Res 2005; 96:442–450.
23. Haworth SG. Pulmonary endothelium in the perinatal period. Pharmacol Rep 2006; 58(suppl):153–164.
24. Wojciak-Stothard B, Haworth SG. Perinatal changes in pulmonary vascular endothelial function. Pharmacol Ther 2006; 109:78–91.
25. Newman JH, Fanburg BL, Archer SL, et al. Pulmonary arterial hypertension: future directions: report of a National Heart, Lung and Blood Institute/Office of Rare Diseases workshop. Circulation 2004; 109:2947–2952.
26. Giaid A, Yanagisawa M, Langleben D, et al. Expression of endothelin-1 in the lungs of patients with pulmonary hypertension. N Engl J Med 1993; 328:1732–1739.
27. Black SM, Bekker JM, Johengen MJ, et al. Altered regulation of the ET-1 cascade in lambs with increased pulmonary blood flow and pulmonary hypertension. Pediatr Res 2000; 47:97–106.
28. Black SM, Mata-Greenwood E, Dettman RW, et al. Emergence of smooth muscle cell endothelin B-mediated vasoconstriction in lambs with experimental congenital heart disease and increased pulmonary blood flow. Circulation 2003; 108:1646–1654.
29. Ovadia B, Reinhartz O, Fitzgerald R, et al. Alterations in ET-1, not nitric oxide, in 1-week-old lambs with increased pulmonary blood flow. Am J Physiol Heart Circ Physiol 2003; 284:H480–H490.
30. Shafique T, Johnson RG, Dai HB, et al. Altered pulmonary microvascular reactivity after total cardiopulmonary bypass. J Thorac Cardiovasc Surg 1993; 106:479–486.
31. Carteaux JP, Roux S, Siaghy M, et al. Acute pulmonary hypertension after cardiopulmonary bypass in pig: the role of endogenous endothelin. Eur J Cardiothorac Surg 1999; 15:346–352.
32. Komai H, Adatia IT, Elliott MJ, et al. Increased plasma levels of endothelin-1 after cardiopulmonary bypass in patients with pulmonary hypertension and congenital heart disease. J Thorac Cardiovasc Surg 1993; 106:473–478.
33. Perloff JK. The Clinical Recognition of Congenital Heart Disease. 5th ed. Philadelphia: W.B. Saunders Co., 2003.
34. Lock JE, Keane JF, Stanton BP. Diagnostic and Interventional Catheterization in Congenital Heart Disease. 2nd ed. Norwell: Kluwer Academic Publishers, 2000.
35. Lindberg L, Olsson AK, Jogi P, et al. How common is severe pulmonary hypertension after pediatric cardiac surgery? J Thorac Cardiovasc Surg 2002; 123:1155–1163.
36. Diller GP, Dimopoulos K, Okonko D, et al. Exercise intolerance in adult congenital heart disease: comparative severity, correlates, and prognostic implication. Circulation 2005; 112:828–835.
37. Dimopoulos K, Okonko DO, Diller GP, et al. Abnormal ventilatory response to exercise in adults with congenital heart disease relates to cyanosis and predicts survival. Circulation 2006; 113:2796–2802.
38. Niwa K, Perloff JK, Kaplan S, et al. Eisenmenger syndrome in adults: ventricular septal defect, truncus arteriosus, univentricular heart. J Am Coll Cardiol 1999; 34:223–232.

39. Wilson W, Taubert KA, Gewitz M, et al. Prevention of infective endocarditis: guidelines from the American Heart Association: a guideline from the American Heart Association Rheumatic Fever, Endocarditis and Kawasaki Disease Committee, Council on Cardiovascular Disease in the Young, and the Council on Clinical Cardiology, Council on Cardiovascular Surgery and Anesthesia, and the Quality of Care and Outcomes Research Interdisciplinary Working Group. J Am Dent Assoc 2007; 138:739–745, 47–60.

40. Fyfe A, Perloff JK, Niwa K, et al. Cyanotic congenital heart disease and coronary artery atherogenesis. Am J Cardiol 2005; 96:283–290.

41. Chugh R, Perloff JK, Fishbein M, et al. Extramural coronary arteries in adults with cyanotic congenital heart disease. Am J Cardiol 2004; 94:1355–1357.

42. Perloff JK. The coronary circulation in cyanotic congenital heart disease. Int J Cardiol 2004; 97(suppl 1):79–86.

43. Dedkov EI, Perloff JK, Tomanek RJ, et al. The coronary microcirculation in cyanotic congenital heart disease. Circulation 2006; 114:196–200.

44. Rosove MH, Perloff JK, Hocking WG, et al. Chronic hypoxaemia and decompensated erythrocytosis in cyanotic congenital heart disease. Lancet 1986; 2:313–315.

45. Ammash N, Warnes CA. Cerebrovascular events in adult patients with cyanotic congenital heart disease. J Am Coll Cardiol 1996; 28:768–772.

46. Aboulhosn J, Castellon YM, Shao E, et al. Quantification of pulmonary artery calcium deposits in patients with pulmonary hypertension using computed tomography. In: American Foundation for Medical Research Western Convention, 2005.

47. Silversides CK, Granton JT, Konen E, et al. Pulmonary thrombosis in adults with Eisenmenger syndrome. J Am Coll Cardiol 2003; 42:1982–1987.

48. Perloff JK, Rosove MH, Child JS, et al. Adults with cyanotic congenital heart disease: hematologic management. Ann Intern Med 1988; 109:406–413.

49. Daliento L, Somerville J, Presbitero P, et al. Eisenmenger syndrome. Factors relating to deterioration and death. Eur Heart J 1998; 19:1845–1855.

50. Gatzoulis MA, Beghetti M, Galie N, et al. Longer-term bosentan therapy improves functional capacity in Eisenmenger syndrome: results of the BREATHE-5 open-label extension study. Int J Cardiol 2008; 127:27–32.

51. Apostolopoulou SC, Manginas A, Cokkinos DV, et al. Long-term oral bosentan treatment in patients with pulmonary arterial hypertension related to congenital heart disease: a 2-year study. Heart 2007; 93:350–354.

52. Schulze-Neick I, Hartenstein P, Li J, et al. Intravenous sildenafil is a potent pulmonary vasodilator in children with congenital heart disease. Circulation 2003; 108(suppl 1,2):167–173.

53. Okyay K, Cemri M, Boyac B, et al. Use of long-term combined therapy with inhaled iloprost and oral sildenafil in an adult patient with Eisenmenger syndrome. Cardiol Rev 2005; 13:312–314.

54. Mukhopadhyay S, Sharma M, Ramakrishnan S, et al. Phosphodiesterase-5 inhibitor in Eisenmenger syndrome: a preliminary observational study. Circulation 2006; 114:1807–1810.

55. Lunze K, Gilbert N, Mebus S, et al. First experience with an oral combination therapy using bosentan and sildenafil for pulmonary arterial hypertension. Eur J Clin Invest 2006; 36(suppl 3):32–38.

56. Ivy DD, Doran AK, Smith KJ, et al. Short- and long-term effects of inhaled iloprost therapy in children with pulmonary arterial hypertension. J Am Coll Cardiol 2008; 51:161–169.

57. Rosenzweig EB, Kerstein D, Barst RJ. Long-term prostacyclin for pulmonary hypertension with associated congenital heart defects. Circulation 1999; 99:1858–1865.

58. Simonneau G, Barst RJ, Galie N, et al. Continuous subcutaneous infusion of treprostinil, a prostacyclin analogue, in patients with pulmonary arterial hypertension: a double-blind, randomized, placebo-controlled trial. Am J Respir Crit Care Med 2002; 165:800–804.

59. Rimensberger PC, Spahr-Schopfer I, Berner M, et al. Inhaled nitric oxide versus aerosolized iloprost in secondary pulmonary hypertension in children with congenital heart disease: vasodilator capacity and cellular mechanisms. Circulation 2001; 103:544–548.

60. Barst RJ, McGoon M, McLaughlin V, et al. Beraprost therapy for pulmonary arterial hypertension. J Am Coll Cardiol 2003; 41:2119–2125.

61. Finer NN, Etches PC, Kamstra B, et al. Inhaled nitric oxide in infants referred for extracorporeal membrane oxygenation: dose response. J Pediatr 1994; 124:302–308.

62. Tworetzky W, Bristow J, Moore P, et al. Inhaled nitric oxide in neonates with persistent pulmonary hypertension. Lancet 2001; 357:118–120.

63. Davidson D, Barefield ES, Kattwinkel J, et al. Inhaled nitric oxide for the early treatment of persistent pulmonary hypertension of the term newborn: a randomized, double-masked, placebo-controlled, dose-response, multicenter study. The I-NO/PPHN Study Group. Pediatrics 1998; 101:325–334.

64. Wessel DL, Adatia I, Thompson JE, et al. Delivery and monitoring of inhaled nitric oxide in patients with pulmonary hypertension. Crit Care Med 1994; 22:930–938.

65. Clark RH, Kueser TJ, Walker MW, et al. Low-dose nitric oxide therapy for persistent pulmonary hypertension of the newborn. Clinical Inhaled Nitric Oxide Research Group. N Engl J Med 2000; 342:469–474.

66. Roberts JD Jr, Fineman JR, Morin FC III, et al. Inhaled nitric oxide and persistent pulmonary hypertension of the newborn. The Inhaled Nitric Oxide Study Group. N Engl J Med 1997; 336:605–610.

67. The Neonatal Inhaled Nitric Oxide Study Group. Inhaled nitric oxide in full-term and nearly full-term infants with hypoxic respiratory failure. N Engl J Med 1997; 336:597–604.

68. Abman SH, Griebel JL, Parker DK, et al. Acute effects of inhaled nitric oxide in children with severe hypoxemic respiratory failure. J Pediatr 1994; 124:881–888.

69. Kinsella JP, Abman SH. Clinical approach to inhaled nitric oxide therapy in the newborn with hypoxemia. J Pediatr 2000; 136:717–726.

70. Davidson D, Barefield ES, Kattwinkel J, et al. Safety of withdrawing inhaled nitric oxide therapy in persistent pulmonary hypertension of the newborn. Pediatrics 1999; 104:231–236.

71. Kerstein D, Levy PS, Hsu DT, et al. Blade balloon atrial septostomy in patients with severe primary pulmonary hypertension. Circulation 1995; 91:2028–2035.

72. Rothman A, Sklansky MS, Lucas VW, et al. Atrial septostomy as a bridge to lung transplantation in patients with severe pulmonary hypertension. Am J Cardiol 1999; 84:682–686.

73. Law MA, Grifka RG, Mullins CE, et al. Atrial septostomy improves survival in select patients with pulmonary hypertension. Am Heart J 2007; 153:779–784.

74. Danon S, Levi DS, Alejos JC, et al. Reliable atrial septostomy by stenting of the atrial septum. Catheter Cardiovasc Interv 2005; 66:408–413.

75. Lammers AE, Derrick G, Haworth SG, et al. Efficacy and long-term patency of fenestrated amplatzer devices in children. Catheter Cardiovasc Interv 2007; 70:578–584.

76. Althoff TF, Knebel F, Panda A, et al. Long-term follow-up of a fenestrated Amplatzer atrial septal occluder in pulmonary arterial hypertension. Chest 2008; 133:283–285.

77. Noyes BE, Kurland G, Orenstein DM. Lung and heart-lung transplantation in children. Pediatr Pulmonol 1997; 23:39–48.

78. Bridges ND, Clark BJ, Gaynor JW, et al. Outcome of children with pulmonary hypertension referred for lung or heart and lung transplantation. Transplantation 1996; 62:1824–1828.

13

Pulmonary Arterial Hypertension and Human Immunodeficiency Virus Infection

BRUNO DEGANO
CHU Rangueil-Larrey, Toulouse; and Hôpital Antoine Béclère, Clamart, France

OLIVIER SITBON
Université Paris Sud 11, Service de Pneumologie et Réanimation Respiratoire, Hôpital Antoine Béclère, Assistance Publique Hôpitaux de Paris, Clamart, France

I. Introduction

Human immunodeficiency virus (HIV) infection has been associated with both infectious and noninfectious complications. With the advent of highly active antiretroviral therapy (HAART) and specific chemoprophylactic drugs, prolonged survival has allowed noninfectious complications of HIV to gain greater recognition and attention. Pulmonary arterial hypertension (PAH), resulting from chronic obstruction of small pulmonary arteries, is one of these complications. Since the first reported case of PAH associated with HIV infection (PAH-HIV) (1), it has been established that HIV infection is one independent risk factor for development of PAH (2,3).

II. Epidemiology of PAH in HIV-infected Patients

A. Demographic Features of Patients with PAH-HIV

PAH-HIV has been described in both HIV-1 and HIV-2 infections (4,5). There is no apparent correlation between the severity of PAH and the stage of HIV infection or the degree of immunodeficiency (4,5). Unlike idiopathic PAH, which is more common in women than in men (ratio of males to females 1:1.7), males are more frequently affected by PAH-HIV (ratio of males to females 1.2:1) (3,5,6). PAH-HIV arises regardless of the route of HIV infection (2,5,7–9). Most studies have reported a higher proportion of patients with HIV acquired from intravenous drug use among PAH-HIV patients compared with HIV-infected patients without PAH (3,7,10). However, the role of intravenous drug use as an independent risk factor of PAH was ruled out (8).

B. Incidence and Prevalence of PAH-HIV in HIV-Infected Patients

In the French PAH Registry, PAH-HIV represented around 7% of all the reported cases of PAH (3). Initial studies in the early 1990s—a time when therapy with HAART was not yet available—indicated a prevalence of 0.5% [95% confidence interval (CI),

0.10–0.90%] (11). In the current HAART era, a prospective study conducted in more than 7500 HIV-infected patients found a prevalence of 0.46% (95% CI, 0.32–0.64%) (7). Although the prevalence of PAH-HIV seems to have not changed in recent years, recent data from the Swiss HIV Cohort Study indicate that the incidence declined from 0.21% in 1995 to only 0.03% in 2006 (10). This decrease in incidence may be related to improvements in HAART leading to higher CD4 cell counts and a decrease in immune activation (10).

III. Pathophysiology

A. Pathology

In PAH-HIV, the pathological aspect of the affected vessels shares broad similarities with all other forms of PAH (12). Plexiform lesions are found in approximately 80% of cases of PAH-HIV (4). By contrast, pulmonary veno-occlusive disease (PVOD) is observed in only approximately 7% of patients (12). There is often a significant inflammatory infiltrate surrounding the pulmonary vessels of patients with PAH-HIV, which is more apparent than that seen in idiopathic PAH (13).

B. Genetic Predisposition in PAH-HIV

Heterozygous germline mutations in the bone morphogenetic protein type 2 receptor (BMPR2) have been identified in more than 70% of patients with familial PAH and also in up to 25% of patients with apparently sporadic idiopathic PAH (14). In PAH-HIV, no BMPR2 mutation of any kind has been identified (5). Of note, the HIV-1 tat (transcriptional transactivator) protein represses *BMPR2* gene expression in human macrophages in vitro, thus interfering with transcriptional regulation of BMP and BMPR2 (15). Therefore, BMPR2 protein downregulation may participate in PAH in HIV-infected individuals.

C. HIV Infection

Although HIV is present in inflammatory cells in the lungs, the virus itself has not been detected in the complex pulmonary lesions seen in patients with PAH-HIV (16,17). The mechanism of PAH-HIV may therefore rely on indirect action of HIV proteins and/or on the associated immune dysregulation present in HIV-infected patients (18).

HIV Infection and Endothelial Dysfunction

HIV itself has never been shown to directly infect pulmonary vascular endothelial cells (16,19). However, HIV viral antigens are present in pulmonary endothelium and may directly stimulate abnormal apoptosis, growth, and proliferation (17). Excessive production of endothelin-1 (ET-1) has been implicated in endothelial cell dysfunction and in pathogenesis of PAH (20). In the setting of HIV infection, HIV-related proteins may affect ET-1 production, not only by endothelial cells but also by inflammatory cells (21). Glycoprotein 120, a viral protein necessary for the binding and entry of HIV into macrophages, has been shown to target human lung endothelial cells, increase markers of apoptosis, and stimulate the secretion of ET-1 (19).

HIV Infection and Pulmonary Inflammation

Inflammation is especially notable in PAH-HIV (21). Infection with HIV induces a chronic inflammatory state and persistent immune activation and dysregulation (22) that induce the release of proinflammatory cytokines and growth factors, which may be implicated in the pathogenesis of PAH (23). Increased expression of platelet-derived growth factor, a potent stimulus of smooth muscle cell and fibroblast growth and migration, has been noted in lung tissue from patients with PAH-HIV (16). Similarly, vascular endothelial growth factor A produced by T cells infected by HIV induces vascular permeability and endothelial cell proliferation and was therefore implicated in the development of vasculopathy in HIV-infected patients (24).

HIV-1 nef Protein

The negative factor (*nef*) antigen, critical for the maintenance of HIV viral loads and for host cell signaling interactions, has been localized to multiple pulmonary and vascular cell types in HIV-infected patients (18). In vitro, human endothelial cells exposed to *nef* demonstrate increased apoptosis followed by proliferation (25). In a comparison of primates infected with a chimeric SHIV *nef* virion [a chimeric viral construct containing the human HIV *nef* gene in a simian immunodeficiency virus (SIV) backbone] and those infected with constructs containing the native SIV *nef* allele, complex plexiform-like lesions were found exclusively in animals infected with SHIV human *nef* (18). In SHIV *nef*–infected animals, *nef* antigen was localized to the endothelium of the lung vasculature (18). The pattern of *nef* expression in patients with PAH-HIV was found to be similar to that seen in SHIV *nef*–infected primates, suggesting that *nef* may play a role in the development of PAH in HIV-infected individuals (18). Voelkel et al. proposed that *nef* taken up by endothelial cells may induce apoptosis in these cells; phagocytosis of such apoptotic bodies by neighboring cells may then initiate the release of growth factors and cytokines, which may lead to the emergence of apoptosis-resistant cells and uncontrolled endothelial proliferation, with the subsequent selection of an apoptosis-resistant angio-proliferative phenotype (26).

Human Herpesvirus 8

Human herpesvirus 8 (HHV-8) has been reported to be associated with idiopathic PAH (27), but this association has not been consistently confirmed (28). Histological studies on the implication of HHV-8 in PAH-HIV are lacking. Results of serological study on a possible link between PAH-HIV and HHV-8 infection are controversial (8,29).

IV. Clinical Presentation and Diagnosis of PAH in HIV-infected Patients

A. Detection

The major presenting symptoms of PAH in HIV-infected patients arise as a result of right ventricular dysfunction (5). These symptoms are nonspecific and could relate to a number of underlying conditions, especially in HIV-infected individuals. A detection algorithm based on dyspnea and transthoracic Doppler echocardiography has been recently validated (Fig. 1) (7).

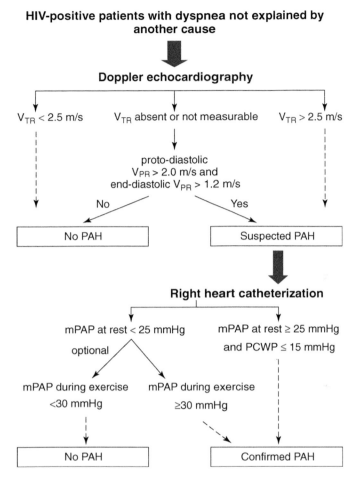

Figure 1 Diagnostic algorithm based on clinical symptoms of dyspnea, transthoracic Doppler echocardiography, and right-heart catheterization. *Abbreviations*: mPAP, mean pulmonary arterial pressure; PAH, pulmonary arterial hypertension; PCWP, pulmonary capillary wedge pressure; V_{PR}, peak velocity of pulmonary regurgitation; V_{TR}, peak velocity of tricuspid regurgitation. *Source*: From Ref. 7.

B. Characterization

Diagnosis of PAH

The false-positive rate from Doppler echocardiography for PAH diagnosis in HIV-infected patients was reported to be as high as 72% (7). Right-heart catheterization is therefore the standard for diagnosing PAH, as well as for evaluating hemodynamic status and response to treatment (Fig. 1) (7).

HIV-Infected Patients with Portal Hypertension

A history of viral hepatitis is found in about half the PAH-HIV patients in many series (30). Some of these patients present with cirrhosis and, therefore, with portal hypertension at the time of PAH diagnosis. As they have two associated risk factors for PAH—namely, portal hypertension and HIV infection—these patients are generally excluded from reports on PAH-HIV (5). This situation is however not unusual, representing about 4% of all PAH patients from the French Registry (3).

Pulmonary Veno-occlusive Disease

PVOD has been described as a cause of PAH in HIV-infected patients (31). Several features in the setting of severe PAH support the diagnosis of PVOD. Examination of lung parenchyma on CT scan provides evidence of septal lines, centrilobular ground-glass opacities, and lymph node enlargement. Low diffusing lung capacity of carbon monoxide is typically measured, and alveolar hemorrhage may be found on broncho-alveolar lavage (32).

V. Survival and Prognostic Factors

Survival data from several studies of patients with PAH-HIV are summarized in Table 1. The presence of PAH is an independent risk factor of mortality in patients with HIV infection (2). Prognosis is particularly poor for patients in New York Heart Association (NYHA) functional class III to IV, with a three-year survival rate of only 28% (5). In a majority of cases, death has been reported to be causally related to PAH rather than to other complications of HIV infection (6). Nunes et al. showed that to have $CD4^+$ counts >212 cells/mm^3 at the time of PAH diagnosis was independently associated with better survival (5).

VI. Treatments

Current guidelines for the treatment of PAH are largely based on data from patients with idiopathic PAH, and caution is recommended if these guidelines are to be extrapolated to other forms of PAH. Treatment guidelines list PAH-HIV as a special condition and stress that evidence to support best management of PAH-HIV is lacking (33).

A. Effects of Antiretroviral Therapy on PAH-HIV

In the HAART era, a large majority of PAH-HIV patients are diagnosed while on HAART (Table 1), showing that although effective against HIV, this treatment does not prevent PAH (10). Most results concerning the effects of HAART on functional and hemodynamic parameters in PAH-HIV are based on indirect and retrospective data, and are somewhat controversial. Pellicelli et al. reported an accelerated course of PAH in two HIV patients receiving HAART (34). In a study by Barbaro et al., significant improvements in exercise capacity were seen in PAH-HIV patients after 12 weeks of HAART alone, but hemodynamic parameters were not improved (35). By contrast,

Table 1 Summary of Data from Studies of Patients with PAH-HIV

Author (Ref.)	Year	Age at diagnosis (yr)	Duration of HIV infection (yr)	CD4$^+$ <200/ mm^3, n (%)	Highly active antiretroviral therapy at diagnosis, n (%)	Median survival (mo)	Survival at 1/2/3 yr (%)
Speich et al. (11)	1991	30 ± 5	–	3 (50)	0	8.5	–
Petitpretz et al. (6)	1994	32 ± 5	5 ± 2	12 (60)	0	–	53/53/24
Opravil et al. (2)	1997	30[a]	–	12 (63)	6 (32)	15.6	58/32/21
Nunes et al. (5)	2003	34 ± 6	6.4 ± 3.7	42 (51)	39 (48)	~36	73/60/47
Zuber et al. (9)	2004	34.4[a]	7.7[a]	28 (60)	19 (40)	32.4	–
Opravil et al. (10)	2008	43	–	–	13 (68)	55.2	90/~75/~65

[a]Median.

Abbreviations: PAH, pulmonary arterial hypertension; HIV, human immunodeficiency virus.

HAART was shown to improve right ventricular systolic pressure over right atrial pressure gradient (evaluated by cardiac echo-Doppler and not measured by right catheterization) in a retrospective analysis of 35 patients from the Swiss HIV Cohort Study (9). In this study, HAART significantly decreased mortality due to PAH as well as to other causes, and the authors therefore recommended treating all patients with PAH-HIV with HAART irrespective of their CD4$^+$ lymphocyte counts (9).

B. Nonspecific Supportive Therapies

Nonspecific supportive therapies in PAH include those which are generally considered to be efficacious and beneficial, but for which there are few clinical data to support their use. Examples include supplemental oxygen, anticoagulants, and oral vasodilators (20). Treatment with oral anticoagulants is recommended as background therapy in patients with idiopathic PAH (33), but their use in PAH-HIV needs to be considered in light of the risk of thrombocytopenia and associated hepatic disease frequently seen in these patients, and of the potential for drug interactions, particularly with some protease inhibitors (36).

Indication for calcium channel blockers (CCBs) treatment in PAH is strictly limited to patients with acute pulmonary vasodilator response, a situation rarely encountered in patients with PAH-HIV (37). The use of CCBs in PAH-HIV has been associated with side effects, and there is potential for drug-drug interaction with antiretroviral therapies (38).

C. Specific PAH Therapies

Prostacyclin and Prostacyclin Analogues

Treatment with intravenous epoprostenol in PAH-HIV was shown to result in a significant and sustained improvement in exercise capacity and hemodynamics (5,39). However, continuous intravenous infusion is associated with a risk of catheter-related sepsis, particularly in HIV-positive patients who present with immunosuppression (40). A further consideration is the use of an intravenous preparation to treat intravenous drug abusers, especially given the high prevalence of such patients in the HIV-infected cohort.

Nebulized prostacyclin analogs may overcome the limitations of intravenous administration, but there are very few data regarding these compounds in PAH-HIV (41). Similarly, subcutaneous treprostinil was shown to be effective on functional parameters in a very limited number of PAH-HIV patients, and its usefulness in this indication remains to be proven (42).

Sildenafil

There are currently no controlled trials of sildenafil in PAH-HIV, and data for its possible effects come from case studies where improvements in mean pulmonary artery pressure (mPAP), dyspnea, NYHA functional class, and exercise capacity have been reported (43–45). Sildenafil is largely metabolized by cytochrome P (CYP)450 3A4, and there is a potential for drug interactions when coadministered with a number of antiretroviral therapies, particularly protease inhibitors, resulting in increases in serum

Table 2 Data of Patients Who Normalized Hemodynamics on Bosentan Monotherapy

$n = 10$	Baseline	32 ± 22 mo
NYHA I:II:III:IV (n)	0:3:5:2	All in class I[a]
6MWD (m)	375 ± 102	532 ± 52[a]
mPAP (mmHg)	51 ± 10	19 ± 4[a]
CI (L/min/m^2)	3.3 ± 0.7	4.1 ± 0.8[a]
PVR (dyne.sec/cm^5)	713 ± 314	159 ± 76[a]
CD4$^+$ (cells.mL)	304 ± 111	539 ± 180[a]

[a]$p < 0.05$ versus baseline.
Abbreviations: NYHA, New York Heart Association; 6MWD, six-minute walk distance; mPAP, mean pulmonary artery pressure; CI, cardiac index; PVR, pulmonary vascular resistance.
Source: Adapted from Ref. 30.

sildenafil levels. The coadministration of sildenafil with potent CYP3A4 inhibitors including ritonavir is contraindicated (46).

Oral Endothelin Receptor Antagonists (ERAs)

In the prospective, open-label BREATHE-4 study, Sitbon et al. showed that treating PAH-HIV patients with the dual ET-1 receptor antagonist bosentan improved functional and hemodynamic parameters compared with baseline (47). Barbaro et al. showed that treatment of PAH-HIV patients with bosentan plus HAART resulted in significant hemodynamic improvements compared with treatment of patients with HAART alone (35). A retrospective study showed a long-term beneficial effect of bosentan on functional and hemodynamic parameters without impacting control of HIV infection (30). Notably, bosentan resulted in functional and hemodynamic normalization in 10 out of the 59 patients of this series (Table 2) (30). The results of the Tracleer post-marketing surveillance (PMS) Database indicated that the incidence of liver enzymes elevations was similar in PAH-HIV and idiopathic PAH patients (8.8% vs. 8.4%, respectively) (48). The use of bosentan is contraindicated in patients with more advanced liver disease (Child-Pugh C). There are currently no data concerning the use of the selective ERAs sitaxsentan or ambrisentan in PAH-HIV.

VII. Summary

PAH is a rare but life-threatening complication of HIV infection. Given the good long-term prognosis of HIV-infected patients in the HAART era, the severity of PAH, and the absence of predictive factors for PAH in HIV-infected patients, screening for PAH according to a precise algorithm is warranted in patients presenting with dyspnea not explained by another identified cause. Beneficial effects of HAART on PAH-HIV still remain to be proven. Although there are increasing data regarding the efficacy of specific PAH therapies in PAH-HIV, evidence to support best management of PAH in HIV-infected patients is still lacking.

References

1. Kim KK, Factor SM. Membranoproliferative glomerulonephritis and plexogenic pulmonary arteriopathy in a homosexual man with acquired immunodeficiency syndrome. Hum Pathol 1987; 18:1293–1296.
2. Opravil M, Pechere M, Speich R, et al. HIV-associated primary pulmonary hypertension. A case control study. Swiss HIV Cohort Study. Am J Respir Crit Care Med 1997; 155:990–995.
3. Humbert M, Sitbon O, Chaouat A, et al. Pulmonary arterial hypertension in France: results from a national registry. Am J Respir Crit Care Med 2006; 173:1023–1030.
4. Mehta NJ, Khan IA, Mehta RN, et al. HIV-Related pulmonary hypertension: analytic review of 131 cases. Chest 2000; 118:1133–1141.
5. Nunes H, Humbert M, Sitbon O, et al. Prognostic factors for survival in human immuno-deficiency virus-associated pulmonary arterial hypertension. Am J Respir Crit Care Med 2003; 167:1433–1439.
6. Petitpretz P, Brenot F, Azarian R, et al. Pulmonary hypertension in patients with human immunodeficiency virus infection. Comparison with primary pulmonary hypertension. Circulation 1994; 89:2722–2727.
7. Sitbon O, Lascoux-Combe C, Delfraissy JF, et al. Prevalence of HIV-related pulmonary arterial hypertension in the current antiretroviral therapy era. Am J Respir Crit Care Med 2008; 177:108–113.
8. Hsue PY, Deeks SG, Farah HH, et al. Role of HIV and human herpesvirus-8 infection in pulmonary arterial hypertension. AIDS 2008; 22:825–833.
9. Zuber JP, Calmy A, Evison JM, et al. Pulmonary arterial hypertension related to HIV infection: improved hemodynamics and survival associated with antiretroviral therapy. Clin Infect Dis 2004; 38:1178–1185.
10. Opravil M, Sereni D. Natural history of HIV-associated pulmonary arterial hypertension: trends in the HAART era. AIDS 2008; 22(suppl 3):S35–S40.
11. Speich R, Jenni R, Opravil M, et al. Primary pulmonary hypertension in HIV infection. Chest 1991; 100:1268–1271.
12. Pietra GG, Capron F, Stewart S, et al. Pathologic assessment of vasculopathies in pulmonary hypertension. J Am Coll Cardiol 2004; 43:25S–32S.
13. Cool CD, Kennedy D, Voelkel NF, et al. Pathogenesis and evolution of plexiform lesions in pulmonary hypertension associated with scleroderma and human immunodeficiency virus infection. Hum Pathol 1997; 28:434–442.
14. Sztrymf B, Coulet F, Girerd B, et al. Clinical outcomes of pulmonary arterial hypertension in carriers of BMPR2 mutation. Am J Respir Crit Care Med 2008; 177:1377–1383.
15. Caldwell RL, Gadipatti R, Lane KB, et al. HIV-1 TAT represses transcription of the bone morphogenic protein receptor-2 in U937 monocytic cells. J Leukoc Biol 2006; 79:192–201.
16. Humbert M, Monti G, Fartoukh M, et al. Platelet-derived growth factor expression in primary pulmonary hypertension: comparison of HIV seropositive and HIV seronegative patients. Eur Respir J 1998; 11:554–559.
17. Mette SA, Palevsky HI, Pietra GG, et al. Primary pulmonary hypertension in association with human immunodeficiency virus infection. A possible viral etiology for some forms of hypertensive pulmonary arteriopathy. Am Rev Respir Dis 1992; 145:1196–1200.
18. Marecki JC, Cool CD, Parr JE, et al. HIV-1 Nef is associated with complex pulmonary vascular lesions in SHIV-nef-infected macaques. Am J Respir Crit Care Med 2006; 174:437–445.
19. Kanmogne GD, Primeaux C, Grammas P. HIV-1 gp120 proteins alter tight junction protein expression and brain endothelial cell permeability: implications for the pathogenesis of HIV-associated dementia. J Neuropathol Exp Neurol 2005; 64:498–505.
20. Humbert M, Sitbon O, Simonneau G. Treatment of pulmonary arterial hypertension. N Engl J Med 2004; 351:1425–1436.

21. Humbert M. Mediators involved in HIV-related pulmonary arterial hypertension. AIDS 2008; 22(suppl 3):S41–S47.
22. Fauci AS, Pantaleo G, Stanley S, et al. Immunopathogenic mechanisms of HIV infection. Ann Intern Med 1996; 124:654–663.
23. Morse JH, Barst RJ, Itescu S, et al. Primary pulmonary hypertension in HIV infection: an outcome determined by particular HLA class II alleles. Am J Respir Crit Care Med 1996; 153:1299–1301.
24. Ascherl G, Hohenadl C, Schatz O, et al. Infection with human immunodeficiency virus-1 increases expression of vascular endothelial cell growth factor in T cells: implications for acquired immunodeficiency syndrome-associated vasculopathy. Blood 1999; 93:4232–4241.
25. Marecki J, Cool C, Voelkel N, et al. Evidence for vascular remodeling in the lungs of macaques infected with simian immunodeficiency virus/HIV NEF recombinant virus. Chest 2005; 128:621S–622S.
26. Voelkel NF, Cool CD, Flores S. From viral infection to pulmonary arterial hypertension: a role for viral proteins? AIDS 2008; 22(suppl 3):S49–S53.
27. Cool CD, Rai PR, Yeager ME, et al. Expression of human herpesvirus 8 in primary pulmonary hypertension. N Engl J Med 2003; 349:1113–1122.
28. Henke-Gendo C, Mengel M, Hoeper MM, et al. Absence of Kaposi's sarcoma-associated herpesvirus in patients with pulmonary arterial hypertension. Am J Respir Crit Care Med 2005; 172:1581–1585.
29. Montani D, Marcelin AG, Sitbon O, et al. Human herpes virus 8 in HIV and non-HIV infected patients with pulmonary arterial hypertension in France. AIDS 2005; 19:1239–1240.
30. Degano B, Yaici A, Le Pavec J, et al. Long-term effects of bosentan in patients with HIV-associated pulmonary arterial hypertension. Eur Respir J 2009; 33:92–98.
31. Escamilla R, Hermant C, Berjaud J, et al. Pulmonary veno-occlusive disease in a HIV-infected intravenous drug abuser. Eur Respir J 1995; 8:1982–1984.
32. Montani D, Achouh L, Dorfmuller P, et al. Pulmonary veno-occlusive disease: clinical, functional, radiologic, and hemodynamic characteristics and outcome of 24 cases confirmed by histology. Medicine (Baltimore) 2008; 87:220–233.
33. Badesch DB, Abman SH, Simonneau G, et al. Medical therapy for pulmonary arterial hypertension: updated ACCP evidence-based clinical practice guidelines. Chest 2007; 131:1917–1928.
34. Pellicelli AM, Palmieri F, D'Ambrosio C, et al. Role of human immunodeficiency virus in primary pulmonary hypertension–case reports. Angiology 1998; 49:1005–1011.
35. Barbaro G, Lucchini A, Pellicelli AM, et al. Highly active antiretroviral therapy compared with HAART and bosentan in combination in patients with HIV-associated pulmonary hypertension. Heart 2006; 92:1164–1166.
36. Bonora S, Lanzafame M, d'Avolio A, et al. Drug interactions between warfarin and efavirenz or lopinavir-ritonavir in clinical treatment. Clin Infect Dis 2008; 46:146–147.
37. Sitbon O, Humbert M, Jais X, et al. Long-term response to calcium channel blockers in idiopathic pulmonary arterial hypertension. Circulation 2005; 111:3105–3111.
38. Glesby MJ, Aberg JA, Kendall MA, et al. Pharmacokinetic interactions between indinavir plus ritonavir and calcium channel blockers. Clin Pharmacol Ther 2005; 78:143–153.
39. Aguilar RV, Farber HW. Epoprostenol (prostacyclin) therapy in HIV-associated pulmonary hypertension. Am J Respir Crit Care Med 2000; 162:1846–1850.
40. Limsukon A, Saeed AI, Ramasamy V, et al. HIV-related pulmonary hypertension. Mt Sinai J Med 2006; 73:1037–1044.
41. Stricker H, Domenighetti G, Mombelli G. Prostacyclin for HIV-associated pulmonary hypertension. Ann Intern Med 1997; 127:1043.
42. Cea-Calvo L, Escribano Subias P, Tello de Menesses R, et al. [Treatment of HIV-associated pulmonary hypertension with treprostinil]. Rev Esp Cardiol 2003; 56:421–425.

43. Alp S, Schlottmann R, Bauer TT, et al. Long-time survival with HIV-related pulmonary arterial hypertension: a case report. AIDS 2003; 17:1714–1715.
44. Carlsen J, Kjeldsen K, Gerstoft J. Sildenafil as a successful treatment of otherwise fatal HIV-related pulmonary hypertension. AIDS 2002; 16:1568–1569.
45. Schumacher YO, Zdebik A, Huonker M, et al. Sildenafil in HIV-related pulmonary hypertension. AIDS 2001; 15:1747–1748.
46. Electronic Medicines Compendium. Summary of product characteristics. Available at: http://emc.medicines.org.uk/emc/assets/c/html/DisplayDoc.asp?DocumentID=17443# CONTRAINDICATIONS.
47. Sitbon O, Gressin V, Speich R, et al. Bosentan for the treatment of human immunodeficiency virus-associated pulmonary arterial hypertension. Am J Respir Crit Care Med 2004; 170:1212–1217.
48. Humbert M, Segal ES, Kiely DG, et al. Results of European post-marketing surveillance of bosentan in pulmonary hypertension. Eur Respir J 2007; 30:338–344.

14
Portopulmonary Hypertension

MICHAEL J. KROWKA
Mayo Clinic, Rochester, Minnesota, U.S.A.

I. Overview

Portopulmonary hypertension (POPH) is a well-recognized type of pulmonary artery hypertension (group 1 in the Dana Point 2008 classification) that occurs in association with portal hypertension (1,2). First recognized by Mantz and Craige in 1951 (3), enhanced recognition and renewed importance of POPH has evolved in the era of liver transplantation (LT) due to the unanticipated complications (increased mortality) when transplantation has been attempted in the setting of *untreated*, moderate to severe pulmonary artery hypertension (4).

II. Clinical Presentation

The usual signs and symptoms of advanced liver disease may mask the clinical suspicion for pulmonary artery hypertension. Ascites, lower extremity edema, fatigue, and exertional dyspnea are commonly present due to portal hypertension alone (5). The existence of clubbing and hypoxemia in the setting of liver disease is *atypical* in POPH and suggests the existence of the distinct hepatopulmonary syndrome (triad of portal hypertension, pulmonary vascular dilatation, and hypoxemia) (2). Chest pain and/or syncope may portend at least moderate to severe POPH and deserve a thorough cardiovascular evaluation.

III. Diagnosis

POPH must be viewed within the greater context of three main categories of pulmonary hemodynamics associated with portal hypertension (6,7). Hyperdynamic (high-flow) circulatory state, excess volume, and obstruction to flow (see following text) within the pulmonary arterial bed can each result in pulmonary hypertension (mean pulmonary artery pressure, MPAP > 25 mmHg). However, the hyperdynamic state is usually flow phenomenon and the calculated pulmonary vascular resistance (PVR) is normal or low due to high cardiac output (CO); there is nothing intrinsically abnormal about the pulmonary arterial bed and no obstruction to pulmonary artery flow. Excess volume may

Table 1 Portopulmonary Hypertension Diagnostic Criteria

1. Existence of portal hypertension (a clinical diagnosis)
2. Right-heart catheterization criteria:

    a. Mean pulmonary artery pressure (MPAP) >25 mmHg
    b. Pulmonary vascular resistance (PVR) >240 dyne.sec/cm^5
    c. Transpulmonary gradient >12 mmHg[a]

[a]Transpulmonary gradient (TPG) = mean pulmonary artery pressure – pulmonary artery occlusion pressure (MPAP – PAOP). TPG replaced initial PAOP <15 mmHg criteria due to the combined presentation of excess volume *and* obstruction to pulmonary arterial flow (increased PVR) that was not infrequent in the setting of portal hypertension.

result from renal dysfunction, diastolic dysfunction, or the inability of the left heart to handle volume loads (as noted in alcoholic cardiomyopathy). Mild pulmonary *venous* hypertension can result in approximately 25% of such patients screened for pulmonary hypertension and is usually associated with an increased pulmonary artery occlusion pressure (same as pulmonary capillary wedge pressure >15 mmHg) (7). The PVR may be slightly increased in this scenario. Finally, pulmonary arterial obstruction to flow characterizes POPH. The MPAP and PVR may be extremely high with CO initially increased, but declining as the PVR increases. Right-heart failure and death inevitably ensue. As mentioned earlier, the importance of identifying the existence and severity of POPH in potential LT candidates cannot be overemphasized. Current diagnostic criteria for POPH, initially put forth by a 2004 European/U.S. Consensus Task Force of hepatologists, transplant surgeons, pulmonologists, cardiologists, and anesthesiologists, slightly modified in 2006, are summarized in Table 1 (2).

IV. Screening

Unfortunately, routine chest radiographs (cardiomegaly with enlarged central pulmonary arteries) and electrocardiograms (right axis, t-wave inversions V1–V4) occur when POPH is moderate to severe (usually MPAP > 35 mm Hg) (5). Because of the adverse effect of POPH during liver transplant surgery, all liver transplant candidates are expected to be screened for all-cause pulmonary hypertension. Transthoracic Doppler echocardiography has emerged as a reasonable screening tool to estimate pulmonary artery systolic pressure, as well as assess right ventricular function in a qualitative manner (8). Such screening is a recognized 2005 practice guideline put forth by the American Association for the Study of Liver Disease (AASLD) (9). At the Mayo Clinic, all LT candidates with right ventricular pressure systolic pressures (RVSP) greater than 50 mmHg (normal less than 30–35 mmHg) undergo outpatient RHC for complete pulmonary hemodynamic characterization to determine if POPH exists. From 1996 to 2005, 1235 liver transplant candidates were screened and 101 went on to RHC. In that cohort 66% had increased PVR (>240 dyne.sec/cm^5) and 34% were noted to have high-flow states (normal PVR) (Fig. 1) (7). Importantly, the latter group would *not* be

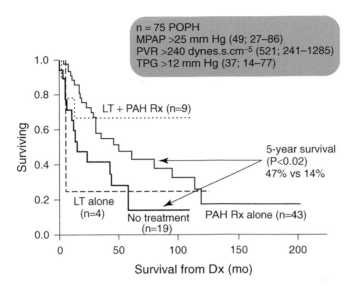

Figure 1 Survival curves from the time of POPH diagnosis in a cohort of 75 patients from the Mayo Clinic (1996–2006). There no significant differences in survival related to the degree of severity as characterized by MPAP, PVR, or CO. *Source*: From Ref. 38.

appropriate recipients of pulmonary vasomodulating therapies, despite the screening echocardiographic findings. This major screening study underscored the importance of RHC to confirm the suspected diagnosis of POPH. Depending on individual screening criteria at a given institution, approximately 10% of all LT candidates will need RHC to either confirm or rule out POPH. Whether *any* patient with chronic liver disease (not just LT candidates) should have screening echocardiography to assess for pulmonary hypertension is a decision most appropriate between a patient and his or her personal physician.

V. Epidemiology

It has been reported that 3.5% to 8.5% of all liver transplant candidates have POPH (7,10,11). Recent data from the REVEAL registry (Registry to Evaluate Early and Long-Term PAH Disease Management), as well as and French and U.S. experiences in pulmonary hypertension clinics, describe POPH frequencies ranging from 5.3% to 10.4% (12–14). Autoimmune liver disease and female gender appear to be correlated to the existence of POPH (15); however, there appears to be no relationship to the type or severity of liver disease as characterized by the Child-Turcotte-Pugh or Model for End-Stage Liver Disease (MELD) scoring systems (5). POPH does appear to be more frequent in patients who have undergone portocaval shunt surgery (16,17). Although quite uncommon, POPH has been reported in the pediatric population (18).

VI. Pathophysiology

The portal hypertension that precedes pulmonary artery hypertension can be for any reason, cirrhosis (from any cause) or any obstruction of blood flow to the liver (such as portal vein thrombosis) that causes increased blood pressure in the venous system that enters the liver (5). It is hypothesized that such increased pressure causes blood from the splanchnic system to bypass the liver and its normal metabolic functions. The pulmonary vascular bed, downstream from the liver, is thus exposed to many potential factors that can adversely affect the pulmonary arterial bed in *genetically susceptible* individuals (15). Such adversity results in obstruction to blood flow caused by pulmonary endo-thelial/smooth muscle proliferation, with or without vasoconstriction, in situ thrombosis possibly caused by platelet dysfunction, and classic plexogenic arteriopathy (5,19,20). The specific reasons how this happens is unclear, but we know deficiencies in endo-thelial prostacyclin synthase (21), excess circulating endothelin-1 (22), and pulmonary artery platelet aggregates (23) have been well documented in POPH patients.

VII. Treatment and Long-Term Survival

Ironically, the exclusion of POPH patients from *all* randomized, controlled pulmonary artery hypertension trials to date has hampered therapeutic understandings (5). Despite this limitation, the pharmacological treatment and liver transplant experience for POPH is evolving. Prospective, multicenter trials enrolling only POPH patients are planned to begin in 2009.

To date, the therapeutic role for prostacyclins, oral endothelin antagonists, and oral phosphodiesterase inhibitors in case reports and small series appear encouraging in POPH. Studies from the United States (48 patients from 5 centers) have demonstrated the significant effectiveness of intravenous prostacyclin administration in reducing MPAP (48 → 36 mmHg) and PVR (550 → 262 dyne.sec/cm^5) and increasing CO (6.3 → 8.7 L/min) with at least 12 weeks of therapy (24–28). Despite potential adverse effects on liver function, case reports and small uncontrolled series from Europe and the United States have demonstrated clinically significant improvement and improved one-year survival in both MPAP and PVR at varying time intervals using the dual endothelin receptor antagonist bosentan (29–33). Improved pulmonary hemodynamics have been reported with the use of the phosphodiesterase inhibitor sildenafil either alone or in combination with a prostacyclin (34–36). Therapeutic use of β-blockers in POPH patients (used to prevent variceal bleeds) has been shown to depress CO (decrease heart rate) and increase PVR with no change in MPAP (37).

Recent Mayo Clinic five-year survival data for POPH in patients who have never received the current regimens for pulmonary artery hypertension or undergone LT was poor at 14% ($n = 19$); five-year survival for those mainly treated with prostanoids (IV or subcutaneous) was 45% ($n = 43$) (38). Cause of death associated with POPH is equally distributed between complications of liver disease (bleeding and infection) and pro-gressive right-heart failure. The recent French experience following 154 POPH patients (51% had Child's A liver disease) from 1984 to 2004 has documented a five-year *overall* survival of 68% with poorest long-term survival in Child B and C patients, as well as those with reduced CO (39). However, specific pulmonary hypertension therapies were administered to 45 of 154 patients, thus complicating interpretation of clinical course versus "natural history" of POPH. These data confirm the initial experience that reduced CO was associated with poor prognosis and the existence and severity of POPH was not correlated to the severity of portal hypertension per se (40). A small U.S. study ($n = 13$) reported a 30% five-year survival ($n = 13$) with 8 of 13 receiving intravenous prostacyclin therapy (41).

Outcome of POPH when LT is attempted continues to be problematic and unpredictable. Mortality during and after the transplant procedure remains a significant clinical problem when pre-LT MPAP is greater than 35 mmHg (14% intraoperative death; 22% during the transplant hospitalization in the largest multicenter series to date ($n = 36$); however, only 1 of 13 patients who died received pre-LT prostacyclin therapy (42). However, there are limited, but encouraging data to suggest that patients who respond to 24-hour continuous intravenous epoprostenol, bosentan, or sildenafil *and* undergo LT have excellent survival and in some cases complete resolution of POPH (26,28,36,38). A 70% five-year survival ($n = 9$) was reported from the Mayo Clinic when prostacyclin was used pre-LT to improve pulmonary hemodynamics months prior to operation (38).

"Earlier" LT following the hemodynamic improvement with pulmonary vaso-modulating therapy may be advised to prevent the long-term right-heart effects of POPH, but additional study is needed to support that conjecture (43).

References

1. Simonneau G, Robbins I, Beghetti M, et al. Updated clinical classification of pulmonary hypertension. J Am Coll Cardiol 2009 (in press).
2. Rodriguez-Roisin R, Krowka MJ, Herve P, et al. Pulmonary-hepatic disorders (PHD). Eur Respir J 2004; 24: 861–880.
3. Mantz FA, Craige E. Portal axis thrombosis with spontaneous portocaval shunt and resultant cor pulmonale. AMA Arch Pathol 1951; 52:91–97.
4. Krowka MJ, Plevak DJ, Findlay JY, et al. Pulmonary hemodynamics and perioperative cardiopulmonary mortality in patients with portopulmonary hypertension undergoing liver transplantation. Liver Transpl 2000; 6:443–450.
5. Golbin JA, Krowka MJ. Portopulmonary hypertension. Clin Chest Med 2007; 28:203–218.
6. Kuo PC, Plotkin JS, Johnson LB, et al. Distinctive clinical features of portopulmonary hypertension. Chest 1997; 112:980–986.
7. Krowka MJ, Swanson KL, Frantz RP, et al. Portopulmonary hypertension; results of a 10-year screening study. Hepatology 2006; 44:1502–1510.
8. Kim WR, Krowka MJ, Plevak DJ, et al. Accuracy of Doppler echocardiography in the assessment of pulmonary hypertension in liver transplant candidates. Liver Transpl 2000; 6(4):453–458.
9. Murray KF, Carithers RL. American Association for the study of liver disease (AASLD) Practice guidelines: evaluation of the patients for liver transplantation. Hepatology 2005; 47:1407–1432.
10. Ramsay MAE, Simpson BR, Nguyen AT, et al. Severe pulmonary hypertension in liver transplant candidates. Liver Transpl Surg 1997; 3:494–500.
11. Kuo PC, Plotkin J, Gaine S, et al. Portopulmonary hypertension and the liver transplant candidate. Transplantation 1999; 67:1087–1093.

12. McGoon MD, Krichman A, Fraber H, et al. Design of the REVEAL registry for US patients with pulmonary artery hypertension. Mayo Clin Proc 2008; 83:923–931.
13. Humbert M, Sitbon O, Chaouat A, et al. Pulmonary artery hypertension in France. Am Rev Respir Crit Care Med 2006; 173:1023–1030.
14. Thenappan T, Shah SJ, Rich S, et al. A USA-based registry for pulmonary arterial hypertension Eur Respir J 2007; 30:1103–1110.
15. Kawut SM, Krowka MJ, Trotter F, et al. Clinical risk factors for portopulmonary hypertension. Hepatology 2008; 48:196–203.
16. Senior RM, Britton RC, Turino GM, et al. Pulmonary hypertension associated with cirrhosis of the liver and portocaval shunts. Circulation 1968; 37:88–96.
17. Lebrec D, Capron JP, Dhubaux D, et al. Pulmonary hypertension complicating portal hypertension. Am Rev Respir Dis 1979; 120:849–855.
18. Condino AA, Ivy DD, O'Connor IA, et al. Portopulmonary hypertension in pediatric patients. J Pediatr 2005; 147:20–26.
19. Krowka MJ, Edwards WD. A spectrum of pulmonary vascular pathology in portopulmonary hypertension. Liver Transpl 2000; 6:241–242.
20. Edwards BS, Weir KE, Edwards WD, et al. Coexistent pulmonary and portal hypertension: morphologic and clinical features. J Am Coll Cardiol 1987; 10:1233–1238.
21. Tuder RM, Cool CD, Geraci MW, et al. Prostacyclin synthase expression is decreased in lungs from patients with severe pulmonary hypertension. Am J Respir Crit Care Med 1999; 159:1925–1932.
22. Benjaminov FS, Prentice M, Sniderman KW, et al. Portopulmonary hypertension in decompensated cirrhosis with refractory ascites. Gut 2003; 52:355–362.
23. Sankey EA, Crow J, Mallet SV, et al. Pulmonary platelet aggregates: possible cause of sudden preoperative death in adults undergoing liver transplantation. J Clin Pathol 1993; 46:222–227.
24. Kuo PC, Johnson JB, Plotkin JS, et al. Continuous intravenous infusion of epoprostenol for the treatment of portopulmonary hypertension. Transplantation 1997; 63:604–606.
25. Krowka MJ, Frantz RP, McGoon MD, et al. Improvement in pulmonary hemodynamics during intravenous epoprostenol (prostacyclin): a study of 15 patients with moderate to severe portopulmonary hypertension. Hepatology; 1999; 30:641–648.
26. Sussman N, Kaza V, Barshes N, et al. Successful liver transplantation following medical management of portopulmonary hypertension: a single center series. Am J Transplant 2006; 6:2177–2182.
27. Fix OK, Bass NM, DeMarco T, et al. Long-term follow-up of portopulmonary hypertension: effect of treatment with epoprostenol. Liver Transpl 2007; 13:875–885.
28. Ashfaq M, Chinnakoatla S, Rogers L, et al. The impact of treatment of portopulmonary hypertension on survival following liver transplantation. Am J Transplant 2007; 7:1258–1264.
29. Halank M, Miehlke S, Hoeffen G, et al. Use of oral endothelin receptor antagonist bosentan in the treatment of portopulmonary hypertension. Transplantation 2004; 77:1775–1776.
30. Hinterhuber L, Graziadei IW, Kahler C, et al. Endothelin-receptor antagonist treatment of POPH. Clin Gastro Hepatol 2004; 2:1039–1042.
31. Kuntzen C, Gulberg V, Gerbes AL. Use of a mixed endothelin receptor antagonist in POPH: a safe and effective therapy? Gastroenterology 2005; 128:164–168.
32. Hoeper MM, Seyfarth HJ, Hoeffken G, et al. Experience with inhaled iloprost and bosentan in portopulmonary hypertension. Eur Respir J 2007; 30:1096–1102.
33. Humbert M, Segal ES, Kiely DG, et al. Results of European post-marketing surveillance of bosentan in pulmonary hypertension. Eur Respir J 2007; 30:338–344.
34. Makisalo H, Koivusalo A, Vakkuri A, et al. Sildenafil for portopulmonary hypertension in patients undergoing liver transplantation. Liver Transpl 2004; 10:945–950.
35. Reichenberger F, Voswinckel R, Steveling E, et al. Sildenafil treatment for portopulmonary hypertension. Eur Respir J 2006; 28:563–567.

36. Hemmes AR, Robbins IM. Sildenafil monotherapy in portopulmonary hypertension can facilitate liver transplantation. Liver Transpl 2009; 15:15–19.
37. Provencher S, Herve P, Jais X, et al. Deleterious effects of beta-blockers on exercise capacity and hemodynamics in patients with portopulmonary hypertension. Gastroenterology 2006; 130:120–126.
38. Swanson KL, Krowka MJ, Wiesner RH, et al. Survival in portopulmonary hypertension: Mayo Clinic experience categorized by treatment groups. Am J Transplant 2008; 8:2445–2453.
39. Le Pavec J, Souza R, Herve P, et al. Portopulmonary hypertension: survival and prognostic factors. Am J Respir Crit Care Med 2008; 178:637–643.
40. Hadengue A, Benhayoun MK, Lebrec D, et al. Pulmonary hypertension complicating portal hypertension: prevalence and relation to splanchnic hemodynamics. Gastroenterology 1991; 100:520–528.
41. Kawut S, Taichman DB, Ahya VN, et al. Hemodynamics and survival in patients with portopulmonary hypertension. Liver Transpl 2005; 11:1107–1111.
42. Krowka MJ, Mandell MS, Ramsay MAE, et al. Hepatopulmonary syndrome and porto-pulmonary hypertension: a report of the multicenter liver transplant database. Liver Transpl 2004; 10:174–182.
43. Krowka MJ, Fallon, MB, Mulligan D, et al. MELD exception and portopulmonary hyper-tension. Liver Transpl 2006; 12(suppl):S114–S116.

15

Pulmonary Hypertension Complicating Schistosomiasis

CAIO J. C. S. FERNANDES, CARLOS JARDIM, and ROGÉRIO SOUZA
University of São Paulo Medical School, São Paulo, Brazil

I. Epidemiology of Schistosomiasis

Schistosomiasis is one of the most prevalent infectious diseases in the world. The disease is most prevalent in sub-Saharan Africa but is endemic in more than 70 countries including major populated areas such as China, India, and Brazil. It is believed that 20% of the endemic area population is at risk of developing schistosomiasis (1). The World Health Organization (WHO) estimates that 200 million people are infected worldwide, 120 million of whom are symptomatic; about 20 million exhibit severe manifestations of the disease (1). Mortality from schistosomiasis is estimated at 11,000 deaths per year, and the burden of disease, at 1.7 million disability-adjusted life years lost per year (2).

Schistosomiasis is caused by a group of parasitic trematode worms; the main ones that infect humans are *Schistosoma mansoni* (present in Africa, Brazil, Venezuela, and the Caribbean), *S. haematobium* (present in Africa), *S. intercalatum* (Africa), *S. japonicum* (China, Indonesia, and Philippines), and *S. mekongi* (Cambodia and Laos, along the Mekong River) (3,4). Nevertheless, the impact of this disease has transcended the traditional geographic limits because of the increasing number of returning travelers and migratory practices. The Center for Disease Control and Prevention and the International Society of Travel Medicine maintain a database—GeoSentinel—related to the morbidity among returning travelers from a network of 25 travel and tropical clinics around the world. According to GeoSentinel, schistosomiasis is one of the ten leading causes of morbidity among travelers, accounting for 6% of the cases related to sub-Saharan Africa. Among travelers to sub-Saharan Africa who maintained direct contact with bodies of freshwater, the rate of symptomatic infections has been estimated at between 55% and 100% (5,6).

The global magnitude of schistosomiasis has led to several attempts of epidemic control worldwide, such as the Schistosomiasis Control Initiative (SCI). The SCI, which has been implemented in seven African countries, is a collaborative program focused on morbidity control that is supported by national health and education ministries and the Bill and Melinda Gates Foundation, through the Imperial College London (7). Similar efforts are pursued by the Special Program for Research and Training in Tropical Diseases of the United Nations Development Program, the World Bank, and the WHO (1).

II. The Parasite Life Cycle

All *Schistosoma* infections follow direct contact with freshwater that harbors free-swimming larval forms of the parasite known as cercariae. Cercariae penetrate the skin of humans or, in the case of *S. japonicum*, humans or other mammalian hosts that act as reservoirs for infection. The cercariae shed their tails, and the resultant schistosomula enter capillaries and lymphatic vessels en route to the lungs. After several days, the worms perforate the alveolar-capillary barrier and go up in the bronchial tree until they reach the gut. Then they migrate to the venous portal venous system, mature, and unite.

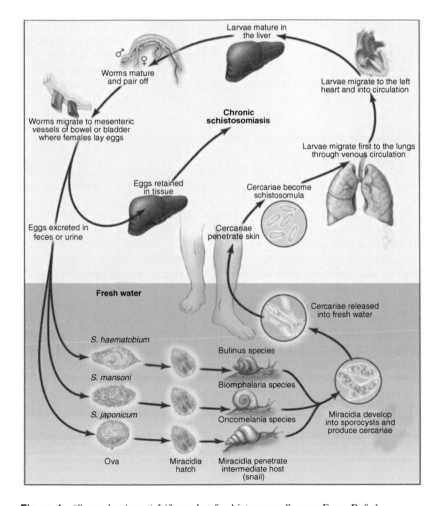

Figure 1 (*See color insert*) Life cycle of schistosome. *Source*: From Ref. 1.

Pairs of worms then migrate to the superior mesenteric veins (in the case of *S. mansoni*), the inferior mesenteric and superior hemorrhoidal veins (*S. japonicum*), or the vesical plexus and veins draining the ureters (*S. haematobium*). Egg production commences four to six weeks after infection and continues for the life of the worm—usually three to five years. Eggs pass from the lumen of blood vessels into adjacent tissues, and many then pass through the intestinal or bladder mucosa and are shed in the feces (*S. mansoni* and *S. japonicum*) or urine (*S. haematobium*). The life cycle is completed when the eggs hatch, releasing miracidia that in turn infect specific freshwater snails (*S. mansoni* infects *Biomphalaria* sp., *S. haematobium* infects *Bulinus* sp., and *S. japonicum* infects *Oncomelania* sp.). After two generations—primary and then daughter sporocysts— within the snails they release cercariae starting the cycle over (Fig. 1) (1,8).

About one-third of the eggs produced by *S. mansoni* and *S. japonicum* spp. do not follow the direction of the intestinal lumen and are deposited instead in the small veins of the liver as a natural consequence of the portal flow (9). There they induce a pre-sinusoidal granulomatous inflammatory response and periportal fibrosis with subsequent portal hypertension. In the presence of this condition, portacaval shunts open and, besides the generation of pulmonary blood overflow, it enables the eggs to be carried to the lung capillaries, where they lodge (10). It should be emphasized that cirrhosis is not a feature of schistosomiasis, even in the presence of advanced hepatosplenic disease.

III. Pulmonary Hypertension and Schistosomiasis

Schistosomiasis results from the host's immune response to schistosome eggs and the granulomatous reaction evoked by the antigen they secrete (11). The intensity and duration of infection determine the amount of antigen released and the severity of chronic fibro-obstructive disease. Most granulomas develop at the sites of maximum accumulation of eggs—intestine and liver (*S. mansoni* and *S. japonicum*) and genito-urinary tract (*S. haematobium*). However, perivascular granulomas have been found in the skin, lung, brain, adrenal glands, and skeletal muscle. The inflammatory response started by the egg migration may assist the passage of the egg to the gut lumen or urinary tract, with various degrees of tissue damage in the way (1,12).

Chronic schistosomiasis may be present in up to 20% of infected patients; a cardial feature is hepatosplenic disease with portal hypertension (*S. mansoni* and *S. japonicum*) (13). About 4% to 8% of patients with schistosomiasis develop hepatosplenic disease (1,14). An autopsy study of 313 cases of *S. mansoni* in the southeastern part of Brazil noted hepatosplenic disease with pulmonary arterial hypertension (PAH) in 7.7% (15). The importance of schistosomiasis-associated PAH in developing countries was underscored by a recent study showing that it may represent up to 30% of all PAH patients followed at reference centers in Brazil (16).

More recently, a prospective study screening patients with hepatosplenic *S. mansoni* for the presence of PAH found a 7.6% prevalence of PAH. More interestingly, about 4.6% were diagnosed via right-heart catheterization as PAH (with pulmonary artery occlusion pressure lower than 15 mmHg), while 3.0% presented postcapillary pulmonary hypertension. This finding reinforces the multifactorial pathophysiology associated with the development of pulmonary hypertension in *S. mansoni*, as well as the importance of invasive hemodynamic measurements for the appropriate diagnosis (17).

Considering the prevalence of hepatosplenic disease and the prevalence of PAH in this subgroup, we may speculate that schistosomiasis-associated PAH represents the most prevalent form of PAH worldwide.

IV. Vascular Lung Pathology and Mechanism of Lesion

The pathophysiology of PAH associated with schistosomiasis is a matter of debate. Previous studies emphasized the mechanical role of the ova in causing vascular obstruction and focal arteritis (18). Later studies evidenced that mechanical obstruction was not the only factor related to the development of PAH; some authors suggested that inflammation also had a significant role in the genesis of the vasculopathy (19–23), as has been observed in other forms of PAH (24). These early works already acknowledged the presence of plexiform lesions unrelated to the angiomatoid lesions characteristically described as the pathological feature of schistosomiasis (21,25). Preliminary results of an ongoing study comparing lung specimens from necropsies of patients with idiopathic and schistosomiasis-associated PAHs support the spectrum of vascular lesions not related to the presence of eggs or granuloma (Fig. 2) (26).

Some authors speculated that schistosomiasis-associated PAH is just another form of portopulmonary hypertension without liver failure (27). In fact, it shares with portopulmonary hypertension many clinical features (e.g., the better hemodynamic profile at diagnosis and the lack of acute response to vasodilator challenge) (28). Recent data (6) suggest that schistosomiasis-associated PAH may be related to multiple mechanisms, including mechanical impaction of *S. mansoni* eggs within the pulmonary vessels (18), the consequent inflammatory process in the lung vasculature (23), and the higher blood flow that occurs in portal hypertension because of arteriovenous shunts (25,29).

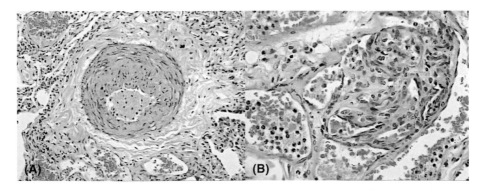

Figure 2 (*See color insert*) (**A**) Vascular granuloma associated with *Schistosoma* egg impaction. (**B**) Plexiform lesion from a patient with schistosomiasis-associated pulmonary hypertension (indistinguishable from those found in patients with idiopathic pulmonary arterial hypertension). *Source*: Courtesy of Prof Thais Mauad, Pathology Department, University of São Paulo Medical School.

V. Classification, Clinical Features, and Treatment

The classification of schistosomiasis in the setting of PAH follows the timeline of better understanding its pathophysiology and clinical course. In 1988, the Evian classification of pulmonary hypertension put schistosomiasis in the inflammatory group along with sarcoidosis, which could have had incorrect implications in terms of treatment (30). The revised classification, from the international symposium held in Venice in 2003 (31), relocated schistosomiasis in the nonthrombotic embolic group, emphasizing the mechanical effect of egg obstruction in the lung vasculature. In 2008, at the last international symposium held in Dana Point, schistosomiasis was reclassified as a form of PAH, reflecting recent findings regarding pathology and hemodynamic presentation. Nevertheless, it is important to reemphasize that schistosomiasis is a multifactorial disease and that the proper diagnosis of PAH associated with its hepatosplenic form is highly dependent on right-heart catheterization.

Clinical presentation of schistosomiasis-associated PAH is indistinguishable from idiopathic PAH (17). The symptoms of progressive dyspnea, chest pain, dry cough, lower-extremity edema, and, eventually, syncope may be present, which worsens progressively over years. The radiological features suggest an insidious process with remarkable vascular dilatations (32). The main pulmonary artery enlargement is more pronounced when compared with idiopathic PAH even considering the severity of the hemodynamic profile (Fig. 3).

Diagnosis of schistosomiasis is based mainly on environmental exposure to the parasite and identification of the parasite eggs in stool examination or in rectal biopsy (9). However, the absence of viable eggs does not exclude the diagnosis. Abdominal ultrasonographic findings such as enlargement of the left lobe of the liver or periportal fibrosis may suggest schistosomiasis and in prevalent areas have a high positive predictive value (33). The presence of hepatosplenic abnormalities may support the

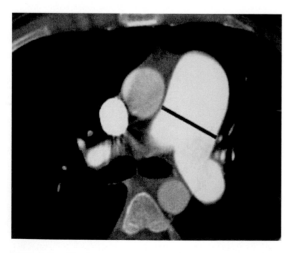

Figure 3 Chest CT scan evidencing prominent enlargement of pulmonary artery trunk. *Source*: Courtesy of Dr Claudia Figueiredo, Radiology Department, Fleury Research Institute.

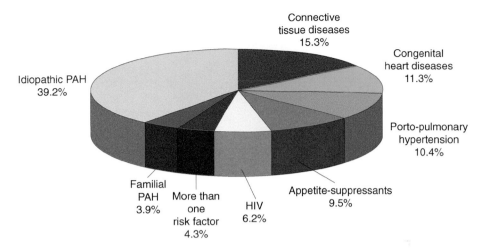

Figure 2.1 Distribution of patients with PAH in the 2002 to 2003 French Registry. *Abbreviations*: HIV, human immunodeficiency virus. *Source*: From Ref. 5 (*see page 11*).

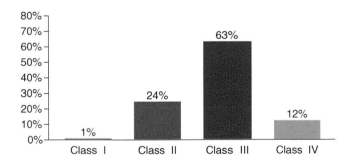

Figure 2.2 NYHA functional class at diagnosis in 674 patients with PAH from the French Registry. *Abbreviation*: NYHA, New York Heart Association. *Source*: From Ref. 5 (*see page 13*).

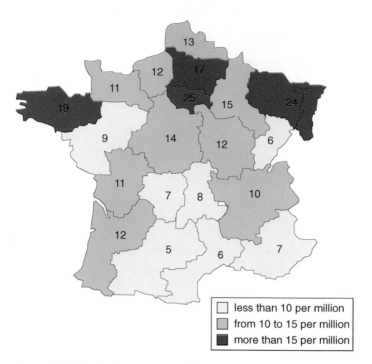

Figure 2.3 Regional prevalence of PAH in France in 2002 to 2003 from the French Registry. Prevalence less than 10 per million inhabitants (*light gray*). Prevalence between 10 and 15 per million (*darker gray*). Prevalence above 15 per million (*most dark area*). *Source*: From Ref. 5 (*see page 15*).

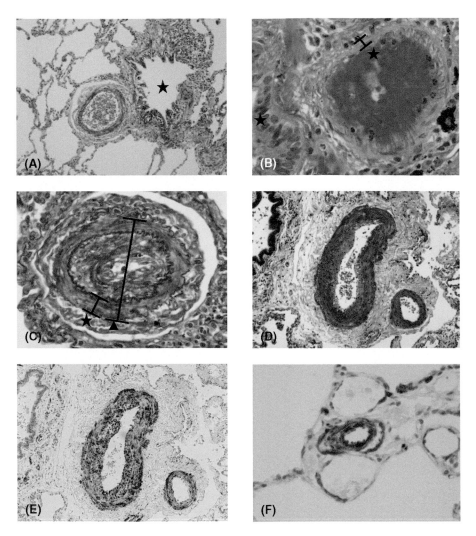

Figure 3.1 Remodelling of the media with proliferation of smooth muscle-cells in pulmonary arteries and arterioles of patients suffering from IPAH and controls. (**A**) Normal muscular pulmonary artery with adjacent bronchiole (asterisk) lacking any signs of remodelling. WHPS (Weigert-Hematoxylin-Phloxin-Saffron) staining, magnification ×40. (**B**) Unaffected, slender medial layer in a congestive pulmonary artery (asterisk). WHPS staining, magnification ×200. (**C**) Medial hypertrophy (and intimal thickening) of a pulmonary artery: the medial thickness is defined as the distance between internal and external elastic lamina (asterisk). Medial hypertrophy is defined as the exceeding of 10 per cent of the arterial cross-sectional diameter (triangle). WHPS staining, magnification ×200. (**D**) Pulmonary artery and a smaller branch, both with hypertrophy of the tunica media, WHPS staining, magnification ×100. (**E**) Same arteries after immunohistochemical reaction with an antibody directed against smooth muscle cell actin highlighting the tunica media. Magnification ×100. (**F**) Muscularized arteriole (<100 μm) with anti-smooth muscle cell actin staining. Magnification ×200 (*see page 22*).

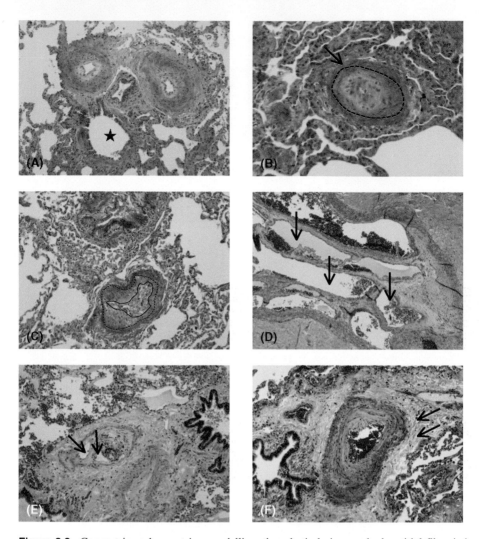

Figure 3.2 Concentric and eccentric remodelling, thrombotic lesions and adventitial fibrosis in pulmonary arteries of patients suffering from IPAH. (**A**) Pulmonary artery (2 branches) and their adjacent bronchiole (asterisk): the arterial lumina are narrowed by intimal concentric non-laminar fibrosis. HES (Hematoxylin-Eosin-Saffron) staining, magnification ×40 (**B**) Another artery with intimal concentric non-laminar fibrosis. The internal elastic lamina (iel, dashed line) delimits the inner boundary of the medial layer and emphasizes the extensive intimal thickening, as compared to the discrete medial hypertrophy (arrow). HES staining, magnification ×100. (**C**) Pulmonary artery with eccentric intimal fibrosis: note the uneven thickening of the intimal layer, which is delimited by the internal elastic lamina (dashed line) and by the lumen (continuous line). HES staining, magnification ×40. (**D**) Large pulmonary artery with remodeled thrombus/embolus in a patient with thromb-embolic disease: note the wide lumina of newly developed vessels within the occlusion (arrows) in an attempt to recanalize the obstructed artery. WHPS staining, magnification ×40. (**E**) Small pulmonary artery with thrombotic lesion, or "colander lesion" in a patient with IPAH: same recanalization phenomenon (arrows) leading sometimes to confusion with plexiform lesions (see beneath). WHPS staining, magnification ×40. (**F**) Pulmonary artery with occluding intimal fibrosis and associated excessive adventitial fibrosis (arrows). WHPS staining, magnification ×40 (*see page 24*).

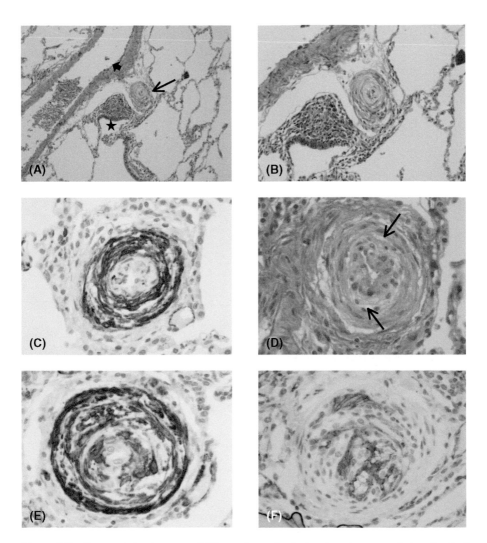

Figure 3.3 Concentric laminar remodelling and complex lesions in pulmonary arteries of patients suffering from IPAH. (**A**) Longitudinally sectioned larger pulmonary artery (arrowhead) with small branch displaying concentric laminar fibrosis (arrow) and adjacent bronchiole (asterisk). HES staining, magnification ×40. (**B**) Magnification of same arterial lesion: note the concentric and laminar arrangement of fibrous layers with a decrease of cellular density in the periphery of the lesion. HES staining, magnification ×100. (**C**) Smooth muscle cell staining in a concentric laminar fibrosis: smooth muscle elements are present within this intimal lesion. Note negativity of the inner, endothelial layer. Magnification ×200. (**D**) Concentric laminar "onion-skin" lesion with near arterial occlusion. This lesion was adjacent to a plexiform lesion and small channels within the occlusion are faintly perceivable (arrows). HES staining, magnification ×200. (**E**) Same lesion after immunohistochemical reaction with an antibody directed against smooth muscle cell actin. Note negativity of the mentioned channels. Magnification ×200. (**F**) Same lesion after immuno-histochemical reaction with an antibody directed against endothelial cells. Note the staining of endothelium-lined channels within the occlusion, probably the "beginning" of a plexiform lesion. Magnification ×200 (*see page 25*).

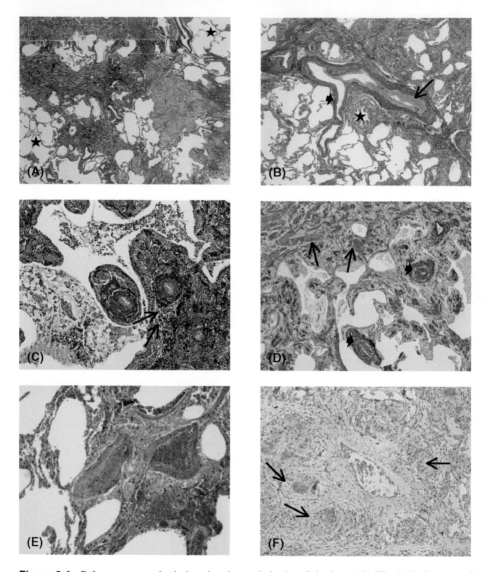

Figure 3.4 Pulmonary vascular lesions in other pathologies of the lung. (**A**) Histological aspect of lungs from a patient with interstitial pulmonary fibrosis (IPF). Note the patchy distribution of parenchymal fibrotic lesions with alternating unaffected parenchyma (asterisks). Elastica van Gieson staining (EvG), magnification ×20. (**B**) Transition zone between diseased and preserved pulmonary parenchyma. Note the pulmonary artery and the adjacent bronchiole (asterisk): Arterial intimal thickening is present within the zone of IPF typical parenchymal remodelling (arrow), while absent in the arterial branch leaving the main artery into the preserved area (arrowhead). EvG staining, magnification ×20. (**C**) Small pulmonary arteries of the same lung displaying concentric intimal fibrosis. Note the close association to inflammatory cells mainly consisting of lymphocytes (arrows). EvG staining, magnification ×40. (**D**) Same lung with smooth muscle actin staining: Smooth muscle cell hyperplasia is present in a remodeled arteries (arrowheads) and in the pulmonary interstitium (arrows). Magnification ×20. (**E**) Pulmonary arteries in a lung resection specimen of a patient with spontaneous idiopathic pneumothorax: intimal thickening is present in the absence of pulmonary hypertension. HES staining, magnification ×40. (**F**) Pulmonary arterial remodeling in a patient with pulmonary hypertension associated with sarcoidosis. The arterial wall displays intense inflammatory infiltrate and numerous epitheloid granulomas with giant cells (arrows), narrowing the arterial lumen considerably. CD68 (macrophages) stain, magnification ×40 (*see page 27*).

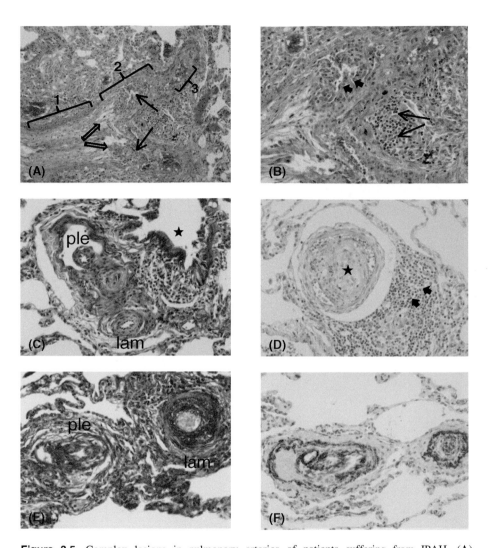

Figure 3.5 Complex lesions in pulmonary arteries of patients suffering from IPAH. (A) Branching point of a pulmonary artery (bold arrows) with 2 complex lesions developing on each of the successive branches (arrows). Typical constellation with 3 segments: 1 = intimal thickening; 2 = plexiform lesion with exuberant endothelial cell proliferation; 3 = dilation lesion. HES staining, magnification ×40. (B) Magnification of the upper plexiform lesion (arrowheads): note the perivascular lymphocytic infiltrate at the arterial bifurcation (arrows). HES staining, magnification ×100. (C) Another small "developing" plexiform lesion forming sinusoidal channels within the original arterial lumen (ple). Note the regular association with concentric laminar intimal thickening (lam). WHPS staining, magnification ×100. (D) Fibrous, scarred aspect of a plexiform lesion (asterisk) surrounded by inflammatory, round cells, corresponding to lymphocytes (arrowheads). HES staining, magnification ×100. (E) Close association of a plexiform and a concentric laminar intimal lesion. WHPS staining, magnification ×100. (F) Same lesions with smooth muscle cell staining: smooth muscle cells/myofibroblasts nicely highlight the remodelling process in both lesions. Magnification ×100 (*see page 29*).

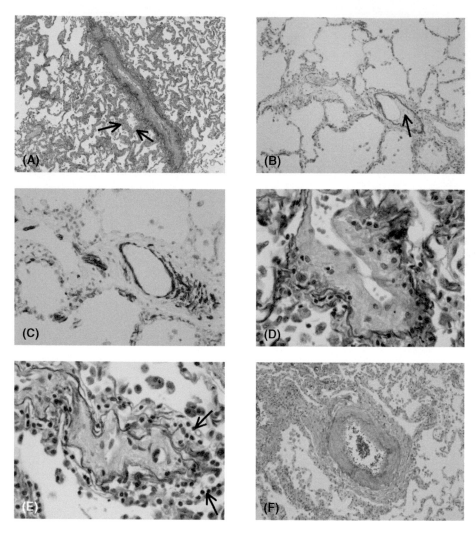

Figure 3.6 Remodeling of pulmonary septal veins and pre-septal venules in patients suffering from PVOD. (**A**) Fibrous intimal thickening in a large septal vein. Note the adjacent broad alveolar septa with capillary multiplication (arrows). WHPS staining, magnification ×20. (**B**) Smaller septal vein with loose intimal fibrosis, partially occluding the lumen (arrow). WHPS staining, magnification ×40. (**C**) Same vein with smooth muscle cell staining, highlighting partial muscularization. Magnification ×100. (**D**) Small pre-septal venule displaying occlusive intimal fibrosis. Note the paucicellular aspect of the occluded venule. WHPS staining, magnification ×200. (**E**) Small pulmonary vein with near occlusion and inflammatory lymphocytic infiltrate (arrows). WHPS staining, magnification ×200. (**F**) Pulmonary artery in a patient with PVOD with medial hypertrophy and adventitial fibrosis: note the typical broadening of alveolar septa and intra-alveolar macrophages. HE (Hematoxylin-Eosin) staining, magnification ×40 (*see page 32*).

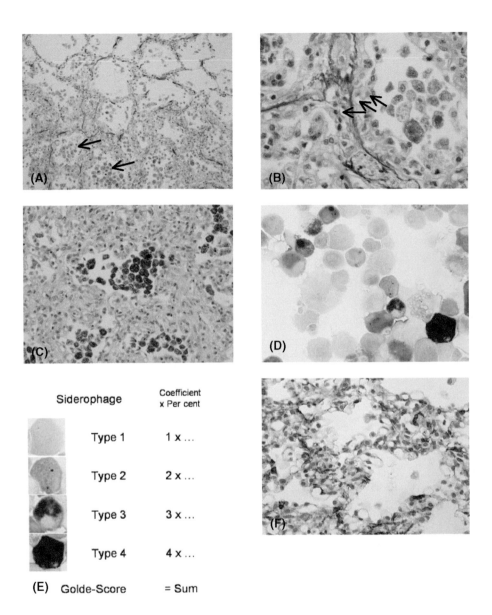

Figure 3.7 Remodeling of alveolar septa and alveolar hemorrhage in patients suffering from PVOD. (**A**) Patchy distribution of alveolar septal thickening. Alveoli within this remodeled area contain numerous macrophages (arrows). HES staining, magnification ×40. (**B**) Capillary multiplication leading to alveolar septal thickening with doubling or even trebling of the capillary lumina (arrows). Note the pigment-rich macrophages to the left of the marked alveolar septum. HES staining, magnification ×400. (**C**) Same area with Perls Prussian Blue staining, revealing siderin-laden macrophages within the alveoli, the morphologic equivalent of persistent hemorrhage. Magnification ×200. (**D**) Broncho-alveolar lavage: numerous siderin-laden macrophages (or siderophages) are present, displaying different degrees of Prussian Blue staining. Magnification ×400. (**E**) Siderophages isolated from figure 6D: typing of macrophagic Prussian Blue staining is performed in order to assess the degree of alveolar hemorrhage: a Golde score above 100 is considered as occult alveolar hemorrhage. (**F**) Pulmonary parenchyma of a patient suffering from PCH: note the capillary proliferation within the alveolar septa leading to a histological pattern very similar to PVOD. Smooth-muscle staining, magnification ×200 (*see page 34*).

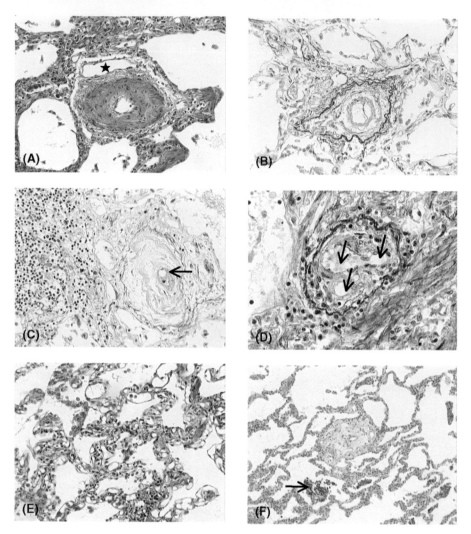

Figure 3.8 Pulmonary vascular lesions found in patients suffering from PAH associated to connective tissue disease. (**A**) Intimal concentric non-laminar fibrosis of a small pulmonary artery. Note the dilated lymphatic vessel adjacent to the artery (asterisk). HE staining, magnification ×100. (**B**) Pre-septal venule with loose occlusive intimal fibrosis. WHPS staining, magnification ×100. (**C**) Occlusive loose fibrotic remodeling of a pre-septal venule (arrow) with peri-vascular lymphocytic infiltrate. WHPS staining, magnification ×100. (**D**) Thrombotic lesion of a pre-septal venule with recanalization channels within the occluded vessel (arrows). WHPS staining, magnification ×200. (**E**) Capillary angiectasia and alveolar septal thickening similar to the histological pattern seen in PVOD (see above). HE staining, magnification ×100. (**F**) Occluded vein (center) and signs of occult alveolar hemorrhage: note the stained siderin-laden macrophages within the adjacent alveoli. Perls Prussian Blue staining, magnification ×40 (*see page 36*).

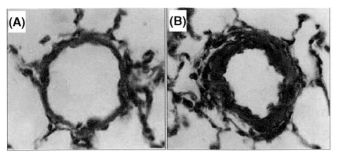

Ppa: 22 mmHg   Ppa: 36 mmHg

Figure 5.2 Pulmonary arterioles and pulmonary artery pressure (Ppa) of normal (**A**) and two-week chronic hypoxia (**B**) exposed rats. Chronic hypoxia induces medial hypertrophy, without any intimal or adventitial alterations. *Source*: From Ref. 22 (*see page 62*).

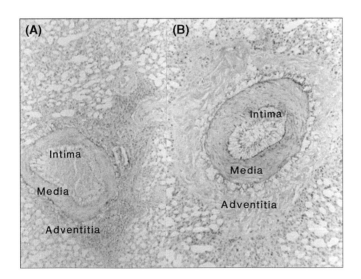

Figure 5.3 Pulmonary arterioles of normal-growing (**A**) and very fast-growing (**B**) chickens after two weeks of hypoxic exposure. There is a marked remodeling of the three layers of the vascular wall in fast-growing chickens. *Source*: From Ref. 27 (*see page 63*).

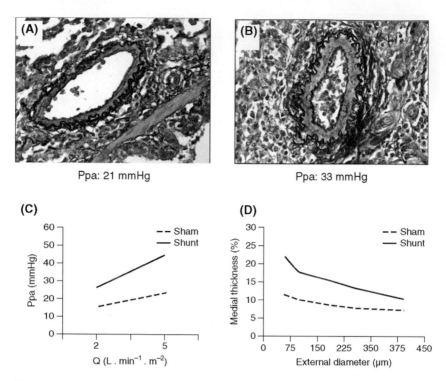

Figure 5.5 Pulmonary arterioles and pulmonary artery pressures (Ppa) of sham-operated (**A**) and shunted (**B**) piglets. Three months of shunting induces a shift of the pulmonary artery pressure (Ppa) versus flow curves (Q) to higher pressures (**C**) and an upward shift of medial thickness versus arteriolar diameter curves (**D**), mainly in smallest pulmonary resistive arterioles. *Source*: From Ref. 86 (*see page 67*).

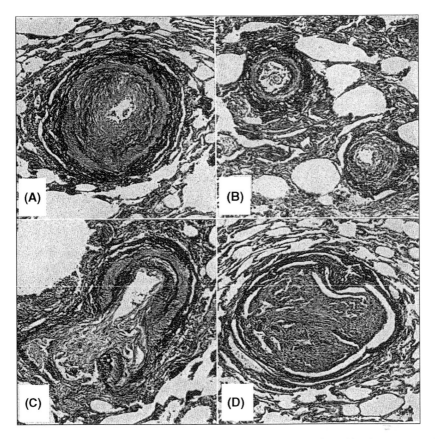

Figure 5.6 Pulmonary sections of long-term (4 years) shunted dogs. (**A**) Transverse section of a muscular pulmonary artery, with medial hypertrophy. The vessel is almost totally occluded by fibrous tissue, most of which is acellular. (**B**) Transverse section of two pulmonary arterioles. In both, there is a thick muscular media between distinct internal and external elastic laminae. The arteriole to the right is partially occluded by acellular fibrous tissue and the underlying muscular media is thinned. There is no intimal fibrosis and no thinning of the media in the arteriole to the left. (**C**) Transverse sections of a muscular pulmonary artery showing medial hypertrophy, severe acellular intimal fibrosis, and a dilated branch that forms a distented sac filled with proliferated cellular endothelium. The appearances are characteristic of those of a "plexiform dilatation" lesion. (**D**) Transverse section of a "plexiform dilatation" lesion that forms a distented sac containing proliferated cellular endothelium arranged in parts in a plexiform pattern. An arc of the remaining media of the parent muscular pulmonary artery can be seen at the periphery of the sac. *Source*: From Ref. 93 (*see page 68*).

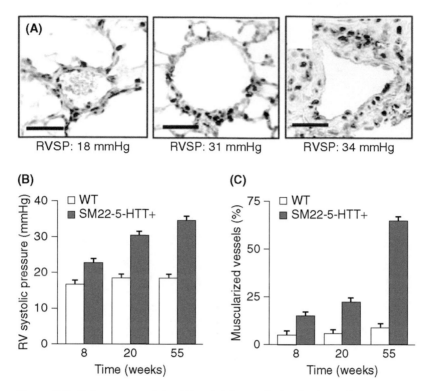

Figure 5.7 Pulmonary arterioles (**A**) and right ventricular (RV) systolic pressure curves (**B**) and morphometry (**C**) of wild-type and transgenic mice overexpressing serotonin transporter (5-HTT) under the control of the SM22 promoter (SM22–5-HTT+) at 20 and 55 weeks of age. *Source*: From Ref. 124 (*see page 71*).

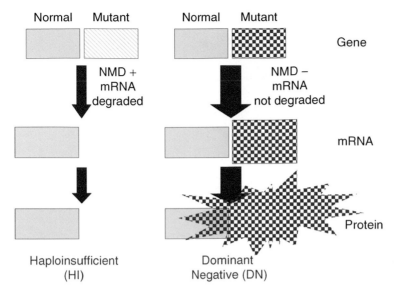

Figure 6.2 Comparison of a heterozygous mutation that results in a haploinsufficient effect versus one that results in a potentially DN effect in the context of NMD. In the case of HI, the heterozygous state results in one normal (wild-type) allele and one mutant allele. The mutant allele is degraded by activation of the NMD pathway, such that the only protein product that results is from the wild-type allele. In contrast, a potentially DN effect occurs when products of a mutant allele interact with and reduce the expression of normal (wild-type) allele products. The potential result is even less normal protein is available to function than in the HI situation. *Abbreviations*: DN, dominant negative; NMD, nonsense-mediated decay; HI, haploinsufficiency (*see page 88*).

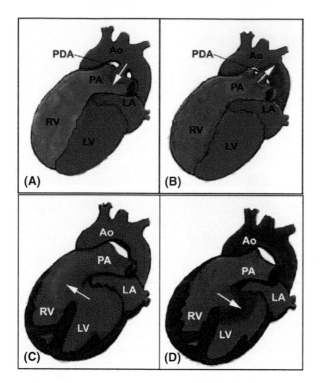

Figure 12.1 (**A**) PDA with left to right shunt (*white arrow*) of oxygenated blood from the Ao to the PA. The RV, LA, and LV are also labeled. (**B**) PDA with Eisenmenger syndrome. Pulmonary vascular resistance is now suprasystemic and the shunt has reversed, deoxygenated blood from the PA is shunted to the Ao via the PDA. Most of this deoxygenated blood flows to the lower extremities given the typical location of a PDA at the distal aortic arch, resulting in differential cyanosis where the upper extremity digits are typically not cyanotic while the lower extremity digits are cyanotic. (**C**) Nonrestrictive ventricular septal defect during infancy, prior to the development of elevated pulmonary vascular resistance. The shunt is left to right (*arrow*) with highly oxygenated pulmonary venous blood entering the LA, to the LV, and thereafter to the Ao as well as shunting to the PA. This leads to LA and LV volume overload and pulmonary edema. (**D**) Gradually over the first few years of life the pulmonary vascular resistance rises to approximate or exceed systemic vascular resistance and the VSD shunt reverses (*arrow*). Now, deoxygenated blood from the RV is shunted leftward to the LV and Ao, resulting in systemic cyanosis and the Eisenmenger complex. Note that the RV is now enlarged and severely hypertrophied. *Abbreviations*: PDA, patent ductus arteriosus; Ao, aorta; PA, pulmonary artery; LV, right ventricle; LA, left atrium; LV, left ventricle; VSD, ventricular septal defect; RV, right ventricle (*see page 177*).

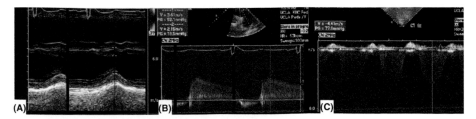

Figure 12.2 (**A**) ECHO M-mode of a patient with a large ASD and PAH. Note the large RV and flattened interventricular septum. (**B**) Pulse-wave Doppler signal form the pulmonary valve of the same patient. There is high-velocity pulmonary insufficiency with a gradient of 52 mmHg in early diastole. (**C**) Estimation of RV pressures by tricuspid regurgitation jet velocity. By the Bernouli's equation, this patient's RV and PA systolic pressure is 79 mmHg plus the central venous pressure. In this case it was suprasystemic. *Abbreviations*: ASD, atrial septal defect; PAH, pulmonary arterial hypertension; PA, pulmonary artery; RV, right ventricle (*see page 185*).

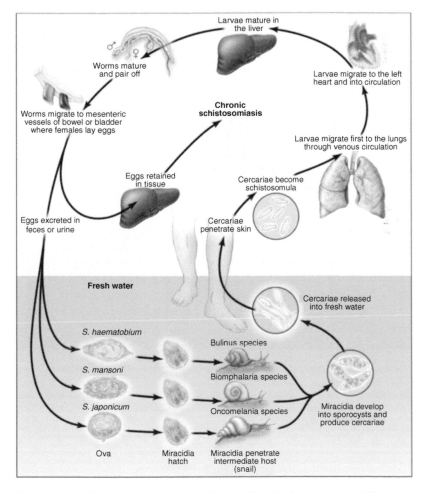

Figure 15.1 Life cycle of schistosome. *Source*: From Ref. 1 (*see page 215*).

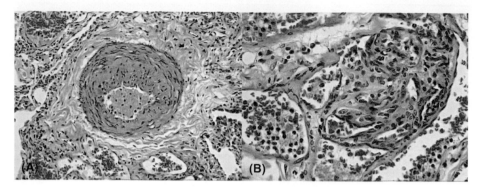

Figure 15.2 (**A**) Vascular granuloma associated with *Schistosoma* egg impaction. (**B**) Plexiform lesion from a patient with schistosomiasis-associated pulmonary hypertension (indistinguishable from those found in patients with idiopathic pulmonary arterial hypertension). *Source*: Courtesy of Prof Thais Mauad, Pathology Department, University of Sâo Paulo Medical School (*see page 217*).

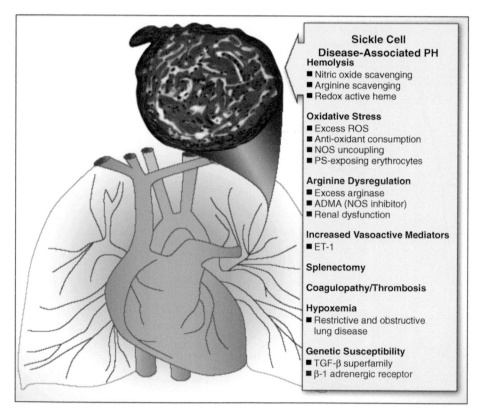

Figure 16.1 Mechanisms identified that contribute to the development of pulmonary hypertension in sickle cell disease. Hemolytic anemia is a dominant mechanism that leads to NO and arginine depletion, oxidant stress, and hypercoagulability (*see page 225*).

Doppler-Echocardiography

Brain Natriuretic Peptide

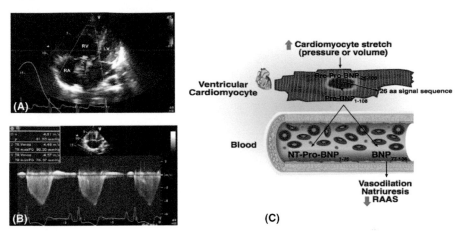

Figure 16.3 Screening modalities for pulmonary hypertension in sickle cell disease. (**A**) Four chamber view of the heart is shown from a patient with sickle cell disease and pulmonary hypertension, illustrating severe right ventricular (RV) and right atrial (RA) dilation and moderate tricuspid regurgitation (blue color Doppler). (**B**) The Doppler tracing reveals severe pulmonary hypertension, which reveals a jet velocity of more than 4 m/sec. (**C**) Mechanism of brain natriuretic peptide release from the cardiomyocyte and endocrine effect of the cleaved hormone on natriuresis, downregulation of the renin-angiotensin-aldosterone axis. This hormone can be quantified and used as a biomarker that reflects right ventricular volume or pressure overload for the diagnosis of pulmonary hypertension in sickle cell disease (*see page 227*).

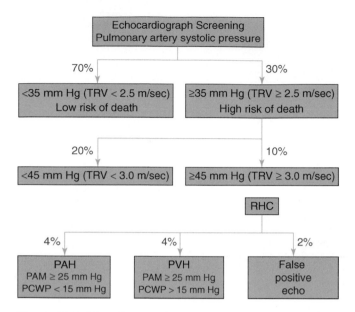

Figure 16.4 Flow diagram of prevalence estimates of pulmonary arterial hypertension and pulmonary venous hypertension diagnosed by right-heart catheterization based on screening data from the NIH. Percentages reflect absolute values from starting 100% of screened patients (*see page 228*).

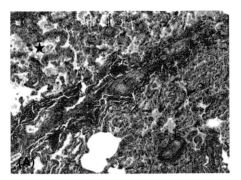
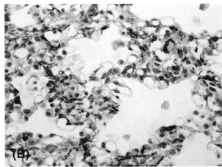

Figure 17.1 Pulmonary veins with obstructive venopathy in lungs of patients with pulmonary veno-occlusive disease and a case of PCH. (**A**) Longitudinally dissected septal vein with asymmetric intimal and partially occlusive fibrosis. Note the hemorrhage (*) due to the postcapillary bloc in the upper half of the photograph. Magnification 100×, Elastica van Gieson staining. (**B**) Excessively proliferating alveolar capillaries in a patient with PCH. Note the protrusion of ectatic lumina into the alveoli. Magnification 200×, anti-CD31 staining. *Abbreviation*: PCH, pulmonary capillary hemangiomatosis (*see page 238*).

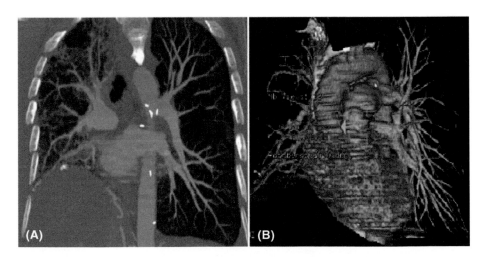

Figure 19.1 Computed tomography angiogram of an idiopathic pulmonary fibrosis patient after left single-lung transplant contrasting the effects of fibrosis on the native lung pulmonary vasculature with the normal vasculature in the allograft. *Source:* Courtesy of Steven D. Nathan, MD (*see page 267*).

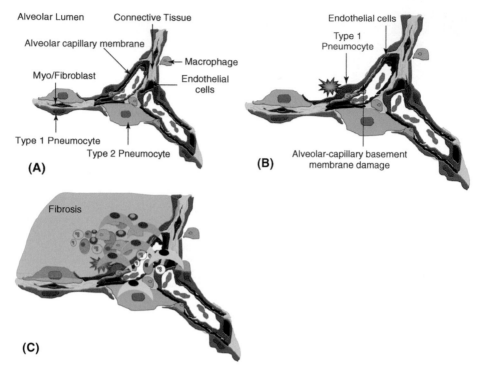

Figure 19.2 Pathogenesis of IPF. (**A**) Normal ACBM. (**B**) Severe injury to the type I pneumocyte and neighboring endothelial cell with loss of the ACBM. (**C**) Inflammation, remodeling, and fibrosis. *Abbreviation:* ACBM, alveolar-capillary basement membrane (*see page 269*).

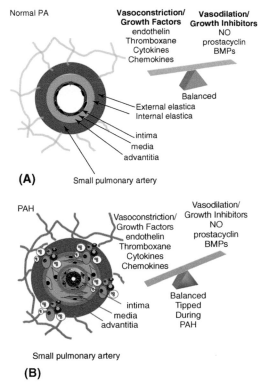

(A) Small pulmonary artery

(B)

Small pulmonary artery

Figure 19.3 Pathogenesis of PAH. (**A**) In the normal lung, there is a delicate balance of mediators that leads to normal vascular turnover (e.g., vasoconstrictors, cytokines, and growth factors vs. vasodilators and anti-inflammatory cytokines). (**B**) When there is some insult to the lung such as a vascular insult or an epithelial/endothelial injury as seen in IPF, there is a disproportionate over-expression of growth factors and vasoconstrictors. This imbalance of growth factors and vaso-constrictors leads to intimal expansion from endothelial cell hyperplasia with migration/proliferation of smooth muscle cells, and myo/fibroblasts as well as the recruitment of inflammatory cells that allows for extracellular matrix deposition. Similarly, the media expands secondary to inflammatory cells and the migration/proliferation of smooth muscle cells, and myo/fibroblasts causing more matrix deposition. The adventitia can also develop chronic inflammatory changes. Ultimately, the combination of these events leads to vessel narrowing and obliteration. *Abbreviations*: PAII, pulmonary arterial hypertension; NO, nitric oxide; BMPs, bone morphogenetic proteins (*see page 270*).

(A)

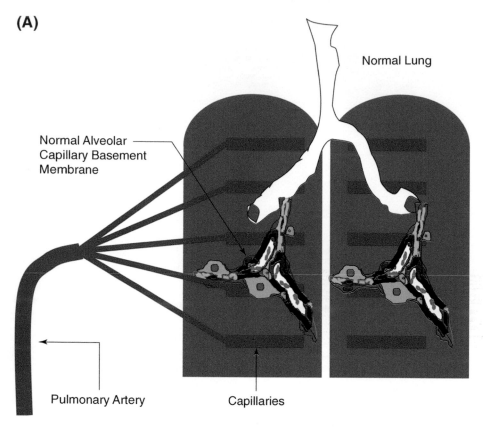

Normal Lung

Normal Alveolar
Capillary Basement
Membrane

Pulmonary Artery   Capillaries

Figure 19.4 Pathogenesis of PAH. (**A**) Normal lung without PAH. (**B**) With IPF there is vascular remodeling with obliteration and thrombosis of capillaries/venules causing a pressure head on the upstream pulmonary vessels (PA). This pressure and shear stress eventually leads to PAH. *Abbreviations*: PAH, pulmonary arterial hypertension; PA, pulmonary arterial; IPF, idiopathic pulmonary fibrosis (*see page 272*).

(B)

ILD with vascular remodeling
and vascular obliteration

Damaged ACBM with capillary
obliteration causing a pressure
head and shear stress on the PA

Pulmonary Artery Hypertension
now being obliterated

Figure 19.4 (*Continued*)

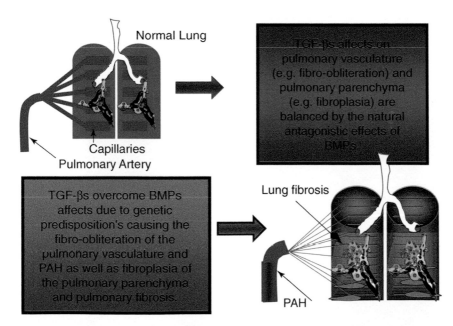

Normal Lung

TGF-βs affects on
pulmonary vasculature
(e.g. fibro-obliteration) and
pulmonary parenchyma
(e.g. fibroplasia) are
balanced by the natural
antagonistic effects of
BMPs

Capillaries
Pulmonary Artery

TGF-βs overcome BMPs
affects due to genetic
predisposition's causing the
fibro-obliteration of the
pulmonary vasculature and
PAH as well as fibroplasia of
the pulmonary parenchyma
and pulmonary fibrosis.

Lung fibrosis

PAH

Figure 19.5 Role of TGF-β superfamily during the pathogenesis of PH-associated ILD. TGF-β released during an initial insult to the lung causes the release of TGF-β that in certain individuals, due to a genetic predisposition, does not allow the BMPs to signal through the appropriate receptor (e.g., BMPR2) allowing for vessel obliteration and lung parenchyma fibroplasia. *Abbreviations*: TGF-β, transforming growth factor β; PAH, pulmonary arterial hypertension; PH, pulmonary hypertension; ILD, interstitial lung disease; BMPs, bone morphogenetic proteins; BMPR2, bone morphogenetic receptor type 2 (*see page 273*).

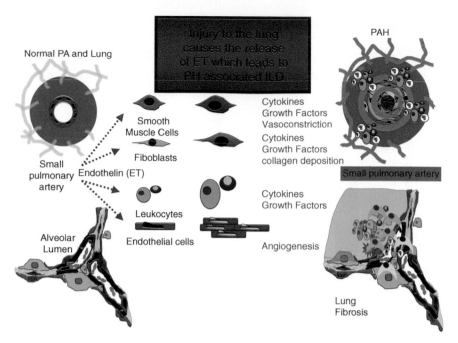

Figure 19.6 The role of receptor/endothelin interactions during PH-associated ILD. Endothelin interaction with specific receptors on smooth muscle cells, fibroblasts, endothelial cells, and leukocytes causes vessel fibro-obliteration and lung parenchyma fibrosis. *Abbreviations*: PH, pulmonary hypertension; ILD, interstitial lung disease; PAH, pulmonary arterial hypertension; ET, endothelin (*see page 275*).

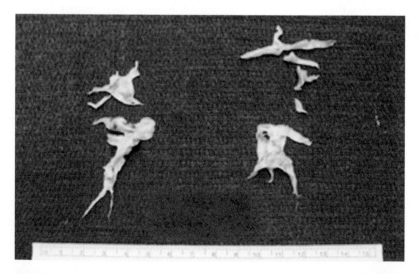

Figure 21.2 Chronic thromboembolic material endarterectomized from the patient whose angiogram is shown in Figure 1. Postoperatively, pulmonary hemodynamics were normal (*see page 316*).

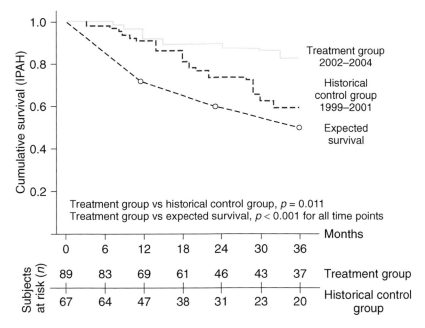

Figure 27.1 Survival of patients with idiopathic pulmonary arterial hypertension with goal-oriented therapy compared with a historical group, and the expected survival as calculated from the National Institutes of Health Registry equation. *Abbreviation*: IPAH, idiopathic pulmonary arterial hypertension (*see page 384*).

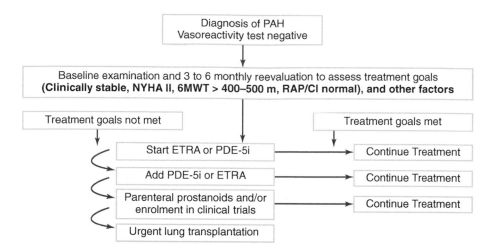

Figure 27.2 Proposal for a goal-oriented approach to PAH as it is currently (2008) used at Hannover Medical School, Hannover, Germany. *Abbreviations*: PAH, pulmonary arterial hypertension; NYHA, New York Heart Association; 6MWT, six-minute walk test; RAP, right atrial pressure; CI, cardiac index; ETRA, endothelin receptor antagonists; PDE-5i, phosphodiesterase-5 inhibitor (*see page 385*).

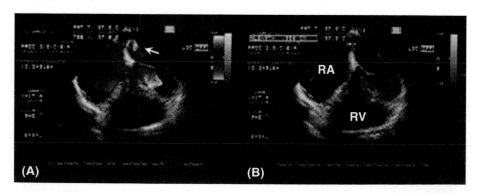

Figure 28.2 Transesophageal echocardiography to confirm (**A**) and measure the diameter (**B**) of the created interatrial defect. Note the right to-left shunt at the level of atrial septum (*arrow*). *Abbreviations*: RA, right atrium; RV, right ventricle (*see page 391*).

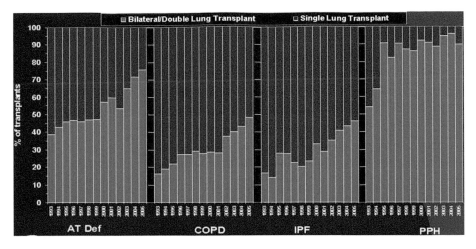

Figure 29.1 Adult lung transplantation: procedure type within indication, by year from 1993 to 2005. *Source*: From Ref. 2, with permission from Elsevier (*see page 402*).

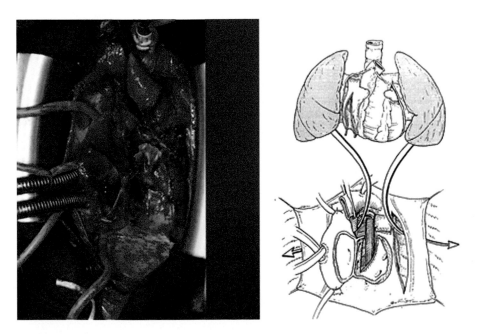

Figure 29.2 Photo and schematic drawing showing the principle of "en bloc" heart-lung transplantation (*see page 403*).

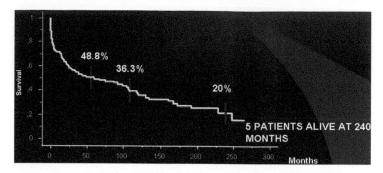

Figure 29.3 Overall survival in transplantation for PAH from 1986 to 2008 concerning 207 transplantations from Paris-Sud University series. *Abbreviation*: PAH, pulmonary arterial hypertension (*see page 404*).

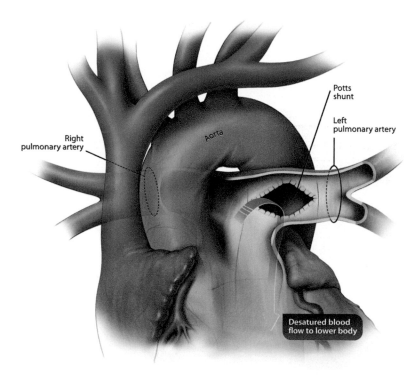

Figure 29.4 Potts procedure consists of performing a direct anastomosis between the left pulmonary artery and the descending thoracic aorta without any prosthetic interposition (*see page 405*).

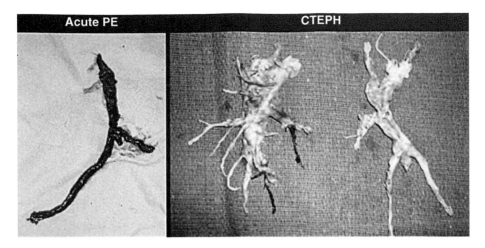

Figure 29.5 Material removed by endarterectomy from the right pulmonary artery (R) and the left one (L) compared with thrombus from acute pulmonary embolism (*see page 406*).

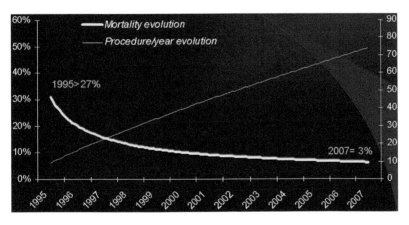

Figure 29.6 Experience and mortality correlated from Paris-Sud University series (*see page 409*).

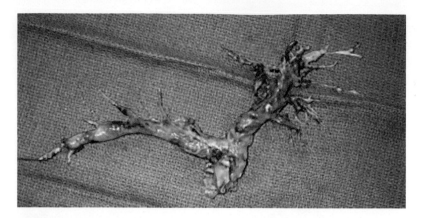

Figure 29.7 Specimen of angiosarcoma resected by endarterectomy (*see page 410*).

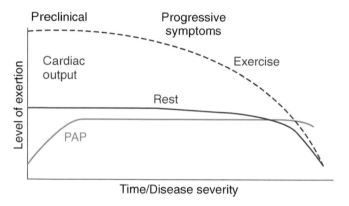

Figure 34.1 In the early phase of the disease, patients have an asymptomatic rise in PAP, with preservation of CO both at rest and on exertion. As the disease progresses, resting cardiac ouput remains stable, but the ability to raise stroke volume and CO on exercise is progressively impaired—resulting in progressive exertional symptoms. In the later stages of the disease, advanced right ventricular failure results in a fall in resting CO with fatigue and breathlessness at rest and right-heart failure. *Abbreviations*: PAP, pulmonary artery pressure; CO, cardiac output (*see page 464*).

association of schistosomiasis with PAH, however, schistosomiasis may also cause PAH in the absence of portal abnormalities. Currently, it is difficult to distinguish schistosomiasis-associated and idiopathic PAHs; even lung biopsy may be inconclusive. Serologies, by means of ELISA technique, may identify previous contact with various forms of *Schistosoma*, but utility is mainly in patients from nonendemic areas, since the massive population exposure lowers the value of serologies as a disease marker (34).

The cardiovascular investigation of schistosomiasis-associated PAH follows the same algorithm established for other forms of PAH. After clinical suspicion, an echocardiogram is performed; when signs of PAH are present, right-heart catheterization is mandatory to confirm an elevated pulmonary artery pressure and determine the main vascular territory implicated (pre or post capillary) (35). A recent study comparing consecutive, newly diagnosed patients with schistosomiasis-related PAH and idiopathic PAH from the same period of time showed that schistosomiasis patients displayed a more preserved hemodynamic profile at diagnosis. Furthermore, none of the schisosomiasis patients displayed acute vasodilation in response to nitric oxide challenge as compared with about 15% response in the idiopathic group (28). The prognosis of schistosomiasis-associated PAH also seems to be better than that of idiopathic PAH. Unpublished data from our group showed that independently of hemodynamic severity at baseline, patients with schistosomiasis-associated PAH had a better three-year survival than what would be expected for patients with idiopathic PAH, suggesting a more benign course of the disease. These findings are similar to what is believed for portopulmonary hypertension, as recently demonstrated by Le Pavec et al. (36), mainly considering the subgroup of patients without liver cirrhosis.

The response of schistosomiasis-associated PAH to specific pulmonary hypertension therapy requires further study. Preliminary reports noted improvement in right ventricular function with sildenafil (assessed by magnetic resonance imaging) (37). Data regarding endothelin receptor antagonists or prostanoids are lacking despite theoretical benefit. The use of high-dosage calcium channel blockers is not advised because of the presence of portal hypertension in virtually all cases. Conventional therapy for PAH such as diuretics and oxygen should be implemented as needed. Anticoagulation should be avoided because of the high potential of life-threatening bleeding due to the presence of esophageal varices.

The effect of antiparasitic treatment is variable. In schistosomiasis-associated hepatosplenic disease, response to antiparasitic treatment is greatly variable, ranging from no effect to resolution of periportal fibrosis (38). Antiparasitic treatment is not believed to have a significant effect on the pulmonary circulation, but at least one case report cited significant improvement in hemodynamics after treatment (39). Nevertheless, as the treatment of the parasite requires one-day treatment with praziquantel, a drug with few side effects, it is reasonable to treat all diagnosed patients, even in the absence of viable worms or eggs.

Schistosomiasis-associated PAH is potentially the leading cause of PAH worldwide. The knowledge about its pathophysiology is increasing, and soon the role of its multiple pathways, from the mechanical impaction of eggs within the pulmonary vessels and passing through inflammatory processes to the hemodynamic abnormalities associated with portal hypertension, may be elucidated, leading to the development of appropriate therapies.

References

1. Ross AGP, Bartley PB, Sleigh AC, et al. Current concepts: schistosomiasis. N Engl J Med 2002; 346(16):1212–1220.
2. Vennervald BJ, Dunne DW. Morbidity in schistosomiasis: an update. Curr Opin Infect Dis 2004; 17:439–447.
3. Gryseels B, Polman K, Clerinx J, et al. Human schistosomiasis. Lancet 2006; 368:1106–1118.
4. Chitsulo L, Engels D, Montresor A, et al. The global status of schistosomiasis and its control. Acta Trop 2000; 77:41–51.
5. Freedman DO, Kozarsky PK, Weld LH, et al. The global emerging infections sentinel network of the international society of travel medicine. J Travel Med 1999; 6:94–98
6. Schwartz E. Pulmonary schistosomiasis. Clin Chest Med 2002; 23:433–443.
7. Schistosomiasis Control Initiative. Home page. Available at: http://www.sci-ntds.org.
8. Webbe G. The parasites. The intermediate hosts and host-parasite relationships. The life-cycles of the parasites. In: Jordan P, Webbe G, eds. Schistosomiasis, Epidemiology, Treatment and Control. Bath, U.K.: The Piman Press, 1982:1–78.
9. Prata A. Esquistossomose mansonica. In: Veronessi R, Foccacia R, Dietze R, eds. Doenças Infecciosas Parasitárias. 8th ed. Rio de Janeiro, RJ, Brazil: Guanabara Koogan, 1991:838–855.
10. Meira JA. Esquistossomose mansônica. In: Meira DA, ed. Clínica De Doenças Tropicais E Infecciosas. Rio de Janeiro: Interlivros Edições, 1991:401–450.
11. Boros DL, Warren KS. Delayed hypersensitivity-type granuloma formation and dermal reaction induced and elicited by a soluble factor isolated from Schistossoma mansoni eggs. J Exp Med 1970; 132:488–507.
12. King CL. Initiation and regulation of disease in schistossomiasis. In: Mahmoud AAF, ed. Schistosomiasis. London: Imperial College Press, 2001:213–264.
13. Pedroso ERP. Alterações pulmonares associadas à esquistossomose mansonica. Mem Inst Oswaldo Cruz 1989; 84(suppl 1):46–57.
14. Conceicao MJ, Borges-Pereira J, Coura JR. A thirty years follow-up study on Schistosomiasis mansoni in a community of Minas Gerais, Brazil. Memorias do Instituto Oswaldo Cruz 2007; 102:1007–1009.
15. Gonçalves EC, Fonseca AP, Pittella JE. Frequency of schistosomiasis mansoni, of its clinicopathological forms and of the ectopic locations of the parasite in autopsies in Belo Horizonte, Brazil. J Trop Med Hyg 1995; 98(5):289–295.
16. Lapa MS, Ferreira EV, Jardim C, et al. Clinical characteristics of pulmonary hypertension patients in two reference centers in the city of Sao Paulo. Rev Assoc Med Bras 2006; 52:139–143.
17. Lapa M, Dias BA, Jardim C, et al. Cardio-pulmonary manifestations of hepatosplenic schistosomiasis. Circulation 2009; 119(11):1518–1523.
18. Shaw AP, Ghareeb A. The pathogenesis of pulmonary schistosomiasis in Egypt with special reference to Ayerza's disease. J Pathol Bacteriol 1938; 46:401–424.
19. Magalhaes Filho A. Pulmonary lesions in mice experimentally infected with Schistosoma mansoni. Am J Trop Med Hyg 1959; 8:527–535.
20. Chaves E. Pulmonary Schistosomiasis arteritis; morphological study of 54 cases with special reference to hypersensitivity reactions. Hospital (Rio J) 1964; 66:1335–1346.
21. Chaves E. Plexiform lesions in chronic cor pulmonale in schistosomiasis. Hospital (Rio J) 1965; 68:635–645.
22. Chaves E. Pathology of pulmonary endarteritis obliterans in Manson's schistosomiasis. An Inst Med Trop (Lisb) 1965; 22:171–177.
23. Chaves E. The pathology of the arterial pulmonary vasculature in manson's schistosomiasis. Dis Chest 1966; 50:72–77.
24. Dorfmuller P, Perros F, Balabanian K, et al. Inflammation in pulmonary arterial hypertension. Eur Respir J 2003; 22:358–363.

25. de CI, Tompson G, de S, et al. Pulmonary hypertension in schistosomiasis. Br Heart J 1962; 24:363–371.
26. Pozzan G, Souza R, Jardim C, et al. Histopathological features of pulmonary vascular disease in chronic Schistosoma mansoni infection are not different from those in idiopathic pulmonary hypertension. In: American Thoracic Society International Conference, Toronto, 2008:A443.
27. Pereira GA Jr., Bestetti RB, Leite MP, et al. Portopulmonary hypertension syndrome in schistosomiasis mansoni. Trans R Soc Trop Med Hyg 2002; 96(4):427–428.
28. Fernandes CJC, Jardim C, Lapa M, et al. Hemodynamics in pulmonary hypertension associated to schistosomiasis. In: European Respiratory Society Annual Congress, 2007:E3281.
29. Zhou YG, Yang Z, Li DJ. The experimental study on pathological changes of pulmonary tissues in portal hypertensive rabbits with schistosomal cirrhosis [Chinese]. Zhonghua Wai Ke Za Zhi 2005; 43(9):587–590.
30. Fishman AP. Clinical classification of pulmonary hypertension. Clin Chest Med 2001; 22:385–391.
31. Simmoneau G, Nazzareno G, Rubin L, et al. Clinical classification of pulmonary hypertension. J Am Coll Cardiol 2004; 43(suppl):5S–12S.
32. Figueiredo C, Souza R, Ota JS, et al. Pulmonary hypertension in Schistosomiasis: a chest CT study. Am J Respir Crit Care Med 2004; 169:A174.
33. Hatz C, Jenkins JM, Ali QM, et al. A review of the literature on the use of ultrasonography in schistosomiasis with special reference to its use in field studies. 2. Schistosoma mansoni. Acta Trop 1992; 51(1):15–28.
34. Igreja RP, Matos JA, Goncalves MM, et al. Schistosoma mansoni-related morbidity in a low-prevalence area of Brazil: a comparison between egg excretors and seropositive non-excretors. Ann Trop Med Parasitol 2007; 101(7):575–584.
35. Galie N, Torbicki A, Barst R, et al. Guidelines on diagnosis and treatment of pulmonary arterial hypertension. The task force on diagnosis and treatment of pulmonary arterial hypertension of the European Society of Cardiology. Eur Heart J 2004; 25:2243–2278.
36. Le Pavec J, Souza R, Herve P, et al. Portopulmonary hypertension: survival and prognostic factors. Am J Respir Crit Care Med 2008; 178(6):637–643.
37. Loureiro R, Mendes A, Bandeira A, et al. Oral sildenafil improves functional status and cardiopulmonary hemodynamics in patientes with severe pulmonary hypertension secondary to chronic pulmonary schistosomiasis: a cardiac magnetic resonance study. New Orleans: American Heart Association, 2004:2569.
38. Richter J. Evolution of schistosomiasis-induced pathology after therapy and interruption of exposure to schistosomes: a review of ultrasonographic studies. Acta Trop 2000; 77:111–131.
39. Bourée P, Piveteau J, Gerbal JL, et al. Pulmonary arterial hypertension due to bilharziasis. Apropos of a case due to Schistosoma haematobium having been cured by praziquantel [French]. Bull Soc Pathol Exot 1990; 83(1):66–71.

16

Pulmonary Hypertension in Sickle Cell Disease

MARK T. GLADWIN

University of Pittsburgh Medical Center, Pittsburgh, Pennsylvania, U.S.A.

I. Introduction

Sickle cell disease (SCD) is one of the most common monogenetic disorders in the world. The autosomal recessive transmission of a single-point mutation in the β-globin gene, namely the substitution of valine for glutamic acid at position 6 in the β-globin chain, results in the production of a mutant hemoglobin called hemoglobin S (1–4). While 8% of the African American population are heterozygotes, approximately 1 out of 600 have homozygous SCD at birth. In sub-Saharan Africa, an estimated 40% to 60% of individuals are heterozygotes suggesting that 1% to 4% of babies born in this region have the disease (5). Hemoglobin mutations producing SCD are also widespread in the southeastern United States, Central and South America, India, and the Arabian Peninsula.

The mutant hemoglobin, Hb S, behaves normally when oxygenated but polymerizes upon deoxygenation. These polymers make the erythrocyte rigid, distort its shape, and produce both oxidant stress and structural membrane damage that alters rheology, impairs blood flow through the microvasculature, and ultimately leads to hemolysis and vaso-occlusive episodes. The rate and extent of hemoglobin S polymerization is a primary determinant of disease severity (6). Polymerization is proportional to the degree of deoxygenation, the time the hemoglobin is deoxygenated, and the intracellular hemoglobin S concentration to the 34th power (2). Fetal hemoglobin does not participate in polymer formation and directly inhibits polymerization, effectively reducing the concentration of hemoglobin S and the extent of polymerization. Understanding these major mechanistic determinants of polymerization informs about the basic principles underlying the medical management of a hospitalized or critically ill patient (Table 1).

While patients with SCD suffer myriad end-organ complications, the two most common acute events are vaso-occlusive pain crisis, caused by physical and adhesive entrapment of the hemoglobin S containing red cells in the microcirculation, and the acute chest syndrome (ACS), a lung injury syndrome analogous to the acute respiratory distress syndrome (ARDS) (7). Patients now living beyond their third decades of life are developing a progressive vasculopathy and accumulating major end-organ chronic complications of SCD such as chronic renal failure, hemorrhagic and nonhemorrhagic stroke, avascular necrosis of the bones, and a remarkably high prevalence of pulmonary arterial hypertension (PAH) (8,9). From a clinical perspective, epidemiological studies indicate that most patients with SCD die of pulmonary complications, namely the ACS and PAH (4,8,10).

Table 1 Therapeutic Modulation of Hemoglobin S Polymerization

Limit hemoglobin S deoxygenation

- Increase hemoglobin S oxygenation by providing therapeutic oxygen
- Increase hemoglobin S oxygen affinity (increasing pH, controlling fever)

Limit the time hemoglobin S is deoxygenated

- Maximize red cell transit time in microcirculation by maintaining an adequate cardiac output
- Limit inflammatory insults, such as infection, that increase erythrocyte adhesion in the microvasculature

Reduce intracellular hemoglobin S concentration

- Maintain red cell hydration (using hypo-osmotic 5% dextrose in water or 5% dextrose in half-normal saline for fluid replacement)
- Increase hemoglobin F levels by pharmacological therapy (hydroxyurea)

II. Etiology of Pulmonary Hypertension in SCD

A. Hemolysis-Associated Endothelial Dysfunction, Vasculopathy, and Hypercoagulability

The release of hemoglobin into plasma during intravascular hemolysis potently scavenges nitric oxide (NO) (11). Nitric oxide is a critical signaling molecule produced by the endothelium that regulates basal vasodilator tone, inhibits platelet and hemostatic activation and inhibits transcriptional expression of adhesion molecules such as vascular cell adhesion molecule 1 (VCAM-1) (12–16). The half-life of NO in the vasculature is very short because of rapid reactions with red cell hemoglobin to form methemoglobin and nitrate (17). In fact, the vasodilator activity of NO is possible only because all of the hemoglobin is compartmentalized within erythrocytes, which creates diffusional barriers for NO entry into the red blood cells and reduces the scavenging of NO with intracellular hemoglobin (18). The release of hemoglobin into plasma during hemolysis disrupts these diffusion barriers and potently inhibits all NO bioactivity, leading to a clinical state of endothelial dysfunction and NO resistance (4,19,20).

Hemolysis also releases erythrocyte arginase-1 into plasma. Arginase metabolizes plasma arginine into ornithine, reducing the required substrate for NO synthesis and compounding the reduction in NO bioavailability in SCD (21) Accordingly, high arginase activity in plasma has been associated with a higher risk of PAH and death in patients with SCD (21).

Chronic NO depletion may contribute to vasoconstriction, proliferative vasculopathy, activation of endothelial adhesion molecules such as VCAM-1, activation of platelets, and the production of the potent vasoconstrictor and mitogen, endothelin (22). Because NO is a potent inhibitor of platelet activation, this pathway is activated in patients with SCD secondary to direct inhibition of NO by plasma hemoglobin and increased intracellular platelet expression of arginase (23,24). Clinical studies of patients with SCD reveal correlations between the intrinsic rate of intravascular hemolysis and the levels of procoagulant factors in blood (25).

A central risk factor for the development of PAH in patients with SCD is the rate of chronic intravascular hemolysis, characterized by low steady state hemoglobin levels, high lactate dehydrogenase (LDH) levels, high bilirubin levels, and high reticulocyte counts (4,8,26). The association between high plasma hemoglobin and arginase-1 levels has now been reported in other hemolytic diseases such as thalassemia, paroxysmal hemoglobinuria, and malaria, suggesting that hemolysis may represent a common mechanism of disease for the chronic hereditary and acquired hemolytic anemias (22,27,28). Pulmonary hypertension is now a recognized frequent complication of all chronic hereditary or acquired hemolytic anemias, including thalassemia intermedia and major, paroxysmal nocturnal hemoglobinuria, spherocytosis, stomatocytosis, pyruvate kinase deficiency, alloimmune hemolytic anemia, glucose 6 phosphate dehydrogenase (G6PD) deficiency, and the microangiopathic hemolytic anemias (22,29). A constellation of complications are more common in patients with SCD who suffer from higher rates of intravascular hemolysis. These complications are also observed to a similar or lesser extent in other hemolytic diseases and include PAH, priapism and cutaneous leg ulceration, suggesting that intravascular hemolysis contributes to a subphenotype of vasculopathic complications (8,9,26,30,31).

A state of resistance to NO mediated by cell-free plasma hemoglobin and the development of PAH has also been shown in transgenic mouse models of SCD and spherocytosis and in mouse models of alloimmune hemolysis and malaria (32,33).

In addition to intravascular hemolysis, other mechanisms contribute to the development of PAH in patients with SCD and should be identified and treated (Fig. 1). Iron overload, hepatitis C, or nodular regenerative hyperplasia produces liver dysfunction, which may lead to portopulmonary hypertension (8). Chronic renal failure, a common complication of SCD, is an additional risk factor for the development of PAH (8,34). In situ thrombosis and pulmonary emboli are often identified clinically and at autopsy (35). This may be a particular risk factor in patients with functional or post-surgical splenectomy (36,37). Chronic thromboembolic pulmonary hypertension occurs in approximately 5% of patients with SCD and severe PAH (Fig. 2) (38). Patients with sickle cell syndromes, such as hemoglobin SC disease (who have a low level of hemolysis, higher hemoglobin levels, and normal LDH levels), should be evaluated carefully for other etiologies for PAH, such as thromboembolic disease, liver disease secondary to iron overload or hepatitis C infection, and human immunodeficiency virus (HIV) infection.

III. Epidemiology and Screening for Pulmonary Hypertension in SCD

A. Echocardiographic Studies in SCD

Pulmonary hypertension is an increasingly recognized complication of SCD. Three prospective adult screening studies have reported that 20% of the population has mild PAH, defined by a pulmonary artery systolic pressure (PASP) greater than 35 mmHg (the upper limit of normal PASP is 32 mmHg); further, 10% of patients with SCD have

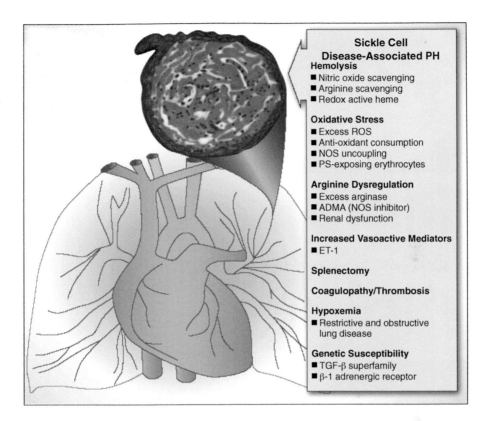

Figure 1 (*See color insert*) Mechanisms identified that contribute to the development of pulmonary hypertension in sickle cell disease. Hemolytic anemia is a dominant mechanism that leads to NO and arginine depletion, oxidant stress, and hypercoagulability.

moderate to severe PAH, defined by a PASP greater than 45 mmHg (8,34,39). Despite pulmonary pressure increases that are much lower than those observed in patients with idiopathic or hereditable PAH, the prospective risk of death associated with even mild PAH is extremely high (8,34,39–42).

It is recommended that adult patients with SCD be screened for PAH using transthoracic Doppler echocardiography (8). The thin body habitus of homozygous hemoglobin S patients along with dilated and hyperdyamic heart chambers allows for facile detection of the regurgitation of blood backward across the tricuspid valve during right ventricular systole (Fig. 3). This tricuspid regurgitant jet velocity (TRV) is used to calculate the right ventricular and pulmonary artery systolic pressures (PASP $\approx$ 4TRV^2) after adding an estimate of the central venous pressure. In patients with SCD, this estimate correlates well with measured PASP by right-heart catheterization (8).

TRV $\geq$2.5 m/sec is approximately two standard deviations above normal. For patients less than 40 years of age the normal reference mean Doppler echocardiographic estimated PASP is 27.5 $\pm$ 4.2 with a 95% confidence interval of 19.3 to 35.5 mmHg

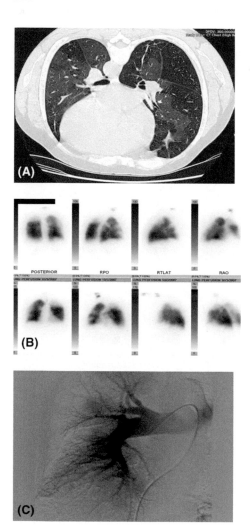

Figure 2 Chronic thromboembolic pulmonary hypertension in a patient with sickle cell disease. Evaluation of a 48-year-old male with sickle cell disease (hemoglobin SC phenotype) revealed a mosaic perfusion pattern on (**A**) a high-resolution CT scan of the chest, (**B**) a high-probability lung perfusion scan, and (**C**) a pulmonary artery angiogram that revealed main pulmonary artery enlargement with peripheral vascular pruning and hypoperfusion.

(4,43). In other populations, a more traditional definition of PAH would be a TRV ≥3.0 m/sec. However, in SCD patients, the risk of death associated with high PASP rises linearly, and even values between 2.5 and 2.9 m/sec are associated with a high risk of death with an odds ratio for death of 4.4 (95% CI, 1.6–12.2; $p < 0.001$); a TRV ≥3 m/sec is associated with an odds ratio for death of 10.6 (95% CI, 3.3–33.6; $p < 0.001$) (8,34,39).

Doppler-Echocardiography   Brain Natriuretic Peptide

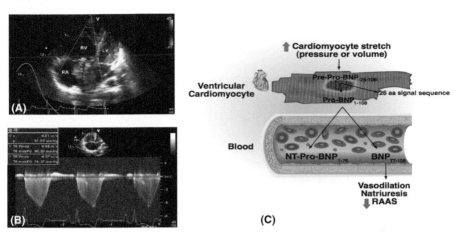

Figure 3 (*See color insert*) Screening modalities for pulmonary hypertension in sickle cell disease. (**A**) Four chamber view of the heart is shown from a patient with sickle cell disease and pulmonary hypertension, illustrating severe right ventricular (RV) and right atrial (RA) dilation and moderate tricuspid regurgitation (blue color Doppler). (**B**) The Doppler tracing reveals severe pulmonary hypertension, which reveals a jet velocity of more than 4 m/sec. (**C**) Mechanism of brain natriuretic peptide release from the cardiomyocyte and endocrine effect of the cleaved hormone on natriuresis, downregulation of the renin-angiotensin-aldosterone axis. This hormone can be quantified and used as a biomarker that reflects right ventricular volume or pressure overload for the diagnosis of pulmonary hypertension in sickle cell disease.

B. Left-Sided Heart Disease in SCD

Left-sided heart disease in SCD is primarily due to diastolic dysfunction (present in ~13% of patients), although cases of systolic dysfunction and mitral or aortic valvular disease can occur as well (the latter present in ~2% of patients) (8). The presence of diastolic dysfunction alone in SCD patients is an independent risk factor for mortality (44). Patients with both pulmonary vascular disease and echocardiographic evidence of diastolic dysfunction are at a particularly high risk of death (odds ratio for death of 12.0; 95% CI, 3.8–38.1; $p < 0.001$) (44).

C. Elevations in Brain Natriuretic Peptide in SCD

A second screening modality utilizes the plasma levels of brain natriuretic peptide (BNP), released from the cardiomyocyte during pressure or volume stretch (Fig. 3) (42). Antibody-based detection assays of the N-terminal fragment or the active BNP have been used to diagnose left-heart disease. In patients with both idiopathic and sickle cell–associated PAH the levels of BNP correlate with increasing pulmonary vascular resistance and prospectively determined risk of death (42). An analysis of the levels of

N-terminal BNP at study entry from both the NIH sickle cell pulmonary hypertension screening study and the Multicenter Study of Hydroxyurea revealed that approximately 30% of patients with SCD in both cohorts had levels above the 75th percentile (>160 ng/mL) and were at greatest risk of death (risk ratio, 5.1; 95% CI, 2.1–12.5; $p < 0.001$) (42).

D. Findings on Right-Heart Catheterization

Right-heart catheterization studies of patients with SCD and PAH reveal a hyperdynamic state similar to the hemodynamics characteristic of portopulmonary hypertension (38). The mean pulmonary artery pressure in patients with SCD and PAH is approximately 40 mmHg and pulmonary vascular resistance approximately 250 dyne.sec/cm^5. The relatively low pulmonary vascular resistance is caused by the high cardiac output of anemia. Approximately 60% of catheterized patients with a TRV greater than 3.0 m/sec meet the definition of PAH, indicating that vasculopathy primarily involves the pulmonary arterial system. In the other 40% of subjects, the left ventricular end-diastolic pressures are greater than 15 mmHg, indicating a component of left ventricular diastolic dysfunction (38).

Figure 4 reveals a flow diagram of prevalence estimates of PAH and pulmonary venous hypertension diagnosed by right-heart catheterization based on screening data from the NIH.

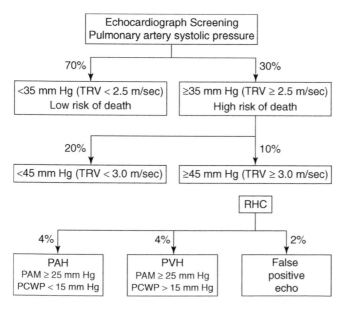

Figure 4 (*See color insert*) Flow diagram of prevalence estimates of pulmonary arterial hypertension and pulmonary venous hypertension diagnosed by right-heart catheterization based on screening data from the NIH. Percentages reflect absolute values from starting 100% of screened patients.

Table 2 Management of the Acute Chest Syndrome

Oxygen therapy to maintain arterial hemoglobin oxygen saturations above 95%
Pain control and incentive spirometry to reduce chest wall splinting and pulmonary atelectasis
Asthma therapy if indicated
Close clinical observation, particularly pO_2/FiO_2 ratio: early diagnosis of worsening respiratory function

Empiric antibiotics

- Considering the high prevalence of atypical bacteria and viral infections, empiric coverage should include a macrolide or quinolone
- Consider the regional and seasonal risk of methicillin-resistant *Staphylococcus aureus* and Influenza A or B and tailor therapy accordingly

Transfusion therapy

- Acute red cell transfusion during the acute chest syndrome increases hemoglobin oxygen saturation and may rapidly resolve the pulmonary event (10, 47).
- The main indication for transfusion therapy in ACS is worsening respiratory function as indicated by falling pO_2/FiO_2 ratio or by some other index of alveolar-arterial oxygen gradient.
- The National Acute Chest Syndrome Study Group found no significant differences in postoperative vaso-occlusive outcomes between simple preoperative transfusion or a pre-operative red cell exchange (erythrocytopheresis), suggesting that either approach is acceptable therapy in mild to moderate ACS cases (10).
- To avoid the effects of viscosity on increasing the risk of vaso-occlusion, it is not recommended to increase the hemoglobin level higher than 11 g/dL after transfusion. However, most Hb SS patients with the acute chest syndrome are anemic with a mean hemoglobin level of 7.7 g/dL (10). This allows for the transfusion of 2–4 units of packed red cells over 24–48 hours without complication. In severely anemic patients, the transfusion of 4 units of packed red cells provides an approximately equivalent reduction in the percentage of blood Hb S as a 5-unit erythrocytopheresis.
- Patients with high initial hemoglobin concentrations (≥ 9 g/dL), or patients with more severe disease should receive erythrocytopheresis. However, while awaiting erythrocytapheresis, severe ACS patients should be given 2 to 3 RBC units as simple transfusions.
- In severe patients, we recommend serial transfusions to maintain a hemoglobin level between 10 and 11.
- The major complication of transfusion therapy is a delayed transfusion reaction (DHTR). Many patients with sickle cell disease have developed alloantibodies directed against minor red cell membrane antigens such as Rh and Kell. The antibodies may not be detectable initially but upon transfusion the memory plasma cells will begin producing antibodies, much like a booster response to a vaccine. This results in delayed hemolytic anemia 3–10 days after transfusion, often accompanied by a phenomenon called bystander hemolysis, which produces severe drops in hemoglobin to levels as low as 2–3 g/dL. The most consistent and earliest symptom of a DHTR in sickle patients is vaso-occlusive pain so that a pain crisis developing in the week or so after transfusions should raise the suspicion of this complication. In an attempt to prevent delayed hemolytic transfusion reactions, most sickle cell centers recommend routine matching for Rh and Kell antigens, which will reduce alloantibody formation by greater than 50%.

Table 2 Management of the Acute Chest Syndrome (*Continued*)

Investigational therapeutic agents

- Treatment with corticosteroids has been shown to reduce the severity of pain and length of hospitalization, but this therapy is complicated by a high rate of rebound hospitalization (48, 49). On-going studies are evaluating strategies to maintain the beneficial effects of corticosteroids while limiting rebound pain and readmission using slow tapering protocols.
- Inhaled nitric oxide (NO) has been shown in case studies to improve oxygenation and reduce pulmonary hypertension in mechanically ventilated patients with severe lung injury and active clinical trials for vaso-occlusive crisis are on-going (50–52).
- Complicating right-heart failure in patients with the acute chest syndrome should be identified and clinically indicated therapy with sildenafil, intravenous prostacyclin, or inhaled NO considered.

Prevention of acute chest syndrome

- Patients with a history of acute chest syndrome should be treated with hydroxyurea in the outpatient setting. The induction of fetal hemoglobin by relatively low doses of hydroxyurea (15–35 mg/kg) has been shown to reduce the risk of developing the acute chest syndrome by ~50% (53, 54).
- In patients failing hydroxyurea, a chronic transfusion program should be considered. The Stroke Prevention (STOP) trial demonstrated that chronic transfusion was highly effective in reducing the incidence of acute chest syndrome compared with the standard of care arm (2.2 vs. 15.7 events per 100 patient-years, $p = 0.0001$) (55).
- Allogeneic bone marrow transplantation is a reasonable option in children with recurrent acute chest syndrome (56)

E. Acute Rises in Pulmonary Pressures During Vaso-occlusive Pain Crisis and During the Acute Chest Syndrome

It is increasingly clear that pulmonary pressures rise acutely during vaso-occlusive crisis and even more during ACS (45). A recent study examined 84 consecutive hospitalized patients with the ACS (46). Remarkably, only 40% had normal PASP (TRV of less than 2.5 m/sec) and in 60% the pressures were elevated. A full 13% of patients manifested right-heart failure, and this subgroup had the highest risk for mechanical ventilation and death. These data suggest that acute PAH and right-heart dysfunction represent a major comorbidity during the ACS, and that right-heart failure should be considered in patients presenting with the ACS. A detailed treatment guide for the ACS is outlined in Table 2.

IV. Treatment

Treatment strategies for PAH in patients with SCD are outlined in Table 3. However, note that evidence-based guidelines for the management of PAH in patients with SCD have not yet been established. Our recommendations are based on the PAH literature, case reports (57,58), and small open-label studies (59,60).

Table 3 Treatment of Pulmonary Hypertension in Sickle Cell Disease

Mild pulmonary hypertension

- Patients with borderline or mild pulmonary hypertension, defined by a tricuspid regurgitant jet velocity of 2.5–2.9 m/sec, are clearly at greater risk of death. Therefore, it is recommended to intensify proven therapies specific for sickle cell disease.
- Because episodes of vaso-occlusive pain crisis and the acute chest syndrome produce acute increases in pulmonary pressures and right-heart failure, patients should be treated with hydroxyurea to increase fetal hemoglobin and reduce these events (45, 53, 54).
- Therapy for iron overload and for nocturnal or exercise hemoglobin oxygen desaturation is recommended.

Moderate to severe pulmonary hypertension

- For patients with a tricuspid regurgitant jet velocity of ≥3.0 m/sec, more aggressive evaluation and therapy is indicated.
- Pulmonary thromboembolism should be excluded and anti-coagulation considered. We have found that ~5% of our patients with pulmonary hypertension have complicating pulmonary embolism and may suffer from thromboembolic pulmonary hypertension (38).
- If coexisting renal insufficiency limits hydroxyurea dosing and efficacy, the addition of erythropoietin to hydroxyurea (use of erythropoietin alone is risky) can increase hydroxyurea responsiveness and hemoglobin levels (61).
- Simple or exchange transfusion therapy should be considered if hydroxyurea therapy is not effective.
- We recommend right-heart catheterization in all patients with moderate to severe pulmonary hypertension as identified on echocardiogram to determine if this is caused by pulmonary vascular disease or left-heart disease, i.e. diastolic dysfunction, systolic dysfunction, or mitral valve disease, or both (44).
- Patients with pulmonary arterial hypertension should be referred for treatment in multicenter trials of specific pulmonary vasodilators. Phase I–II trials of sildenafil in patients with sickle cell disease and pulmonary hypertension show that this agent reduces pulmonary pressures, reduces N-terminal brain natriuretic peptide levels, and increases six-minute walk distance (59). An NHLBI-sponsored multicenter trial of sildenafil is currently underway in the United States and the European Union.
- Other agents such as endothelin receptor antagonists; intravenous, inhaled, and subcutaneous prostanoids; and L-arginine have all been used and appear efficacious (62).
- It is critical to develop close collaborations between hematologists expert in sickle cell disease and pulmonary hypertension specialists for the comprehensive management of these medically complicated patients.

General recommendations include the intensification of specific hematological therapy for SCD, treatment of causal factors or associated diseases, general supportive measures, and use of PAH-specific pharmacological agents (4)

In the absence of clinical guidelines and placebo-controlled therapeutic trials for the evaluation and treatment of PAH in the sickle cell population, a diagnostic and therapeutic approach based on expert opinion is summarized below.

A. Patients with Mild PAH (TRV 2.5–2.9 m/sec)

On the basis of the fact that pulmonary pressures rise during acute vaso-occlusive pain crisis and during the ACS, proven treatments that control these complications are warranted.

Hydroxyurea treatment at the maximum tolerated dose, as defined by the Multicenter Study of Hydroxyurea, with erythropoietin therapy considered if reticulocytopenia limits hydroxyurea therapy. Erythropoietin is often needed in combination with hydroxyurea because many of the adult patients presenting with PAH have coexistent renal insufficiency that limits hydroxyurea dose escalation (61).

Monthly transfusion therapy may be considered for patients with poor responses to hydroxyurea, accompanied by iron-chelation therapy, if indicated.

Consultation with a pulmonologist or a cardiologist experienced in PAH is recommended, the latter especially if the echocardiogram shows evidence of left or right ventricular dysfunction.

Identify and treat risk factors associated with PAH such as rest, exercise and nocturnal hypoxemia, sleep apnea, pulmonary thromboembolic disease, restrictive lung disease/fibrosis, left ventricular systolic and diastolic dysfunction, severe anemia, and iron overload.

B. Patients with TRV ≥ 3 m/sec

Follow Recommendations for TRV 2.5–2.9 m/sec

Right-heart catheterization to confirm diagnosis and to directly assess left ventricular diastolic and systolic function.

Rule out chronic thromboemolic pulmonary hypertension with a CT pulmonary angiogram, ventilation/perfusion (V/Q) scan, and/or pulmonary angiogram.

Consider systemic anticoagulation based on data that this improves outcomes in patients with primary PAH with in situ thrombosis and the fact that at autopsy patients with SCD often have in situ thrombosis.

Consider specific therapy with selective pulmonary vasodilator and remodeling drugs if the patient has PAH defined by right-heart catheterization and exercise limitation defined by a low six-minute walk distance. Drugs that are FDA approved for primary PAH include the endothelin receptor antagonists (bosentan and ambrisentan), prostaglandin-based therapy (epoprostenol, treprostinol, and iloprost), and the phosphodiesterase 5 inhibitors (sildenafil). Treatment with oral sildenafil improved exercise tolerance and PAH in patients with SCD (59,60) and thalassemia (57,58). No published randomized studies in the SCD population exist for any of these agents, although a multicenter placebo-controlled trial of sildenafil for PAH of SCD is currently underway (Walk-PHaSST).

V. Conclusions

Pulmonary hypertension has now been identified as the leading cause of death in adult patients with SCD. It is also now appreciated that patients who die of the ACS often develop acute increases in pulmonary pressures and develop right-heart failure, indicating a major interaction between these clinical entities. Identification, prevention, and expert management of these complications by both hematologists and pulmonologists represents a new challenge for the medical field as this population ages and expands worldwide.

References

1. Platt OS. The acute chest syndrome of sickle cell disease. N Engl J Med 2000; 342: 1904–1907.
2. Bunn HF. Pathogenesis and treatment of sickle cell disease. N Engl J Med 1997; 337: 762–769.
3. Steinberg MH. Management of sickle cell disease. N Engl J Med 1999; 340:1021–1030.
4. Gladwin MT, Vichinsky E. Pulmonary complications of sickle cell disease. N Engl J Med 2008; 359:2254–2265.
5. Aliyu ZY, Gordeuk V, Sachdev V, et al. Prevalence and risk factors for pulmonary artery systolic hypertension among sickle cell disease patients in Nigeria. Am J Hematol 2008; 83:485–490.
6. Brittenham GM, Schechter AN, Noguchi CT. Hemoglobin S polymerization: primary determinant of the hemolytic and clinical severity of the sickling syndromes. Blood 1985; 65:183–189.
7. Platt OS, Brambilla DJ, Rosse WF, et al. Mortality in sickle cell disease. Life expectancy and risk factors for early death [see comments]. N Engl J Med 1994; 330:1639–1644.
8. Gladwin MT, Sachdev V, Jison ML, et al. Pulmonary hypertension as a risk factor for death in patients with sickle cell disease. N Engl J Med 2004; 350:886–895.
9. Kato GJ, Gladwin MT, Steinberg MH. Deconstructing sickle cell disease: reappraisal of the role of hemolysis in the development of clinical subphenotypes. Blood Rev 2007; 21: 37–47.
10. Vichinsky EP, Neumayr LD, Earles AN, et al, National Acute Chest Syndrome Study Group. Causes and outcomes of the acute chest syndrome in sickle cell disease. N Engl J Med 2000; 342:1855–1865.
11. Reiter CD, Wang X, Tanus-Santos JE, et al. Cell-free hemoglobin limits nitric oxide bio-availability in sickle-cell disease. Nat Med 2002; 8:1383–1389.
12. Furchgott RF, Zawadzki JV. The obligatory role of endothelial cells in the relaxation of arterial smooth muscle by acetylcholine. Nature 1980; 288:373–376.
13. Ignarro LJ, Buga GM, Wood KS, et al. Endothelium-derived relaxing factor produced and released from artery and vein is nitric oxide. Proc Natl Acad Sci U S A 1987; 84:9265–9269.
14. Palmer RM, Ashton DS, Moncada S. Vascular endothelial cells synthesize nitric oxide from L-arginine. Nature 1988; 333:664–666.
15. Panza JA, Casino PR, Kilcoyne CM, et al. Role of endothelium-derived nitric oxide in the abnormal endothelium-dependent vascular relaxation of patients with essential hypertension. Circulation 1993; 87:1468–1474.
16. De Caterina R, Libby P, Peng HB, et al. Nitric oxide decreases cytokine-induced endothelial activation. Nitric oxide selectively reduces endothelial expression of adhesion molecules and proinflammatory cytokines. J Clin Invest 1995; 96:60–68.
17. Doherty DH, Doyle MP, Curry SR, et al. Rate of reaction with nitric oxide determines the hypertensive effect of cell-free hemoglobin. Nat Biotechnol 1998; 16:672–676.
18. Schechter AN, Gladwin MT. Hemoglobin and the paracrine and endocrine functions of nitric oxide. N Engl J Med 2003; 348:1483–1485.
19. Reiter CD, Gladwin MT. An emerging role for nitric oxide in sickle cell disease vascular homeostasis and therapy. Curr Opin Hematol 2003; 10:99–107.

20. Yu B, Raher MJ, Volpato GP, et al. Inhaled nitric oxide enables artificial blood transfusion without hypertension. Circulation 2008; 117:1982–1990.
21. Morris CR, Kato GJ, Poljakovic M, et al. Dysregulated arginine metabolism, hemolysis-associated pulmonary hypertension, and mortality in sickle cell disease. JAMA 2005; 294:81–90.
22. Rother RP, Bell L, Hillmen P, et al. The clinical sequelae of intravascular hemolysis and extracellular plasma hemoglobin: a novel mechanism of human disease. JAMA 2005; 293:1653–1662.
23. Raghavachari N, Xu X, Harris A, et al. Amplified expression profiling of platelet transcriptome reveals changes in arginine metabolic pathways in patients with sickle cell disease. Circulation 2007; 115:1551–1562.
24. Villagra J, Shiva S, Hunter LA, et al. Platelet activation in patients with sickle disease, hemolysis-associated pulmonary hypertension, and nitric oxide scavenging by cell-free hemoglobin. Blood 2007; 110:2166–2172.
25. Ataga KI, Moore CG, Hillery CA, et al. Coagulation activation and inflammation in sickle cell disease-associated pulmonary hypertension. Haematologica 2008; 93:20–26.
26. Kato GJ, McGowan VR, Machado RF, et al. Lactate dehydrogenase as a biomarker of hemolysis-associated nitric oxide resistance, priapism, leg ulceration, pulmonary hypertension and death in patients with sickle cell disease. Blood 2006; 107(6):2279–2285 [Epub November 15, 2005].
27. Hillmen P, Muus P, Duhrsen U, et al. Effect of the complement inhibitor eculizumab on thromboembolism in patients with paroxysmal nocturnal hemoglobinuria. Blood 2007; 110:4123–4128.
28. Yeo TW, Lampah DA, Gitawati R, et al. Impaired nitric oxide bioavailability and L-arginine reversible endothelial dysfunction in adults with falciparum malaria. J Exp Med 2007; 204:2693–2704.
29. Machado RF, Gladwin MT. Chronic sickle cell lung disease: new insights into the diagnosis, pathogenesis and treatment of pulmonary hypertension. Br J Haematol 2005; 129:449–464.
30. Nolan VG, Adewoye A, Baldwin C, et al. Sickle cell leg ulcers: associations with haemolysis and SNPs in Klotho, TEK and genes of the TGF-beta/BMP pathway. Br J Haematol 2006; 133:570–578.
31. Nolan VG, Wyszynski DF, Farrer LA, et al. Hemolysis associated priapism in sickle cell disease. Blood 2005; 106(9):3264–3267 [Epub June 28, 2005].
32. Hsu LL, Champion HC, Campbell-Lee SA, et al. Hemolysis in sickle cell mice causes pulmonary hypertension due to global impairment in nitric oxide bioavailability. Blood 2007; 109:3088–3098.
33. Gramaglia I, Sobolewski P, Meays D, et al. Low nitric oxide bioavailability contributes to the genesis of experimental cerebral malaria. Nat Med 2006; 12:1417–1422.
34. De Castro LM, Jonassaint JC, Graham FL, et al. Pulmonary hypertension associated with sickle cell disease: clinical and laboratory endpoints and disease outcomes. Am J Hematol 2008; 83:19–25.
35. Haque AK, Gokhale S, Rampy BA, et al. Pulmonary hypertension in sickle cell hemoglobinopathy: a clinicopathologic study of 20 cases. Hum Pathol 2002; 33:1037–1043.
36. Hayag-Barin JE, Smith RE, Tucker FC Jr. Hereditary spherocytosis, thrombocytosis, and chronic pulmonary emboli: a case report and review of the literature. Am J Hematol 1998; 57:82–84.
37. Vichinsky EP. Pulmonary hypertension in sickle cell disease. N Engl J Med 2004; 350: 857–859.
38. Anthi A, Machado RF, Jison ML, et al. Hemodynamic and functional assessment of patients with sickle cell disease and pulmonary hypertension. Am J Respir Crit Care Med 2007; 175:1272–1279.

39. Ataga KI, Moore CG, Jones S, et al. Pulmonary hypertension in patients with sickle cell disease: a longitudinal study. Br J Haematol 2006; 134:109–115.
40. Castro OL, Hoque M, Brown BD. Pulmonary hypertension in sickle cell disease: cardiac catheterization results and survival. Blood 2002; 3:3.
41. Ataga KI, Sood N, De Gent G, et al. Pulmonary hypertension in sickle cell disease. Am J Med 2004; 117:665–669.
42. Machado RF, Anthi A, Steinberg MH, et al. N-terminal pro-brain natriuretic peptide levels and risk of death in sickle cell disease. JAMA 2006; 296:310–318.
43. McQuillan BM, Picard MH, Leavitt M, et al. Clinical correlates and reference intervals for pulmonary artery systolic pressure among echocardiographically normal subjects. Circulation 2001; 104:2797–2802.
44. Sachdev V, Machado RF, Shizukuda Y, et al. Diastolic dysfunction is an independent risk factor for death in patients with sickle cell disease. J Am Coll Cardiol 2007; 49:472–479.
45. Machado RF, Kyle Mack A, Martyr S, et al. Severity of pulmonary hypertension during vaso-occlusive pain crisis and exercise in patients with sickle cell disease. Br J Haematol 2007; 136:319–325.
46. Mekontso Dessap A, Leon R, Habibi A, et al. Pulmonary hypertension and cor pulmonale during severe acute chest syndrome in sickle cell disease. Am J Respir Crit Care Med 2008; 177:646–653.
47. Styles LA, Vichinsky E. Effects of a long-term transfusion regimen on sickle cell-related illnesses. J Pediatr 1994; 125:909–911.
48. Bernini JC, Rogers ZR, Sandler ES, et al. Beneficial effect of intravenous dexamethasone in children with mild to moderately severe acute chest syndrome complicating sickle cell disease. Blood 1998; 92:3082–3089.
49. Strouse JJ, Takemoto CM, Keefer JR, et al. Corticosteroids and increased risk of readmission after acute chest syndrome in children with sickle cell disease. Pediatr Blood Cancer 2008; 50(5):1006–1012.
50. Oppert M, Jorres A, Barckow D, et al. Inhaled nitric oxide for ARDS due to sickle cell disease. Swiss Med Wkly 2004; 134:165–167.
51. Gladwin MT, Schechter AN, Shelhamer JH, et al. The acute chest syndrome in sickle cell disease. Possible role of nitric oxide in its pathophysiology and treatment. Am J Respir Crit Care Med 1999; 159:1368–1376.
52. Atz AM, Wessel DL. Inhaled nitric oxide in sickle cell disease with acute chest syndrome. Anesthesiology 1997; 87:988–990.
53. Charache S, Terrin ML, Moore RD, et al. Effect of hydroxyurea on the frequency of painful crises in sickle cell anemia. Investigators of the multicenter study of hydroxyurea in sickle cell anemia. N Engl J Med 1995; 332:1317–1322.
54. Platt OS. Hydroxyurea for the treatment of sickle cell anemia. N Engl J Med 2008; 358:1362–1369.
55. Miller ST, Wright E, Abboud M, et al. Impact of chronic transfusion on incidence of pain and acute chest syndrome during the Stroke Prevention Trial (STOP) in sickle-cell anemia. J Pediatr 2001; 139:785–789.
56. Walters MC, Patience M, Leisenring W, et al. Bone marrow transplantation for sickle cell disease. N Engl J Med 1996; 335:369–376.
57. Derchi G, Forni GL, Formisano F, et al. Efficacy and safety of sildenafil in the treatment of severe pulmonary hypertension in patients with hemoglobinopathies. Haematologica 2005; 90:452–458.
58. Littera R, La Nasa G, Derchi G, et al. Long-term treatment with sildenafil in a thalassemic patient with pulmonary hypertension. Blood 2002; 100:1516–1517.
59. Machado RF, Martyr S, Kato GJ, et al. Sildenafil therapy in patients with sickle cell disease and pulmonary hypertension. Br J Haematol 2005; 130:445–453.

60. Little J, Hauser KP, Martyr S, et al. Hematologic, biochemical, and cardiopulmonary effects of L-arginine supplementation or phosphodiesterase 5 inhibition in patients with sickle cell disease who are on hydroxyurea therapy. Eur J Haematol 2009; 82(4):315–321 [Epub February 10, 2008].
61. Little JA, McGowan VR, Kato GJ, et al. Combination erythropoietin-hydroxyurea therapy in sickle cell disease: experience from the National Institutes of Health and a literature review. Haematologica 2006; 91:1076–1083.
62. Morris CR, Morris SM Jr., Hagar W, et al. Arginine therapy: a new treatment for pulmonary hypertension in sickle cell disease? Am J Respir Crit Care Med 2003; 168:63–69.

17

Pulmonary Veno-occlusive Disease and Pulmonary Capillary Hemangiomatosis

DAVID MONTANI
Université Paris Sud 11, Service de Pneumologie et Réanimation Respiratoire, Hôpital Antoine Béclère, Assistance Publique Hôpitaux de Paris, Clamart, France

I. Introduction

Pulmonary veno-occlusive disease (PVOD) and pulmonary capillary hemangiomatosis (PCH) are classified as a distinct subgroup of pulmonary arterial hypertension (PAH) and account for 5% to 10% of histological forms of cases initially considered as idiopathic PAH. Even though the first well-documented case of PVOD was described more than 70 years ago and the first case of PCH more than 30 years ago, the characteristics and pathophysiology of this disease remain poorly understood (1–3). While the pulmonary vascular pathology of idiopathic or familial PAH is characterized by major remodeling of small precapillary pulmonary arteries with typical plexiform lesions, PVOD and PCH preferentially affect the postcapillary pulmonary vessels: the small pulmonary veins and capillaries, respectively (4–6). Despite this histological difference, PVOD and PCH have a clinical presentation very similar to PAH but are characterized by a worse prognosis and the possibility of developing severe pulmonary edema with specific PAH therapy, justifying the importance of diagnosing this disease. A definitive diagnosis of PVOD and PCH require histological analysis of a lung sample (7,8); however, surgical lung biopsy is a high-risk procedure in these patients, and the recent improved characterization of these diseases has permitted to propose a less invasive diagnostic approach (2,9–13).

II. Classification and Definition

It has been hypothesized that PAH, PVOD, and PCH may represent different forms of the same disease spectrum, with lesions in different components of the vascular tree (predominantly arteriolar, venous, or capillary lesions) (5). Because of the differences in pathological assessment, responsiveness to specific PAH therapy, and its poorer prognosis, PVOD and PCH are now clearly identified as a specific subgroup of PAH, and this should be reflected in the future revised classification of the 4th World Symposium on Pulmonary Hypertension (Simonneau et al., personal communication). Additionally, occlusive venopathy and capillary proliferation may also occur in PAH associated with different conditions, and this has been recently demonstrated to be frequently observed in PAH associated with connective tissue diseases (14,15). Pulmonary venopathy has also been reported in virtually all conditions associated with PAH.

III. Pathological Assessment

In PVOD, the observed postcapillary lesions target septal veins and preseptal venules and frequently consist of loose, fibrous remodeling of the intima, which may totally occlude the lumen (Fig. 1A). The tunica media may be muscularized in septal veins and preseptal venules. Fibrous occlusion of large septal veins may be seen in many forms of secondary pulmonary venous hypertension, and the involvement of preseptal venules should be considered as necessary for the diagnosis of PVOD. Pleural and pulmonary lymphatic vessels are usually dilated (16). Occult pulmonary hemorrhage regularly occurs in patients displaying PVOD. Even if vascular lesions in PVOD predominate

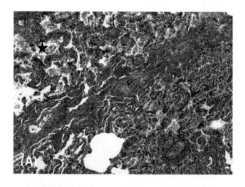

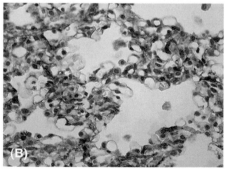

Figure 1 (*See color insert*) Pulmonary veins with obstructive venopathy in lungs of patients with pulmonary veno-occlusive disease and a case of PCH. (**A**) Longitudinally dissected septal vein with asymmetric intimal and partially occlusive fibrosis (*arrows*). Note the hemorrhage (*) due to the postcapillary block in the upper half of the photograph. Magnification 100×, Elastica van Gieson staining. (**B**) Excessively proliferating alveolar capillaries in a patient with PCH. Note the protrusion of ectatic lumina into the alveoli. Magnification 200×, anti-CD31 staining. *Abbreviation*: PCH, pulmonary capillary hemangiomatosis.

within the pulmonary veins, lesions frequently affect capillaries and arteries (4,6). Thrombotic occlusion of small postcapillary microvessels may be present, corresponding to "colander-like" lesions. Arterial lesions of patients displaying PVOD mainly consist of intimal thickening and medial hypertrophy, but complex lesions are absent. Focal capillary angioproliferations are frequently observed in the lungs of PVOD patients, and it has been suggested that this could be the consequence of chronic postcapillary obstruction (4,5). In PCH, the abnormal proliferating capillaries extend into bronchovascular bundles and infiltrate the walls of arterioles, arteries, venules, and veins (Fig. 1B) (4). After histological review of 35 patients originally classified as PVOD and PCH, Lantuejoul et al. found that PCH-like lesions were found in 24 out of 30 PVOD patients; conversely, 4 out of 5 PCH patients showed significant venous involvement. The capillary involvement in PVOD has raised questions concerning a possible overlap between PVOD and PCH (5). This hypothesis is consistent with similar clinical and radiological presentations of PVOD and PCH (10,12,17,18). Dorfmuller et al. have recently reported frequent involvement of pulmonary veins and capillaries in a PVOD-like pattern in patients displaying PAH associated with connective tissue diseases, suggesting a clinically relevant effect of postcapillary occlusion in this subset of PAH (14).

In conclusion, these latest insights into the pathology of PVOD and PCH may indicate a new approach to the disease with a less rigid perception of pre- and post-capillary and capillary lesions in patients with pulmonary hypertension. The most clinically relevant information is the presence of postcapillary involvement, which may lead to a very different clinical outcome and a different management.

IV. Pulmonary Veno-occlusive Disease

A. Epidemiology

A very wide range for age at diagnosis has been reported in case report and series, from the first weeks of life to the seventh decade (2,7,8). In contrast with idiopathic PAH, which has a clear female predominance, PVOD occurs equally in men and women (2,7).

The true incidence of PVOD is probably underestimated as many cases may be classified as idiopathic PAH. Usually, PVOD is considered to account for 5% to 10% of histological forms of cases initially thought to be "idiopathic" (8,12). However, PVOD can also occur in patients with associated diseases including connective tissue diseases (14,15,19), sarcoidosis (20), pulmonary Langerhans cell granulomatosis (8,21,22), HIV infection (23–25), bone marrow transplantation (26–32), and idiopathic pulmonary fibrosis (33–35), suggesting that PVOD could have a much higher prevalence. In national registries, PAH associated with connective diseases represents 15% to 30% of PAH patients (36,37), but the true prevalence of venopathy in PAH associated with connective tissue diseases is difficult to estimate as no study include systematic assessments of venous involvement in these patients. Johnson et al. described a series of probable PVOD in four patients with scleroderma-associated PAH (15). Dorfmuller et al. studied lung samples from eight patients with end-stage PAH associated with connective tissue disease and demonstrated that significant pulmonary vascular lesions predominating in veins or preseptal venules were more frequent in PAH associated with connective tissue disease (75%) compared with idiopathic PAH (17.2%) (14).

B. Risk Factors

In contrast to idiopathic PAH where it has been clearly demonstrated that the risk of developing PAH is increased after exposure to anorexigens (38–40), the association of risk factors with PVOD was reported only in one series (2). Chemical exposures have been suggested to play a role in the development of the disease. PVOD has been associated with various chemotherapy regimens including bleomycin, BCNU, and mitomycin (41–44) and after bone marrow transplantation (26–32,45).

We have recently reported a higher tobacco exposure and an increased proportion of smokers in PVOD as compared with PAH (2). It is not clear why tobacco exposure would be a specific risk factor for PVOD and why it was not found in idiopathic PAH (39). This relationship is also supported by the described association between PVOD and pulmonary Langerhans cell granulomatosis, a pulmonary disease occurring almost exclusively in smokers (21,22,46,47).

C. Hereditable PVOD

Genetic risk in the development of PVOD has been previously suggested by reports of occurrence in siblings (48,49), and several bone morphogenetic protein type 2 receptor (*BMPR2*) mutations were reported (2,50–52). These reports demonstrate a probable role of the BMPR2 pathway in the development of PVOD and support systematic screening for a familial history of pulmonary vascular disease and genetic counseling in PVOD patients.

D. Clinical Features

PVOD and idiopathic PAH share the same clinical presentation, and clinical examination is unhelpful to distinguish them. As observed in PAH, most of the patients have severe exertional dyspnea at the time of the diagnosis (2,7). Auscultatory crackles may occur in PVOD patients with predominant pulmonary infiltrates (7). Clubbing and Raynaud's phenomenon have been reported in PVOD, but our recent series suggested that Raynaud's phenomenon (8% of PVOD patients) and clubbing (16%) remain rare in PVOD and can also be found in idiopathic PAH (2).

E. Hemodynamic Characteristics

A large recent series comparing patients with biopsy-proven idiopathic PAH and PVOD indicated that PVOD and PAH share broadly similar hemodynamic characteristics and confirmed that PVOD patients were characterized by severe precapillary PAH on right-heart catheterization (2,12).

Even if PVOD is histologically characterized by postcapillay obstruction, pulmonary capillary wedge pressure (PCWP) is normal in PVOD patients (2,7,9,12). PCWP reflects the pressure in a pulmonary vein of diameter similar to that of the pulmonary artery occluded by the inflated balloon. This vein is larger than the small veins affected by the occlusive venopathy, and the pressure measured by PCWP is therefore distal to the site affected by the disease, explaining why PWCP is normal in these patients (2,4).

An acute vasodilator response has been reported in some PVOD cases (12). In a recent series, one patient with PVOD responded to NO. However, within 24 hours of initiation of calcium channel blockers (CCBs) therapy, severe pulmonary edema developed.

An acute vasodilator response in PVOD was not predictive of a long-term response to CCBs and should not be used in the context of a positive acute test. However, acute testing with 10 ppm NO for a short period (5–10 minutes) is thought to be safe in patients with suspected PVOD but is unable to predict those patients in whom the initiation of PAH-specific therapy was associated with pulmonary edema (2).

F. Noninvasive Tools

In PVOD, histological proof is usually lacking as surgical lung biopsy is a high-risk procedure that should not be performed. Recent data have shown that a noninvasive approach including arterial blood gases, pulmonary function tests, bronchoalveolar lavage (BAL), and high-resolution computed tomography (HRCT) of the chest was helpful to screen for patients with high probability of PVOD (2,12).

Pulmonary Function Tests

With the exception of occlusive venopathy associated with respiratory diseases, PVOD patients had generally normal pulmonary function tests analyzed during spirometry and plethysmography (2). Even if low diffusing capacity of lung for carbon monoxide (D_LCO) is observed in PAH patients, D_LCO was significantly reduced in PVOD compared with idiopathic PAH, suggesting that D_LCO may be helpful to identify PVOD patients (2).

Oxygenation Parameters

Montani et al. have shown that baseline partial pressure of arterial oxygen (PaO_2) at rest is significantly lower in PVOD patients than that in idiopathic PAH (61 ± 17 and 75 ± 14 mmHg, respectively) (2). Furthermore, even though PVOD patients had similar six-minute walk distance (6MWD) at baseline when compared with idiopathic PAH, Montani et al. showed that PVOD patients had a significantly lower nadir on pulse oxygen saturation (SpO_2) during 6MWD (80 ± 9 and 87 ± 7%, respectively) (2).

Bronchoalveolar Lavage

Bronchoscopy is not a routine investigation in PAH, but there may be a role for BAL in patients with suspected PVOD (9). It has been described that bronchoscopic airway inspection may show hyperemia of the lobar and segmental bronchi because of vascular engorgement (53). Compared with PAH, Rabiller et al. found a significantly elevated percentage of hemosiderin-laden macrophages and a higher Golde score in keeping with the hypothesis of an occult alveolar hemorrhage in PVOD (9).

High-Resolution Computed Tomography of the Chest

Chest radiographs and HRCT of the chest may show Kerley B lines or pleural effusions when pulmonary edema occurs after initiation of specific PAH therapy (2,7,17,54,55). With the exception of this situation, HRCT showed a significantly higher frequency of centrilobular ground-glass opacities, septal lines, and mediastinal lymph node enlargement in PVOD as compared with idiopathic PAH (Fig. 2) (2,7,10,17). Montani et al. demonstrated that the presence of two or three of these radiological abnormalities were observed in 75% of PVOD patients but may also be present in idiopathic PAH (15%) (2). In contrast, the absence of radiological abnormalities on HRCT could not rule out PVOD (2).

These findings suggest that noninvasive testing could be helpful to suggest the diagnosis of PVOD in patients with precapillary pulmonary hypertension. A low resting

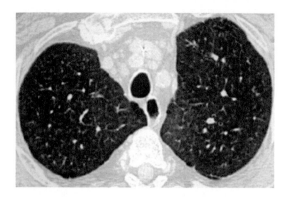

Figure 2 HRCT of the chest in pulmonary veno-occlusive disease. HRCT of the chest showing marked ground-glass opacities with centrilobular pattern, poorly defined nodular opacities, and septal lines. *Abbreviation*: HRCT, high-resolution computed tomography.

PaO_2, low SpO_2 during 6MWD, low D_LCO, presence of an occult alveolar hemorrhage, and radiological abnormalities on HRCT of the chest may identify a subgroup of patients with a high probability of PVOD and therefore avoidance of hazardous and invasive surgical procedures in these patients.

G. Treatments

Even if baseline hemodynamics, New York Heart Association (NYHA) functional class, and 6MWD are similar to those observed in PAH patients, PVOD patients have a poorer outcome. Data suggest that the one-year mortality rate may be as high as 72% in PVOD (7), and the most recent series of a group of 24 histologically confirmed severe PVOD patients found a mean time from diagnosis to death or lung transplantation of 11.8 ± 16.4 months compared with 42.3 ± 29.9 months in idiopathic PAH patients (2). These data suggest that the worse outcome of patients displaying PAH associated with connective tissue diseases may be due, at least in part, to the frequent pulmonary venous involvement in these conditions (14). Excluding lung transplantation, treatment options are unfortunately limited in PVOD, highlighting the relevance of noninvasive approach to screen for PVOD and consideration of lung transplantation earlier in the course of the disease.

Conventional Therapy

Severe resting hypoxemia and exertional desaturation are frequently observed in PVOD patients, justifying oxygen therapy to maintain saturation above 90% (56). Conventional therapy includes high-dose diuretics to decrease the risk of pulmonary edema. Even if there is no specific data in PVOD, the rationale for anticoagulation is present because of the subsequent in situ thrombosis (4). However, anticoagulation is not indicated if there is a history of severe hemoptysis.

No evidence supports a possible role of immunosuppressive therapy in PVOD except in the context of venous involvement associated with connective tissue disease (57). In this context, PAH patients with mixed connective tissue disease and systemic lupus erythematosus (but not scleroderma) may improve with immunosuppressive therapy (58,59).

Specific PAH Therapy

The major concern with specific PAH therapy in PVOD is the risk of severe pulmonary edema, which has been reported with all specific PAH therapies (prostacyclin and its derivatives, endothelin receptor antagonists, phosphodiesterase-5 inhibitors, and CCBs). The mechanism is thought to be due to the relative vasodilatation of the precapillary vessels more than the pulmonary capillaries and veins, associated with an increase in blood flow, resulting in an increase in transcapillary hydrostatic pressure and transudation of fluid into the pulmonary interstitium and alveoli (12).

In our recent cohort of histologically confirmed PVOD patients, 7 out of 16 patients who received specific PAH therapy developed pulmonary edema. None of the clinical, functional, or hemodynamic characteristics were predictive of the development of pulmonary edema after initiation of specific therapy (2). However, clinical improvement or at least stabilization has been observed in some patients with continuous intravenous prostacyclin, oral sildenafil monotherapy, and even chronic inhaled NO or iloprost therapy (7,60–67). While pulmonary vasodilators such as intravenous prostacyclin have established efficacy in PAH (68,69), benefits of these treatments in patients with PVOD are still unclear. Continuous intravenous epoprostenol therapy has been shown to improve hemodynamics in some cases of PVOD (7,62,65,66) and should be considered in these patients because of their very poor prognosis (2). Cautious use of PAH-specific therapy may be of interest in PVOD, as a bridge to lung transplantation. In our experience, continuous intravenous epoprostenol can be initiated in the most severe patients with a slowly increasing dose along with high-dose diuretics under close medical monitoring. Since 2003, we have proposed this approach as a bridge therapy to lung transplantation in several severe highly probable PVOD patients. In these patients, epoprostenol may improve hemodynamics at three months without major adverse complications (Montani et al., personal communication). In less severe patients, one may consider oral or inhaled agents associated with high-dose diuretics as bridge therapy to lung transplantation.

Lung Transplantation

Lung transplantation remains the treatment of choice for PVOD and still offers the only real possibility of cure for the disease (56,70,71). Of note, there has been one reported case of PVOD recurrence three months following transplantation with similar symptoms, worsening PAH and radiographic pulmonary congestion (72). Because of the worse prognosis of PVOD patients, it may be necessary to discuss lung transplantation early in the course of PVOD. At our center, eligible PVOD patients in functional class III or IV are now listed for lung transplantation at the time of diagnosis (12).

V. Pulmonary Capillary Hemangiomatosis

PCH is defined by its pathological assessment showing localized capillary proliferation with possible infiltration of vascular, bronchial, and interstitial pulmonary structures that is usually associated with PAH. However, similar pathological findings have been described in patients without evidence of pulmonary hypertension (73). Havlik et al.

reported, at autopsy, PCH-like foci findings in 5.7% (8/140) of patients without symptoms of PAH (73). These authors suggested that these PCH-like foci at autopsy should be considered as incidental findings with uncertain significance (73).

Lantuejoul et al. reported that capillary proliferation was observed in 73% of cases diagnosed as PVOD and that venous involvement is present in 80% of cases initially diagnosed as PCH (5). The authors suggested that the majority of cases of PCH are a secondary angioproliferative process in response to a postcapillary obstruction (5). They proposed to use the term "secondary PCH" for PCH-like changes associated with different disorders, including PVOD, and to reserve the term "primary PCH" for the rare case of isolated PCH without an identified cause (5). Indeed, PCH shares the same clinical and radiological characteristics of idiopathic PAH, and PCH can also be complicated by occult alveolar hemorrhage and severe pulmonary edema with specific therapy. These findings raise the hypothesis that PVOD and PCH may be two parts of the same spectrum of disease.

Very few data are available regarding patients with histologically confirmed PCH. Almagro et al. reported two cases of PCH and reviewed the characteristics of 35 PCH patients from the literature (13). Similar to PVOD, no female predominance was observed (55% of PCH patients were male), and PCH occurred at ages from 2 to 71 years (mean age of 29 years). Even if PCH appears to be sporadic in most of the cases, rare familial PCH was described (74). PCH may also occur in association with different conditions, and PCH has been associated with systemic lupus erythematosus (75) and Takayasu's arteritis (76).

As observed in idiopathic PAH or PVOD, dyspnea and signs of right-heart failure were the most frequent clinical signs observed in PCH patients, highlighting the severity of PCH patients at the time of diagnosis. Almagro et al. reported in PCH, a high frequency of hemoptysis (one-third of the PCH patients) and pleural effusions (one quarter of PCH patients) (13). The pleural effusion was hemorrhagic in four of the nine PCH patients with pleural effusions (13). These findings suggest that pleural effusion and hemoptysis might have a higher prevalence than that observed in idiopathic PAH or PVOD (2,13) even if no study compared characteristics of patients with histologically confirmed PVOD and PCH. As described in PVOD, clubbing and auscultatory crackles have been reported but remain relatively uncommon (13). Almagro et al. reported in their literature review that 28 patients died with a median survival of three years from the first clinical manifestation (13). These results confirm a very poor prognosis in PCH, broadly similar to that described in PVOD and worse than that in idiopathic PAH (2,36).

The hemodynamic characteristics confirm that PCWP is usually normal in PCH (14 out of 16 patients in this series) (13). As explained above, PCWP reflects the pressure in the large pulmonary veins, and even the presence of a capillary obstruction in PCH remains normal. Therefore, hemodynamics cannot help to discriminate between PCH, PVOD, and idiopathic PAH.

Several reports found that in PCH the same radiological abnormalities are present on HRCT of the chest as that described in PVOD. These abnormalities were nonspecific and include septal lines, centrolobular ground-glass opacities, lymph node enlargement, and pleural effusion (13,17,66). Few specific data are available on pulmonary function tests in PCH. Almagro et al. reported diminished D_LCO and hypoxemia in PCH patients, but these findings may also be found in PVOD and idiopathic PAH (2,13).

Few PCH patients treated with prostaglandins are reported in the literature. In the vast majority of cases, prostaglandins had to be withdrawn because of hemodynamic intolerance or pulmonary edema (13,77). Furthermore, prostaglandins seem to be incriminated directly in the death for some of these patients (13). Even if the prostacyclin was used without specific cautions in these reported cases, its use seems to be associated with a very high frequency of clinical deterioration and pulmonary edema. No data are available about the recent specific PAH therapies, particularly with oral therapy (e.g., phosphodiesterase-5 inhibitors and endothelin receptor antagonists). Glucocorticosteroids have been initiated in some PCH patients, without any effect on the evolution of the disease (13). Clinical improvements have been reported in PCH with interferon α-2a (78,79). However, these results involve only a few patients, and these results need to be confirmed in a larger series. As observed in idiopathic PAH (80), an overexpression of platelet-derived growth factor (PDGF)-B gene and PDGF receptor β gene have been demonstrated in the nodules of proliferating capillaries in PCH patients (81,82), suggesting a possible interest of tyrosine kinase inhibitors inhibiting the PDGF pathway in PCH. Specific studies in PCH are needed to confirm this hypothesis. However, because of the worse prognosis of PCH, the treatment of choice for PCH remains urgent lung transplantation. To the best of our knowledge, no case of PCH recurrence was reported in the transplanted lungs.

In conclusion, PVOD and PCH share similar clinical, functional, and radiological characteristics and can be associated with occult alveolar hemorrhage. Clinical examination and hemodynamics are not helpful to discriminate PVOD and PCH from idiopathic PAH. A stepwise noninvasive approach including pulmonary function tests (low D_LCO, hypoxemia at rest, low SpO_2 during 6MWD), CT of the chest (septal lines, centrilobular ground-glass opacities, and lymph node enlargement) and BAL may be helpful to screen patients displaying PVOD or PCH. Indeed, PVOD and PCH are characterized by a very poor prognosis and the possibility of severe pulmonary edema after initiation of specific PAH therapies. All these similarities associated with the recent description of a frequent association of venous and capillary involvement in PCH and PVOD suggest that these two diseases could be two manifestations of the same disease. Even if some specific PAH therapies might be useful in PVOD, lung transplantation remains the treatment of choice and the only curative treatment of these two devastating diseases.

References

1. Höra J. Zur histologie der klinischen "primaren pulmonal-sklerose." Frankf Z Pathol 1934; 47:100–118.
2. Montani D, Achouh L, Dorfmuller P, et al. Pulmonary veno-occlusive disease: clinical, functional, radiologic, hemodynamic characteristics and outcome of 24 cases confirmed by histology. Medicine (Baltimore) 2008; 87(4):220–233.
3. Wagenvoort CA, Beetstra A, Spijker J. Capillary haemangiomatosis of the lungs. Histopathology 1978; 2(6):401–406.
4. Pietra GG, Capron F, Stewart S, et al. Pathologic assessment of vasculopathies in pulmonary hypertension. J Am Coll Cardiol 2004; 43(12 suppl S):25S–32S.
5. Lantuejoul S, Sheppard MN, Corrin B, et al. Pulmonary veno-occlusive disease and pulmonary capillary hemangiomatosis: a clinicopathologic study of 35 cases. Am J Surg Pathol 2006; 30(7):850–857.

6. Wagenvoort CA, Wagenvoort N. The pathology of pulmonary veno-occlusive disease. Virchows Arch A Pathol Anat Histol 1974; 364(1):69–79.
7. Holcomb BW Jr., Loyd JE, Ely EW, et al. Pulmonary veno-occlusive disease: a case series and new observations. Chest 2000; 118(6):1671–1679.
8. Mandel J, Mark EJ, Hales CA. Pulmonary veno-occlusive disease. Am J Respir Crit Care Med 2000; 162(5):1964–1973.
9. Rabiller A, Jais X, Hamid A, et al. Occult alveolar haemorrhage in pulmonary veno-occlusive disease. Eur Respir J 2006; 27 (1):108–113.
10. Resten A, Maitre S, Humbert M, et al. Pulmonary hypertension: CT of the chest in pulmonary venoocclusive disease. AJR Am J Roentgenol 2004; 183(1):65–70.
11. Rambihar VS, Fallen EL, Cairns JA. Pulmonary veno-occlusive disease: antemortem diagnosis from roentgenographic and hemodynamic findings. Can Med Assoc J 1979; 120(12): 1519–1522.
12. Montani D, Price LC, Dorfmuller P, et al. Pulmonary veno-occlusive disease. Eur Respir J 2009; 33(1):189–200.
13. Almagro P, Julia J, Sanjaume M, et al. Pulmonary capillary hemangiomatosis associated with primary pulmonary hypertension: report of 2 new cases and review of 35 cases from the literature. Medicine (Baltimore) 2002; 81(6):417–424.
14. Dorfmuller P, Humbert M, Perros F, et al. Fibrous remodeling of the pulmonary venous system in pulmonary arterial hypertension associated with connective tissue diseases. Hum Pathol 2007; 38(6):893–902.
15. Johnson SR, Patsios D, Hwang DM, et al. Pulmonary veno-occlusive disease and scleroderma associated pulmonary hypertension. J Rheumatol 2006; 33(11):2347–2350.
16. Heath D, Edwards JE. The pathology of hypertensive pulmonary vascular disease: a description of six grades of structural changes in the pulmonary arteries with special reference to congenital cardiac septal defects. Circulation 1958; 18(4 part 1):533–547.
17. Dufour B, Maitre S, Humbert M, et al. High-resolution CT of the chest in four patients with pulmonary capillary hemangiomatosis or pulmonary venoocclusive disease. AJR Am J Roentgenol 1998; 171(5):1321–1324.
18. Simonneau G, Galie N, Rubin LJ, et al. Clinical classification of pulmonary hypertension. J Am Coll Cardiol 2004; 43(12 suppl S):5S–12S.
19. Zhang L, Visscher D, Rihal C, et al. Pulmonary veno-occlusive disease as a primary cause of pulmonary hypertension in a patient with mixed connective tissue disease. Rheumatol Int 2007; 27(12):1163–1165.
20. Nunes H, Humbert M, Capron F, et al. Pulmonary hypertension associated with sarcoidosis: mechanisms, hemodynamics and prognosis. Thorax 2006; 61(1):68–74.
21. Fartoukh M, Humbert M, Capron F, et al. Severe pulmonary hypertension in histiocytosis X. Am J Respir Crit Care Med 2000; 161(1):216–223.
22. Hamada K, Teramoto S, Narita N, et al. Pulmonary veno-occlusive disease in pulmonary Langerhans' cell granulomatosis. Eur Respir J 2000; 15(2):421–423.
23. Escamilla R, Hermant C, Berjaud J, et al. Pulmonary veno-occlusive disease in a HIV-infected intravenous drug abuser. Eur Respir J 1995; 8(11):1982–1984.
24. Hourseau M, Capron F, Nunes H, et al. [Pulmonary veno-occlusive disease in a patient with HIV infection. A case report with autopsy findings]. Ann Pathol 2002; 22(6):472–475.
25. Ruchelli ED, Nojadera G, Rutstein RM, et al. Pulmonary veno-occlusive disease. Another vascular disorder associated with human immunodeficiency virus infection? Arch Pathol Lab Med 1994; 118(6):664–666.
26. Williams LM, Fussell S, Veith RW, et al. Pulmonary veno-occlusive disease in an adult following bone marrow transplantation. Case report and review of the literature. Chest 1996; 109(5):1388–1391.

27. Kuga T, Kohda K, Hirayama Y, et al. Pulmonary veno-occlusive disease accompanied by microangiopathic hemolytic anemia 1 year after a second bone marrow transplantation for acute lymphoblastic leukemia. Int J Hematol 1996; 64(2):143–150.

28. Troussard X, Bernaudin JF, Cordonnier C, et al. Pulmonary veno-occlusive disease after bone marrow transplantation. Thorax 1984; 39(12):956–957.

29. Salzman D, Adkins DR, Craig F, et al. Malignancy-associated pulmonary veno-occlusive disease: report of a case following autologous bone marrow transplantation and review. Bone Marrow Transplant 1996; 18(4):755–760.

30. Seguchi M, Hirabayashi N, Fujii Y, et al. Pulmonary hypertension associated with pulmonary occlusive vasculopathy after allogeneic bone marrow transplantation. Transplantation 2000; 69(1):177–179.

31. Hackman RC, Madtes DK, Petersen FB, et al. Pulmonary venoocclusive disease following bone marrow transplantation. Transplantation 1989; 47(6):989–992.

32. Bunte MC, Patnaik MM, Pritzker MR, et al. Pulmonary veno-occlusive disease following hematopoietic stem cell transplantation: a rare model of endothelial dysfunction. Bone Marrow Transplant 2008; 41(8):677–686.

33. Nathan SD, Noble PW, Tuder RM. Idiopathic pulmonary fibrosis and pulmonary hypertension: connecting the dots. Am J Respir Crit Care Med 2007; 175(9):875–880.

34. Patel NM, Lederer DJ, Borczuk AC, et al. Pulmonary hypertension in idiopathic pulmonary fibrosis. Chest 2007; 132(3):998–1006.

35. Colombat M, Mal H, Groussard O, et al. Pulmonary vascular lesions in end-stage idiopathic pulmonary fibrosis: histopathologic study on lung explant specimens and correlations with pulmonary hemodynamics. Hum Pathol 2007; 38(1):60–65.

36. Humbert M, Sitbon O, Chaouat A, et al. Pulmonary arterial hypertension in France: results from a national registry. Am J Respir Crit Care Med 2006; 173(9):1023–1030.

37. Peacock AJ, Murphy NF, McMurray JJ, et al. An epidemiological study of pulmonary arterial hypertension. Eur Respir J 2007; 30(1):104–109.

38. Humbert M, Nunes H, Sitbon O, et al. Risk factors for pulmonary arterial hypertension. Clin Chest Med 2001; 22:459–475.

39. Abenhaim L, Moride Y, Brenot F, et al. Appetite-suppressant drugs and the risk of primary pulmonary hypertension. International Primary Pulmonary Hypertension Study Group. N Engl J Med 1996; 335(9):609–616.

40. Souza R, Humbert M, Sztrymf B, et al. Pulmonary arterial hypertension associated with fenfluramine exposure: report of 109 cases. Eur Respir J 2008; 31(2):343–348.

41. Joselson R, Warnock M. Pulmonary veno-occlusive disease after chemotherapy. Hum Pathol 1983; 14(1):88–91.

42. Knight BK, Rose AG. Pulmonary veno-occlusive disease after chemotherapy. Thorax 1985; 40(11):874–875.

43. Swift GL, Gibbs A, Campbell IA, et al. Pulmonary veno-occlusive disease and Hodgkin's lymphoma. Eur Respir J 1993; 6(4):596–598.

44. Waldhorn RE, Tsou E, Smith FP, et al. Pulmonary veno-occlusive disease associated with microangiopathic hemolytic anemia and chemotherapy of gastric adenocarcinoma. Med Pediatr Oncol 1984; 12(6):394–396.

45. Trobaugh-Lotrario AD, Greffe B, Deterding R, et al. Pulmonary veno-occlusive disease after autologous bone marrow transplant in a child with stage IV neuroblastoma: case report and literature review. J Pediatr Hematol Oncol 2003; 25(5):405–409.

46. Wright JL, Tai H, Churg A. Cigarette smoke induces persisting increases of vasoactive mediators in pulmonary arteries. Am J Respir Cell Mol Biol 2004; 31(5):501–509.

47. Wright JL, Tai H, Churg A. Vasoactive mediators and pulmonary hypertension after cigarette smoke exposure in the guinea pig. J Appl Physiol 2006; 100(2):672–678.

48. Davies P, Reid L. Pulmonary veno-occlusive disease in siblings: case reports and morphometric study. Hum Pathol 1982; 13(10):911–915.
49. Voordes CG, Kuipers JR, Elema JD. Familial pulmonary veno-occlusive disease: a case report. Thorax 1977; 32(6):763–766.
50. Runo JR, Vnencak-Jones CL, Prince M, et al. Pulmonary veno-occlusive disease caused by an inherited mutation in bone morphogenetic protein receptor II. Am J Respir Crit Care Med 2003; 167(6):889–894.
51. Machado RD, Aldred MA, James V, et al. Mutations of the TGF-beta type II receptor BMPR2 in pulmonary arterial hypertension. Hum Mutat 2006; 27(2):121–132.
52. Aldred MA, Vijayakrishnan J, James V, et al. BMPR2 gene rearrangements account for a significant proportion of mutations in familial and idiopathic pulmonary arterial hypertension. Hum Mutat 2006; 27(2):212–213.
53. Matthews AW, Buchanan R. A case of pulmonary veno-occlusive disease and a new bronchoscopic sign. Respir Med 1990; 84(6):503–505.
54. Palmer SM, Robinson LJ, Wang A, et al. Massive pulmonary edema and death after prostacyclin infusion in a patient with pulmonary veno-occlusive disease. Chest 1998; 113(1): 237–240.
55. Swensen SJ, Tashjian JH, Myers JL, et al. Pulmonary venoocclusive disease: CT findings in eight patients. AJR Am J Roentgenol 1996; 167(4):937–940.
56. Humbert M, Sitbon O, Simonneau G. Treatment of pulmonary arterial hypertension. N Engl J Med 2004; 351(14):1425–1436.
57. Dorfmuller P, Perros F, Balabanian K, et al. Inflammation in pulmonary arterial hypertension. Eur Respir J 2003; 22(2):358–363.
58. Jais X, Launay D, Yaici A, et al. Management of lupus and mixed connective tissue disease-associated pulmonary arterial hypertension. Arthritis Rheum 2008; 58:521–531.
59. Sanchez O, Sitbon O, Jais X, et al. Immunosuppressive therapy in connective tissue diseases-associated pulmonary arterial hypertension. Chest 2006; 130(1):182–189.
60. Barreto AC, Franchi SM, Castro CR, et al. One-year follow-up of the effects of sildenafil on pulmonary arterial hypertension and veno-occlusive disease. Braz J Med Biol Res 2005; 38(2):185–195.
61. Creagh-Brown BC, Nicholson AG, Showkathali R, et al. Pulmonary veno-occlusive disease presenting with recurrent pulmonary oedema and the use of nitric oxide to predict response to sildenafil. Thorax 2008; 63(10):933–934.
62. Davis LL, deBoisblanc BP, Glynn CE, et al. Effect of prostacyclin on microvascular pressures in a patient with pulmonary veno-occlusive disease. Chest 1995; 108(6):1754–1756.
63. Hoeper MM, Eschenbruch C, Zink-Wohlfart C, et al. Effects of inhaled nitric oxide and aerosolized iloprost in pulmonary veno-occlusive disease. Respir Med 1999; 93(1):62–64.
64. Kuroda T, Hirota H, Masaki M, et al. Sildenafil as adjunct therapy to high-dose epoprostenol in a patient with pulmonary veno-occlusive disease. Heart Lung Circ 2006; 15(2):139–142.
65. Okumura H, Nagaya N, Kyotani S, et al. Effects of continuous IV prostacyclin in a patient with pulmonary veno-occlusive disease. Chest 2002; 122(3):1096–1098.
66. Resten A, Maitre S, Humbert M, et al. Pulmonary arterial hypertension: thin-section CT predictors of epoprostenol therapy failure. Radiology 2002; 222(3):782–788.
67. Shackelford GD, Sacks EJ, Mullins JD, et al. Pulmonary venoocclusive disease: case report and review of the literature. AJR Am J Roentgenol 1977; 128(4):643–648.
68. Barst RJ, Rubin LJ, Long WA, et al. A comparison of continuous intravenous epoprostenol (prostacyclin) with conventional therapy for primary pulmonary hypertension. The Primary Pulmonary Hypertension Study Group. N Engl J Med 1996; 334(5):296–302.
69. Sitbon O, Humbert M, Nunes H, et al. Long-term intravenous epoprostenol infusion in primary pulmonary hypertension: prognostic factors and survival. J Am Coll Cardiol 2002; 40(4):780–788.

70. Sitbon O, Humbert M, Simonneau G. Primary pulmonary hypertension: current therapy. Prog Cardiovasc Dis 2002; 45(2):115–128.
71. Cassart M, Gevenois PA, Kramer M, et al. Pulmonary venoocclusive disease: CT findings before and after single-lung transplantation. AJR Am J Roentgenol 1993; 160(4):759–760.
72. Izbicki G, Shitrit D, Schechtman I, et al. Recurrence of pulmonary veno-occlusive disease after heart-lung transplantation. J Heart Lung Transplant 2005; 24(5):635–637.
73. Havlik DM, Massie LW, Williams WL, et al. Pulmonary capillary hemangiomatosis-like foci. An autopsy study of 8 cases. Am J Clin Pathol 2000; 113(5):655–662.
74. Langleben D, Heneghan JM, Batten AP, et al. Familial pulmonary capillary hemangiomatosis resulting in primary pulmonary hypertension. Ann Intern Med 1988; 109(2):106–109.
75. Fernandez-Alonso J, Zulueta T, Reyes-Ramirez JR, et al. Pulmonary capillary hemangiomatosis as cause of pulmonary hypertension in a young woman with systemic lupus erythematosus. J Rheumatol 1999; 26(1):231–233.
76. Kakkar N, Vasishta RK, Banerjee AK, et al. Pulmonary capillary haemangiomatosis as a cause of pulmonary hypertension in Takayasu's aortoarteritis. Respiration 1997; 64(5):381–383.
77. Humbert M, Maitre S, Capron F, et al. Pulmonary edema complicating continuous intravenous prostacyclin in pulmonary capillary hemangiomatosis. Am J Respir Crit Care Med 1998; 157(5 pt 1):1681–1685.
78. White CW, Sondheimer HM, Crouch EC, et al. Treatment of pulmonary hemangiomatosis with recombinant interferon alfa-2a. N Engl J Med 1989; 320(18):1197–1200.
79. White CW, Wolf SJ, Korones DN, et al. Treatment of childhood angiomatous diseases with recombinant interferon alfa-2a. J Pediatr 1991; 118(1):59–66.
80. Perros F, Montani D, Dorfmuller P, et al. Platelet-derived growth factor expression and function in idiopathic pulmonary arterial hypertension. Am J Respir Crit Care Med 2008; 178(1):81–88.
81. Kawut SM, Assaad AM, Arcasoy SM, et al. Pulmonary capillary hemangiomatosis: results of gene expression analysis. Chest 2005; 128(6 suppl):575S–5766S.
82. Assaad AM, Kawut SM, Arcasoy SM, et al. Platelet-derived growth factor is increased in pulmonary capillary hemangiomatosis. Chest 2007; 131(3):850–855.

18

Pulmonary Hypertension in Chronic Obstructive Pulmonary Disease

EMMANUEL WEITZENBLUM
Service de Pneumologie, Nouvel Hôpital Civil, Strasbourg, France

ARI CHAOUAT
Service des Maladies Respiratoires et de Réanimation Respiratoire, Centre Hospitalier Universitaire Nancy, Vandoeuvre les Nancy, France

I. Introduction

Chronic obstructive pulmonary disease (COPD) is a major cause of morbidity and mortality worldwide, with an increasing prevalence during the past decade (1). One well-known complication of COPD is pulmonary hypertension (PH), a condition that was denominated "cor pulmonale" in the past (2–4). Owing to its frequency, COPD is by far the most common cause of PH, far more common than interstitial lung disease, obesity-hypoventilation syndrome, pulmonary thromboembolic disease, and idiopathic pulmonary arterial hypertension (PAH). It should be emphasized that PH is only one among other complications of advanced COPD and that the prognosis of COPD is linked to the severity of respiratory insufficiency rather than to the occurrence of PH, which is essentially a "marker" of long-standing hypoxemia (5). This does not apply to severe or "disproportionate" PH, but very few COPD patients exhibit this severe form of PH (6). This chapter gives an overview of PH resulting from COPD and tries to cover all aspects from epidemiology to treatment.

II. Definition

PH complicating chronic respiratory disease and particularly COPD was generally defined as pulmonary artery mean pressure (PAP) >20 mmHg at rest, which is slightly different from the definition of PAH, that is, PAP >25 mmHg. The reason for setting a threshold at 20 mmHg is that in healthy subjects, PAP is always <20 mmHg at rest. However, in some recent studies, PH in COPD was defined by PAP >25 mmHg (7,8), and these various definitions should be kept in mind when comparing studies (9).

There are few data on the prevalence of PH resulting from COPD. The main reason is that right-heart catheterization (RHC) cannot be performed on a large scale for ethical reasons. An alternative is the use of Doppler echocardiography, but echocardiographic measurements are often inaccurate in COPD patients (10). Only studies based on samples of hospitalized patients are presently available, and they have no epidemiological value. The prevalence of PH defined by PAP >20mmHg ranges between 35% and >90% in these series of severe COPD (6,7,11–13).

The study of Williams and Nicholl (14) aimed to determine the prevalence of COPD patients at risk of developing PH, that is, hypoxemic patients. They found that in Sheffield (United Kingdom), an estimated 0.3% of the population aged ≥45 years had both a partial pressure of arterial oxygen (PaO_2) <55 mmHg and a FEV_1 <50%. For England and Wales, this would represent 60,000 subjects at risk of PH. Extrapolating these results to the United States, one obtains a figure of 300,000. These data were obtained more than 20 years ago, and taking into account the marked increase of prevalence of COPD in recent years, these estimates should be increased by at least 100%.

The prevalence of COPD among adults in European cities has been estimated to be ~6% (15), and 5% to 6% of patients have severe or very severe disease (FEV_1 < 50%). It is estimated that 1% of these severe patients are likely to have PAP >40 mmHg (6). Accordingly, the prevalence of PH is probably high, and there are also a significant number of patients with severe (>40 mmHg) PH (9).

III. Pathophysiology: Mechanisms of PH in COPD

PH may result from an increased cardiac output, an increased pulmonary "capillary" wedge pressure (PCWP), or an increased pulmonary vascular resistance (PVR). In COPD the roles of an elevated cardiac output and of an increase of the wedge pressure are almost negligible. During exercise an almost constant increase of PCWP has been observed in COPD patients of the emphysematous type and has been attributed to dynamic hyperinflation (16). At rest, during a steady state of the disease, wedge pressure is most often normal in COPD and PH is precapillary (Fig. 1), almost exclusively accounted for by the increased PVR (4,17).

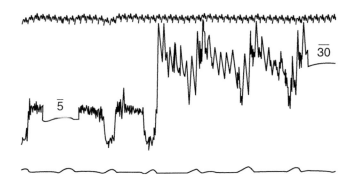

Figure 1 In COPD pulmonary hypertension is "precapillary": the pulmonary "capillary" wedge pressure (left part of the trace) is normal (5 mmHg), whereas pulmonary artery mean pressure (right part of the trace) is elevated (30 mmHg) owing to the elevation of pulmonary vascular resistance. In COPD patients, important swings of systolic and diastolic pulmonary artery pressure from inspiration to expiration are observed, which reproduce the elevated intrathoracic pressure changes. *Abbreviation*: COPD, chronic obstructive pulmonary disease.

The factors leading to an increased PVR in COPD are numerous (3,4,9), but alveolar hypoxia is by far the predominant one (2–4,18). Two distinct mechanisms of action of alveolar hypoxia must be considered: acute hypoxia causes pulmonary vaso-constriction, and chronic hypoxia induces with time structural changes in the pulmonary vascular bed, the so-called "remodeling" of the pulmonary vasculature.

Acute alveolar hypoxia induces in humans and in almost all species of mammals a rise of PVR and PAP that is accounted for by hypoxic pulmonary vasoconstriction. Hypoxic vasoconstriction is observed in normal subjects as well as in patients with chronic respiratory disease (19). This vasoconstriction is localized in small precapillary arteries, and its mechanism is now better understood (20). In fact, the reactivity of the pulmonary circulation to acute hypoxia varies from one individual to another, and this interindividual variability is also found in COPD patients (21).

Chronic alveolar hypoxia induces in healthy people living at altitudes >3500 m precapillary PH, nearly identical to that observed in COPD (22), and morphological studies have shown remodeling of the pulmonary vascular bed, somewhat similar to the structural changes observed in COPD patients with PH (muscularization of pulmonary arterioles, intimal thickening in muscular pulmonary arteries and arterioles).

It is accepted that remodeling of the pulmonary vasculature induced by chronic alveolar hypoxia is the major cause of elevated PVR and PAP in COPD, but it should be emphasized that chronic alveolar hypoxia is not the only cause of an elevated PVR: these patients have marked morphological changes of the lung parenchyma particularly when emphysema is severe and these changes, including the loss of pulmonary capil-laries, could partly account for the increased PVR (23).

Finally, it has been known for many years that pulmonary vascular remodeling is present not only in end-stage COPD patients but also in patients with mild COPD (24). It has been shown more recently that smokers with normal lung function may also develop intimal thickening in pulmonary muscular arteries (25). These structural abnormalities could be the consequences of an endothelial dysfunction of pulmonary arteries caused by cigarette smoke (25). However, the clinical relevance of these early abnormalities is presently unknown.

IV. Main Features of PH in COPD

A. At Rest During the Stable State of COPD

PH in COPD is precapillary, with an increased pressure difference between PAP and PCWP (Fig. 1) reflecting the increased PVR. In almost all COPD patients, marked oscillations of systolic and diastolic pulmonary pressures are observed with respiration (Fig. 1); these oscillations reflect the elevated intrapressure changes due to increased airway resistance.

The main characteristic of PH in COPD is probably its mild to moderate degree, resting PAP in a stable state of the disease ranging usually between 20 and 35 mmHg (6,12). This modest degree of PH, also observed in other chronic respiratory diseases, is very different from other causes of PH such as pulmonary thromboembolic disease and in particular idiopathic PAH in which PAP is usually >40 mmHg and may exceed 80 mmHg in some patients. In a series of COPD patients, the average PAP is generally 25 to 30 mmHg (6,12), which corresponds to a mild level of PH. A PAP >40 mmHg is thus unusual in COPD except when the patients are investigated during an acute exacerbation or when there is an associated cardiopulmonary disease (6). Special attention will be paid to severe or disproportionate PH in COPD, which has been investigated in recent studies (6,7) (see below). The consequences of the (generally) modest degree of PH in COPD include the absence or late occurrence of right-heart failure (RHF).

B. Worsening of PH During Exercise, Sleep, and Exacerbations

During steady-state exercise, PAP increases markedly in advanced COPD patients with resting PH (11,26). As illustrated in Figure 2, a COPD patient whose baseline mean PAP is modestly elevated (25–30 mmHg) may exhibit severe PH (50–60 mmHg) during moderate (30–40 W) exercise. This is explained by the fact that PVR does not decrease during exercise in these advanced patients (11,26), whereas it does decrease in healthy subjects. From a practical viewpoint, this means that daily activities such as climbing stairs or even walking can induce profound PH.

Acute increases of PAP during sleep have been observed in "advanced" COPD patients with daytime hypoxemia and PH (27,28). They are principally observed in REM sleep during which dips of O_2 desaturation are more severe, with a fall of SaO_2 from its baseline value (wakefulness), which may be as high as 20% to 25%. These episodes of sleep-related desaturation are not due to apneas but to alveolar hypoventilation and/or

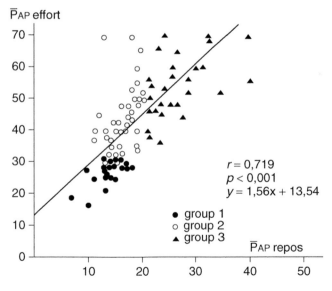

Figure 2 "Resting and exercising PAPs in a large series of chronic obstructive pulmonary disease patients ($n = 92$). Group 1, no resting pulmonary hypertension and exercising PAP <30 mmHg; group 2, no resting pulmonary hypertension but exercising PAP >30 mmHg; and group 3, resting pulmonary hypertension. PAP repos, resting PAP; PAP effort, exercising PAP. Level of exercise: 30 to 40 W, steady state. For comments see text (personal data). *Abbreviation*: PAP, pulmonary artery mean pressure; r, correlation coefficient; p, statistical coefficient; y, exercising PAP; x, resting PAP.

ventilation-perfusion mismatching (28). PAP can increase by as much as 20 mmHg from its baseline value (27). These acute increases of PAP reflect hypoxic pulmonary vasoconstriction.

In advanced COPD, severe exacerbations can lead to acute respiratory failure, characterized by a worsening of hypoxemia and hypercapnia. There is simultaneously a marked increase in PAP from its baseline value (29). There is a parallel between changes in PaO_2 and PAP, illustrating the effects of hypoxic pulmonary vasoconstriction (4). PAP may increase by as much as 20 mmHg but usually returns to its baseline after recovery (30).

Thus, even though PH is usually mild (20–35 mmHg) in COPD patients, it may increase markedly during exercise, sleep, and exacerbations. These acute increases of afterload can favor the development of RHF, especially during exacerbations of the disease (31).

V.   Severe or Disproportionate PH in COPD

As mentioned above, PH in COPD is usually mild to moderate. A minority of patients exhibit severe PH, which can be defined by a resting PAP >35 to 40 mmHg. This level of PH, considered as severe or disproportionate, has promoted recent studies (6,7), which aimed to evaluate its frequency and understand its mechanisms.

Our group has observed that of 998 COPD patients undergoing RHC during a period of disease stability, only 27 had a resting PAP $\geq$40 mmHg (6). Of these 27 patients, 16 had another disease possibly causing PH (e.g., severe obesity plus obstructive sleep apneas). Only 11 patients (1.1% of this series) had COPD as the *only* cause of PH. It is clear that severe PH is very uncommon in COPD. Table 1 indicates that these patients had less severe bronchial obstruction than the remainder (COPD patients with "usual" PH, COPD patients without PH), and their mean FEV_1 was 50%; they had profound hypoxemia, hypocapnia, and a severe reduction of diffusion capacity of lung for carbon monoxide ($D_L CO$). Thabut et al. (7) have identified a similar subgroup of COPD patients in whom pulmonary vascular disease is predominant, and interestingly, this "atypical" subgroup of 16 patients is very similar to our subgroup of 11 patients with severe COPD.

How can the presence of severe PH in COPD patients with moderate airflow obstruction (but with severe hypoxemia) be explained? Two hypotheses can at least be proposed. Some COPD patients could have an increased reactivity of the pulmonary circulation to hypoxia: the "high responders" to hypoxia (21) could develop a marked vascular remodeling when exposed to persistent alveolar hypoxia. The pulmonary vascular response to hypoxia may be inherited, and a study has suggested a role for genetic predisposition to PH in COPD patients (32). The second hypothesis is the fortuitous coexistence of COPD and a pulmonary vascular disease somewhat similar to idiopathic PAH (6).

It seems necessary to detect these COPD patients with severe PH because they have a poor prognosis when compared with COPD patients with usual PH (20–40 mmHg) or without PH (<20 mmHg) (6). These patients should be referred to an expert center of pulmonary vascular disease and should be included in registries and clinical trials (9).

Table 1 Comparison of Three Subgroups of Chronic Obstructive Pulmonary Disease Patients Classified According to the Presence and Severity of Pulmonary Hypertension

	Severe PH without associated disease ($n = 11$)	Control subgroup (PAP > 20 mmHg) ($n = 16$)	Control subgroup (PAP < 20 mmHg) ($n = 16$)
Age (yr)	67 (62–68)	66 (63–73)	62 (53–75)
FEV_1 (% predicted)	50 (44–56)	27 (23–34)	35 (29–50)
FEV_1/VC (%)	49 (39–53)	34 (26–38)	39 (31–52)
$D_L CO$ (mL/min/mmHg)	4.6 (4.2–6.7)	10.3 (8.9–12.8)	13 (11–17)
PaO_2 (mmHg)	46 (41–53)	56 (54–64)	72 (68–76)
$PaCO_2$ (mmHg)	32 (28–37)	47 (44–49)	40 (37–42)
$A\text{-}aO_2$ (mmHg)	56 (50–68)	30 (27–37)	28 (25–34)
PAP (mmHg)	48 (46–50)	25 (22–37)	16 (13–18)
PCWP (mmHg)	6 (4–7)	7 (6.5–7.5)	7.5 (7–7.5)
Q (L/min/m^2)	2.3 (1.8–2.5)	2.8 (2.4–3.1)	3.3 (2.9–4)
TPR (IU/m^2)	21.3 (17.6–36.6)	9 (7.4–9.9)	4 (3.7–5.5)

Values are median (interquartile range).

Severe PH (group 1) is defined by PAP $\geq$40 mmHg. In group 2, PAP ranges between 20 and 40 mmHg (usual PH). In group 3, PAP is <20 mmHg (no PH).

Group 1 is characterized by less severe bronchial obstruction, marked decrease of $D_L CO$, profound hypoxemia, and marked hypocapnia; the differences are statistically significant with the two other subgroups.

Abbreviations: PH, pulmonary hypertension; $A\text{-}aO_2$, alveolar-arterial partial pressure of arterial oxygen difference; $D_L CO$, diffusion capacity for carbon monoxide; FEV_1, forced expiratory volume in one second; $PaCO_2$, partial pressure of arterial carbon dioxide; PaO_2, partial pressure of arterial oxygen; PAP, pulmonary artery mean pressure; PCWP, pulmonary capillary wedge pressure; Q, cardiac output; TPR, total pulmonary resistance; VC, vital capacity.

Source: Adapted from Ref. 6.

VI. Diagnosis of PH in COPD

Symptoms and physical signs are of little help in the diagnosis of PH in COPD. Dyspnea on exertion and fatigue are generally present in advanced COPD patients with or without PH; they are essentially the consequence of airflow limitation and hyperinflation rather than PH.

Physical signs that are observed in severe PH, particularly in idiopathic PAH [e.g., pansystolic murmur owing to tricuspid regurgitation (TR)] are rarely present in COPD patients with PH. This can be explained by the modest degree of PH in most patients and by the late occurrence (or no occurrence at all) of RHF. Peripheral edema occurs rather late in the course of COPD and is not synonymous with RHF (31).

The sensitivity of the electrocardiogram (ECG) for the diagnosis of PH is poor (20–40%), whereas the specificity of signs of right ventricular hypertrophy is high (33). The radiological prediction of PH is even more problematic since radiological signs lack both sensitivity and specificity (33). Magnetic resonance imaging may prove useful for the diagnosis of PH and altered right ventricular structure and function, but it is not routinely used in COPD patients suspected of exhibiting PH.

Doppler echocardiography is by far the best method for the noninvasive diagnosis of PH (34). The maximum velocity of the TR jet allows the calculation of the right ventricular–right atrial pressure gradient from the Bernoulli's equation (4 V^2, where V is the maximum velocity of TR). The calculated gradient is added to the (estimated) right atrial pressure to give an estimated value of right ventricular systolic pressure that is equal to the pulmonary artery systolic pressure. With the same technique, it is possible to estimate the pulmonary artery diastolic pressure.

In COPD patients, the chance of obtaining TR signals of sufficient quality is generally low (35). Arcasoy et al. (10) investigated a large series ($n = 374$) of patients who were candidates for lung transplantation, most of them exhibiting COPD. The estimation of systolic PAP by Doppler echocardiography was possible in only 44% of the patients, and 52% of pressure estimations were found to be inaccurate (>10 mmHg difference compared with pressure measured during RHC).

In spite of technical difficulty in COPD patients, Doppler echocardiography remains the best noninvasive method for PH diagnosis and it may compliment RHC when the latter is mandatory, by providing additional information (34).

Plasma brain natriuretic peptide (BNP) release is due to increased wall stretch of atria and ventricles and may have a relatively good sensitivity and specificity for the assessment of PH in COPD patients (36). However, further studies are needed to determine whether BNP is a useful diagnostic tool in COPD patients.

RHC continues to be the gold standard for the diagnosis of PH (3). It allows the direct measurement of PAP, PCWP, right-heart filling pressures, and cardiac output (by thermodilution or according to the Fick's principle). Measurements are performed at rest in the supine position and can be obtained during steady-state exercise and after therapeutic interventions (O_2, NO, vasodilatators). PVR is calculated according to the formula

$$PVR = \frac{PAP - PCWP}{Q}$$

where Q is the cardiac output.

RHC has two main drawbacks: first, it is an invasive procedure, has some risks, and cannot be routinely performed in COPD patients. The second drawback is the inherent methodological limitation of this technique, which is incapable of measuring instantaneous pressures and does not give information about the natural pulsatility of the pulmonary circulation (34). Micromanometer-tipped, high-fidelity catheters have been developed to overcome this problem (37).

In COPD patients, Doppler echocardiography should be attempted when PH is suspected. The indications for RHC should be limited to the cases when a severe PH is suspected (systolic pressure estimated from Doppler echocardiography >50–60 mmHg).

VII. Evolution and Prognosis of PH in COPD

A. "Natural History" of PH in COPD

The progression of PH is slow in COPD patients, and several studies have shown that PAP may remain stable over periods of two to five years (30,38). In a study in which 93 patients were followed for 5 to 12 years, the changes in PAP were rather small: +0.5 mmHg/yr for the group as a whole (39); the evolution of PAP was identical in the patients with and without initial PH. A study on the natural history of pulmonary hemodynamics in COPD patients with an initial PAP <20 mmHg showed that only 33 out of 121 developed PH after a mean interval of 6.8 ± 2.9 years (40) (Table 2).

Table 2 Long-Term Evolution of Resting and Exercising PAP in 131 Chronic Obstructive Pulmonary Disease Patients Without Resting Pulmonary Hypertension

	T_0	T_1	p value (T_0 vs. T_1)
Resting PAP (mmHg)			
All patients ($n = 131$)	15.2 ± 2.7	17.8 ± 6.6	0.001
Group 1 ($n = 55$)	14.1 ± 2.8	16.0 ± 5.2	0.005
Group 2 ($n = 76$)	16.0 ± 2.3	19.0 ± 7.3	0.001
Exercising PAP (mmHg)			
All patients ($n = 79$)	30.7 ± 7.3	33.3 ± 8.9	0.004
Group 1 ($n = 36$)	25.1 ± 4.1	30.1 ± 8.8	0.001
Group 2 ($n = 43$)	37.2 ± 4.3	37.2 ± 7.4	NS

Group 1, no resting or exercising pulmonary hypertension at T_0; group 2, no resting but exercising pulmonary hypertension at T_0. The mean interval between T_0 and T_1 is 6.8 ± 2.9 years.
Values are mean $\pm$SD.
Abbreviations: PAP, pulmonary artery mean pressure; T_0, time of first right-heart catheterization; T_1, time of second right-heart catheterization.
Source: Adapted from Ref. 40.

Nevertheless, a minority ($\sim 30\%$) of advanced COPD patients exhibit a marked worsening of PAP during follow-up (39). These patients do not differ from the others at the onset, but they are characterized by a progressive deterioration of PaO_2 and partial pressure of arterial carbon dioxide ($PaCO_2$) during the evolution (30,39) and there is a significant correlation between the changes in PaO_2 and PAP (39). The longitudinal evolution of PH is favorably influenced by long-term oxygen therapy (LTOT) (see following text).

B. From PH to RHF

The classic view of the development of RHF in COPD patients is the following (3): PH increases the work of the right ventricle, which leads to right ventricular enlargement (hypertrophy plus dilatation), which can result in right ventricular dysfunction (systolic, diastolic). Later, RHF, characterized by the presence of peripheral edema, can be observed in some COPD patients. There is a relationship between the severity of PH and the development of RHF.

Peripheral edema is frequently observed in advanced COPD patients and is considered to reflect RHF, but the possible occurrence of RHF in these patients has been questioned (41) in particular because the degree of PH is most often mild in COPD. Peripheral edema may simply indicate the presence of secondary hyperaldosteronism induced by functional renal insufficiency (42). In COPD patients, the presence of edema is not synonymous with heart failure (3,41).

The role of pressure overload in the development of RHF in these patients has been debated. MacNee et al. (43), comparing COPD patients with and without clinical (edema) and hemodynamic signs of RHF concluded that RHF was probably due to other causes than PH. A study from our group has led to different conclusions (31): in 9 out of 16 patients with marked peripheral edema, hemodynamic signs of RHF were present during the episode of edema and were probably accounted for by a significant worsening of PH (from 27 ± 5 to 40 ± 6 mmHg, $p < 0.001$), which in turn was explained by a worsening of hypoxemia (Table 3).

Table 3 Evolution of Arterial Blood Gases and Hemodynamic Variables Before and During an Episode of Peripheral Edema in Severe Chronic Obstructive Pulmonary Disease Patients

	RVEDP (mmHg)		PAP (mmHg)		Q (L/min/m^2)		PaO$_2$ (mmHg)		PaCO$_2$ (mmHg)	
	T_1	T_2	T_1	T_2	T_1	T_2	T_1	T_2	T_1	T_2
Group 1 ($n = 9$)	7.5 ± 3.9	13.4 ± 1.2[a]	27 ± 5	40 ± 6[a]	3.23 ± 0.82	3.19 ± 1.07	63 ± 4	49 ± 7[a]	46 ± 7	59 ± 14[a]
Group 2 ($n = 7$)	5.5 ± 2.4	5.1 ± 1.5	20 ± 6	21 ± 5	3.63 ± 0.36	3.29 ± 1.32	66 ± 7	59 ± 7	42 ± 6	45 ± 6

Values are mean ±SD.

Group 1, patients with hemodynamic signs of right-heart failure (elevated RVEDP); group 2, patients without hemodynamic signs of right-heart failure.

[a]Difference between T_1 and T_2 statistically significant, $p < 0.001$.

Abbreviations: PAP, pulmonary artery mean pressure; Q, cardiac output; RVEDP, right ventricular end diastolic pressure; PaCO$_2$, partial pressure of arterial carbon dioxide; PaO$_2$, partial pressure of arterial oxygen; T_1, time of stable state of the disease; T_2, time of episode of edema.

Source: Adapted from Ref. 31.

The best way of assessing right ventricular performance is to measure right ventricular contractility (end-systolic pressure–volume relationship of the right ventricle), but indeed, this cannot be done in routine. Right ventricular contractility is near normal in COPD patients with PH investigated in a stable state but has been found decreased during severe exacerbations with marked peripheral edema (43). On the other hand, right ventricular ejection fraction (RVEF) is not a good index of right ventricular contractility since a decreased RVEF is most often the consequence of an increased afterload (increased PAP or PVR or both).

Thus, many patients with advanced COPD will never develop RHF, and on the other hand, at least some patients experience episodes of "true" RHF during exacerbations of the disease accompanied by a worsening of PH (31).

C. Prognosis of PH in COPD

The level of PAP is a good indicator of prognosis (12,44). The prognosis is worse in patients with PH compared with patients without PH and is particularly poor for patients with a severe degree of PH (>35–40 mmHg) (44) including patients with disproportionate PH (6).

The five-year survival rate of COPD patients with PH (PAP > 20 mmHg) is about 50% (12,44). LTOT significantly improves the survival of markedly hypoxemic COPD patients, most of them exhibiting PH (45,46). Consequently, it can be expected that the prognosis of PH will improve with LTOT. PAP is still an excellent prognostic indicator in COPD patients treated with LTOT, which can be explained by the fact that it is a good marker of both the duration and the severity of alveolar hypoxia in these patients (5).

VIII. Treatment of PH in COPD

The treatment of PH includes oxygen therapy and vasodilators. An important question is: is it necessary to treat PH in COPD? We have seen that PH is mild to moderate in COPD, and the necessity for treatment can be questioned. The best argument in favor of treatment is that PH may worsen particularly during acute exacerbations and these acute increases in PAP can contribute to the development of RHF (31).

A. Long-Term Oxygen Therapy

Alveolar hypoxia is considered to be the major determinant of the elevation of PVR and PAP in COPD patients. One of the aims of LTOT is the improvement in PH induced by chronic alveolar hypoxia. The well-known Noctural Oxygen Therapy Trial (NOTT) and Medical Research Council (MRC) studies (45,46) were not principally devoted to pulmonary hemodynamics, but RHC was performed at the onset in all patients and follow-up data were available in a relatively high number of patients. In the MRC study (46) from 42 patients who survived >500 days from the onset of the study, those ($n = 21$) who were given LTOT had a stable PAP, whereas PAP increased significantly (+2.8 mmHg/yr) in the control group of 21 patients. In the NOTT study (45), hemodynamic data at the onset and after six months of LTOT were available in 117 patients. Continuous ($\geq$18 hr/day) LTOT decreased slightly (3 mmHg) but significantly resting PAP and PVR, whereas nocturnal oxygen therapy (10–12 hr/day) did not.

Further studies more specifically devoted to the pulmonary hemodynamic evolution under LTOT (47,48) have shown either a tendency to the reversal of the progression of PH (47) or a stabilization of PH under LTOT (48) over periods of two to six years. However, PAP seldom returns to normal. It must be emphasized that the best hemodynamic results have been obtained in the studies in which the daily duration of LTOT was the longest ($\geq$17–18 hr/day) (45,47). Accordingly, one should recommend continuous oxygen therapy.

B. Vasodilator Drugs

Treatment of PAH has shown a dramatic change in the past few years. Epoprostenol, prostacyclin analogues, endothelin receptor antagonists, and phosphodiesterase-5 inhibitors were tested in randomized controlled trials, leading to the approval of several drugs. It is tempting to use these drugs in PH complicating COPD, particularly in the (rare) cases of disproportionate PH. Unfortunately, there have been very few studies in this field. A recent study, having included COPD patients with mild resting PH or no PH, treated with bosentan (endothelin receptor antagonist) or placebo, has shown no improvement in pulmonary hemodynamics but a worsening of gas exchange abnormalities (49).

Nitric oxide (NO) is a selective and potent pulmonary vasodilator. One long-term study (50) on 40 patients already on LTOT has shown that the addition of NO produced a significant improvement in PAP, PVR, and cardiac output. However, the technological and toxicological problems related to the prolonged use of inhaled NO are far from being solved.

It is presently recommended not to treat COPD patients with drugs dedicated to PAH outside trials. More randomized controlled studies are required in this area.

IX. Conclusions

PH is frequently observed in patients with advanced COPD, but its actual prevalence is still unknown. PH is probably more a marker of both the duration and the severity of chronic alveolar hypoxia than a true complication of COPD. The main characteristic of PH in COPD is probably its mild to moderate degree, resting PAP in a stable state of the disease usually ranging between 20 and 35 mmHg. However, PH may worsen during exercise, sleep, and exacerbations of the disease, and these acute increases in afterload can favor the development of RHF, which is observed in some COPD patients, most often during acute exacerbations.

At present, LTOT is the logical treatment of PH since alveolar hypoxia is considered to be the major determinant of the elevation of PVR and PAP in COPD. LTOT stabilizes or at least attenuates and sometimes reverses the progression of PH. The longer the daily duration of LTOT, the better are the pulmonary hemodynamic results. Vasodilators used for the treatment of PAH (prostacyclin, endothelin receptor antagonists, sildenafil) have rarely been prescribed to patients with severe (>35–40 mmHg) PH who are probably <5% of patients with advanced COPD, and we need randomized controlled trials in these patients with disproportionate PH.

References

1. Celli BR, MacNee W. Standards for the diagnosis and treatment of patients with COPD: a summary of the ATS/ERS position paper. Eur Respir J 2004; 23:932–946.
2. Fishman AP. Chronic cor pulmonale. Am Rev Respir Dis 1976; 114:775–794.
3. MacNee W. Pathophysiology of cor pulmonale in chronic obstructive pulmonary disease. Am J Respir Crit Care Med 1994; 150:833–852, 1158–1168.
4. Weitzenblum E. Chronic cor pulmonale. Heart 2003; 89:225–230.
5. Oswald-Mammosser M, Weitzenblum E, Quoix E, et al. Prognostic factors in COPD patients receiving long-term oxygen therapy. Chest 1995; 107:1193–1198.
6. Chaouat A, Bugnet AS, Kadaoui N, et al. Severe pulmonary hypertension and chronic obstructive pulmonary disease. Am J Respir Crit Care Med 2005; 172:189–194.
7. Thabut G, Dauriat G, Stern JB, et al. Pulmonary hemodynamics in advanced COPD candidates for lung volume reduction surgery or lung transplantation. Chest 2005; 127:1531–1536.
8. Fisher MR, Criner GJ, Fishman AP, et al. Estimating pulmonary artery pressures by echocardiography in patients with emphysema. Eur Respir J 2007; 30:914–921.
9. Chaouat A, Naeije R, Weitzenblum E. Pulmonary hypertension in COPD. Eur Respir J 2008; 32:1371–1385.
10. Arcasoy SM, Christie JD, Ferrari VA, et al. Echocardiographic assessment of pulmonary hypertension in patients with advanced lung disease. Am J Respir Crit Care Med 2003; 167:735–740.
11. Burrows B, Kettel LJ, Niden AH, et al. Patterns of cardiovascular dysfunction in chronic obstructive lung disease. N Engl J Med 1972; 286:912–991.
12. Weitzenblum E, Hirth C, Ducolone A, et al. Prognostic value of pulmonary artery pressure in chronic obstructive pulmonary disease. Thorax 1981; 36:752–758.
13. Scharf S, Igbal M, Keller C, et al. Hemodynamic characterization of patients with severe emphysema. Am J Respir Crit Care Med 2002; 166:314–322.
14. Williams BT, Nicholl JP. Prevalence of hypoxaemic chronic obstructive lung disease with reference to long-term oxygen therapy. Lancet 1985; 1:369–372.
15. Boutin-Forzano S, Moreau D, Kalaboka S, et al. Reported prevalence and comorbidity of asthma, chronic bronchitis and emphysema: a pan-European estimation. Int J Tuberc Lung Dis 2007; 11:695–702.
16. Butler J, Schrijen F, Henriquez A, et al. Cause of the raised wedge pressure on exercise in chronic obstructive pulmonary disease. Am Rev Respir Dis 1988; 138:350–354.
17. Barbera JA, Peinado VI, Santos S. Pulmonary hypertension in chronic obstructive pulmonary disease. Eur Respir J 2003; 21:892–905.
18. Fishman AP. Hypoxia on the pulmonary circulation. How and where it acts. Circ Res 1976; 38:221–231.
19. Fishman AP, McClement J, Himmelstein A, et al. Effects of acute anoxia on the circulation and respiration in patients with chronic pulmonary disease studied during the steady state. J Clin Invest 1952; 31:770–781.
20. Archer S, Michelakis E. The mechanism(s) of hypoxic pulmonary vasoconstriction: potassium channels, redox O_2 sensors, and controversies. News Physiol Sci 2002; 17:131–137.
21. Weitzenblum E, Schrijen F, Mohan-Kumar T, et al. Variability of the pulmonary vascular response to acute hypoxia in chronic bronchitis. Chest 1988; 94:772–778.
22. Penaloza D, Sime F, Banchero N, et al. Pulmonary hypertension in healthy men born and living at high altitude. Med Thorac 1962; 19:449–460.
23. Wilkinson M, Langhome CA, Heath D, et al. A pathophysiological study of 10 cases of hypoxic cor pulmonale. Q J Med 1988; 66:65–85.

24. Wright JL, Lawson L, Pare PD, et al. The structure and function of the pulmonary vasculature in mild chronic obstructive pulmonary disease. The effect of oxygen and exercise. Am Rev Respir Dis 1983; 128:702–707.

25. Santos S, Peinado VI, Ramirez J, et al. Characterization of pulmonary vascular remodelling in smokers and patients with mild COPD. Eur Respir J 2002; 19:6.

26. Horsfield K, Segel N, Bishop JM. The pulmonary circulation in chronic bronchitis at rest and during exercise breathing air and 80% oxygen. Clin Sci 1968; 43:473–483.

27. Coccagna G, Lugaresi E. Arterial blood gases and pulmonary and systemic arterial pressure during sleep in chronic obstructive pulmonary disease. Sleep 1978; 1:117–124.

28. Fletcher EC, Levin DC. Cardiopulmonary hemodynamics during sleep in subjects with chronic obstructive pulmonary disease: the effect of short and long-term oxygen. Chest 1984; 85:6–14.

29. Abraham AS, Cole RB, Green ID, et al. Factors contributing to the reversible pulmonary hypertension of patients with acute respiratory failure studied by serial observations during recovery. Circ Res 1969; 24:51–60.

30. Weitzenblum E, Loiseau A, Hirth C, et al. Course of pulmonary hemodynamics in patients with chronic obstructive pulmonary disease. Chest 1979; 75:656–662.

31. Weitzenblum E, Apprill A, Oswald M, et al. Pulmonary hemodynamics in patients with chronic obstructive pulmonary disease before and during an episode of peripheral edema. Chest 1994; 105:1377–1382.

32. Eddahibi S, Chaouat A, Morrell N, et al. Polymorphism of the serotonin transporter gene and pulmonary hypertension in chronic obstructive pulmonary disease. Circulation 2003; 108:1839–1844.

33. Oswald-Mammosser M, Oswald T, Nyankiye E, et al. Non-invasive diagnosis of pulmonary hypertension in chronic obstructive pulmonary disease. Comparison of ECG, radiological measurements, echocardiography and myocardial scintigraphy. Eur J Respir Dis 1987; 71:419–429.

34. Naeije R, Torbicki A. More on the noninvasive diagnosis of pulmonary hypertension: Doppler echocardiography revisited. Eur Respir J 1995; 8:1445–1449.

35. Tramarin R, Torbicki A, Marchandise B, et al. Doppler echocardiographic evaluation of pulmonary artery pressure in chronic obstructive pulmonary disease. A European multicentre study. Eur Heart J 1991; 12:103–111.

36. Leuchte HH, Baumgartner RA, Nounou ME, et al. Brain natriuretic peptide is a prognostic parameter in chronic lung disease. Am J Respir Crit Care Med 2006; 173:744–750.

37. Raeside D, Peacock A. Making measurements in the pulmonary circulation: when and how? Thorax 1997; 52:9–11.

38. Schrijen F, Uffholtz H, Polu JM, et al. Pulmonary and systemic hemodynamic evolution in chronic bronchitis. Am Rev Respir Dis 1978; 117:25–23.

39. Weitzenblum E, Sautegeau A, Ehrhart M, et al. Long-term course of pulmonary arterial pressure in chronic obstructive pulmonary disease. Am Rev Respir Dis 1984; 130:993–998.

40. Kessler R, Faller M, Weitzenblum E, et al. "Natural history" of pulmonary hypertension in a series of 131 patients with chronic obstructive lung disease. Am J Respir Crit Care Med 2001; 164:219–224.

41. Richens JM, Howard P. Oedema in cor pulmonale. Clin Sci 1982; 62:255–259.

42. Farber MO, Weinberger MH, Robertson GL, et al. Hormonal abnormalities affecting sodium and water balance in acute respiratory failure due to chronic obstructive lung disease. Chest 1984; 85:49–54.

43. MacNee W, Wathen C, Flenley DC, et al. The effects of controlled oxygen therapy on ventricular function in patients with stable and decompensated cor pulmonale. Am Rev Respir Dis 1988; 137:1289–1295.

44. Bishop JM, Cross KW. Physiological variables and mortality in patients with various categories of chronic respiratory disease. Bull Eur Physiopathol Respir 1984; 20:495–500.
45. Nocturnal Oxygen Therapy Trial Group. Continuous or nocturnal oxygen therapy in hypoxemic chronic obstructive lung disease. Ann Intern Med 1980; 93:391–398.
46. Report of the Medical Research Council Working Party. Long-term domiciliary oxygen therapy in chronic hypoxic cor pulmonale complicating chronic bronchitis and emphysema. Lancet 1981; 1:681–686.
47. Weitzenblum E, Sautegeau A, Ehrhart M, et al. Long term oxygen therapy can reverse the progression of pulmonary hypertension in patients with chronic obstructive pulmonary disease. Am Rev Respir Dis 1985; 131:493–498.
48. Zielinski J, Tobiasz M, Hawrylkiewicz I, et al. Effects of long-term oxygen therapy on pulmonary hemodynamics in COPD patients. A 6-year prospective study. Chest 1998; 113:65–70.
49. Stolz D, Rasch H, Linka A, et al. A randomised controlled trial of bosentan in severe COPD. Eur Respir J 2008; 32:619–628.
50. Vonbank K, Ziesche R, Higenbottam TW, et al. Controlled prospective randomised trial on the effects on pulmonary haemodynamics of the ambulatory long-term use of nitric oxide and oxygen in patients with severe COPD. Thorax 2003; 58:289–293.

19

Pulmonary Hypertension Complicating Interstitial Lung Disease

DAVID A. ZISMAN, JOHN A. BELPERIO, RAJAN SAGGAR, RAJEEV SAGGAR, MICHAEL C. FISHBEIN, and JOSEPH P. LYNCH III
David Geffen School of Medicine at UCLA, Los Angeles, California, U.S.A.

I. Introduction

The interstitial lung diseases (ILDs) are a varied group of conditions characterized by inflammation and fibrosis of the lung parenchyma. Pulmonary hypertension (PH) has been described in most of these conditions. In ILD, the term PH is preferred over pulmonary arterial hypertension (PAH) as PAH refers to World Health Organization (WHO) group 1, that is, idiopathic pulmonary arterial hypertension (IPAH) and connective tissue disease (CTD)-associated pulmonary hypertension. PH complicating ILD is included under WHO class 3 (hypoxia-associated PH) (1). PH has been described in nearly all patients with advanced pulmonary Langerhans cell histiocytosis (PLCH) (2–4), in advanced cases of lymphangioleiomyomatosis (LAM), hypersensitivity pneumonitis (HP), amyloidosis, drugs, asbestosis, pneumoconioses, bronchoalveolar carcinoma, lymphangitic carcinomatosis, and radiation (5–12). This chapter will focus on PH complicating idiopathic pulmonary fibrosis (IPF) and sarcoidosis since most of the investigations have focused on these two conditions. Given that CTD-associated PH patients commonly have a primary vasculopathic component, this group will be the topic of a separate discussion.

II. Prevalence

The prevalence of PH in ILD varies depending on how PH was defined and the method of detection employed. PH has been defined by using different mean pulmonary artery pressure (MPAP) cutoffs (e.g., >17, 20, or 25 mmHg) and diagnosed either by right-heart catheterization (RHC) or transthoracic echocardiography (TTE). In IPF, PH has been reported in 8% to 80% of patients (13–15). In a prospective analysis of 78 consecutive IPF patients undergoing initial workup with RHC, PH (defined as MPAP > 25 mmHg) was detected in only six patients (8.1%) (13). It is possible that the lower prevalence of PH in that study could be explained by the fact that those patients as a whole were in relatively early stages of IPF when they underwent their initial RHC. Investigations in patients referred for lung transplantation (LT) have included patients with more severe IPF and have consistently shown a higher prevalence of PH. In one retrospective analysis of 79 consecutive patients with IPF undergoing pretransplantation RHC, PH was present in 32% of patients (16). In a subsequent cross-sectional study of 61 patients with IPF evaluated for LT, PH (defined as MPAP from RHC >25 mmHg) was present in 39% of patients (17). PH may more prevalent in IPF patients with coexistent emphysema. In a study of 61 patients with combined pulmonary fibrosis and emphysema, PH was present in 47% of patients at diagnosis and 55% during follow-up; further, 11 patients (18%) developed right-sided cardiac failure during follow-up (18). The prevalence of PH in IPF is higher (80%) when patients are exercised (15). In one study, the mean MPAP at rest was 22 mmHg; at maximal exercise, the mean MPAP increased to 45 mmHg (15). In that study, when PH was absent at rest, it developed in two-thirds of patients when exercised. The prevalence of PH in IPF also increases as patients are followed over time. In one study of 44 IPF patients with serial RHC data, the baseline prevalence of PH was 40% and increased to 80% at follow-up; in that study, the baseline mean MPAP was 23 mmHg and increased to 33 mmHg on follow-up evaluation (14). The MPAP in IPF follows a Gaussian distribution; most cases have an MPAP between 20 and 30 mmHg; a minority (10%) present with MPAP >30 mmHg (16). The optimal MPAP cut point to define PH in ILD remains under investigation. By using receiver operating characteristic (ROC) analysis, one group of investigators identified the "optimal" cut point MPAP in association with mortality to be 17 mmHg; however, this finding awaits confirmation in future investigations (13). In patients with non-specific interstitial pneumonia (NSIP), PH was described in 40% of cases (19). PH has been noted in 1% to 12% of patients with pulmonary sarcoidosis (20–23), but the incidence is considerably higher among patients with advanced fibrocystic sarcoidosis (24–29). One study of 30 patients with pulmonary sarcoidosis noted normal pulmonary artery pressure in patients with stages I and II, but progressive elevation in pulmonary artery pressure was noted in radiographic stage III. All patients with stage III disease exhibited PH with exercise (30). In a separate study, PH was present in 3 of 24 patients (12.5%) with pulmonary sarcoidosis at rest and in 18 patients (75%) with exercise (31). Sulica et al. reported 106 patients with sarcoidosis who had TTE, chest radiographs, and pulmonary function tests (PFTs) from a single center (32). Overall, 54 patients (51%) had PH (defined as RVSP $\geq$ 40 mmHg) by TTE; 9 patients had RVSP >75 mmHg. The United Network for Organ Sharing (UNOS) database identified 363 patients with sarcoidosis listed for LT in the United States between January 1995 and December 2002, who had undergone RHC (33). PH (defined as MPAP > 25 mmHg) was present in 74%: MPAP exceeded 36 mmHg in 36%.

PH is common in patients with severe PLCH and likely represents intrinsic pulmonary vascular disease (4). In a series of 21 patients with advanced PLCH referred for LT, all patients had PH (MPAP, 59 mmHg); PH was disproportionate to the degree of pulmonary functional impairment or hypoxemia (4). Histopathology demonstrated proliferative vasculopathy involving muscular arteries and veins, with prominent venular involvement. Epoprostenol precipitated pulmonary edema in two patients with PH complicating PLCH, possibly reflecting the impact of downstream venular obstruction (4). A fatal case of veno-occlusive disease complicating PLCH has also been described (34). A retrospective series from the Mayo Clinic reported 123 patients with PLCH (3). PH was present in 15 of 17 patients who had TTE; 7 had RVSP >65 mmHg and an enlarged RV and impaired systolic function. An inverse correlation was found between the FVC and RVSP ($r = -0.61; p = .03$); no correlation was found between RVSP and other pulmonary function parameters. The presence of PH markedly increased mortality (hazard ratio, 28.8), $p < 0.01$ (3).

III. Prognosis

PH in ILD portends a poor prognosis. In a study of 99 patients with well-documented IPF, the median survival of those with TTE-estimated pulmonary artery systolic pressure (SPAP) >50 mmHg was less than one year (35). In patients with IPF referred for LT, an RHC-measured MPAP > 25 mmHg was associated with a median survival of two years (16). Therefore, patients with ILD and PH should be referred for LT. In addition, PH in ILD is associated with limited functional capacity. In a study of 79 IPF patients listed for LT, those with PH (RHC-measured MPAP >25 mmHg) walked on average <150 m during a six-minute walk test (6MWT); by contrast, those without PH walked on average >350 m (16). In a recent study, 34 patients with pulmonary fibrosis underwent exercise testing. Patients with PH showed a significantly impaired exercise tolerance and worsened ventilatory inefficiency (36).

Several studies found that PH in sarcoid patients was associated with increased mortality. One study of 22 sarcoid patients with PH cited two- and five-year survival rates of 74% and 59%, respectively (37). In contrast, five-year survival among sarcoid controls without PH was 96.4%. A retrospective review of the UNOS database from 1995 to 2000 identified 404 sarcoid patients listed for LT in the United States (38). Three factors were associated with increased mortality: (*i*) the presence of PH, (*ii*) the amount of supplemental oxygen needed, and (*iii*) African American race. The MPAP of survivors was 31.7 mmHg compared with 41.4 mmHg among nonsurvivors ($p < 0.001$) (38). Another study of 43 patients with sarcoidosis awaiting LT found that MPAP $\geq$ 35 mmHg, CI < 2 L/min/m^2, and RAP > 15 mmHg were associated with a higher mortality risk (39). By multivariate analysis, MRAP >15 mmHg was the only independent prognostic variable [5.2-fold odds ratio (OR) for mortality]. Hence, PH in sarcoidosis is also associated with poor prognosis and should prompt consideration for LT (38).

IV. Etiology

PH in ILD may result from (*i*) the fibrotic process itself, (*ii*) the intrinsic vascular abnormalities, (*iii*) the underlying pathogenic process, and (*iv*) the presence of comorbid conditions.

A. The Fibrotic Process

As the pulmonary capillaries fenestrate the interstitium of the lung, inflammation and fibrosis of the interstitium may affect the vascular bed. In early honeycomb lung, the vascular disease consists largely of muscularization. As the honeycomb lung develops, there is a stage of fibrous vascular atrophy and ablation. This is characterized by pronounced intimal fibrosis and recanalization of thrombus. Subsequently, there is fibrous atrophy of the media and finally fibrous ablation of affected vessels (40). In some cases, there is a plexus of thin-walled vessels, which may be the histological counterpart of

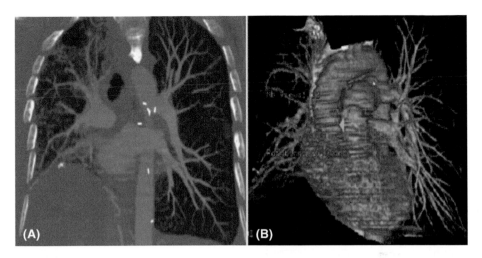

Figure 1 (*See color insert*) Computed tomography angiogram of an idiopathic pulmonary fibrosis patient after left single-lung transplant contrasting the effects of fibrosis on the native lung pulmonary vasculature with the normal vasculature in the allograft. *Source:* Courtesy of Steven D. Nathan, MD.

pulmonary-systemic anastomoses demonstrated radiologically in this condition (40). Vascular ablation and redistribution of blood vessels in areas of interstitial thickening are evident in the lungs of patients with IPF. In a study of open lung biopsies from eight patients with IPF, vessel density was markedly reduced in IPF compared with controls. In that study, fibroblastic foci were characterized by almost complete absence of blood vessels. However, immediately adjacent to fibroblastic foci, an increase in microvessels was evident (41). The vascular ablation reduces the conductance of the vascular bed, augments the pulmonary vascular resistance, and generates PH. Furthermore, the perivascular fibrosis may influence the distensibility of the pulmonary vessels, possibly augmenting the pulmonary vascular resistance and pulmonary artery pressure. The location of the fibrotic process may also play a role in the genesis of PH; for instance in IPF, the fibrotic process occurs mainly in a subpleural distribution with a basilar predilection, whereas in sarcoidosis, the fibrotic process has a peribronchovascular distribution affecting the proximal pulmonary arteries and upper lobes vessels. Figure 1 depicts the abnormal pulmonary vasculature of a patient with IPF who underwent a left single-lung transplant. This figure highlights some of the macroscopic lesions that the fibrotic process may impose on the pulmonary arteries. The pulmonary arteries of the right native lung are irregular with a "moth-eaten" appearance; by contrast, the right-lung allograft is perfused by normal vessels with smooth borders.

B. Intrinsic Vascular Abnormalities

The blood vessels themselves may participate in the genesis of PH via intrinsic mechanisms independent of the fibrotic process. This notion has been suggested by the poor correlations between MPAP and various measures of lung fibrosis (17,27,42). For instance, aberrant neovascularization in IPF may alter vascular compliance or increase the vascular resistance of the pulmonary vessels leading to PH. There is evidence of regional heterogeneity with some areas demonstrating increased vascularity and others demonstrating decreased vascularity (41,43–46). While fibroblastic foci are notable for the absence of blood vessels, they are surrounded by a rich network of vessels (47); this finding may explain why there is no correlation between extent of fibrosis and MPAP (17,27,42). Human and animal investigations of lung injury and fibrosis demonstrate upregulation of protease inhibitors (48), leading to hypercoagulability, suppression of fibrinolysis, and, possibly, thrombotic events; hence, patients with pulmonary fibrosis have a prothrombotic tendency with a propensity to form microthrombi that in turn may contribute to the genesis of PH (48,49). Further, as in other forms of PH, shear stress of the vessel may lead to endothelial cell dysfunction that may perpetuate the PH (50). Similar cytokine derrangements have been described in pulmonary fibrosis and primary vascular disease [e.g., transforming growth factor β (TGF-β), connective tissue growth factor (CTGF), endothelin-1 (ET-1)], suggesting that these disorders share pathogenic features and that one may influence, generate, or perpetuate the other. The dysfunction of the pulmonary endothelial cell in ILD may manifest as enhanced synthesis of ET-1 (51), TGF-β (52), and platelet-derived growth factor (PDGF), or decreased synthesis of vasodilators and antismooth muscle cell proliferation molecules such as nitric oxide (NO) or prostacyclin (51,53). NO is a potent vasodilator detectable in the exhaled air of humans. When compared with normal subjects, patients with pulmonary fibrosis have lower levels of resting NO and show no significant increase in response to exercise. Failure to increase NO during exercise in IPF may reflect an inability to recruit the capillary bed and pulmonary endothelial dysfunction (54). Microarray analysis performed on 13 patients with IPF and PH revealed that underexpressed genes included angiogenic factors such as vascular endothelial growth factor (VEGF) and platelet endothelial cell adhesion molecule, as well as factors affecting vessel tone such as angiotensin-converting enzyme and ET-1. Overexpressed genes included phospholipase A_2 and other factors that mediate remodeling. The decrease in angiogenic factors and the increase in inflammatory and remodeling genes may reflect a fundamental alteration in the vascular cell phenotype in IPF that may contribute to the development of PH (55).

V.   Pathogenesis

A.   Overall Review of the Pathogenesis of ILD

ILD involves an initial lung injury either from the inhalation of noxious agents damaging the epithelium or through an immune injury to the pulmonary vasculature (46,56–64). When either injury is aggressive enough to cause significant damage to the alveolar-capillary basement membrane (ACBM), pulmonary fibrosis will occur (Fig. 2). The commonality between an inhalation and vascular injury causing pulmonary fibrosis has to do with the inseparability of the alveolus epithelium and endothelium that fuse together creating the ACBM (Fig. 2A). Thus, injury to one cell type (epithelium) also causes injury to its neighboring cell (endothelium) (Fig. 2B). Injury to the ACBM begins a cascade of events including the extravasation of red blood cells, heme, platelets, and plasma. This is followed by the activation of the coagulation cascade resulting in platelet activation/ degranulation and fibrin deposition creating provisional matrix deposition (highly vascularized immature matrix made up of fibrin, fibronectin, and collagen-type III > I)

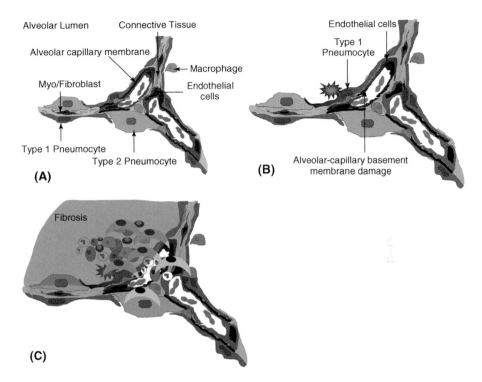

Figure 2 (*See color insert*) Pathogenesis of IPF. (**A**) Normal ACBM. (**B**) Severe injury to the type I pneumocyte and neighboring endothelial cell with loss of the ACBM. (**C**) Inflammation, remodeling, and fibrosis. *Abbreviation:* ACBM, alveolar-capillary basement membrane.

within the alveolus. Furthermore, a stress response from each cellular component of the ACBM augments local inflammation [e.g., lipid mediators, cytokines, chemokines, growth factors, and matrix metalloproteinases (MMPs)]. This new inflammatory milieu triggers the recruitment/activation of immune, nonimmune, and progenitor/stem cells to the site of injury (Fig. 2C). The combination of new mediators, new cell to cell interactions, and new cell to matrix interactions leads to a change in phenotype of multiple cells. For instance, normally inflammatory mediators and cells work together to cause a repair with resolution of immature matrix allowing for the dissolution of fibrosis (e.g., repair-resolution-dissolution). However, with pulmonary fibrosis there are phenotypic changes (e.g., antiapoptotic and fibroproliferative phenotypes) of multiple cell types causing aberrant repair/remodeling resulting in a fibrotic lung (e.g., aberrant repair-remodeling-fibrosis) (Fig. 2C).

B. Pathogenesis of PH during ILD

The typical pulmonary artery (PA) is made up of three layers of delicate tissue. The innermost layer is called the intima and consists of endothelial cells surrounded by rare smooth muscle cells (SMCs) and fibroblasts that are contained within a border called the

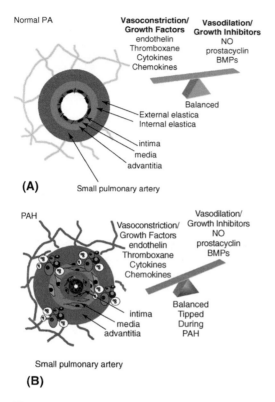

Figure 3 (*See color insert*) Pathogenesis of PAH. (**A**) In the normal lung, there is a delicate balance of mediators that leads to normal vascular turnover (e.g., vasoconstrictors, cytokines, and growth factors vs. vasodilators and anti-inflammatory cytokines). (**B**) When there is some insult to the lung such as a vascular insult or an epithelial/endothelial injury as seen in IPF, there is a disproportionate overexpression of growth factors and vasoconstrictors. This imbalance of growth factors and vasoconstrictors leads to intimal expansion from endothelial cell hyperplasia with migration/proliferation of smooth muscle cells, and myo/fibroblasts as well as the recruitment of inflammatory cells that allows for extracellular matrix deposition. Similarly, the media expands secondary to inflammatory cells and the migration/proliferation of smooth muscle cells, and myo/fibroblasts causing more matrix deposition. The adventitia can also develop chronic inflammatory changes. Ultimately, the combination of these events leads to vessel narrowing and obliteration. *Abbreviations*: PAH, pulmonary arterial hypertension; NO, nitric oxide; BMPs, bone morphogenetic proteins.

internal elastica (Fig. 3A). Then there is a media predominately made up of SMCs, few fibroblasts, some matrix, and rare immune cells that is bordered by the external elastica (Fig. 3A). The adventitia is the final layer and predominantly made up of connective tissue with rare immune cells (Fig. 3A). The pathogenesis of PH during ILD is multifactorial and likely involves all three layers of the PA (Fig. 3). Numerous factors all cause capillary/arterial/venular obliteration and intraluminal thrombosis/fibrosis that eventually leads to an increased pressure head and shearing of the feeding pulmonary arterial walls (Figs 3 and 4). The specific factors causing PH-associated ILD include (*i*) injury to the ACBM causing a loss of pulmonary capillary/arterial bed, (*ii*) altered immune response during ILD via molecular mimicry where the immune system injuries the pulmonary vessels causing obliteration and thrombosis/fibrosis, (*iii*) altered immune response with excess release of vasoconstrictive compounds (e.g., ET-1, serotonin, thromboxane A_2) and exhaustion/deficiency of pulmonary arterial vaso-dilators (e.g., prostacyclin, NO), (*iv*) altered immune response with excess fibroplasia/fibroproliferation/fibro-obliteration of pulmonary vessels (Figs 3 and 4). Overall each of these processes affects the intima causing endothelial cell hyperplasia/thrombosis/fibrosis with SMC and myofibroblast proliferation/recruitment resulting in vessel narrowing (Figs 3 and 4). In addition, the media will also develop inflammation with SMC and myofibroblast proliferation/recruitment, which contributes to vessel narrowing, while the adventitia can also develop inflammatory changes that can also lead directly or indirectly to luminal narrowing (1,65,66) (Figs 3 and 4). Importantly, the same mediators (cytokines, chemokines, growth factors, and MMPs) that are involved in the pathogenesis of ILD are also involved in the vascular remodeling of PH (1,65,67–71). In this review, we will focus on available data, which demonstrate an overlap of specific cytokines, chemokines, and growth factors that are associated with both PH and ILD.

C. TGF-β Superfamily Involvement in PH and ILD

TGF-β isoforms (e.g., TGF-$β_1$, TGF-$β_2$, and TGF-$β_3$) are involved in vascular remod-eling, SMC proliferation, immune cell regulation, and myo/fibroblast matrix deposition (72–100). Bone morphogenetic proteins (e.g., BMP2, BMP4, BMP6, and BMP7), named because they were first discovered to be involved in cartilage and bone growth/repair, interact with the specific receptor, bone morphogenetic receptor type 2 (BMPR2), which tends to have the opposite physiological effects of TGF- βs (101–103).

Concerning ILD, TGF-β protein levels in BALF and lung tissue homogenates were elevated in IPF patients, compared with normal control lungs (104–108). Proof of concept studies using a rodent model of bleomycin-induced ILD demonstrated that passive immunization of bleomycin-treated mice with neutralizing antibodies to both TGF-$β_1$ and TGF-$β_2$ resulted in a significant reduction in total lung collagen content (109). Similarly, using a knockout of the TGF-β downstream signaler Smad 3 led to less lung fibrosis in response to bleomycin compared with wild-type controls (110). Fur-thermore, the role of TGF-β and lung fibrosis was emphasized when transient over-expression of active TGF-$β_1$ resulted in prolonged and severe interstitial/pleural fibrosis (111). Moreover, mice deficient of αvβ6 (αvβ6 binds to and activates latent TGF-$β_1$) develop exaggerated inflammation but are protected from the development of fibrosis in response to bleomycin (112,113). These studies illustrate the importance of TGF-β in the promotion of fibrosis and support the contention that TGF-β may be an important mediator of pulmonary fibrosis in humans.

Studies demonstrating an involvement of the TGF-β superfamily and vessels injury make the case for a possible connection between the TGF-β superfamily and PH-associated ILD. Vessel restenosis secondary to angioplasty/stenting have demonstrated that TGF-β stimulates neointimal hyperplasia and extracellular matrix accumulation via

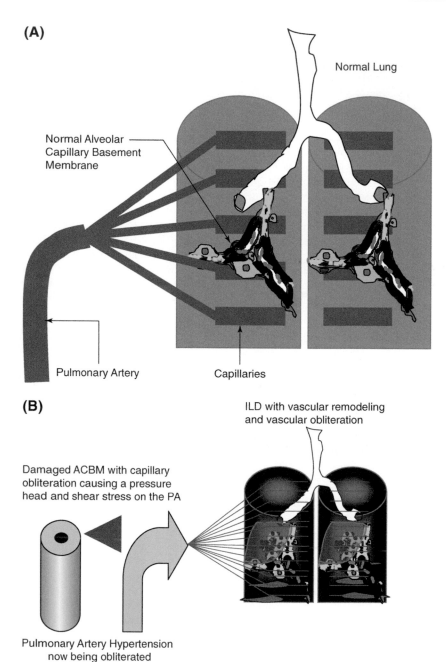

Figure 4 (*See color insert*) Pathogenesis of PAH. (**A**) Normal lung without PAH. (**B**) With IPF there is vascular remodeling with obliteration and thrombosis of capillaries/venules causing a pressure head on the upstream pulmonary vessels (PA). This pressure and shear stress eventually leads to PAH. *Abbreviations*: PAH, pulmonary arterial hypertension; PA, pulmonary arterial; IPF, idiopathic pulmonary fibrosis.

direct/indirect interaction with endothelial cells, immune cells, fibroblasts, and SMCs (72). Importantly, studies have shown TGF-β polymorphisms that increase TGF-β activity modulate age at diagnosis and penetrance of familial PAH (114). Moreover, the mutation that is associated with idiopathic PAH (IPAH) occurs in the gene for BMP receptor type 2 (BMPR2). All BMPR2 mutations (>100) cause loss of receptor function, thus reducing the ability of BMPs to regulate cell growth or other functions during IPAH (115). BMPR2 is activated predominantly by BMP2, BMP4, and BMP7 and does not respond to TGF-$β_1$. While not expected to have a role in PAH until genetic studies showed the link, data suggests that BMPR2-related PAH is secondary to the failure of BMPR2 signaling (e.g., patients with the BMPR2 gene mutation no longer have the normal physiological ability to offset the effects of TGF-β on endothelial cells/SMC/ fibroblasts), eventually leading to pulmonary vessel fibro-obliteration. The imbalance of increased signaling of TGF-β (considered the accelerator of vascular remodeling) compared with the decreased activation of BMPR2 signaling (considered the inhibitor of vascular remodeling) ultimately results in PH. Collectively these studies suggest a link between the imbalance of TGF-β and BMP signaling in the development of PH-associated ILD (Fig. 5).

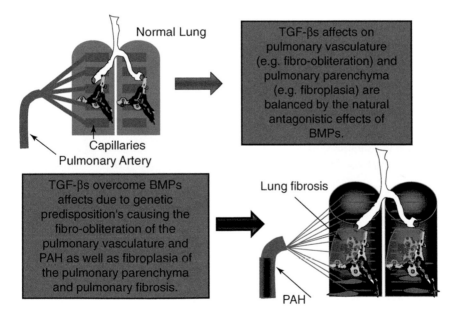

Figure 5 (*See color insert*) Role of TGF-β superfamily during the pathogenesis of PH-associated ILD. TGF-β released during an initial insult to the lung causes the release of TGF-β that in certain individuals, due to a genetic predisposition, does not allow the BMPs to signal through the appropriate receptor (e.g., BMPR2) allowing for vessel obliteration and lung parenchyma fibro-plasia. *Abbreviations*: TGF-β, transforming growth factor β; PAH, pulmonary arterial hypertension; PH, pulmonary hypertension; ILD, interstitial lung disease; BMPs, bone morphogenetic proteins; BMPR2, bone morphogenetic receptor type 2.

D. Endothelin/Receptors Involvement in PH and ILD

ET-1 plays an important physiological role in the regulation of vascular tone and matrix deposition via its interaction with its receptors ET_A and ET_B. ET-1 has been shown to be critical in the pathogenesis of PAH and more recently was found to induce fibroblast proliferation/chemotaxis and extracellular matrix production, and stimulates the generation of local mediators (e.g., interleukins, NO, prostacyclins, and platelet-activating factors) all of which suggest a role in PH-associated ILD (116–123).

ET-1 in BALF was found to be responsible, in part, for the increase in lung fibroblast proliferation in patients with scleroderma (124). Translational studies using a rodent model of bleomycin-induced pulmonary fibrosis demonstrated increased ET-1 immunoreactivity that correlated with collagen deposition (125,126). Furthermore, in rodents, treatment with bosentan (a combined ET_A and ET_B receptor antagonist) significantly attenuated pulmonary fibrosis (127). However, the most striking evidence for a role of ET-1 in lung fibrosis comes from a transgenic mouse model in which overexpression of the ET-1 gene resulted in significant pulmonary fibrosis (128,129).

Patients with PH and higher plasma levels of ET-1 have a shorter life expectancy than patients with lower levels of ET-1, and these levels correlated with important parameters of pulmonary vascular hemodynamics (130). Proof of concept studies in a rat model of PH demonstrated that oral treatment of rats with bosentan protected against the development of chronic hypoxic PH (131). Furthermore, sitaxsentan, a selective ET_A receptor blockade, reversed hypoxic vasoconstriction in an acute setting of PH. In a chronic model of PH, selective ET_A receptor blockade attenuated the effects of hypoxia and even late treatment, starting after two weeks of hypoxia, partially reversed already established hemodynamic and structural sequela of hypoxia-induced PH (132). Collectively, these studies suggest that endothelin/receptor biology may be a key biologic to target during the pathogenesis of PH-associated ILD (Fig. 6).

E. The Involvement of Inflammation via Cytokines/Growth Actors/ Chemokines During the Pathogenesis of PH and ILD

Multiple studies have demonstrated a link between inflammation and lung fibrosis (60,133–143) and inflammation and PAH (65,144–151). In this chapter, we will focus on the relevant studies involving similar inflammatory mediators associated with both PH and ILD.

One of the most important and proximal inflammatory mediators is the interleukin-1 family of cytokines (152–155). This family consists of two agonists, IL-1α and IL-1β, and one antagonist, interleukin-1 receptor antagonist (IL-1ra) (152). Piguet and associates have shown that exogenous IL-1ra can inhibit IL-1 biology and attenuate bleomycin- or silica-induced pulmonary fibrosis (153). Furthermore, the transient expression of IL-1 using an adenoviral vector causes progressive pulmonary fibrosis in a rodent model (155). These studies demonstrate a critical role of IL-1 biology during the pathogenesis of ILD.

With regard to PH multiple studies cited elevated plasma levels of IL-1 associated with PH or PH-associated POEMS disease (145,147,156,157). Importantly, using a rodent model of monocrotoline-induced PH, the inhibition of IL-1 biology attenuated the PH (158). These studies suggest the IL-1 cytokine family may be important during the development of PH-associated ILD.

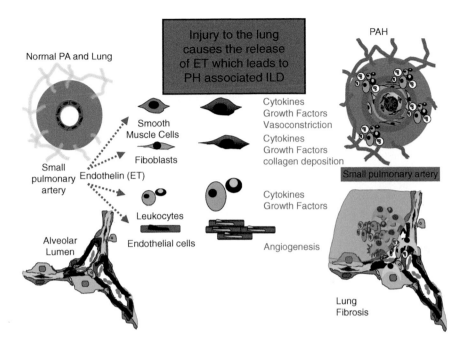

Figure 6 (*See color insert*) The role of receptor/endothelin interactions during PH-associated ILD. Endothelin interaction with specific receptors on smooth muscle cells, fibroblasts, endothelial cells, and leukocytes causes vessel fibro-obliteration and lung parenchyma fibrosis. *Abbreviations*: PH, pulmonary hypertension; ILD, interstitial lung disease; PAH, pulmonary arterial hypertension; ET, endothelin.

The PDGFs are chemotaxins for myo/fibroblasts and SMCs. Alveolar macrophages recovered by bronchoalveolar lavage (BAL) from patients with IPF have markedly greater spontaneous release of PDGF-like activity than alveolar macrophages isolated from normal subjects (159). In lung tissues with early-stage IPF, PDGF was localized in alveolar macrophages, mononuclear phagocytes, fibroblasts, type II pneumocytes, vascular endothelial cells, and vascular smooth muscle cells (159). PDGF has been found in BAL from rodents with bleomycin-induced pulmonary fibrosis (160). Using a vanadium pentoxide model of lung injury (161), inhibition of autophosphorylation of the PDGF-receptor is 90% effective in preventing lung fibrosis (162). Taken together these findings suggest an important role for PDGF in the development of pulmonary fibrosis.

In a recent study, the expression of PDGF-A, PDGF-B, PDGFR-α, and PDGFR-β was found to be increased in small pulmonary arteries [e.g., mainly localized to pulmonary artery smooth muscle cell (PASMCs) and endothelial cells] from patients with IPAH, compared with control subjects (67). This suggests that PDGF may play an important role in human IPAH and together with the above studies suggests that receptor/PDGF biology may be a novel target for PH-associated ILD.

Several studies have found CC chemokines in ILD. CCL3 is elevated in BALF from patients with ILD (163). In addition, BALF CCL3 levels correlated with increased monocyte chemotactic activity (163). The predominant cellular sources of CCL3 within the lungs of these patients, by immunolocalization, were both alveolar and interstitial macrophages and pulmonary fibroblasts (163). Similar to the findings for CCL3, CCL2 is significantly elevated in ILD (163,164). These findings suggest that both CCL3 and CCL2 are expressed in increased amounts within the airspace and interstitium of patients with ILD, and that these chemokines may be important mediators of mononuclear cell recruitment that propagate ILDs.

Translational studies involving rodent models of bleomycin-induced lung fibrosis have noted associations between increased expression of CCL2, CCL3, CCL5, lung infiltrating mononuclear cells, and lung fibrosis (165–169). Passive immunization of animals with either neutralizing antibodies to murine CCL2, CCL3, or CCR1 (one of the main mononuclear cell receptors for both CCL3 and CCL5) or CCR2 (the receptor for CCL2) ablation resulted in a reduction of infiltrating cells into the lungs of bleomycin-treated animals and attenuated lung fibrosis (165–170).

Similarly CX_3CL1, CCL3, and CCL5 expression were elevated in lung samples from PH patients compared with controls (149–151,171). While animal studies evaluating the true biological function of these chemokines during the pathogenesis of PH are lacking, we speculate that the above studies will focus investigators' attention to specific chemokines that are likely to be important in PH-associated ILD.

Overall, there is an overlap between the inflammatory and fibroproliferative mediators during the pathogenesis of both PAH and ILD. These overlapping mediators (TGF-β superfamily, endothelin, IL-1, PDGF, CCL2, CCL3, and CX_3CL1) may be appropriate targets to improve dyspnea and survival in patients with PH-associated ILD.

VI. Pathological Changes

Intimal proliferation, medial smooth muscle hypertrophy, and adventitial changes are commonly observed in patients with PH and IPF (172). Intimal fibrosis is a very common lesion and may be an expression of a variety of conditions. It is very prominent in patients with pulmonary fibrosis, mainly in or near the areas of fibrosis. In most forms of intimal fibrosis, the cells within the thickened subendothelial layer are indistinguishable from ordinary SMCs and are thought to be derived from medial SMCs (173). These changes are no different than those seen in most primary or secondary vascular disorders; however, reduplication of the basement membrane may a specific change seen in pulmonary fibrosis (22). Vascular smooth muscle cell hyperplasia is the main pulmonary vascular finding in PH of ILD (174). Pulmonary veno-occlusive disease, that is, PH secondary to obliteration of the lumina of pulmonary veins and venules may be present as well (172,175). In a retrospective study on lung explant specimens from 26 patients with IPF, occlusion of venules and small pulmonary veins in nonfibrotic areas was present in 65% of patients (172). Muscularization of the terminal portions of the pulmonary arterial tree (pulmonary arterioles) is common to all forms of hypertensive pulmonary vascular disease (176). This muscularization of the pulmonary arterioles is the initial basis for increased pulmonary vascular resistance, but secondary occlusive changes in the intima of pulmonary arteries and arterioles may augment this resistance and transform it into a fixed form (176).

VII. Clinical Manifestations

Patients with ILD and PH present with insidious and progressive dyspnea on exertion and dry cough. These symptoms are similarly reported by patients with primary vascular disorders (IPAH) and ILD without PH; hence, these symptoms, although sensitive, are not specific for diagnosing ILD-associated PH. Physical examination findings of increased second heart sound, hepatomegaly, and peripheral edema are evident in patients with advanced ILD and cor pulmonale; these findings are specific but not sensitive in diagnosing PH in ILD.

VIII. Diagnosis

RHC remains the "gold standard" method to diagnose PH in ILD. RHC allows quantification of right-sided pressures as well as identification of the cause of PH, that is, intrinsic vascular disease as evidenced by an elevated PVR, or pulmonary venous hypertension as seen in patients with left-sided heart disease [left ventricular (LV) systolic or diastolic dysfunction]. Echocardiography (TTE) is commonly used to screen for PH in ILD; however, it is not a reliable method to diagnose PH in these conditions. In a study of 374 patients with advanced lung disease referred for LT (COPD, 68%; various ILDs, 28%; pulmonary vascular disease, 4%), PH was present in 59% of cases [defined by RHC-determined SPAP $\geq$ 45 mmHg]. In that study, there was a good correlation between the Doppler echocardiography (DE)-estimated SPAP and the RHC-measured SPAP ($r = 0.69$; $p < 0.0001$); however, roughly 50% of DE-estimated SPAPs were accurate (within 10 mmHg of the measured SPAP by RHC). When PH was absent, echocardiography often overestimated the true SPAP; when patients had PH by RHC, echocardiography under- or overestimated the true SPAP with similar frequency. In that study, the performance characteristics of echocardiography in diagnosing PH in ILD were unacceptable: sensitivity, 85%; specificity, 17%; positive predictive value (PPV), 60%; and negative predictive value (NPV), 44%. Lastly, SPAP estimation by echocardiography was possible in only 54% of patients who underwent the procedure (177). In a subsequent study of 110 patients with well-characterized IPF referred for LT with available TTE and RHC data, we showed that SPAP was reported in only 55% of patients who underwent TTE (178). Importantly, one-third of these patients were shown to have PH by RHC; therefore, a lack of a reported SPAP from TTE does not imply that the patient does not have PH. As shown previously, in our study, 40% of the TTE-estimated SPAP were accurate when compared with RHC-measured values. Similarly, the performance characteristics of this method were unacceptably low for it to be used as a stand-alone test to screen for PH in IPF (using TTE-estimated SPAP > 45 mmHg as a cut point, the sensitivity was 59%, specificity 53%, PPV 40%, and NPV 71%). Combining echoestimated SPAP with physiological data (PFT, 6MWT) improved on specificity at the expense of sensitivity (178).

Similarly, chest computed tomography (CT) findings do not predict PH in IPF. We performed a cross-sectional study of 65 patients with IPF and available RHC and high-resolution chest computed tomography (HRCT); an expert radiologist scored lung parenchyma changes using a Likert scale (0–4) to quantify ground-glass, fibrosis, and honeycombing changes. The main pulmonary artery diameter (MPAD) and the aorta diameter (AD) were measured as well. No correlations were found between various HRCT measures of lung parenchymal abnormality (ground-glass, fibrotic, or honeycomb change scores) and RHC-measured MPAP and other hemodynamic variables. Ground-glass, fibrotic, or honeycomb change scores were similar between those with and without PH. MPAP and MPAD/AD ratio did not correlate with MPAP; further, these parameters did not discriminate patients with or without PH (42). A subsequent study of patients with pulmonary fibrosis with available CT and RHC data confirmed our original findings (179). In that study, the investigators reported that PA dilatation occurs in the absence of PH in patients with pulmonary fibrosis and is therefore an unreliable sign of PH in these patients. Hence, we do not recommend TTE or chest CT to screen for PH in patients with ILD.

Brain natriuretic peptide (BNP) is secreted by the cardiac ventricles and has been found elevated in the sera of patients with LV failure, acute dyspnea evaluated in the emergency department, idiopathic pulmonary hypertension, and right ventricular overload from pulmonary embolism (180). In a study of 39 patients with various causes of pulmonary fibrosis [IPF ($n = 28$); sarcoidosis ($n = 4$); HP ($n = 4$); connective tissue disease ($n = 3$)] without LV failure or renal insufficiency, the mean MPAP and PVR were higher and the cardiac index (CI) and six-minute walk distance (6MWD) were lower in those with elevated BNP levels (180). Strong correlations in the expected directions were observed between BNP and MPAP, PVR, cardiac output (CO), CI, and 6MWD. In agreement with other studies (17,27), there were no correlations between BNP and lung volume measurements. In patients with BNP levels >18 pg/mL, the mean MPAP was 41 mmHg; by contrast, those with BNP levels <18 pg/mL had a mean MPAP of 23 mmHg. In a follow-up study by the same investigators, 176 patients with chronic lung disease were studied (55 with IPF). In that study, a BNP >33 pg/mL had a sensitivity of 87%, and a specificity of 81% for MPAP >35 mmHg by RHC (181). Although the performance characteristics of BNP are satisfactory in identifying patients with MPAP >35 mmHg, the sensitivity to detect mild to moderate PH (MPAP 26–34 mmHg) is unknown, and this method has not been validated. We do not recommend its routine use in clinical practice until further confirmatory studies become available.

Physiological data has been used to noninvasively identify patients with IPF and PH. Lettieri and associates combined the need for supplemental oxygen (yes/no) with diffusion capacity for carbon monoxide (D_LCO) <40% of predicted; patients with that combination of findings were 10 times more likely to have PH (16). However, PH was present in 32% of their sample, and the predicted prevalence by using that combination was only 15%; hence a prediction based on that combination would miss half the PH cases (16). The forced vital capacity (FVC) to D_LCO ratio (FVC/D_LCO) identifies patients with systemic sclerosis (SSc) and pulmonary vascular disease. FVC/D_LCO >1.4 was reported in 70% of SSc patients with PH (182). In a separate study, FVC/D_LCO >1.8 identified patients with SSc with pulmonary fibrosis and PH (183). Hypoxia is a well-known stimulus for pulmonary vasoconstriction and is strongly correlated to MPAP (17,184,185). On the basis of these findings, we sought to determine whether those two variables (FVC/D_LCO ratio and room air oxygen saturation (SpO_2)] could be combined to improve the prediction of PH in IPF. In the initial derivation study, we regressed MPAP on SpO_2 and the percentage of predicted FVC/ percentage of predicted D_LCO (% FVC/% D_LCO) ratio (17). The linear regression formula [MPAP $= -11.9 + 0.272 \times SpO_2 + 0.0659 \times (100 - SpO_2)^2 + 3.06 \times$ (% FVC/% D_LCO)] explained 57% of the variability of MPAP. Subsequently, we validated this method in a separate group of patients with IPF (external validation) and demonstrated that this method could be used to screen for PH in IPF patients (we selected the 21 mmHg cut point from the formula, as it was associated with a sensitivity of 95% and NPV of 96%) (186). We use this formula to screen for PH in IPF. Those with a formula-predicted MPAP $\leq$ 21 mmHg do not undergo RHC and are followed serially; however, in all patients with a formula-predicted MPAP >21 mmHg, we perform confirmatory RHC (PPV of 51%).

There is no consensus with regard to the clinical and physiological variables that predict PH in patients with sarcoidosis. In one study, PH was associated with male gender, advanced chest radiographic (CXR) changes, reduced arterial oxygen saturation, and decreased % FVC, percentage of predicted forced expiratory volume in one second (% FEV_1), and percentage of predicted total lung capacity (% TLC) (187). In that study, % TLC was independently associated with PH and all patients with % TLC below 60% of predicted had PH. Similarly, Sulica et al. found that PH was associated with lower % FVC, % FEV_1, and more advanced CXR findings (32). By contrast, Shorr and colleagues showed no associations between gender, arterial oxygen saturation, 6MWD, and RHC-measured hemodynamic variables. In that study, % D_LCO was lower in those with PH (33). Likewise, Nunes and associates showed correlation between hemodynamic variables and % D_LCO but with no other pulmonary function variables (37).

IX. Therapy

Therapies targeting PH include vasodilators, anticoagulants, prostacyclin analogues, NO, endothelin-1 receptor antagonists (ETRAs), phosphodiesterase (PDE) inhibitors, and oxygen (for patients with hypoxemia) (188–190). These therapies have been extensively studied in IPAH and other disorders associated with PAH (e.g., CTD, CHD, chronic pulmonary thromboemboli, HIV, dexfenfluramine), but limited data are available among patients with PH complicating ILDs. LT may be an option for patients with severe PH failing medical therapy (all causes) (discussed in chap. 30) (191,192).

Treatment of the underlying condition with immunosuppressant therapy (e.g., sarcoidosis) and management of comorbid conditions may improve pulmonary hemodynamics in patients with ILD-associated PH. The role of anticoagulation in the treatment of these patients is unknown. Therapy with vasodilators is controversial because benefits are unproven and vasodilator therapy in patients with ILD may worsen oxygenation (increase shunt fraction) or cause pulmonary edema if PVOD-like lesions coexist. Currently, there are no large (well-powered), prospective, randomized, double-blind, placebo-controlled studies to assert whether one should treat PH in ILD with vasodilators. However, several small studies suggest that vasodilator therapy may be safe and benefit some patients with ILD-associated PH. In one study, German investigators randomized 16 patients with RHC-confirmed PH due to diverse ILDs to receive either a single oral dose of sildenafil (50 mg) or intravenous (IV) epoprostenol. Sildenafil therapy was associated with reduced PVR (one-third of the baseline value) and increased blood oxygen tension (mean 14 mmHg). Treatment with sildenafil was safe, as it did not increase the shunt fraction [maintained ventilation/perfusion (V/Q) matching]. By contrast, although IV epoprostenol-treated patients demonstrated similar hemodynamic benefits, IV epoprostenol increased the shunt fraction and reduced the oxygen tension (193). The authors concluded that sildenafil is not only a pulmonary "selective" agent (preferentially vasodilates the pulmonary circulation over the systemic circulation) but a "supraselective" drug (preferentially vasodilates well-ventilated areas of the lung). To test whether those hemodynamic benefits would translate into improvements in functional capacity, we conducted an open-label study of 14 patients with IPF and well-documented PH. Patients had 6MWD measured at baseline and after three months of daily therapy with sildenafil. In that study, we observed a mean improvement in 6MWD of 49.0 m, and 57% of the patients were classified as "responders" ($\geq$20% improvement in 6MWD); the drug was generally well tolerated; diarrhea and headaches were the most commonly reported adverse effects (194). These preliminary results await confirmation in a large ($n = 170$) multicenter, prospective, double-blind, placebo-controlled study sponsored by the National Institutes of Health (www.clinicaltrials.gov). In an attempt to overcome the risk of worsening V/Q matching observed with IV prostacyclin therapy, German investigators tested the inhaled route of prostaglandin therapy (PGI_2). They performed a randomized controlled study of eight patients with PH and pulmonary fibrosis [New York Heart Association (NYHA) class III–IV]. In that study, IV prosta-glandin (PGI_2) therapy was associated with reduced MPAP, but it led to reduced sys-temic blood pressure, worsening shunt, and hypoxemia. By contrast, inhaled PGI_2 was associated with reductions in MPAP and PVR and improvement in blood oxygenation (no change in shunt fraction); in one patient with severe disease (NYHA class IV), inhaled PGI_2 improved the 6MWD (195). By contrast, in a double-blind, randomized, placebo-controlled subsequent study of 51 patients with IPF, inhaled iloprost was not found to be superior to placebo in improving exercise tolerance (6MWD) (19). In a more recent study of 19 patients with PH and fibrotic ILD (IPF, 8; sarcoidosis, 6; CVD-associated ILD, 5), IV epoprostenol (10 subjects) and bosentan (9 subjects) were reported to be beneficial. In that study, 79% of patients improved their 6MWD by >50 m (responders); however, at one year of follow-up, 47% of initial responders deteriorated, suggesting that the benefits of vasodilator therapy in ILD-associated PH may be transient (196).

Data regarding treatment of PH complicating sarcoidosis are limited. In a study of 24 patients with sarcoidosis, sildenafil treatment (150 mg/day for 4 months) was asso-ciated with reductions in MPAP (-8 mmHg) and PVR (-4.9 Wood units) as well as increases in CO; however, there were no changes in 6MWD (197). In a retrospective study of 22 sarcoid patients with PAH, no patients exhibited short-term responses to vasodilators (37). However, hemodynamic improvement was noted in 3 of 10 patients treated with corticosteroids (37). In a study of 24 patients with pulmonary sarcoidosis treated with corticosteroids, chest radiographs and PFTs improved at one year in 22 (92%) but hemodynamics improved in only three patients (12%) (131). However, only three patients had PAH at rest in that study. Favorable response to corticosteroids was noted in a single case report (198). Short- and long-term responses to vasodilators have been noted in case reports (199) or small series (197,200–202). A study of eight sarcoid patients with PAH noted favorable short-term responses ($\geq$20% decrease in PVR) in seven of eight patients receiving inhaled nitric oxide (iNO), four of six receiving epo-prostenol, and two of five receiving calcium channel blockers (CCB) (200). Long-term iNO was associated with improved 6MWD in five of five treated patients, three of whom later died. Both patients treated with CCB died. Fisher et al cited favorable responses to epoprostenol in six of seven sarcoid patients with PAH (203). Five patients were alive on chronic epoprostenol therapy at long-term follow-up (mean of 29 months); all had improved WHO class. Baughman cited favorable short-term responses in five sarcoid patients with PH treated with bosentan; two died during follow-up (202). Favorable responses to bosentan were noted in two sarcoid patients with PH (204,205). Danish investigators retrospectively reviewed 25 patients with end-stage pulmonary sarcoidosis referred for LT (197). PAH (mPAP > 25 mmHg) was present in 19 (79%). Sildenafil (daily dose 75–150 mg) was administered to 12 patients and was associated with hemodynamic improvement without adverse effects; however, 6MWD did not change. In a recent retrospective study of patients with sarcoidosis and PH at two referral centers, 22 sarcoidosis patients treated with PH-specific therapies were identified. After a median of 11 months of follow-up, NYHA class was improved in nine subjects. Mean 6MWD ($N = 18$) increased by 59 m ($p = 0.032$). Patients with a higher FVC experienced a greater increment in exercise capacity. Among 12 patients with follow-up hemodynamic data, MPAP was reduced from 48.5 ± 4.3 to 39.4 ± 2.8 mmHg ($p = 0.008$). The one- and three-year transplant–free survival was 90% and 74%, respectively. The authors concluded that PH-specific therapy may improve functional class, exercise capacity, and hemodynamics in PH associated with sarcoidosis (206). These various studies suggest that a subset of sarcoid patients with PH may respond to vasodilator therapy, but appropriate indications, dose, and duration are not known. Prospective controlled trials of PH therapies in sarcoidosis are warranted to verify this apparent benefit.

References

1. Farber HW, Loscalzo J. Pulmonary arterial hypertension. N Engl J Med 2004; 351(16): 1655–1665.
2. Dauriat G, Mal H, Thabut G, et al. Lung transplantation for pulmonary Langerhans' cell histiocytosis: a multicenter analysis. Transplantation 2006; 81(5):746–750.
3. Chaowalit N, Pellikka PA, Decker PA, et al. Echocardiographic and clinical characteristics of pulmonary hypertension complicating pulmonary Langerhans cell histiocytosis. Mayo Clin Proc 2004; 79(10):1269–1275.
4. Fartoukh M, Humbert M, Capron F, et al. Severe pulmonary hypertension in histiocytosis X. Am J Respir Crit Care Med 2000; 161(1):216–223.
5. Lupi-Herrera E, Sandoval J, Bialostozky D, et al. Extrinsic allergic alveolitis caused by pigeon breeding at a high altitude (2,240 meters). Hemodynamic behavior of pulmonary circulation. Am Rev Respir Dis 1981; 124(5):602–607.
6. Dingli D, Utz JP, Gertz MA. Pulmonary hypertension in patients with amyloidosis. Chest 2001; 120(5):1735–1738.
7. Eder L, Zisman D, Wolf R, et al. Pulmonary hypertension and amyloidosis—an uncommon association: a case report and review of the literature. J Gen Intern Med 2007; 22(3): 416–419.
8. Odeh M, Oliven A, Misselevitch I, et al. Acute cor pulmonale due to tumor cell microemboli. Respiration 1997; 64(5):384–387.
9. Tomasini M, Chiappino G. Hemodynamics of pulmonary circulation in asbestosis: study of 16 cases. Am J Ind Med 1981; 2(2):167–174.
10. Evers H, Liehs F, Harzbecker K, et al. Screening of pulmonary hypertension in chronic obstructive pulmonary disease and silicosis by discriminant functions. Eur Respir J 1992; 5(4):444–451.

11. Akkoca Yildiz O, Eris Gulbay B, Saryal S, et al. Evaluation of the relationship between radiological abnormalities and both pulmonary function and pulmonary hypertension in coal workers' pneumoconiosis. Respirology 2007; 12(3):420–426.
12. Kramer MR, Estenne M, Berkman N, et al. Radiation-induced pulmonary veno-occlusive disease. Chest 1993; 104(4):1282–1284.
13. Hamada K, Nagai S, Tanaka S, et al. Significance of pulmonary arterial pressure and diffusion capacity of the lung as prognosticator in patients with idiopathic pulmonary fibrosis. Chest 2007; 131(3):650–656.
14. Nathan SD, Shlobin OA, Ahmad S, et al. Serial development of pulmonary hypertension in patients with idiopathic pulmonary fibrosis. Respiration 2008; 76(3):288–294.
15. Weitzenblum E, Ehrhart M, Rasaholinjanahary J, et al. Pulmonary hemodynamics in idiopathic pulmonary fibrosis and other interstitial pulmonary diseases. Respiration 1983; 44(2):118–127.
16. Lettieri CJ, Nathan SD, Barnett SD, et al. Prevalence and outcomes of pulmonary arterial hypertension in advanced idiopathic pulmonary fibrosis. Chest 2006; 129(3):746–752.
17. Zisman DA, Ross DJ, Belperio JA, et al. Prediction of pulmonary hypertension in idiopathic pulmonary fibrosis. Respir Med 2007; 101(10):2153–2159.
18. Cottin V, Nunes H, Brillet PY, et al. Combined pulmonary fibrosis and emphysema: a distinct underrecognised entity. Eur Respir J 2005; 26(4):586–593.
19. Nathan SD. Pulmonary hypertension in interstitial lung disease. Int J Clin Pract 2008; 62(suppl 160):21–28.
20. Girgis RE, Mathai SC. Pulmonary hypertension associated with chronic respiratory disease. Clin Chest Med 2007; 28(1):219–232, x.
21. Kawut SM, Taichman DB, Archer-Chicko CL, et al. Hemodynamics and survival in patients with pulmonary arterial hypertension related to systemic sclerosis. Chest 2003; 123(2):344–350.
22. Patel NM, Lederer DJ, Borczuk AC, et al. Pulmonary hypertension in idiopathic pulmonary fibrosis. Chest 2007; 132(3):998–1006.
23. Simonneau G, Galie N, Rubin LJ, et al. Clinical classification of pulmonary hypertension. J Am Coll Cardiol 2004; 43(12 suppl S):5S–12S.
24. Kuhn KP, Byrne DW, Arbogast PG, et al. Outcome in 91 consecutive patients with pulmonary arterial hypertension receiving epoprostenol. Am J Respir Crit Care Med 2003; 167(4):580–586.
25. MacNee W. Pathophysiology of cor pulmonale in chronic obstructive pulmonary disease. Part one. Am J Respir Crit Care Med 1994; 150(3):833–852.
26. McLaughlin V, Oudiz R, Robbins I, al. A randomized, double-blind, placebo-controlled study of iloprost inhalation as add-on therapy to bosentan in pulmonary arterial hypertension. Chest 2005; 128(4):160S.
27. Nathan SD, Shlobin OA, Ahmad S, et al. Pulmonary hypertension and pulmonary function testing in idiopathic pulmonary fibrosis. Chest 2007; 131(3):657–663.
28. Shorr AF, Wainright JL, Cors CS, et al. Pulmonary hypertension in patients with pulmonary fibrosis awaiting lung transplant. Eur Respir J 2007; 30(4):715–721.
29. Sitbon O, Humbert M, Nunes H, et al. Long-term intravenous epoprostenol infusion in primary pulmonary hypertension: prognostic factors and survival. J Am Coll Cardiol 2002; 40(4):780–788.
30. Fell CD, Martinez FJ. The impact of pulmonary arterial hypertension on idiopathic pulmonary fibrosis. Chest 2007; 131(3):641–643.
31. Gluskowski J, Hawrylkiewicz I, Zych D, et al. Effects of corticosteroid treatment on pulmonary haemodynamics in patients with sarcoidosis. Eur Respir J 1990; 3(4):403–407.
32. Sulica R, Teirstein AS, Kakarla S, et al. Distinctive clinical, radiographic, and functional characteristics of patients with sarcoidosis-related pulmonary hypertension. Chest 2005; 128(3):1483–1489.

33. Shorr AF, Helman DL, Davies DB, et al. Pulmonary hypertension in advanced sarcoidosis: epidemiology and clinical characteristics. Eur Respir J 2005; 25(5):783–788.
34. Hamada K, Teramoto S, Narita N, et al. Pulmonary veno-occlusive disease in pulmonary Langerhans' cell granulomatosis. Eur Respir J 2000; 15(2):421–423.
35. Nadrous HF, Pellikka PA, Krowka MJ, et al. Pulmonary hypertension in patients with idiopathic pulmonary fibrosis. Chest 2005; 128(4):2393–2399.
36. Glaser S, Noga O, Koch B, et al. Impact of pulmonary hypertension on gas exchange and exercise capacity in patients with pulmonary fibrosis. Respir Med 2009; 103(2):317–324.
37. Nunes H, Humbert M, Capron F, et al. Pulmonary hypertension associated with sarcoidosis: mechanisms, haemodynamics and prognosis. Thorax 2006; 61(1):68–74.
38. Shorr AF, Davies DB, Nathan SD. Predicting mortality in patients with sarcoidosis awaiting lung transplantation. Chest 2003; 124(3):922–928.
39. Arcasoy SM, Christie JD, Pochettino A, et al. Characteristics and outcomes of patients with sarcoidosis listed for lung transplantation. Chest 2001; 120(3):873–880.
40. Heath D, Gillund TD, Kay JM, et al. Pulmonary vascular disease in honeycomb lung. J Pathol Bacteriol 1968; 95:423.
41. Renzoni EA, Walsh DA, Salmon M, et al. Interstitial vascularity in fibrosing alveolitis. Am J Respir Crit Care Med 2003; 167(3):438–443.
42. Zisman DA, Karlamangla AS, Ross DJ, et al. High-resolution chest CT findings do not predict the presence of pulmonary hypertension in advanced idiopathic pulmonary fibrosis. Chest 2007; 132(3):773–779.
43. Keane MP, Arenberg DA, Lynch JP III, et al. The CXC chemokines, IL-8 and IP-10, regulate angiogenic activity in idiopathic pulmonary fibrosis. J Immunol 1997; 159(3): 1437–1443.
44. Keane MP. Angiogenesis and pulmonary fibrosis: feast or famine? Am J Respir Crit Care Med 2004; 170(3):207–209.
45. Cosgrove GP, Brown KK, Schiemann WP, et al. Pigment epithelium-derived factor in idiopathic pulmonary fibrosis: a role in aberrant angiogenesis. Am J Respir Crit Care Med 2004; 170(3):242–251.
46. Ebina M, Shimizukawa M, Shibata N, et al. Heterogeneous increase in CD34-positive alveolar capillaries in idiopathic pulmonary fibrosis. Am J Respir Crit Care Med 2004; 169(11):1203–1208.
47. Cool CD, Groshong SD, Rai PR, et al. Fibroblast foci are not discrete sites of lung injury or repair: the fibroblast reticulum. Am J Respir Crit Care Med 2006; 174(6):654–658.
48. Olman MA, Mackman N, Gladson CL, et al. Changes in procoagulant and fibrinolytic gene expression during bleomycin-induced lung injury in the mouse. J Clin Invest 1995; 96(3): 1621–1630.
49. Zisman DA, Kawut SM. Idiopathic pulmonary fibrosis: a shot through the heart? Am J Respir Crit Care Med 2008; 178(12):1192–1193.
50. Nathan SD, Noble PW, Tuder RM. Idiopathic pulmonary fibrosis and pulmonary hypertension: connecting the dots. Am J Respir Crit Care Med 2007; 175(9):875–880.
51. Giaid A, Yanagisawa M, Langleben D, et al. Expression of endothelin-1 in the lungs of patients with pulmonary hypertension. N Engl J Med 1993; 328(24):1732–1739.
52. Botney MD, Bahadori L, Gold LI. Vascular remodeling in primary pulmonary hypertension. Potential role for transforming growth factor-beta. Am J Pathol 1994; 144(2):286–295.
53. Tuder RM. Am J Respir Crit Care Med 1997; 155:A627.
54. Riley MS, Porszasz J, Miranda J, et al. Exhaled nitric oxide during exercise in primary pulmonary hypertension and pulmonary fibrosis. Chest 1997; 111(1):44–50.
55. Gagermeier J, Dauber J, Yousem S, et al. Abnormal vascular phenotypes in patients with idiopathic pulmonary fibrosis and secondary pulmonary hypertension. Chest 2005; 128(6 suppl):601S.

56. American Thoracic Society; European Respiratory Society. American Thoracic Society/ European Respiratory Society International Multidisciplinary Consensus Classification of the Idiopathic Interstitial Pneumonias. This joint statement of the American Thoracic Society (ATS), and the European Respiratory Society (ERS) was adopted by the ATS board of directors, June 2001 and by the ERS Executive Committee, June 2001. Am J Respir Crit Care Med 2002; 165(2):277–304.

57. Corrin B, Dewar A, Rodriguez-Roisin R, et al. Fine structural changes in cryptogenic fibrosing alveolitis and asbestosis. J Pathol 1985; 147(2):107–119.

58. Flaherty KR, Travis WD, Colby TV, et al. Histopathologic variability in usual and non-specific interstitial pneumonias. Am J Respir Crit Care Med 2001; 164(9):1722–1727.

59. Hunninghake GW, Lynch DA, Galvin JR, et al. Radiologic findings are strongly associated with a pathologic diagnosis of usual interstitial pneumonia. Chest 2003; 124(4):1215–1223.

60. Keane MP, Strieter RM, Lynch JP III, et al. Inflammation and angiogenesis in fibrotic lung disease. Semin Respir Crit Care Med 2006; 27(6):589–599.

61. Peao MN, Aguas AP, de Sa CM, et al. Neoformation of blood vessels in association with rat lung fibrosis induced by bleomycin. Anat Rec 1994; 238(1):57–67.

62. Selman M, Pardo A. The epithelial/fibroblastic pathway in the pathogenesis of idiopathic pulmonary fibrosis. Am J Respir Cell Mol Biol 2003; 29(3 suppl):S93–S97.

63. Turner-Warwick M. Precapillary systemic-pulmonary anastomoses. Thorax 1963; 18: 225–237.

64. Zuo F, Kaminski N, Eugui E, et al. Gene expression analysis reveals matrilysin as a key regulator of pulmonary fibrosis in mice and humans. Proc Natl Acad Sci U S A 2002; 99(9): 6292–6297.

65. Tuder RM, Marecki JC, Richter A, et al. Pathology of pulmonary hypertension. Clin Chest Med 2007; 28(1):23–42, vii.

66. Runo JR, Loyd JE. Primary pulmonary hypertension. Lancet 2003; 361(9368):1533–1544.

67. Perros F, Montani D, Dorfmuller P, et al. Platelet-derived growth factor expression and function in idiopathic pulmonary arterial hypertension. Am J Respir Crit Care Med 2008; 178(1):81–88.

68. Klinger JR. Pulmonary arterial hypertension: an overview. Semin Cardiothorac Vasc Anesth 2007; 11(2):96–103.

69. Strauss WL, Edelman JD. Prostanoid therapy for pulmonary arterial hypertension. Clin Chest Med 2007; 28(1):127–142; ix.

70. Sztrymf B, Coulet F, Girerd B, et al. Clinical outcomes of pulmonary arterial hypertension in carriers of BMPR2 mutation. Am J Respir Crit Care Med 2008; 177(12):1377–1383.

71. Terrier B, Tamby MC, Camoin L, et al. Identification of target antigens of antifibroblast antibodies in pulmonary arterial hypertension. Am J Respir Crit Care Med 2008; 177(10): 1128–1134.

72. Bobik A. Transforming growth factor-betas and vascular disorders. Arterioscler Thromb Vasc Biol 2006; 26(8):1712–1720.

73. Goumans MJ, Liu Z, Ten Dijke P. TGF-beta signaling in vascular biology and dysfunction. Cell Res 2009; 19:116–127.

74. Reddi AS, Bollineni JS. Selenium-deficient diet induces renal oxidative stress and injury via TGF-beta1 in normal and diabetic rats. Kidney Int 2001; 59(4):1342–1353.

75. Sluijter JP, Verloop RE, Pulskens WP, et al. Involvement of furin-like proprotein convertases in the arterial response to injury. Cardiovasc Res 2005; 68(1):136–143.

76. Gordon KJ, Blobe GC. Role of transforming growth factor-beta superfamily signaling pathways in human disease. Biochim Biophys Acta 2008; 1782(4):197–228.

77. ten Dijke P, Hill CS. New insights into TGF-beta-Smad signalling. Trends Biochem Sci 2004; 29(5):265–273.

78. Ebisawa T, Fukuchi M, Murakami G, et al. Smurf1 interacts with transforming growth factor-beta type I receptor through Smad7 and induces receptor degradation. J Biol Chem 2001; 276(16):12477–12480.
79. Nohe A, Hassel S, Ehrlich M, et al. The mode of bone morphogenetic protein (BMP) receptor oligomerization determines different BMP-2 signaling pathways. J Biol Chem 2002; 277(7):5330–5338.
80. Goumans MJ, Valdimarsdottir G, Itoh S, et al. Balancing the activation state of the endothelium via two distinct TGF-beta type I receptors. EMBO J 2002; 21(7):1743–1753.
81. Ota T, Fujii M, Sugizaki T, et al. Targets of transcriptional regulation by two distinct type I receptors for transforming growth factor-beta in human umbilical vein endothelial cells. J Cell Physiol 2002; 193(3):299–318.
82. Watabe T, Nishihara A, Mishima K, et al. TGF-beta receptor kinase inhibitor enhances growth and integrity of embryonic stem cell-derived endothelial cells. J Cell Biol 2003; 163(6):1303–1311.
83. Valdimarsdottir G, Goumans MJ, Rosendahl A, et al. Stimulation of Id1 expression by bone morphogenetic protein is sufficient and necessary for bone morphogenetic protein-induced activation of endothelial cells. Circulation 2002; 106(17):2263–2270.
84. Hocevar BA, Prunier C, Howe PH. Disabled-2 (Dab2) mediates transforming growth factor beta (TGFbeta)-stimulated fibronectin synthesis through TGFbeta-activated kinase 1 and activation of the JNK pathway. J Biol Chem 2005; 280(27):25920–25927.
85. Samarakoon R, Higgins CE, Higgins SP, et al. Plasminogen activator inhibitor type-1 gene expression and induced migration in TGF-beta1-stimulated smooth muscle cells is pp60(c-src)/ MEK-dependent. J Cell Physiol 2005; 204(1):236–246.
86. Seay U, Sedding D, Krick S, et al. Transforming growth factor-beta-dependent growth inhibition in primary vascular smooth muscle cells is p38-dependent. J Pharmacol Exp Ther 2005; 315(3):1005–1012.
87. Ashcroft GS. Bidirectional regulation of macrophage function by TGF-beta. Microbes Infect 1999; 1(15):1275–1282.
88. Ashcroft GS, Yang X, Glick AB, et al. Mice lacking Smad3 show accelerated wound healing and an impaired local inflammatory response. Nat Cell Biol 1999; 1(5):260–266.
89. Wahl SM, Allen JB, Weeks BS, et al. Transforming growth factor beta enhances integrin expression and type IV collagenase secretion in human monocytes. Proc Natl Acad Sci U S A 1993; 90(10):4577–4581.
90. Wahl SM, Costa GL, Corcoran M, et al. Transforming growth factor-beta mediates IL-1-dependent induction of IL-1 receptor antagonist. J Immunol 1993; 150(8 pt 1):3553–3560.
91. Wahl SM, Costa GL, Mizel DE, et al. Role of transforming growth factor beta in the pathophysiology of chronic inflammation. J Periodontol 1993; 64(5 suppl):450–455.
92. Sato K, Kawasaki H, Nagayama H, et al. TGF-beta 1 reciprocally controls chemotaxis of human peripheral blood monocyte-derived dendritic cells via chemokine receptors. J Immunol 2000; 164(5):2285–2295.
93. Turner M, Chantry D, Feldmann M. Transforming growth factor beta induces the production of interleukin 6 by human peripheral blood mononuclear cells. Cytokine 1990; 2(3):211–216.
94. Dai Y, Datta S, Novotny M, et al. TGFbeta inhibits LPS-induced chemokine mRNA stabilization. Blood 2003; 102(4):1178–1185.
95. Mitani T, Terashima M, Yoshimura H, et al. TGF-beta1 enhances degradation of IFN-gamma-induced iNOS protein via proteasomes in RAW 264.7 cells. Nitric Oxide 2005; 13(1):78–87.
96. Werner F, Jain MK, Feinberg MW, et al. Transforming growth factor-beta 1 inhibition of macrophage activation is mediated via Smad3. J Biol Chem 2000; 275(47):36653–36658.

97. Murphy KM, Reiner SL. The lineage decisions of helper T cells. Nat Rev Immunol 2002; 2(12):933–944.
98. Schramm C, Huber S, Protschka M, et al. TGFbeta regulates the CD4+CD25+ T-cell pool and the expression of Foxp3 in vivo. Int Immunol 2004; 16(9):1241–1249.
99. Rosenzweig BL, Imamura T, Okadome T, et al. Cloning and characterization of a human type II receptor for bone morphogenetic proteins. Proc Natl Acad Sci U S A 1995; 92(17): 7632–7636.
100. Urist MR. Bone: formation by autoinduction. Science 1965; 150(698):893–899.
101. Dorai H, Vukicevic S, Sampath TK. Bone morphogenetic protein-7 (osteogenic protein-1) inhibits smooth muscle cell proliferation and stimulates the expression of markers that are characteristic of SMC phenotype in vitro. J Cell Physiol 2000; 184(1):37–45.
102. Kiyono M, Shibuya M. Bone morphogenetic protein 4 mediates apoptosis of capillary endothelial cells during rat pupillary membrane regression. Mol Cell Biol 2003; 23(13): 4627–4636.
103. Sorescu GP, Song H, Tressel SL, et al. Bone morphogenic protein 4 produced in endothelial cells by oscillatory shear stress induces monocyte adhesion by stimulating reactive oxygen species production from a nox1-based NADPH oxidase. Circ Res 2004; 95(8):773–779.
104. Smith DR, Kunkel SL, Standiford TJ, et al. Increased interleukin-1 receptor antagonist in idiopathic pulmonary fibrosis. A compartmental analysis. Am J Respir Crit Care Med 1995; 151(6):1965–1973.
105. Khalil N, O'Connor RN, Unruh HW, et al. Increased production and immunohistochemical localization of transforming growth factor-beta in idiopathic pulmonary fibrosis. Am J Respir Cell Mol Biol 1991; 5(2):155–162.
106. Khalil N, Greenberg AH. The role of TGF-beta in pulmonary fibrosis. Ciba Found Symp 1991; 157:194–207; discussion 207–111.
107. Khalil N, Corne S, Whitman C, et al. Plasmin regulates the activation of cell-associated latent TGF-beta 1 secreted by rat alveolar macrophages after in vivo bleomycin injury. Am J Respir Cell Mol Biol 1996; 15(2):252–259.
108. Khalil N, O'Connor RN, Flanders KC, et al. TGF-beta 1, but not TGF-beta 2 or TGF-beta 3, is differentially present in epithelial cells of advanced pulmonary fibrosis: an immunohistochemical study. Am J Respir Cell Mol Biol 1996; 14(2):131–138.
109. Giri SN, Hyde DM, Hollinger MA. Effect of antibody to transforming growth factor beta on bleomycin induced accumulation of lung collagen in mice. Thorax 1993; 48(10):959–966.
110. Bonniaud P, Margetts PJ, Ask K, et al. TGF-beta and Smad3 signaling link inflammation to chronic fibrogenesis. J Immunol 2005; 175(8):5390–5395.
111. Sime PJ, Xing Z, Graham FL, et al. Adenovector-mediated gene transfer of active transforming growth factor-beta1 induces prolonged severe fibrosis in rat lung. J Clin Invest 1997; 100(4):768–776.
112. Pittet JF, Griffiths MJ, Geiser T, et al. TGF-beta is a critical mediator of acute lung injury. J Clin Invest 2001; 107(12):1537–1544.
113. Munger JS, Huang X, Kawakatsu H, et al. The integrin alpha v beta 6 binds and activates latent TGF beta 1: a mechanism for regulating pulmonary inflammation and fibrosis. Cell 1999; 96(3):319–328.
114. Phillips JA III, Poling JS, Phillips CA, et al. Synergistic heterozygosity for TGFbeta1 SNPs and BMPR2 mutations modulates the age at diagnosis and penetrance of familial pulmonary arterial hypertension. Genet Med 2008; 10(5):359–365.
115. Machado RD, Pauciulo MW, Thomson JR, et al. BMPR2 haploinsufficiency as the inherited molecular mechanism for primary pulmonary hypertension. Am J Hum Genet 2001; 68(1):92–102.
116. Ito S, Juncos LA, Nushiro N, et al. Endothelium-derived relaxing factor modulates endothelin action in afferent arterioles. Hypertension 1991; 17(6 pt 2):1052–1056.

117. Ito H, Hirata Y, Hiroe M, et al. Endothelin-1 induces hypertrophy with enhanced expression of muscle-specific genes in cultured neonatal rat cardiomyocytes. Circ Res 1991; 69(1): 209–215.

118. Ito T, Kato T, Iwama Y, et al. Prostaglandin H2 as an endothelium-derived contracting factor and its interaction with endothelium-derived nitric oxide. J Hypertens 1991; 9(8):729–736.

119. Belloni AS, Rossi GP, Andreis PG, et al. Endothelin adrenocortical secretagogue effect is mediated by the B receptor in rats. Hypertension 1996; 27(5):1153–1159.

120. Kahaleh MB. Endothelin, an endothelial-dependent vasoconstrictor in scleroderma. Enhanced production and profibrotic action. Arthritis Rheum 1991; 34(8):978–983.

121. Schiffrin EL. Endothelin and endothelin antagonists in hypertension. J Hypertens 1998; 16 (12 pt 2):1891–1895.

122. Peacock AJ, Dawes KE, Shock A, et al. Endothelin-1 and endothelin-3 induce chemotaxis and replication of pulmonary artery fibroblasts. Am J Respir Cell Mol Biol 1992; 7(5): 492–499.

123. Rizvi MA, Katwa L, Spadone DP, et al. The effects of endothelin-1 on collagen type I and type III synthesis in cultured porcine coronary artery vascular smooth muscle cells. J Mol Cell Cardiol 1996; 28(2):243–252.

124. Cambrey AD, Harrison NK, Dawes KE, et al. Increased levels of endothelin-1 in bronchoalveolar lavage fluid from patients with systemic sclerosis contribute to fibroblast mitogenic activity in vitro. Am J Respir Cell Mol Biol 1994; 11(4):439–445.

125. Mutsaers SE, Marshall RP, Goldsack NR, et al. Effect of endothelin receptor antagonists (BQ-485, Ro 47-0203) on collagen deposition during the development of bleomycin-induced pulmonary fibrosis in rats. Pulm Pharmacol Ther 1998; 11(2–3):221–225.

126. Mutsaers SE, Foster ML, Chambers RC, et al. Increased endothelin-1 and its localization during the development of bleomycin-induced pulmonary fibrosis in rats. Am J Respir Cell Mol Biol 1998; 18(5):611–619.

127. Park SH, Saleh D, Giaid A, et al. Increased endothelin-1 in bleomycin-induced pulmonary fibrosis and the effect of an endothelin receptor antagonist. Am J Respir Crit Care Med 1997; 156(2 pt 1):600–608.

128. Kaisers U, Busch T, Wolf S, et al. Inhaled endothelin A antagonist improves arterial oxygenation in experimental acute lung injury. Intensive Care Med 2000; 26(9):1334–1342.

129. Hocher B, Thone-Reineke C, Rohmeiss P, et al. Endothelin-1 transgenic mice develop glomerulosclerosis, interstitial fibrosis, and renal cysts but not hypertension. J Clin Invest 1997; 99(6):1380–1389.

130. Rubens C, Ewert R, Halank M, et al. Big endothelin-1 and endothelin-1 plasma levels are correlated with the severity of primary pulmonary hypertension. Chest 2001; 120(5): 1562–1569.

131. Eddahibi S, Raffestin B, Clozel M, et al. Protection from pulmonary hypertension with an orally active endothelin receptor antagonist in hypoxic rats. Am J Physiol 1995; 268(2 pt 2): H828–835.

132. Tilton RG, Munsch CL, Sherwood SJ, et al. Attenuation of pulmonary vascular hypertension and cardiac hypertrophy with sitaxsentan sodium, an orally active ET(A) receptor antagonist. Pulm Pharmacol Ther 2000; 13(2):87–97.

133. Belperio JA, Dy M, Burdick MD, et al. Interaction of IL-13 and C10 in the pathogenesis of bleomycin-induced pulmonary fibrosis. Am J Respir Cell Mol Biol 2002; 27(4):419–427.

134. Belperio JA, Dy M, Murray L, et al. The role of the Th2 CC chemokine ligand CCL17 in pulmonary fibrosis. J Immunol 2004; 173(7):4692–4698.

135. Keane MP, Belperio JA, Arenberg DA, et al. IFN-gamma-inducible protein-10 attenuates bleomycin-induced pulmonary fibrosis via inhibition of angiogenesis. J Immunol 1999; 163(10):5686–5692.

136. Keane MP, Belperio JA, Burdick MD, et al. ENA-78 is an important angiogenic factor in idiopathic pulmonary fibrosis. Am J Respir Crit Care Med 2001; 164(12):2239–2242.
137. Keane MP, Belperio JA, Burdick MD, et al. IL-12 attenuates bleomycin-induced pulmonary fibrosis. Am J Physiol Lung Cell Mol Physiol 2001; 281(1):L92–L97.
138. Keane MP, Belperio JA, Moore TA, et al. Neutralization of the CXC chemokine, macrophage inflammatory protein-2, attenuates bleomycin-induced pulmonary fibrosis. J Immunol 1999; 162(9):5511–5518.
139. Keane MP, Donnelly SC, Belperio JA, et al. Imbalance in the expression of CXC chemokines correlates with bronchoalveolar lavage fluid angiogenic activity and procollagen levels in acute respiratory distress syndrome. J Immunol 2002; 169(11):6515–6521.
140. Keane MP, Standiford TJ, Strieter RM. Chemokines are important cytokines in the pathogenesis of interstitial lung disease [editorial; comment]. Eur Respir J 1997; 10(6): 1199–1202.
141. Weinberger SE, Kelman JA, Elson NA, et al. Bronchoalveolar lavage in interstitial lung disease. Ann Intern Med 1978; 89(4):459–466.
142. Zhang L, Keane MP, Zhu LX, et al. Interleukin-7 and transforming growth factor-beta play counter-regulatory roles in protein kinase C-delta-dependent control of fibroblast collagen synthesis in pulmonary fibrosis. J Biol Chem 2004; 279(27):28315–28319.
143. Huang M, Sharma S, Zhu LX, et al. IL-7 inhibits fibroblast TGF-beta production and signaling in pulmonary fibrosis. J Clin Invest 2002; 109(7):931–937.
144. Lesprit P, Godeau B, Authier FJ, et al. Pulmonary hypertension in POEMS syndrome: a new feature mediated by cytokines. Am J Respir Crit Care Med 1998; 157(3 pt 1):907–911.
145. Feinberg L, Temple D, de Marchena E, et al. Soluble immune mediators in POEMS syndrome with pulmonary hypertension: case report and review of the literature. Crit Rev Oncog 1999; 10(4):293–302.
146. Sanchez O, Humbert M, Sitbon O, et al. Treatment of pulmonary hypertension secondary to connective tissue diseases. Thorax 1999; 54(3):273–277.
147. Isern RA, Yaneva M, Weiner E, et al. Autoantibodies in patients with primary pulmonary hypertension: association with anti-Ku. Am J Med 1992; 93(3):307–312.
148. Cool CD, Kennedy D, Voelkel NF, et al. Pathogenesis and evolution of plexiform lesions in pulmonary hypertension associated with scleroderma and human immunodeficiency virus infection. Hum Pathol 1997; 28(4):434–442.
149. Dorfmuller P, Perros F, Balabanian K, et al. Inflammation in pulmonary arterial hypertension. Eur Respir J 2003; 22(2):358–363.
150. Dorfmuller P, Zarka V, Durand-Gasselin I, et al. Chemokine RANTES in severe pulmonary arterial hypertension. Am J Respir Crit Care Med 2002; 165(4):534–539.
151. Tuder RM, Groves B, Badesch DB, et al. Exuberant endothelial cell growth and elements of inflammation are present in plexiform lesions of pulmonary hypertension. Am J Pathol 1994; 144(2):275–285.
152. Dinarello CA. Biologic basis for interleukin-1 in disease. Blood 1996; 87(6):2095–2147.
153. Piguet PF, Vesin C, Grau GE, et al. Interleukin 1 receptor antagonist (IL-1ra) prevents or cures pulmonary fibrosis elicited in mice by bleomycin or silica. Cytokine 1993; 5(1):57–61.
154. Gasse P, Mary C, Guenon I, et al. IL-1R1/MyD88 signaling and the inflammasome are essential in pulmonary inflammation and fibrosis in mice. J Clin Invest 2007; 117(12): 3786–3799.
155. Kolb M, Margetts PJ, Anthony DC, et al. Transient expression of IL-1beta induces acute lung injury and chronic repair leading to pulmonary fibrosis. J Clin Invest 2001; 107(12): 1529–1536.
156. Balabanian K, Foussat A, Dorfmuller P, et al. CX(3)C chemokine fractalkine in pulmonary arterial hypertension. Am J Respir Crit Care Med 2002; 165(10):1419–1425.

157. Humbert M, Monti G, Brenot F, et al. Increased interleukin-1 and interleukin-6 serum concentrations in severe primary pulmonary hypertension. Am J Respir Crit Care Med 1995; 151(5):1628–1631.
158. Voelkel NF, Tuder R. Interleukin-1 receptor antagonist inhibits pulmonary hypertension induced by inflammation. Ann N Y Acad Sci 1994; 725:104–109.
159. Homma S, Nagaoka I, Abe H, et al. Localization of platelet-derived growth factor and insulin-like growth factor I in the fibrotic lung. Am J Respir Crit Care Med 1995; 152(6 pt 1):2084–2089.
160. Maeda A, Hiyama K, Yamakido H, et al. Increased expression of platelet-derived growth factor A and insulin-like growth factor-I in BAL cells during the development of bleomycin-induced pulmonary fibrosis in mice. Chest 1996; 109(3):780–786.
161. Bonner JC, Lindroos PM, Rice AB, et al. Induction of PDGF receptor-alpha in rat myofibroblasts during pulmonary fibrogenesis in vivo. Am J Physiol 1998; 274(1 pt 1):L72–L80.
162. Lindroos PM, Wang YZ, Rice AB, et al. Regulation of PDGFR-alpha in rat pulmonary myofibroblasts by staurosporine. Am J Physiol Lung Cell Mol Physiol 2001; 280(2):L354–L362.
163. Standiford TJ, Rolfe MW, Kunkel SL, et al. Macrophage inflammatory protein-1 alpha expression in interstitial lung disease. J Immunol 1993; 151(5):2852–2863.
164. Antoniades HN, Neville-Golden J, Galanopoulos T, et al. Expression of monocyte chemoattractant protein 1 mRNA in human idiopathic pulmonary fibrosis. Proc Natl Acad Sci U S A 1992; 89(12):5371–5375.
165. Smith RE, Strieter RM, Phan SH, et al. TNF and IL-6 mediate MIP-1alpha expression in bleomycin-induced lung injury. J Leukoc Biol 1998; 64(4):528–536.
166. Smith RE, Strieter RM, Phan SH, et al. Production and function of murine macrophage inflammatory protein-1 alpha in bleomycin-induced lung injury. J Immunol 1994; 153(10):4704–4712.
167. Smith RE, Strieter RM, Zhang K, et al. A role for C-C chemokines in fibrotic lung disease. J Leukoc Biol 1995; 57(5):782–787.
168. Tokuda A, Itakura M, Onai N, et al. Pivotal role of CCR1-positive leukocytes in bleomycin-induced lung fibrosis in mice. J Immunol 2000; 164(5):2745–2751.
169. Zhang K, Gharaee-Kermani M, Jones ML, et al. Lung monocyte chemoattractant protein-1 gene expression in bleomycin-induced pulmonary fibrosis. J Immunol 1994; 153(10):4733–4741.
170. Moore BB, Paine R III, Christensen PJ, et al. Protection from pulmonary fibrosis in the absence of CCR2 signaling. J Immunol 2001; 167(8):4368–4377.
171. Raychaudhuri B, Bonfield TL, Malur A, et al. Circulating monocytes from patients with primary pulmonary hypertension are hyporesponsive. Clin Immunol 2002; 104(2):191–198.
172. Colombat M, Mal H, Groussard O, et al. Pulmonary vascular lesions in end-stage idiopathic pulmonary fibrosis: Histopathologic study on lung explant specimens and correlations with pulmonary hemodynamics. Hum Pathol 2007; 38(1):60–65.
173. Balk AG, Dingemans KP, Wagenvoort CA. The ultrastructure of the various forms of pulmonary arterial intimal fibrosis. Virchows Arch A Pathol Anat Histol 1979; 382(2):139–150.
174. Tuder RM, Lee SD, Cool CC. Histopathology of pulmonary hypertension. Chest 1998; 114(1 suppl):1S–6S.
175. McDonnell PJ, Summer WR, Hutchins GM. Pulmonary veno-occlusive disease. Morphological changes suggesting a viral cause. JAMA 1981; 246(6):667–671.
176. Heath D, Edwards JE. The pathology of hypertensive pulmonary vascular disease. Circulation 1958; 18:533.
177. Arcasoy SM, Christie JD, Ferrari VA, et al. Echocardiographic assessment of pulmonary hypertension in patients with advanced lung disease. Am J Respir Crit Care Med 2003; 167(5):735–740.
178. Nathan SD, Shlobin OA, Barnett SD, et al. Right ventricular systolic pressure by echocardiography as a predictor of pulmonary hypertension in idiopathic pulmonary fibrosis. Respir Med 2008; 102(9):1305–1310.

179. Devaraj A, Wells AU, Meister MG, et al. The effect of diffuse pulmonary fibrosis on the reliability of CT signs of pulmonary hypertension. Radiology 2008; 249(3):1042–1049.

180. Leuchte HH, Neurohr C, Baumgartner R, et al. Brain natriuretic peptide and exercise capacity in lung fibrosis and pulmonary hypertension. Am J Respir Crit Care Med 2004; 170(4):360–365.

181. Leuchte HH, Baumgartner RA, Nounou ME, et al. Brain natriuretic peptide is a prognostic parameter in chronic lung disease. Am J Respir Crit Care Med 2006; 173(7):744–750.

182. Steen VD, Graham G, Conte C, et al. Isolated diffusing capacity reduction in systemic sclerosis. Arthritis Rheum 1992; 35(7):765–770.

183. Chang B, Wigley FM, White B, et al. Scleroderma patients with combined pulmonary hypertension and interstitial lung disease. J Rheumatol 2003; 30(11):2398–2405.

184. McQuillan LP, Leung GK, Marsden PA, et al. Hypoxia inhibits expression of eNOS via transcriptional and posttranscriptional mechanisms. Am J Physiol 1994; 267(5 pt 2): H1921–H1927.

185. Wang J, Juhaszova M, Rubin LJ, et al. Hypoxia inhibits gene expression of voltage-gated K+ channel alpha subunits in pulmonary artery smooth muscle cells. J Clin Invest 1997; 100(9): 2347–2353.

186. Zisman DA, Karlamangla AS, Kawut SM, et al. Validation of a method to screen for pulmonary hypertension in advanced idiopathic pulmonary fibrosis. Chest 2008; 133(3): 640–645.

187. Handa T, Nagai S, Miki S, et al. Incidence of pulmonary hypertension and its clinical relevance in patients with sarcoidosis. Chest 2006; 129(5):1246–1252.

188. Alam S, Palevsky HI. Standard therapies for pulmonary arterial hypertension. Clin Chest Med 2007; 28(1):91–115, viii.

189. O'Callaghan D, Gaine SP. Combination therapy and new types of agents for pulmonary arterial hypertension. Clin Chest Med 2007; 28(1):169–185, ix.

190. Humbert M, Sitbon O, Simonneau G. Treatment of pulmonary arterial hypertension. N Engl J Med 2004; 351(14):1425–1436.

191. Saggar R, Ross D, Lynch III J, et al. Pulmonary arterial hypertension and lung transplantation. In: Lynch JP III and Ross DJ, eds. Lung and Heart-Lung Transplantation, New York, NY: Taylor & Francis Group, 2006:147–165.

192. Nathan S, Saggar R III JL. Lung transplantation for interstitial lung disorders. In: Lynch JP III, Ross DJ, eds. Lung and Heart-Lung Transplantation, New York, NY: Taylor & Francis Group, 2006:165–204.

193. Ghofrani HA, Wiedemann R, Rose F, et al. Sildenafil for treatment of lung fibrosis and pulmonary hypertension: a randomised controlled trial. Lancet 2002; 360(9337):895–900.

194. Collard HR, Anstrom KJ, Schwarz MI, et al. Sildenafil improves walk distance in idiopathic pulmonary fibrosis. Chest 2007; 131(3):897–899.

195. Olschewski H, Ghofrani HA, Walmrath D, et al. Inhaled prostacyclin and iloprost in severe pulmonary hypertension secondary to lung fibrosis. Am J Respir Crit Care Med 1999; 160(2):600–607.

196. Minai OA, Sahoo D, Chapman JT, et al. Vaso-active therapy can improve 6-min walk distance in patients with pulmonary hypertension and fibrotic interstitial lung disease. Respir Med 2008; 102(7):1015–1020.

197. Milman N, Burton CM, Iversen M, et al. Pulmonary hypertension in end-stage pulmonary sarcoidosis: therapeutic effect of sildenafil? J Heart Lung Transplant 2008; 27(3):329–334.

198. Rodman DM, Lindenfeld J. Successful treatment of sarcoidosis-associated pulmonary hypertension with corticosteroids. Chest 1990; 97(2):500–502.

199. Barst RJ, Ratner SJ. Sarcoidosis and reactive pulmonary hypertension. Arch Intern Med 1985; 145(11):2112–2114.

200. Preston IR, Klinger JR, Landzberg MJ, et al. Vasoresponsiveness of sarcoidosis-associated pulmonary hypertension. Chest 2001; 120(3):866–872.
201. Jones K, Higenbottam T, Wallwork J. Pulmonary vasodilation with prostacyclin in primary and secondary pulmonary hypertension. Chest 1989; 96(4):784–789.
202. Baughman RP. Pulmonary hypertension associated with sarcoidosis. Arthritis Res Ther 2007; 9(suppl 2):S8.
203. Fisher KA, Serlin DM, Wilson KC, et al. Sarcoidosis-associated pulmonary hypertension: outcome with long-term epoprostenol treatment. Chest 2006; 130(5):1481–1488.
204. Foley RJ, Metersky ML. Successful treatment of sarcoidosis-associated pulmonary hypertension with bosentan. Respiration 2008; 75(2):211–214.
205. Sharma S, Kashour T, Philipp R. Secondary pulmonary arterial hypertension: treated with endothelin receptor blockade. Tex Heart Inst J 2005; 32(3):405–410.
206. Barnett CF, Bonura EJ, Nathan SD, et al. Treatment of sarcoidosis-associated pulmonary hypertension: a two-center experience. Chest 2008; [Epub ahead of print].

20
Pulmonary Hypertension in Chronic Mountain Sickness

DANTE PENALOZA and FRANCISCO SIME
University Cayetano Heredia, Lima, Peru

I. Introduction

Peruvian investigators were the first to describe the pathogenesis of chronic hypoxic pulmonary hypertension (PH) in humans (1–4). PH is a common finding in healthy people living at high altitudes. The mean pulmonary arterial pressure (mPAP) is related to the level of altitude. There is a direct relationship represented by a parabolic line, so that above 3500 m there are mild to moderate degrees of PH in comparison with the normal values described at sea level. PH in healthy highlanders is an asymptomatic feature and is associated with physiological and adaptive levels of hypoxemia and polycythemia. Despite PH, hypoxemia, and polycythemia, healthy highlanders are able to perform physical activities similar to and often even more strenuous than those of people living at sea level.

After many years of residence at high altitude, some highlanders may lose their adaptation, become symptomatic, and develop chronic mountain sickness (CMS), a clinical entity associated with marked hypoxemia, exaggerated polycythemia, and increased PH, evolving in some cases to heart failure. CMS was originally described in the Peruvian Andes. Later on, chronic high-altitude diseases resulting from loss of adaptation have also been described in China and Kyrgyzstan with the names high-altitude heart disease (HAHD) and high-altitude cor pulmonale (HACP), respectively. These terms, used by Chinese and Kyrgyz investigators, emphasize the right ventricular hypertrophy (RVH) and overload as a consequence of hypoxic PH. This chapter will focus on pulmonary hemodynamics in chronic high-altitude diseases.

II. Historical Highlights

CMS was first described in 1928 by Professor Monge who placed emphasis on excessive polycythemia (5). Afterward, Professor Hurtado pointed out that alveolar hypoventilation is the primary mechanism in CMS, leading to severe hypoxemia and hence to exaggerated polycythemia (6). Rotta et al. carried out the first cardiac catheterization in one patient with CMS (7). Penaloza et al. were the first to describe the evolution from adaptive PH in healthy highlanders to chronic cor pulmonale and heart failure as a consequence of loss of altitude adaptation (8,9). Wu et al. were the first in China to describe HAHD (10). A similar clinical picture, with the name HACP, was described by Mirrakhimov in Kyrgyzstan (11). A review on pulmonary circulation in chronic high-altitude diseases has recently been published by Penaloza and Arias-Stella (4).

III. CMS: A Clinical Complex Syndrome

Penaloza et al. described CMS as a variety of chronic alveolar hypoventilation that results in a complex syndrome integrating four main components. Respiratory features are characterized by alveolar hypoventilation, relative hypercapnea, ventilation/perfusion ($\dot{V}/\dot{Q}$) mismatch, widened alveolar-arterial (A-a) PO_2 gradient, and increased hypoxemia. Hematological features are excessive polycythemia, increased blood viscosity, and expanded total and lung blood volume. Cardiopulmonary abnormalities include moderate to severe PH and right ventricular enlargement, which may evolve to hypoxic cor pulmonale and heart failure. Neuropsychic symptoms include sleep disorders, headaches, dizziness, and mental fatigue (9).

IV. Current Definition of CMS

According to an international consensus statement published in 2005, CMS is defined as follows:

> A clinical syndrome that occurs in native or long-life residents above 2500 m. It is characterized by excessive erythrocytosis (females, hemoglobin (Hb) $\geq$ 19 g/dL; males, Hb $\geq$ 21 g/dL), severe hypoxemia, and in some cases moderate or severe PH, which may evolve to cor pulmonale, leading to congestive heart failure. The clinical picture of CMS gradually disappears after descending to low altitude and reappears after returning to high altitude. (12)

V. Primary and Secondary CMS

CMS may be classified as primary, without identified cause, or secondary due to underlying conditions. The primary type of CMS is diagnosed after exclusion of lung diseases by pulmonary function testing. The secondary variety of CMS is associated with lung diseases, excessive obesity, neuromuscular disorders, or chest wall deformities. However, most cases represent unrecognized respiratory abnormalities because it is not easy to rule out the influence of smoking and environmental pollution, factors often mentioned in papers dealing with CMS (4,9,11,13).

VI. Pulmonary Hemodynamics in CMS

A. Hemodynamic Studies of CMS at the Altitude of Residence

Studies with cardiac catheterization in patients with CMS at the altitude of their residence have been carried out in Peru, Bolivia, and China (Table 1). Peruvian investigators

Table 1 Pulmonary Arterial Pressure in Chronic High-Altitude Diseases (CMS, HAHD, HACP)

First author (Ref.)	Location	Altitude (m)	Diagnosis	mPAP (mmHg) (n)
Rotta (7)	Morococha Peru	4540	CMS	35 (1)
Penaloza (8)	Cerro de Pasco Peru	4340	CMS	47 ± 17 (10)
Ergueta (14)	La Paz Bolivia	3600	CMS	51 (2)
Manier (15)	La Paz Bolivia	3600	CMS	27 ± 10 (8)
Pei (13)	Lhasa Tibet	3600	CMS	40 ± 11 (5)
Yang (16)	Chengdou Qinghai, China	3950	CMS	31 (6)
Wu (23)	Qinghai-Tibetan Plateau, China[a]	3000–5000	HAHD	36 ± 3 (108)
Cheng (24)	Qinghai-Tibetan Plateau, China[a]	3000–5000	HAHD	28 ± 4 (10)
Sarybaeb (25)	Tien-Shan & Pamir Mountains, Kyrgyzstan[b]	3200–4200	HACP	38 ± 3 (8)
Aldashev (26)	Tien-Shan & Pamir Mountains, Kyrgyzstan[b]	2800–3100	HACP	32 ± 4 (11)

Values for mPAP are mean or mean ± SD
[a]Doppler echocardiography in Xining, 2260 m
[b]Cardiac catheterization in Bishkek, 760 m.
Abbreviations: CMS, chronic mountain sickness; HAHD, high-altitude heart disease; HACP, high-altitude cor pulmonale.

were pioneers in this field. Rotta et al. were the first to perform a cardiac catheterization in one case of CMS living in Morococha, Peru, at 4540 m. This patient had mPAP 35 mmHg, Hb 26 g/dL, and oxygen saturation (SaO_2) 78% (7). Afterward, our group performed cardiac catheterization studies in 10 cases of CMS residing in Cerro de Pasco (4340 m). The mPAP was 47 ± 17 mmHg, and the individual values were all higher than 25 mmHg, the highest value being 85 mmHg (range 31–85 mmHg), SaO_2 was 70 ± 5.0 % (range 61–78), Hb 25 ± 2.0 g/dL (range 20–27), and hematocrit (Hct) 79 ± 4.0 % (range 73–86) (8,9).

Table 2 shows hemodynamic data obtained in patients with CMS living in Cerro de Pasco (4540 m) in comparison with healthy highlanders living in the same location and also compared with sea level residents. Figure 1 shows mPAP as related to SaO_2 in patients with CMS, so that patients with the lowest SaO_2 values have the highest values of mPAP. By comparison, data obtained in healthy highlanders are also shown.

Bolivian investigators carried out two studies with cardiac catheterization in La Paz, Bolivia (3600 m). Ergueta et al. studied 20 patients with CMS, and 2 of them were submitted to cardiac catheterization with the following results: mPAP 51 mmHg, Hb 26 g/dL, and SaO_2 84% (14). Manier et al. studied eight patients with a mean Hb of 21 g/dL and a mPAP of 27 mmHg (15).

Chinese investigators have undertaken two studies with cardiac catheterization. Pei et al. studied 17 patients with CMS in Lhasa, Tibet (3600 m), most of them were men of Chinese Han origin and all were smokers. Five patients had cardiac catheterization and the average mPAP was 39.6 ± 11.1 mmHg, greatly exceeding the normal value for healthy highlanders (13). Yang et al. reported a mPAP value of 31 mmHg in six Han male patients with CMS studied at Chengdou (3950 m), in contrast with 26 mmHg found in healthy natives at the same altitude (16).

Table 2 Hemodynamic Values in CMS in Comparison with Healthy Highlanders (4300 m) and Sea Level Subjects

	SL controls (n = 25; age 17–23 yr)	Healthy highlanders controls (n = 12; age 19–38 yr)	CMS subjects (n = 10; age 22–51 yr)	p, CMS vs. healthy highlanders
Hb (g/dL)	14.7 ± 0.88	20.1 ± 1.69	24.7 ± 2.36	<0.001
Hct (%)	44.1 ± 2.59	59.4 ± 5.4	79.3 ± 4.2	<0.001
SaO$_2$ (%)	95.7 ± 2.07	81.1 ± 4.61	69.6 ± 4.92	<0.001
RAP (mmHg)	2.6 ± 1.31	2.9 ± 1.4	3.9 ± 1.8	NS
mPAP (mmHg)	12 ± 2.2	23 ± 5.1	47 ± 17.7	<0.001
PWP (mmHg)	6.2 ± 1.71	6.9 ± 1.4	5.7 ± 2.3	NS
PVR (dyne.sec/cm^5)	69 ± 25.3	197 ± 57.6	527 ± 218.1	<0.001
CI (L/min/m^2)	3.9 ± 0.97	3.8 ± 0.62	4.0 ± 0.93	NS

Values are mean ± SD.
Abbreviations: CMS, chronic mountain sickness; Hct, hematocrit; RAP, right atrial pressure; PWP, pulmonary wedge pressure; CI, cardiac index; NS, nonsignificant.
Source: From Refs. 2, 4, and 8.

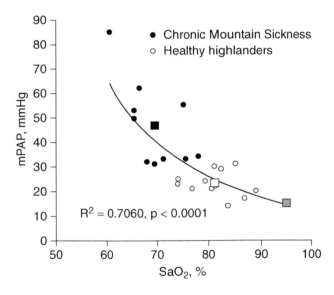

Figure 1 mPAP as related to SaO$_2$ in patients with CMS. There is an inverse relationship between these two variables. As SaO$_2$ decreases, mPAP increases and the patient with the lowest SaO$_2$ has the highest mPAP (*filled circles*). By comparison, values in healthy highlanders are shown (*open circles*). The average values of mPAP for both groups and for sea level residents are also shown (*square symbols*). *Abbreviation*: mPAP, mean pulmonary arterial pressure. *Source*: From Refs. 4, 8, and 9.

B. Hemodynamic Studies of CMS During the Recovery Period at Lower Altitude

These studies have been performed by Chinese investigators. There are two studies in patients with CMS who came from the Guolok area (3700–4200 m) and were then studied in Xining (2100 m), 7 to 10 days after their arrival for recovery. One of the studies was carried out with cardiac catheterization, and the mean value of mPAP was 18 mmHg, an unexpectedly low value, which was incompatible with the evidence of RVH found by electrocardiogram (ECG) and chest X ray in the same patients. The authors ascribed the low mPAP value to the lower altitude where the study was undertaken (17). The second study was performed with a noninvasive procedure ("an equation related to the alveolar air") and the calculated mPAP was 39 mmHg (18). There is an unexplained discrepancy between both studies carried out by the same research group in patients who came from the same high altitude and studied at the same lower altitude.

C. Hemodynamic Studies of CMS with Doppler Echocardiography

These investigations were carried out by Bolivian investigators in La Paz (3600 m) and the results are displayed in Table 3. From the systolic PAP (sPAP) values reported in these publications, we calculated the corresponding mPAP values by using a new European formula (19). Antezana et al. studied a group of patients with an average age of 40 years and excessive polycythemia (Hb 22 g/dL), and the mPAP was 26 mmHg (sPAP 42 mmHg) (20). Vargas and Spielvogel studied two groups of patients with CMS, elderly and young patients, with Hb values of 24 g/dL and 19 g/dL, respectively. The mPAP value in both groups was 22 mmHg (sPAP 35 mmHg), a value similar to the mPAP of healthy people living in La Paz. These data in CMS patients are incompatible with the ECG finding in the same patients of RVH (21). The wrong hemodynamic data have been rectified in a recent paper where some of the same patients appear in a table exhibiting concordance between RVH detected by ECG and PH assessed by Doppler echocardiography (22). It is surprising, however, that the values of mPAP in this chapter are not shown in the column entitled mPAP mmHg and, instead, have been replaced by the abbreviation PH.

Table 3 Pulmonary Arterial Pressure in CMS

First author (Ref.)	Number of cases	Age (yr)	Hemoglobin (g/dL)	sPAP (mmHg)	mPAP[a] (mmHg)
Antezana (20)	17	40	22	42	26
Vargas (21)	28	47	24	35	22
	30	22	19	35	22

Data obtained by Doppler echocardiography at the altitude of residence, La Paz, Bolivia (3600 m).
[a]Calculated mPAP values.
Abbreviation: mPAP, mean pulmonary arterial pressure.

VII. Pulmonary Hemodynamics in Chronic High-Altitude Diseases Described in China and Kyrgyzstan

A. Studies on High-Altitude Heart Disease (China)

The so-called HAHD has been described in adults living in the Qinghai-Tibetan plateau as a consequence of loss of altitude adaptation. Initial descriptions were confused and there was a great overlapping with the polycythemic variety of high-altitude chronic disease (CMS). Most publications on HAHD included a variable degree of polycythemia. The original description included 22 cases with average values of Hb of 21.1 g/dL and Hct of 73% (10), and the last original publication recorded 202 cases with an average Hb of 23.3 g/dL (23). Wu et al. have recognized that publications on HAHD, most of them from their own group, actually correspond to CMS (18).

There are no measurements of PAP obtained by cardiac catheterization in the so-called HAHD. Review of the literature only found two reports of PAP obtained by Doppler echocardiography after one week of residence at the lower altitude of Xining (2261 m). The calculated mPAP values in these studies were 36 ± 3 and 28 ± 4 mmHg, respectively, values similar to or somewhat lower than most of those reported in CMS (23,24) (Table 1). On the other hand, the ECG, vectorcardiogram (VCG), and chest X ray findings described in patients with HAHD are similar to those described in patients with CMS in Peru (8,9) and China (13). In short, as asserted by Wu, the adult type of HAHD actually corresponds to CMS.

B. Studies in High-Altitude Cor Pulmonale (Kyrgyzstan)

Kyrgyz investigators do not have publications with the name CMS. Several decades ago Mirrakhimow described a clinical picture named HACP observed in the Tien-Shan and Pamir Mountains (2800–4200 m). HACP is characterized by clinical evidence (auscultation, ECG, and X ray) of PH, which may evolve to heart failure (11). Sarybaeb and Mirrakhimov found a mPAP of 38 ± 3.2 mmHg in a group of patients with HACP living at 3200 to 4200 m (25). Recently, Aldashev et al. reported a mPAP of 32 ± 4 mmHg (range 20–64 mmHg) in 11 subjects with HACP living at the moderate altitudes of 2800 to 3100 m (26). It should be noted that all cardiac catheterization studies reported by Kyrgyz investigators were performed after one week of residence at low altitude (Bishkek, 750 m) (Table 1), which may explain the absence of significant hypoxemia and polycythemia. There are sparse data on SaO_2, Hb, and Hct in Kyrgyzian investigations. It is well known that SaO_2 improves promptly after descending to low levels and becomes normal or near normal in reported cases (8,9). Clinical and hemodynamic features suggest that HACP is actually a variety of CMS.

VIII. PH: A Common Feature of Chronic High-Altitude Diseases

There are six studies with cardiac catheterization carried out in patients with CMS at their altitude of residence. The average value of mPAP is 39 mmHg with a range from 27 to 51 mmHg. There is a severe degree of PH (≥ 40 mmHg) in three of the six studies (Table 1). There are two studies on pulmonary hemodynamics in Chinese patients with the so-called HAHD, and two studies in Kyrgyzian patients with the so-called HACP, all of them undertaken at low altitudes. The average mPAP of these four studies is 33.5 mmHg with a range from 28 to 38 mmHg. No study with severe PH has been reported (Table 1).

There is strong evidence that CMS, HAHD, and HACP are different shades of the same disease. Differences in PH are not significant. Moreover, there are no differences in the clinical evidence of PH as assessed by auscultation, ECG, and X rays. CMS, HAHD, and HACP are chronic high-altitude diseases resulting from loss of adaptation to an environment of chronic hypoxia. Therefore, it is difficult to assume different mechanisms of disease. However, lesser degrees of hypoxemia and polycythemia have been described in HAHD (China) and HACP (Kyrgyzstan) in comparison to CMS. Differences in the degree of hypoxemia and polycythemia may have two alternative explanations. Lower levels of hypoxemia and polycythemia in Asian patients with HAHD and HACP may be ascribed to the fact that they are generally studied after 7 to 10 days of recovery at lower altitude. Alternatively, higher levels of hypoxemia and polycythemia in Andean patients with CMS may be due to the fact that they are generally living in an environment of industrial pollution as seen in the Andean mining towns.

IX. CMS and Classifications of PH

A. CMS in the Current Clinical Classification of PH

The Evian classification of PH placed "chronic exposure to high altitude" in category 3: "PH associated with disorders of the respiratory system and/or hypoxemia" (27). This categorization was confirmed during the Third World Symposium on PAH held in Venice, Italy (28). "Chronic exposure to high altitude" is a nonspecific name that may be applied to healthy highlanders and chronic high-altitude diseases.

B. CMS in the Classification of the ISMM Consensus Statement

A consensus statement on "chronic and subacute high-altitude diseases" was published in 2005 by an ad hoc committee of the International Society of Mountain Medicine (ISMM) (12). This document recognizes two main groups of high-altitude diseases: (*i*) CMS as a separate entity, and (*ii*) high-altitude pulmonary hypertension (HAPH), which includes other chronic high-altitude diseases resulting from loss of altitude adaptation: HAHD described in China and HACP described in Kyrgyzstan. Subacute infantile mountain sickness (SIMS) was also included in group B. The main rationale for this classification was the assumption that PH was always present and often severe in group B, in contrast to CMS.

At the time when the consensus statement was elaborated, most information from China on HAHD in adults was based on clinical and anecdotal information but reliable data on pulmonary hemodynamics were lacking. The consensus statement has many references from Wu et al., who described HAHD in adults in 1965; however, most references from these authors are related to CMS, but none deals with PH in HAHD. Moreover, as mentioned before, Wu et al. have recognized that publications on HAHD, most of them from their own group, actually correspond to CMS and are associated with a variable degree of polycythemia (18). On the other hand, the exclusion of CMS from the group named HAPH is disconcerting in an era when PH is the target of recent clinical trials for the management of CMS.

A recent review of worldwide literature has demonstrated that PH is a common feature, in different magnitude, of all chronic high-altitude diseases. Differences of mPAP among these diseases are not significant. However, most studies on pulmonary hemodynamics have shown that the degree of PH in CMS is somewhat greater than in the so-called HAHD and HACP. Moreover, severe degrees of PH have only been reported in CMS. Therefore, there is no basis on which to exclude CMS from the diseases associated to PH. Chronic high-altitude diseases (CMS, HAHD, and HACP) should be integrated in only one group. Subacute and acute high-altitude diseases should be considered separately.

C. CMS in a New Classification of High-Altitude Diseases

HAPH is a descriptive term indicating the presence of PH at high altitudes. PH is a frequent feature in healthy highlanders and people with high-altitude diseases. The combination of PH and the time course of HA diseases following a chronic, subacute, or acute evolution is the natural and logical criteria for the classification of HA diseases. For those interested in high-altitude medicine, we propose a more detailed classification of high-altitude clinical conditions associated with HAPH as follows:

1. Healthy highlanders living above 3500 m
2. Chronic high-altitude diseases

   a. Chronic mountain sickness

   b. High-altitude heart disease (described in China)

   c. High-altitude cor pulmonale (described in Kyrgyzstan)

3. Subacute mountain sickness (SMS or subacute HAHD)

   a. Subacute infantile mountain sickness (SIMS or pediatric HAHD)

   b. Subacute adult mountain sickness

4. High-altitude pulmonary edema (HAPE)

We envisage HAPH as a true pathophysiological spectrum. At one end of the spectrum are healthy highlanders with mild PH and at the other end is SIMS (or pediatric HAHD) with severe PH. HAPE, an acute high-altitude disease, is also at this end of the spectrum. In the middle of the spectrum are the chronic high-altitude diseases (CMS, HAHD, and HACP).

X. Reappraisal of the ISMM Consensus Statement on CMS

The introduction of this document includes a warning on the possible evolution of the consensus as a result of new knowledge. This warning coincides with the prophetic words of the renowned investigator John Reeves who, two days before his tragic death, wrote to one of the authors of this chapter the following: "Thanks for your hard work on the CMS score. In Xining, I perceived that no one thought that result was perfect, but that the majority thought it should be floated publicly as a target to shoot at. No doubt at the next reconsideration, there will be numerous bullet holes in the target, but hopefully something will remain."

In accordance with the current knowledge on pulmonary hemodynamics in chronic high-altitude diseases, a revision of the consensus on CMS would be reasonable on the basis of the following issues.

A. Limits of the Consensus Statement on CMS

The ISMM Consensus was originally designed for CMS and, later on other chronic high-altitude diseases described in China and Kyrgyzstan were included. Finally, subacute high-altitude diseases were also added. However, chronic and subacute high-altitude diseases are quite different entities. SIMS is a subacute disease that occurs mainly in infants and results from an inadequate adaptation to high altitude. On the other hand, chronic high-altitude diseases occur in adults and result from loss of altitude adaptation. Therefore, chronic and subacute HA diseases should be considered separately. The scoring system of CMS should be extended to other chronic high-altitude diseases such as HAHD and HACP since PH is a common feature to all of them, without significant differences. Moreover, most of the symptoms and signs are also similar with the exception of the levels of hemoglobin and hypoxemia, which, however, should always be considered at the altitude of residence.

B. Main Scope of the Consensus: Chronic High-Altitude Diseases

CMS and related diseases, resulting from loss of altitude adaptation, are the main scope of the ISMM Consensus. These diseases have been described with different names (CMS, HAHD, and HACP) in various geographic regions. Their clinical picture and pulmonary hemodynamics are somewhat similar. However, some differences in the degree of polycythemia and hypoxemia have been described between Andean and Asian populations, and the probable causes for this variation have been postulated. The score system should be only one for all chronic high-altitude diseases, and PH as well as hypoxemia should be included in the score system.

C. Scoring System for Diagnosis of CMS and Related Diseases

In the last two decades, epidemiological studies of CMS have been performed in Peru, China, and Kyrgyzstan and several scoring systems for its diagnosis have been proposed. However, it is not easy to develop a unique scoring system because of individual characteristics (ethnicity, gender, age) and dissimilar geographical areas and altitudes.

The Qinghai score proposed by Chinese investigators was approved by the CMS Consensus Group during the VI World Congress on Mountain Medicine (Xining, China, 2004) (9). This score system is somewhat empirical and has some limitations (29).

D. PH and the Score System

PH, a major component of all chronic high-altitude diseases, should be included in the scoring system. Clinical evidence of PH assessed by auscultation, chest X ray, and ECG has been advised as the initial methodology for diagnosis of PH in recently approved guidelines (30,31). Following these guidelines, the clinical evidence of PH in chronic high-altitude diseases may be scored as 1 (mild), 2 (moderate), and 3 (severe), in comparison with the normal values described at sea level. Quantification of PH by Doppler echocardiography or right-heart catheterization could be carried out in selected cases of CMS when these procedures are available in the altitude of residence (29).

E. Hypoxemia Levels and the Score System

Hypoxemia is a key player of CMS and is an essential part of the current definition of CMS. It was considered in previous scoring systems. However, hypoxemia does not appear among the parameters of the current score system. Variable threshold values for SaO_2 as <82%, <85%, and <90% were proposed by Peruvian, Chinese, and Kyrgyzian investigators, respectively. These values could be scored as 3, 2, and 1, respectively. It is strongly recommended to measure SaO_2 at the level of residence and not at lower levels during the recovery period.

F. Hemoglobin Threshold Values

Hemoglobin concentration is the parameter with the highest weight in the current score system for CMS. However, the Hb threshold value of 21 g/dL for males (18.3 ± 2SD) was derived from a review of the clinical records of healthy miners living in Cerro de Pasco (4300 m). It was found that values of Hb increased with increasing age, and the cutoff value of 21 g/dL was particularly valid for the age 20 to 29 years living at 4340 m (32,33). This threshold value may not be valid for lower altitudes and the diagnosis of CMS may be missed.

Bolivian investigators working in La Paz (3600 m) found Hb values of 17 g/dL in healthy people, 19.5 g/dL in a group of young patients with CMS and 24 g/dL in a group of elderly patients with CMS (21). A Chinese epidemiological study in more than 5000 normal subjects at three levels of altitude showed that Hb values are related to the level of altitude and ethnicity (Tibetans and Hans), and consequently the threshold values are not the same (34). Therefore, we must be cautious when a unique Hb threshold value is proposed for different conditions (altitude, age, ethnicity, pollution). It is recommended that values of Hb in patients with CMS and related diseases should be measured at the level of residence and not at lower levels during the recovery period.

XI. Prevention and Management Of CMS

Preventive measures are directed toward modifiable risk factors of CMS, such as smoking, obesity, domestic and industrial air pollution, and lung diseases. The definitive treatment of CMS is descending to lower altitudes or sea level. Following this, subjective symptoms and sleep disorders disappear. Alveolar hypoxia, hypoxemia, and cyanosis promptly disappear. Polycythemia decreases progressively. PH and RVH regress gradually and disappear after one or two years (8,9).

Bleeding is a palliative procedure that reduces the excessive polycythemia with partial improvement of signs and symptoms (35). Other procedures are directed to improve ventilation by using stimulant drugs such as acetozolamide. The increased ventilation reduces hypoxemia and hematocrit and as a consequence improves symptomatology (36). Vasodilator therapy is being tested to reduce PH in patients with CMS. Sildenafil, a phosphodiesterase-5 inhibitor and selective pulmonary vasodilator, was tested and after several months improvement in pulmonary hemodynamics and exercise tolerance was observed (37).

Acknowledgments

This chapter is dedicated to the memory of Profs Carlos Monge and Alberto Hurtado, who were pioneers in the investigation of CMS. It is also dedicated to the memory of Carlos Monge Jr., MD, for his valuable contribution to this field. We would like to express our gratitude to all who were our collaborators at the Cardiovascular Laboratory of the High-Altitude Research Institute, Peruvian University Cayetano Heredia. We are grateful to Hector Villagarcia, BSc, for his diligence in the diagramming support for this article.

References

1. Reeves JT, Grover RF. Insights by Peruvian scientists into the pathogenesis of human chronic hypoxic pulmonary hypertension. J Appl Physiol 2005; 98:384–389.
2. Penaloza D, Sime F, Banchero N, et al. Pulmonary hypertension in healthy men born and living at high altitudes. Am J Cardiol 1963; 11:150–157.
3. Arias-Stella J, Saldaña M. The terminal portion of the pulmonary arterial tree in people native to high altitude. Circulation 1963; 28:915–925.
4. Penaloza D, Arias-Stella J. The heart and pulmonary circulation at high altitude. Healthy highlanders and chronic mountain sickness. Circulation 2007; 115:1132–1146.
5. Monge, MC. La Enfermedad de los Andes. Síndromes eritrémicos. Anales de la Facultad de Medicina de Lima, Peru, 1929.
6. Hurtado A. Animals in high altitude: resident man. In: Handbook of Physiology. Adaptation to the Environment. Sect 4, Vol 1. Washington D.C.: Am Physiol Soc 1964:843–860.
7. Rotta A, Cánepa A, Hurtado A, et al.. Pulmonary circulation at sea level and at high altitude. J Appl Physiol 1956; 9:328–336.
8. Penaloza D, Sime F. Chronic cor pulmonale due to loss of altitude acclimatization (chronic mountain sickness). Am J Med 1971; 50:728–743.
9. Penaloza D, Sime F, Ruiz L. Cor pulmonale in chronic mountain sickness: present concept of Monge's disease. In: Porter R, Knight J, eds. High Altitude Physiology: Cardiac and Respiratory Aspects. Edinburgh and London: Churchill Livingstone, 1971:41–60.
10. Wu TY, Li CH, Wang ZW. Adult high altitude heart disease; an analysis of 22 cases. Chin Int Med J 1965; 13:700–702.
11. Mirrakhimov MM. Chronic high-altitude cor pulmonale. In: Transactions of the International Symposium on Pulmonary Arterial Hypertension. Frunze, Kyrgyzstan: Kyrgyz Institute of Cardiology, 1985:267–287.
12. León-Velarde F, Maggiorini M, Reeves JT, et al. Consensus statement on chronic and subacute high altitude diseases. High Alt Med Biol 2005; 6:147–157.
13. Pei SX, Chen XJ, Si Ren BZ, et al. Chronic mountain sickness in Tibet. QJ Med 1989; 266:555–574.

14. Ergueta J, Spielvogel H, Cudkowitz L. Cardio-respiratory studies in chronic mountain sickness (Monge's syndrome). Respiration 1979; 28:485–517.
15. Manier G, Guénard H, Castaing Y, et al. Pulmonary gas exchange in Andean natives with excessive polycythemia-effect of hemodilution. J Appl Physiol 1988; 65:2107–2117.
16. Yang Z, He ZQ, Liu XL. Pulmonary hypertension and high altitude. Chin Cardiovasc Dis 1985; 13:32–34.
17. Wu TY, Miao CY, Li WS, et al. Studies on high altitude pulmonary hypertension. Chin J High Alt Med 1999; 9:1–8.
18. Wu TY, Zhang Q, Jin B, et al. Chronic mountain sickness (Monge's disease): an observation in Qinghai-Tibet Plateau. In: Ueda G, Reeves JT, Sekiguchi M, eds. High Altitude Medicine. Matsumoto, Japan: Shinshu University Press, 1992:314–324.
19. Chemla D, Castelain V, Humbert M, et al. New formula for predicting mean pulmonary artery pressure using systolic pulmonary artery pressure. Chest 2004; 126:1313–1317.
20. Antezana AM, Antezana G, Aparicio O, et al. Pulmonary hypertension in high-altitude chronic hypoxia: response to nifedipine. Eur Respir J 1998; 12:1181–1185.
21. Vargas E, Spielvogel H. Chronic mountain sickness, optimal hemoglobin and heart disease. High Alt Med Biol 2006; 7:138–149.
22. Moore LG, Niermeyer S, Vargas E. Does chronic mountain sickness (CMS) have perinatal origins? Respir Physiol Neurobiol 2007; 158:180–189.
23. Wu TY, Jing BS, Xu FD, et al. Clinical features of adult high altitude heart disease. An analysis of 202 cases (Chinese with English abstract). Acta Cardiovasc Pulm Dis 1990; 9:32–35.
24. Cheng DS, Yang YX, Bian HP, et al. A study on altitude hypoxic pulmonary hypertension by Doppler echocardiography (1996). Chin J High Alt Med 1996; 6:8–31 [Chinese with English abstract].
25. Sarybaeb A, Mirrakhimov M. Prevalence and natural course of high altitude pulmonary hypertension and high altitude cor pulmonale. In: Ohno H, Kobayashi T, Masuyama S, et al, eds. Progress in Mountain Medicine and High Altitude Physiology. Matsumoto, Japan: Dogura & Co., 1998:126–131.
26. Aldashev A, Sarybaev AS, Sydkykov AS, et al. Characterization of high-altitude pulmonary hypertension in the Kyrgyz: association with angiotensin-converting enzyme genotype. Am J Respir Crit Care Med 2002; 166:1396–1402.
27. Rich S, Rubin LJ, Abenhail L, et al. Executive summary from the World Symposium on Primary Pulmonary Hypertension (Evian, France, 1998). WHO publication. Available at: http://www.who.int/ncd/cvd/pph.html.
28. Simmoneau G, Galie N, Rubin LJ, et al. Clinical classification of pulmonary hypertension. J Am Coll Cardiol 2004; 43:5S–12S.
29. Penaloza D. Chronic mountain sickness: an open debate of scoring systems used for its diagnosis. In: Ge Ri-Li, Hackett P, eds. Life on the Qinghai-Tibetan Plateau. Beijing: Beijing University Medical Press, 2007:161–169.
30. Barst RJ, McGoon M, Torbicki A, et al. Diagnosis and differential assessment of pulmonary arterial hypertension. J Am Coll Cardiol 2004; 43:40S–47S.
31. McGoon M, Gutterman D, Steen V, et al. Screening, early detection and diagnosis of pulmonary arterial hypertension. ACCP Evidence-Based Clinical Practice Guidelines. Chest 2004; 126:14S–34S.
32. Monge CC, Leon-Velarde F, Arregui A. Increasing prevalence of excessive erythrocytosis with age among healthy high-altitude miners (letter). N Engl J Med 1989; 321:1271.
33. Monge-C C, León Velarde F, Arregui A. Chronic mountain sickness. In: Horbein TF, Schoene RB, eds. High Altitude. An Exploration of Human Adaptation. New York, NY: Marcel Dekker Inc., 2001:815–838.
34. Wu TY, Li W, Wei L, et al. A preliminary study on the diagnosis of chronic mountain sickness in Tibetan populations. In: Ohno H, Kobayashi T, Masuyama S, et al., eds. Progress

in Mountain Medicine and High Altitude Physiology. Matsumoto, Japan: Dogura & Co., 1998:337–342.

35. Winslow RM, Monge-CC, Brown EG, et al. Effects of hemodilution on O2 transport in high altitude polycythemia. J Appl Physiol 1985; 59:1495–1502.

36. Richalet JP, Rivera M, Maignan M, et al. Acetozolamide for Monge's disease. Efficiency and tolerance of 6-month treatment. Am J Respir Crit Care Med 2008; 177:1370–1376.

37. Aldashev AA, Kojonorazov BK, Amatov TA, et al. Phosphodiesterase type 5 and high altitude pulmonary hypertension. Thorax 2005; 60:683–687.

21
Chronic Thromboembolic Pulmonary Hypertension

WILLIAM R. AUGER and PETER F. FEDULLO
University of California, San Diego, California, U.S.A.

I. Introduction

The initial descriptions of the clinical syndrome of chronic thrombotic obstruction of the major pulmonary arteries appeared during the 1950s (1–4). Later that same decade, Hurwitt et al. reported the first surgical attempt to remove adherent thrombus from the pulmonary vessels, thereby establishing a distinction between acute and chronic thromboembolic disease and suggesting that an endarterectomy would be necessary if surgery for this unusual disease was to be successful (5).

A few years later, the first successful, bilateral pulmonary thromboendarterectomy (PTE) using a sternotomy approach and cardiopulmonary bypass was reported by Houk and colleagues (6). This was followed by several small series describing surgical successes, which underscored the concept that chronic thromboembolic pulmonary hypertension (CTEPH) need not be a fatal diagnosis (7–11). Over the subsequent years, and particularly over the past two decades, the syndrome of CTEPH has been better characterized, and as a result, more widely recognized as a potentially curable form of pulmonary hypertension. With improvements in diagnostic capabilities, surgical techniques, and postoperative management, the mortality risk of surgical thromboendarterectomy has steadily declined. Most dramatic of all have been reports from clinical centers around the world that thromboendarterectomy for selected patients with CTEPH can result in a substantial improvement in pulmonary hemodynamics, functional status, and long-term survival.

II. Chronic Thromboembolic Disease: Incidence and Risk Factors

The incidence of CTEPH as a complication of acute pulmonary embolic disease is unknown. Early suggestions that 0.1% to 0.5% of acute embolic survivors might develop CTEPH was likely an underestimate (12). A recent study by Pengo and colleagues described a two-year cumulative incidence of symptomatic CTEPH of 3.8% following a single episode of pulmonary embolism (median follow-up of 94.3 months in 223 patients) and 13.4% following recurrent venous thromboembolism (13). However, two prospective series subsequently reported a somewhat lower incidence. In a group of 259 patients followed over an average period of 46 months, Becattini and colleagues diagnosed two patients with CTEPH for an incidence of 0.8% (14). Miniati et al. reported a CTEPH incidence of 1.5% in a group of 320 pulmonary embolic survivors followed for a minimum of one year (15). Even if a 1% incidence is used, and one assumes that 210,000 acute pulmonary embolic patients in the United States have long-term survival potential (16), over 2000 patients might be expected to develop CTEPH. With the number of thromboendarterectomy procedures performed annually in the United States estimated to be in the range of 300, either an approximate incidence of 1% is excessive or the disease is being substantially underdiagnosed or CTEPH patients are not coming to the attention of centers capable of surgical intervention.

There is also limited information as to what might predispose patients to develop CTEPH. Recent observational studies have provided some insights about possible risk factors. The overall extent of pulmonary vascular obstruction at presentation may place patients at risk for the development of CTEPH. In Pengo's study, it was suggested that larger perfusion defects at the time of the initial pulmonary embolus diagnosis was a risk factor for developing CTEPH (13). They also showed that a history of multiple pulmonary embolic events, a younger age at presentation, and an idiopathic pulmonary embolic event placed patients at greater risk. In a report where massive pulmonary embolism was defined as >50% obstruction of the pulmonary vascular bed, the incidence of CTEPH was 20.2% despite the use of thrombolytic therapy (17). The presence of pulmonary hypertension when an acute pulmonary embolism is diagnosed might be important "risk factor" and should alert the clinician to the possibility that CTEPH may be a potential problem. In patients presenting with an acute pulmonary embolus, Ribeiro and colleagues reported that those with pulmonary artery systolic pressures >50 mmHg were apt to experience persistent pulmonary hypertension after one year (18).

The presence of a prothombotic condition has been examined in patients with chronic thromboembolic disease. Though hereditary thrombophilic states (deficiencies of antithrombin III, protein C, or protein S, or factor II and factor V Leiden mutations) represent risk factors for venous thromboembolism, their prevalence in patients with established CTEPH has been shown to be no different than that seen in patients with primary pulmonary hypertension or in control subjects (19,20). However, the presence of antiphospholipid antibodies (with or without an accompanying lupus anticoagulant) has been found to be one of the most common prothrombotic states associated with the development of CTEPH. The antiphospholipid antibodies can be found in up to 21% of patients with CTEPH (19). Bonderman and colleagues also demonstrated increased levels of factor VIII in 41% of 122 patients with CTEPH, levels that were substantially higher compared with patients with nonthromboembolic pulmonary arterial hypertension, and which remained elevated following successful pulmonary thromboendarterectomy surgery (21). In a small series of 24 patients, hyperhomocysteinemia was demonstrated in 7 of 14 patients with CTEPH, while 12 of the 24 patients were reported to have antiphospholipid antibodies (20).

There may also be an association between certain medical conditions and the development of chronic thromboembolic disease. Bonderman and colleagues compared 109 consecutive CTEPH patients with 187 patients who did not develop chronic thromboembolic disease after experiencing an acute pulmonary embolism. Multivariate analysis revealed that prior splenectomy, the presence of a ventriculoatrial shunt to treat hydrocephalus, and certain chronic inflammatory disorders, such as osteomyelitis and inflammatory bowel disease, were associated with an increased risk for CTEPH (22).

III. Natural History of CTEPH

Despite the considerable advancements in the diagnosis and management of patients with CTEPH, the pathophysiologic basis for this disease is incompletely understood. The mechanisms by which an acute pulmonary embolus evolves to chronic thromboembolic residua incorporated into the wall of the pulmonary vessel have been difficult to define. The presence of coexisting cardiopulmonary disease, the initial embolic burden, and the age of the thrombus at the time of embolization may all contribute. Under normal physiologic conditions, Rosenhek and colleagues showed that the pulmonary artery demonstrates increased fibrinolytic capabilities compared with the aorta (23). This appears to be based on higher levels of tissue plasminogen activator (TPA) expression versus plasminogen activator inhibitor (PAI-1). However, a TPA–PAI-1 imbalance that would favor incomplete thrombus dissolution has not been found to be operational in CTEPH patients studied (24). More recently, preliminary data suggest that certain patients may have fibrinogen variants that render them resistant to lysis (25).

There is growing body of evidence that suggests mechanical obstruction of the central pulmonary vasculature with chronic thromboembolic residua as the sole basis for elevation of the pulmonary vascular resistance (PVR), whether it be related to recurrent embolic events or in situ pulmonary artery thrombosis, seems to occur in a minority of CTEPH patients. It appears that the progressive rise in pulmonary vascular resistance in the majority of patients results from pathophysiologic changes in the distal pulmonary vascular bed, seemingly those lung regions *not* involved with chronic thromboemboli. There are several important observations to support this line of reasoning. Moser and Bloor described the findings in lung biopsies obtained at the time of PTE surgery and from postmortem tissue in CTEPH patients. They demonstrated the presence of histopathologic changes in the microvasculature similar to that seen in other forms of small vessel pulmonary hypertension, though distal to both obstructed and nonobstructed central arteries (26). In a large percentage of patients, there also appears to be a poor correlation between the scintigraphic and angiographic extent of central thromboembolic obstruction and the severity of pulmonary hypertension (27,28). Furthermore, in patients with sequential perfusion scans available for review, pulmonary hypertension has progressed in the absence of perfusion scan change or clinical evidence of embolic recurrence. And finally, approximately 10% to 15% of CTEPH patients will experience persistent postoperative pulmonary hypertension despite what is considered a satisfactory surgical endarterectomy of major vessel chronic thromboemboli. The pathophysiologic factors responsible for these vasculature changes are unknown. Though speculative, circulating vasoconstrictors, immune-related events, "local" upregulation of vascular growth factors, or an individual genetic predisposition may, individually or in some combination, be operative in the development of this hypertensive pulmonary arteriopathy (29–33).

IV. Clinical Presentation

The most common complaint of patients with CTEPH is exertional dyspnea, which physiologically appears related to a limitation in cardiac output and, in some individuals, to increased dead-space ventilation. Patients accustomed to higher levels of activity recognize the decline in exercise capacity at an earlier point in time than those who lead a sedentary lifestyle. As right ventricular function and coronary perfusion become incapable of responding to increased metabolic demands, symptoms of lightheadedness, exertion-related presyncope, syncopal events, and exertional chest pain may develop. Other symptoms are reported with varying frequencies such as a nonproductive cough (especially with exertion), hemoptysis, and palpitations. A change in voice quality or hoarseness may result from vocal cord dysfunction due to compression of the recurrent laryngeal nerve between the aorta and an enlarged left main pulmonary artery. Chest discomfort is often pleuritic in nature, presumptively due to peripherally infarcted lung. However, exertion-related chest pain can also occur, often prompting an evaluation for coronary artery disease.

Consideration of chronic thromboembolic disease as a diagnostic possibility is frequently delayed, often months to years, following symptom onset. Though this diagnosis is an appropriate concern in patients having experienced previous acute thromboembolic events, up to 40% to 50% of CTEPH patients provide no such history (34,35). As exam findings of pulmonary hypertension are also difficult to discern early in the disease, alternative explanations for a patient's exertional dyspnea, such as physical deconditioning or exercise-induced reactive airways disease are frequently entertained. When coexisting disorders are present, such as coronary artery disease, a modest degree of parenchymal or obstructive lung disease, or minimal left ventricular dysfunction, such presenting complaints can be attributed to these problems. However, exertional dyspnea or a progressive decline in exercise capabilities out of proportion to that expected with these coexisting medical conditions should raise the possibility of pulmonary vascular disease.

Physical examination findings reflect the stage at which a patient with CTEPH presents for evaluation. In the absence of significant right-heart dysfunction, physical findings in the CTEPH patients may be unremarkable. Even in the setting of severe pulmonary hypertension, patients can appear relatively well. The exam findings of pulmonary hypertension such as a right ventricular lift, a pronounced pulmonic component of the second heart sound, a right ventricular S4 gallop, and a tricuspid regurgitation murmur should be carefully sought after. It is not until the development of right-heart failure will jugular venous distention, a right ventricular S3 gallop, severe tricuspid regurgitation, hepatomegaly, ascites, and/or peripheral edema become evident. In the absence of coexisting parenchymal lung disease or airflow obstruction, the lung exam of the CTEPH patient can be unexceptional. In approximately 30% of patients with CTEPH, pulmonary flow murmurs can be appreciated (36). These bruits, which appear to result from turbulent flow across narrowed or partially obstructed pulmonary vessels, are high-pitched in quality. They are auscultated over the lung fields rather than the precordium, can accentuate following inspiration, and may require the patient to hold breath to be clearly heard. However, this exam finding is not specific to chronic thromboembolic disease, and can be heard in other diseases that feature large pulmonary vessel narrowing, such as congenital pulmonary branch stenosis or major vessel pulmonary arteritis. Their importance when discovered in the pulmonary hypertensive patient is that they have not been described in patients with idiopathic or small vessel pulmonary arterial disease. Additional exam findings in the CTEPH patient might include peripheral cyanosis, alerting the clinician to the possibility of a right to left shunt through a patent foramen ovale. Examination of the lower extremities may disclose superficial varicosities and venous stasis skin discoloration in those individuals who have experienced prior venous thrombosis.

V. Evaluation of Patients with Suspected Chronic Thromboembolic Disease

The goals in the evaluation of patients with suspected chronic thromboembolic disease are to confirm the diagnosis; to assess the degree of pulmonary hypertension and right ventricular dysfunction present, which are critical factors in prognosis and operative mortality risk; to determine surgical accessibility of the chronic thromboembolic lesions, thereby establishing a patient as a candidate for PTE surgery; and to assess the extent of coexisting small vessel pulmonary vascular disease.

Information to be gathered from general laboratory testing is important in defining the severity of disease in patients suffering from CTEPH. For those with severe right ventricular dysfunction and coexisting liver congestion, elevation of transaminase and bilirubin levels can be expected. It is this same subgroup of patients where renal blood flow and glomerular perfusion may be compromised, either from a low cardiac output or the use of diuretics (or both). Elevation of serum creatinine and blood urea nitrogen may occur as a result. In this patient population the identification of a prothrombotic state is important. In the absence of heparin anticoagulation, an elevated activated partial thromboplastin time (aPTT) may be the first indication that a lupus anticoagulant is present. It is particularly important to detect antiphospholipid antibodies (anticardiolipin antibodies, lupus anticoagulant) in those CTEPH patients undergoing PTE surgery, as they appear to be at higher risk for postoperative thrombosis. For these patients, more aggressive post-PTE anticoagulation may be warranted.

Chest radiography in patients with CTEPH may be deceptively unremarkable in the early stages of the disease process. However, with the development of significant pulmonary hypertension, enlargement of the proximal pulmonary vascular bed typically occurs. If chronic thromboemboli involve the main or lobar pulmonary arteries, there may be asymmetry to the central pulmonary artery (PA) enlargement, which is not typically seen in those patients with small vessel disease (37). As the right ventricle adapts to the rise in pulmonary vascular resistance, radiographic signs of chamber enlargement, such as obliteration of the retrosternal space and prominence of the right-heart border, can be seen. Without coexisting parenchymal lung disease, interstitial-alveolar markings within the lung fields are atypical. However, relatively avascular lung regions can be appreciated if a large organized thrombus is compromising blood flow to that area. The sequela of lung injury such as peripheral alveolar opacities, linear scar-like lesions, and pleural thickening may also be observed.

Pulmonary function testing is most useful in evaluating for coexisting parenchymal lung disease or airflow obstruction. CTEPH by itself will not significantly impact spirometric or lung volume measurements. For those patients with parenchymal scarring from prior lung infarction, a mild to moderate restrictive defect may be detected (38). Similarly, a modest reduction in single-breath diffusing capacity of lung for carbon monoxide (D_LCO) may be present in some CTEPH patients, though a normal value does not exclude the diagnosis (39). A severe reduction in D_LCO should raise concerns that the distal pulmonary vascular bed is significantly compromised, making it imperative that an alternative diagnosis other than CTEPH be considered.

Patients with CTEPH will frequently exhibit normal resting arterial oxygenation (PaO_2), although dead-space ventilation may be elevated. With exercise, patients with extensive chronic thromboembolic disease will often experience a decline in PaO_2 and an inappropriate rise in dead-space ventilation. These findings reflect the ventilation-perfusion mismatch in CTEPH and an inadequate cardiac output response to exercise, which results in a low mixed venous oxygen saturation (40). Hypoxemia at rest implies severe right-heart dysfunction or the presence of a considerable right to left shunt, such as through a patent foramen ovale.

Transthoracic echocardiography has become an extremely valuable noninvasive tool in the evaluation of the pulmonary hypertensive patient. Available technology allows for estimates of pulmonary artery systolic pressure (using Doppler analysis of the degree of tricuspid regurgitation), along with cardiac output and right ventricular (RV) performance (41). Enlargement of the right heart chambers, tricuspid regurgitation as a result of this chamber enlargement, flattening or paradoxical motion of the interventricular septum, encroachment of an enlarged right ventricle on the left ventricular cavity, and impaired left ventricular diastolic filling that it is not the result of primary left ventricular diastolic dysfunction or valvular heart disease are findings in patients with significant pulmonary hypertension (42,43). Contrast echocardiography using intravenous agitated saline can detect the presence of an intracardiac shunt, such as a patent foramen ovale or a previously undetected septal defect. Identification preoperatively is important as it can be surgically repaired at the time of an endarterectomy. Should an echocardiogram obtained at rest demonstrate minimally elevated pulmonary artery pressures or only modest right ventricular compromise in a patient experiencing cardiopulmonary symptoms with exertion, obtaining a study with exercise may allow to document a substantial rise in pulmonary artery pressures with dilatation of the right ventricle.

Though ventilation-perfusion (V/Q) scintigraphy has seen a diminishing role in the evaluation of suspected acute pulmonary embolic disease, it still provides essential information in the pulmonary hypertensive patient. In these patients, the V/Q scan often is the first indication that chronic thromboembolic disease should be considered. In chronic thromboembolic disease, at least one, and more commonly several segmental or larger mismatched perfusion defect are present (44,45). In disorders of the distal pulmonary vascular bed, perfusion scans either are normal or exhibit a "mottled" appearance characterized by nonsegmental defects. Possible exceptions to this observation include pulmonary veno-occlusive disease and pulmonary capillary hemangiomatosis in which segmental defects have been reported (46,47). Furthermore, the magnitude of the perfusion defects in chronic thromboembolic disease often understates the extent the actual degree of pulmonary vascular obstruction determined angiographically or at surgery (27). During the process of organization, proximal vessel thromboemboli may recannalize, or narrow the vessel, in such a manner that radiolabeled macroaggregated albumin may traverse the area of partial obstruction, creating regions of relative hypoperfusion on the perfusion scan. Therefore, the presence of even a single, mismatched segmental perfusion defect or hypoperfused lung regions in a patient with pulmonary hypertension should raise the possibility of chronic thromboembolic disease.

Though a V/Q scan is useful to differentiate large from small vessel pulmonary vascular pathology, segmental or larger defects in a pulmonary hypertensive patients are not specific for chronic thromboembolic disease. Extrinsic pulmonary vascular compression from mediastinal adenopathy or fibrosis, primary pulmonary vascular tumors, and large vessel pulmonary arteritis may result in a V/Q scan appearance indistinguishable from that seen in CTEPH (48–50). Consequently, additional imaging modalities are necessary to complete the diagnostic evaluation. Computed tomographic (CT) scanning is valuable in detecting disorders of the pulmonary parenchyma, chest wall, and mediastinum. A variety of CT findings have been described in patients with chronic thromboembolic disease, including mosaic perfusion of the lung parenchyma, central pulmonary artery enlargement, with variability in the size of lobar and segmental-level vessels, an abrupt reduction in size of those vessels involved with chronic thrombi, the presence of collateral vessels arising from the systemic arterial circulation (aorta, coronary arteries), and peripheral, scar-like lesions in poorly perfused lung regions (51,52). With appropriate contrast enhancement of the pulmonary vasculature during CT imaging, organized thrombus can be seen to line the pulmonary vessels, often in an eccentric fashion. Narrowing of pulmonary arteries, web strictures, and other irregularities of the intima may also be appreciated. These CT findings are distinct from the intraluminal filling defects of acute thromboemboli or primary pulmonary vascular tumors (48). However, the absence of some of these findings, particularly lining thrombus or thickened intima of the central vessels, does not exclude the diagnosis of chronic thromboembolic disease or the possibility of surgical intervention. This observation has been underscored in a recent series where V/Q scintigraphy was demonstrated to be more sensitive (96% vs. 51%) in detecting chronic thromboembolic disease than multidetector CT pulmonary angiography (53). Conversely, central thrombi have been described in processes other than CTEPH such as idiopathic pulmonary hypertension, Eisenmenger syndrome, and chronic obstructive pulmonary disease (54–56).

Once the possibility of chronic thromboembolic disease has been suggested by preliminary studies, both confirmation of the diagnosis through detailed evaluation of the pulmonary vascular anatomy and hemodynamic assessment should follow. Right-heart catheterization in the evaluation of patients with suspected CTEPH objectively defines the severity of pulmonary hypertension and degree of cardiac dysfunction at rest. This hemodynamic assessment is important in discussions with patients as to perioperative risks, should they prove to be surgical candidates. For symptomatic CTEPH patients with modest pulmonary hypertension at rest, exercise hemodynamic measurements may be obtained. In these cases it is likely that the normal compensatory mechanisms of recruitment and dilation of the pulmonary vasculature have been overcome, and with exercise, a linear elevation in pulmonary artery pressure as cardiac output increases can be observed. This hemodynamic information provides objective evidence to explain an individual's symptoms, and likely reflects a clinically relevant stage in the development of severe CTEPH in which there is coexisting small vessel hypertensive changes.

Furthermore, right-heart catheterization has the potential to provide objective data in analyzing the degree of this small vessel disease, information that may help predict post-PTE outcomes. Partitioning the different elements (proximal vs. distal) of the pulmonary vascular resistance in CTEPH has been investigated. In a small series of 26 CTEPH patients, Kim and colleagues, utilizing pulmonary artery occlusion waveform analysis, demonstrated excellent inverse correlation between the percent upstream resistance and postoperative mean pulmonary artery pressure and pulmonary vascular resistance. In addition, all four deaths in this series occurred in patients in whom the upstream resistance was <60% (57). If future investigations validate these preliminary observations, this information may identify a subgroup of CTEPH patients who should be excluded from surgical consideration.

Confirmation of the diagnosis and assessment of the proximal extent of chronic thromboembolic lesions are essential in evaluating patients for endarterectomy surgery.

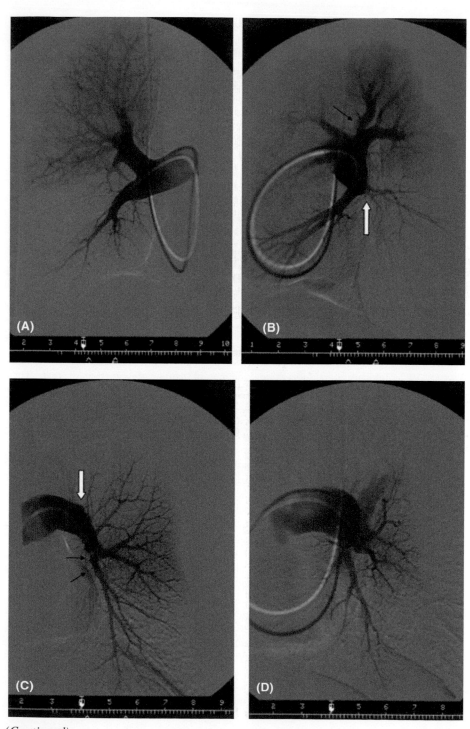

(Continued)

Often considered the "gold standard" for achieving these diagnostic goals, conventional pulmonary angiography can be safely performed, when taking proper precautions, even in severely pulmonary hypertensive patients (58). The angiographic appearance of chronic thromboembolic disease bears little resemblance to that of acute pulmonary embolism. Well-defined, intraluminal filling defects found in acute disease are not present. Instead, the angiographic patterns encountered in chronic thromboembolic disease reflect the complex patterns of organization and recanalization that occur following an acute thromboembolic event. Several angiographic patterns have been described in chronic thromboembolic disease, which correlate with the material removed at the time of surgery (59). These include pouch defects, pulmonary artery webs or bands, intimal irregularities, abrupt and often angular narrowing of the major pulmonary arteries, and complete obstruction of main, lobar, or segmental vessels at their point of origin (Fig. 1). In most patients with extensive chronic thromboembolic disease, two or more of these angiographic findings are present, typically involving both lungs.

For centers where conventional pulmonary angiography is either unavailable or felt to be too risky to perform, there is an expanding experience using magnetic resonance (MR) imaging and magnetic resonance angiography (MRA) as an alternative means to determine surgical candidacy for CTEPH patients (60). Kreitner and colleagues have shown that contrast-enhanced MRA is able to demonstrate the vascular changes typical for CTE disease. In a study of 34 CTEPH patients, wall-adherent thromboembolic material involving the central pulmonary arteries down to the segmental level could be demonstrated; intraluminal webs and bands, as well as abnormal vessel tapering and "cutoffs" were also detected. Further they showed that MRA was superior to digital subtraction angiography in determining the proximal location of resectable chronic thromboembolic material (61). An additional study comparing MR techniques with conventional contrast angiography involved 29 patients with either CTEPH or idiopathic pulmonary arterial hypertension (IPAH). Nikolaou and colleagues showed that the combined interpretation of MR perfusion imaging and MR angiography led to a correct diagnosis of IPAH or CTEPH in 26 (90%) of 29 patients when compared to the reference diagnosis based on V/Q scintigraphy, digital subtraction angiography, or CT angiography. The interpretation of MR angiography alone had a sensitivity of 71% for wall-adherent thrombi, 50% for webs and bands, and between 83% and 86% for detection of complete vessel obstruction and free-floating thrombi when compared to DSA or CT angiography (62). Furthermore, there are other features of MRI that can be useful in the evaluation of CTEPH patients. Cine imaging allows an assessment of RV and left ventricular (LV) function, providing data on end-systolic and end-diastolic volumes, ejection fraction, and muscle mass (63,64). Furthermore, phase contrast imaging may be used to measure cardiac output, along with pulmonary and systemic arterial flow. In CTEPH patients undergoing PTE, this technique has been used to measure changes in aortic and pulmonary arterial blood flow before and after surgery (61,65).

Figure 1 Pulmonary angiogram in a CTEPH patient. (**A**) Narrowing of the right descending PA, with a hypovascular right lower lobe. (**B**) Lateral view: proximal occlusion of the right descending PA (*white arrow*), and narrowing of the proximal apical vessel (*thin arrow*). (**C**) Proximal "pouch" occlusion of a left upper lobe artery (*white arrow*), with narrowing and intimal irregularities of the left descending PA (*thin arrows*). (**D**) Lateral view: better demonstrates an occluded lingular artery and anteromedial left lower lobe vessel. *Abbreviation*: CTEPH, chronic thromboembolic pulmonary hypertension.

VI. Selection of CTEPH Patients for Endarterectomy Surgery

Regardless of the diagnostic study, the critical determinant as to whether or not a patient with chronic thromboembolic disease might be a candidate for PTE surgery is the presence of surgically accessible lesions. However, the differentiation of operable from nonoperable CTEPH remains one of the most problematic issues in the management of these patients. The basis for this controversy is that no precise anatomic definition of "operable" disease has been established. Surgical experience also dictates the extent of material that can be safely removed at the time of endarterectomy. There is general consensus that current surgical techniques allow removal of organized thrombi whose proximal extent is in the main and lobar arteries. For those with more extensive surgical experience, successful endarterectomy of organized thrombi involving the segmental arteries can be achieved.

Additionally, the preoperative pulmonary hemodynamic profile and the anticipated improvement in these hemodynamics with endarterectomy surgery weighs heavily in the decision to proceed with PTE surgery for any CTEPH patient. Identification of those CTEPH patients who are unlikely to benefit hemodynamically from a thromboendarterectomy is a particular challenge. The basis for this concern is that the increased pulmonary vascular resistance associated with chronic thromboembolic disease arises not only from the central, surgically accessible chronic thromboembolic obstruction but also from the resistance arising from a secondary, small vessel arteriopathy. Thromboendarterectomy will relieve only that portion of the pulmonary hypertension that arises from the accessible component of chronic thromboembolic disease. Therefore, a major focus of the preoperative evaluation is an attempt to partition the proximal component of the elevated vascular resistance from the coexisting distal arteriopathy. Though this determination is an essential one, it remains relatively subjective. Failure to lower pulmonary vascular resistance, especially in patients with severe pulmonary hypertension and right ventricular dysfunction, may be associated with severe hemodynamic instability and death in the early postoperative period. In a series by Jamieson and colleagues involving 500 consecutive operated patients in whom the overall mortality rate was 4.4%, 77% of deaths were related to residual high pulmonary artery pressures. Patients with a postoperative PVR >500 dyne.sec/cm^5 had a mortality rate of 30.6% compared to 0.9% in patients with a postoperative PVR <500 dyne.sec/cm^5 (66).

Beyond debate, however, is that long-term survivorship in the absence of appropriate treatment is poor and, as in other forms of pulmonary hypertension, proportional to the degree of pulmonary hypertension and right ventricular dysfunction at the time of diagnosis. In one study, the five-year survival rate in patients with CTEPH was 30% when the mean pulmonary artery pressure was >40 mmHg and 10% when it was >50 mmHg (67). In another study, a mean pulmonary artery pressure >30 mmHg appeared to serve as a threshold value portending a poor prognosis (68).

In general, patients who undergo PTE exhibit a PVR >300 dyne.sec/cm^5. At centers reporting their experience with PTE surgery, mean preoperative PVR is typically in the range of 700 to 1100 dyne.sec/cm^5 (66,69–82).

However, certain patients may present with significant dyspnea and normal or minimally abnormal resting pulmonary hemodynamics. Such patients include those with involvement of one main pulmonary artery and those with unusually vigorous lifestyle expectations. Thromboendarterectomy is effective in these patients by alleviating the exercise impairment associated with their high dead-space and minute ventilatory demands. Surgery has also been offered to patients with normal pulmonary hemodynamics or only mild levels of pulmonary hypertension at rest who exhibit exercise-associated pulmonary hypertension. Though there was a previous inclination to avoid or postpone surgery in this subgroup of chronic thromboembolic patients, given what is currently known about the potential for advancing pulmonary hypertension due to the development of a small vessel arteriopathy, and with the relatively low perioperative mortality risk for PTE in this patient group (1–2% at experienced centers), early surgical intervention seems to be more acceptable. If the decision is made to defer surgery, then careful follow-up is required to assure that progressive pulmonary hypertension does not occur.

The presence of comorbid conditions that may adversely affect perioperative mortality or morbidity must be considered in the evaluation of CTEPH patients for surgery. Advanced age, morbid obesity, and the presence of certain coexisting disorders, such as renal insufficiency and hepatic dysfunction, do not represent absolute contraindications to PTE, although they do influence risk assessment.

VII. Pulmonary Thromboendarterectomy Surgery and Postoperative Outcomes

A detailed description of PTE surgery is beyond the scope of this article, though can be found in referenced manuscripts (66,83,84). However, there are several features of this remarkable operation, which warrant discussion here. Surgical success is based on the concept that a true endarterectomy, not an embolectomy, is necessary. Organized thromboembolic material is fibrotic in nature, incorporated into the native vascular intima (Fig. 2). An adequate endarterectomy involves identification of this "pseudointima" and meticulously establishing a dissection plane to free the thrombotic residua from the native vessel wall. Considerable surgical experience with this procedure is required to identify the correct operative plane. The removal of nonadherent, partially organized thrombus within the lumen of the central pulmonary arteries will be ineffective in reducing right ventricular afterload, while creation of a dissection plane too deep in the vessel wall poses the risk of pulmonary artery perforation. Therefore, optimal exposure of the pulmonary vasculature intima becomes critically important to the outcome of this procedure. Cardiopulmonary bypass with periods of circulatory arrest provides this exposure in a bloodless operative field. It is during these circulatory arrest periods that dissection of thromboembolic residua from the lobar, segmental, and, to a degree, subsegmental arteries can be achieved.

Maintaining tissue integrity during intermittent circulatory arrest periods then becomes the critical challenge for surgical success. Although standard flow for cardiopulmonary bypass is practiced, deep hypothermia is established where the patient is systemically cooled to 18°C to 20°C. Additional measures designed to minimize tissue injury during circulatory arrest periods include hemodilution to a hematocrit in the range of 18% to 25% in an effort to decrease blood viscosity during hypothermia and to optimize capillary blood flow. Cerebral protection is provided by surrounding the head with an ice-cooled "blanket"; following aortic cross-clamping, thiopental is administered until the electroencephalogram becomes isoelectric; and phenytoin is administered intravenously during the cooling period to reduce the risk of perioperative seizure

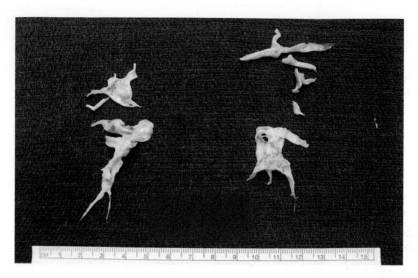

Figure 2 (*See color insert*) Chronic thromboembolic material endarterectomized from the patient whose angiogram is shown in Figure 1. Postoperatively, pulmonary hemodynamics were normal.

activity. Myocardial protection is achieved with the administration of a single dose of cold cardioplegic solution following cross-clamping, and wrapping the heart in a cooling jacket. When the patient is cooled to the optimal level of hypothermia, periods of circulatory arrest can be safely initiated. The endarterectomy can proceed at this point, usually first on the right side, then on the left. After completion of the endarterectomy, cardiopulmonary bypass is resumed and rewarming is commenced.

Modifications of this approach intended to avoid deep hypothermia and/or circulatory arrest have been described and include the use of normothermic cardiopulmonary bypass or moderate hypothermia (28–32°C), aortic bronchial artery occlusion with a balloon catheter, antegrade cerebral artery perfusion with and without total circulatory arrest, and application of negative pressure in the left ventricle (85–88). Implementation of these modifications was primarily designed to avoid deep hypothermic circulatory arrest, and the potential for neurologic complications that may occur when the period of circulatory arrest exceeds 20 to 25 minutes. It has not yet been demonstrated that any of these modifications provides substantive benefit when compared with the traditional technique.

For the majority of patients undergoing PTE surgery, the restoration of blood flow to previously occluded lung regions results in an immediate reduction in pulmonary vascular resistance, with a consequent increase in cardiac output. Since 1997, this immediate hemodynamic benefit from surgery has been reported by numerous groups throughout the world (66,71–82), noting that normalization of the pulmonary artery pressure and pulmonary vascular resistance can be achieved. An improvement in right ventricular function determined by echocardiography has also been shown to occur immediately after endarterectomy (41,89). Similarly encouraging has been reports that this immediate hemodynamic benefit is sustained for months to years following PTE surgery. This is accompanied by substantial gains in gas exchange, functional status, and quality of life (81,82,90–94). Most patients initially in New York Heart Association (NYHA) functional class III or IV return to NYHA class I or II functional class postoperatively and are able to resume normal activities (92,93).

Though the hemodynamic and functional results following PTE are often dramatic, two patient subgroups having undergone this surgery at the University of California, San Diego have been identified. Approximately 10% to 15% of postoperative patients exhibit residual pulmonary hypertension, which has been arbitrarily defined as a postsurgical PVR ≥500 dyne.sec/cm^5. However, a large percentage of these patients experienced pulmonary hemodynamic benefit from surgery, the residual pulmonary hypertension, a function of extensive small vessel disease with or without a component of distal, "unendarterectomized" chronic thromboemboli. A second subgroup of operated patients show minimal to no hemodynamic benefit from surgery due to the severity of their distal vasculopathy, which is unaffected by removal of the central portion of their disease (95). As the ability to identify this "high-risk" group preoperatively has improved over the years, only 2% to 4% of the patients undergoing PTE surgery at this one institution experience this outcome.

In-hospital mortality rates following PTE surgery have steadily declined over the past decades. Since 1996, patient series of widely different numbers have reported postoperative mortality rates between 4.4% and 24% (66,71–82). More practiced and larger-volume programs however, have mortality rates below 7%. Several factors appear to have contributed to this outcome including a clearer understanding of the natural history of the disease, better diagnostic techniques, more selective surgical referral, and advances in operative and postoperative care. Attributable causes of death following PTE surgery are variable and similar to those associated with other open-heart procedures. Cardiac arrest, multiorgan failure, uncontrollable mediastinal bleeding, sepsis syndrome, and massive pulmonary hemorrhage are among the causes of death cited (75,76,78,79,96,97). In larger patient series, residual pulmonary hypertension with right-heart dysfunction and acute lung injury (98,99) represent the major causes for postoperative deaths (66,76). However, long-term survivorship after hospital discharge is significantly better relative to what could be expected in the absence of appropriate surgical intervention (67). Examining a cohort of 532 patients followed for up to 19 years postendarterectomy, in which all causes of death were included, Archibald and colleagues showed a 75% probability of survivorship beyond six years (92).

VIII. CTEPH: Use of Pulmonary Hypertension–Specific Medical Therapy

Medical therapies developed for use in IPAH, including prostacyclin analogues, endothelin receptor antagonists, and phosphodiesterase-5 inhibitors have been studied in patients with CTEPH (100). Although indications for their use in CTEPH and associated efficacy have not been clearly established, the prescription of these medications, even in operable CTEPH, has grown over the past several years. In a retrospective review of patients undergoing PTE at University of California, San Diego in 2007, 37% of patients had been prescribed pulmonary hypertension–specific medical therapy at the time of referral; this is a substantial increase compared with approximately 20% of patients in

2005 (101). Analysis revealed no discernible pulmonary hemodynamic benefit in the patients receiving medical therapy prior to surgery; there appeared to be a resultant delay to referral for surgical consideration, and post-PTE hemodynamic outcomes were similar whether or not medical therapy had been used preoperatively.

The majority of data with pulmonary hypertension–specific medical therapy for CTEPH comes from small, uncontrolled studies, retrospective evaluations, and trials in which patients with inoperable CTEPH and residual postendarterectomy pulmonary hypertension are mixed. Furthermore, existing data does not define whether one class of drugs is superior to another or whether combination therapy is the optimal approach. Despite these limitations, data are emerging that are encouraging for certain subgroups of patients with CTEPH.

In a double-blind, placebo-controlled pilot study comparing sildenafil to placebo for 12 weeks in 19 patients with inoperable CTEPH, Suntharalingam and colleagues found no significant difference between groups in terms of exercise capacity (102). However, there was a significant difference in World Health Organization (WHO) class and in pulmonary vascular resistance (a decrease of 179 $\pm$ 245 compared with an increase of 18 $\pm$ 76 dyne.sec/cm^5). Control patients were then transferred to open-label sildenafil use and follow-up was obtained at 12 months. At that time, significant differences were noted in six-minute walk distance (6MWD), symptom score, and pulmonary vascular resistance (722 $\pm$ 383 to 573 $\pm$ 330 dyne.sec/cm^5). In a larger patient group, Reichenberger and colleagues conducted an open-label study of sildenafil (50 mg three times a day) in 104 patients with inoperable CTEPH. They were able to demonstrate a decrease in pulmonary vascular resistance from 863 $\pm$ 38 dyne.sec/cm^5 to 759 $\pm$ 62 dyne.sec/cm^5 after three months. After 12 months of treatment, 6MWD increased from 310 $\pm$ 11 to 366 $\pm$ 18 m (103).

Bosentan has also been studied in various subgroups of CTEPH patients. In an open-label, national study (BOCTEPH-Study), 15 patients with CTEPH not eligible or awaiting surgery were treated with bosentan. At six months, the pulmonary vascular resistance decreased from 852 $\pm$ 319 to 657 $\pm$ 249 dyne.sec/cm^5; 6MWD increased from 389 $\pm$ 78 to 443 $\pm$ 79 m, with 4 patients improving and 11 patients maintaining their WHO functional class during the treatment period (104). In an open-label study involving 47 patients (39 with inoperable CTEPH and 8 with persistent pulmonary hypertension after PTE) evaluating the long-term efficacy and safety of bosentan in CTEPH, Hughes and colleagues (105) reported a significant improvement in 6MWD (49 $\pm$ 8 m) at one-year follow-up. Twenty-eight subjects had repeated right-heart catheterization at one year; this documented notable improvement in CI (0.2 $\pm$ 0.07 L/min/m^2) and a decrease in total pulmonary resistance (139 $\pm$ 42 dyne.sec/cm^5). In this study, patients with persistent pulmonary hypertension after endarterectomy demonstrated the greatest hemodynamic benefit with bosentan. Though patient subgroups were again mixed, the results of the first randomized, placebo-controlled study examining the effects of bosentan in CTEPH have been recently reported (106). One hundred and fifty-seven patients deemed to have either inoperable CTEPH or persistent/recurrent pulmonary hypertension post PTE were enrolled. Jais and colleagues showed a statistically significant treatment effect of bosentan over placebo on PVR, a decline of 24.1% from baseline. However, despite the positive effect on hemodynamics, no improvement in exercise capacity was observed, 6MWD increasing only by 2.2 m in treated patients.

For patients felt to have inoperable CTEPH, prostanoids have also been administered. Cabrol and colleagues retrospectively reviewed 27 patients with inoperable CTEPH treated with epoprostenol. Following three months of therapy, a decrease in mean pulmonary artery pressure (56 ± 9 to 51 ± 8 mmHg), total pulmonary resistance (29.3 ± 7.0 to 23.0 ± 5.0 U/m^2), and an increase in 6 MWD of 66 m were noted. Out of 23 patients, 11 experienced an improvement in NYHA functional status by one class. In 18 patients evaluated after 20 ± 8 months of therapy (though at higher doses of epoprostenol), NYHA functional class was better in nine patients, while improvements in 6MWD and hemodynamics were sustained (107). In a single-center uncontrolled observational study, 28 patients with severe inoperable CTEPH were treated with subcutaneous treprostinil. Follow-up catheterization was performed in 19 patients after 19 ± 6.3 months. Treprostinil therapy was associated with a significant improvement in pulmonary vascular resistance (924.6 ± 347 to 808.1 ± 372.5 dyne.sec/cm^5), though primarily as a function of an improved cardiac output. Five-year survival rate was 53% compared with 16% in an untreated historical control group (108).

These data would suggest some benefit from the use of pulmonary hypertension–specific medical therapy in certain CTEPH patient subgroups. However, for those patients with inoperable CTEPH, the degree of clinical improvement to be expected from pharmacotherapies appears modest at best. It is therefore imperative that the chronic thromboembolic disease is truly inoperable and the patient is a poor surgical candidate, a determination best established at a clinical center specializing in the treatment of patients with CTEPH. For postendarterectomy patients with residual pulmonary hypertension, the level of pulmonary vascular resistance that requires medical therapy has not been adequately defined. Ongoing investigation is required to establish the optimal care plan for this challenging group of patients.

References

1. Carroll D. Chronic obstruction of major pulmonary arteries. Am J Med 1950; 9:175–185.
2. Owen WR, Thomas WA, Castleman B, et al. Unrecognized emboli to the lungs with subsequent cor pulmonale. N Engl J Med 1953; 249:919–926.
3. Ball KP, Goodwin JF, Harrison CV. Massive thrombotic occlusion of the large pulmonary arteries. Circulation 1956; 14:766–783.
4. Hollister LE, Cull VL. The syndrome of chronic thrombosis of the major pulmonary arteries. Am J Med 1956; 21:312–320.
5. Hurwitt FS, Schein CJ, Rifkin II, et al. A surgical approach to the problem of chronic pulmonary artery obstruction due to thrombosis or stenosis. Ann Surg 1958; 147:157–165.
6. Houk VN, Hufnagel CH, McClenathan JE, et al. Chronic thrombotic obstruction of major pulmonary arteries: report of a case successfully treated by thromboendarterectomy and a review of the literature. Am J Med 1963; 35:269–282.
7. Moser KM, Houk VN, Jones RC, et al. Chronic, massive thrombotic obstruction of pulmonary arteries: analysis of four operated cases. Circulation 1965; 32:377–385.
8. Cabrol C, Cabrol A, Acar J, et al. Surgical correction of chronic postembolic obstructions of the pulmonary arteries. J Thorac Cardiovasc Surg 1978; 76:620–628.
9. Sabiston DC Jr., Wolfe WG, Oldham HN Jr., et al. Surgical management of chronic pulmonary embolism. Ann Surg 1977; 185:699–712.

10. Utley JR, Spragg RG, Long WB, et al. Pulmonary endarterectomy for chronic thromboembolic obstruction: recent surgical experience. Surgery 1982; 92:1096–1102.
11. Moser KM, Daily PO, Peterson K, et al. Thromboendarterectomy for chronic, major-vessel thromboembolic pulmonary hypertension: immediate and long-term results in 42 patients. Ann Intern Med 1987; 107:560–565.
12. Fedullo PF, Auger WR, Kerr KM, et al. Chronic thromboembolic pulmonary hypertension. Semin Resp Crit Care Med 2003; 24:273–285.
13. Pengo V, Lensing AWA, Prins MH, et al. Incidence of chronic thromboembolic pulmonary hypertension after pulmonary embolism. N Engl J Med 2004; 350:2257–2264.
14. Becattini C, Agnelli G, Pesavento R, et al. Incidence of chronic thromboembolic pulmonary hypertension after a first episode of pulmonary embolism. Chest 2006; 130:172–175.
15. Miniati M, Monti S, Bottai M, et al. Survival and restoration of pulmonary perfusion in a long-term follow-up of patients after pulmonary embolism. Medicine 2006; 85:253–262.
16. Silverstein MD, Heit JA, Mohr DN, et al. Trends in the incidence of deep vein thrombosis and pulmonary embolism: a 25-year population-based study. Arch Intern Med 1998; 158:585–593.
17. Liu P, Meneveau N, Schiele F, et al. Predictors of long-term clinical outcome in patients with acute massive pulmonary embolism after thrombolytic therapy. Chin Med J (Engl) 2003; 116:503–509.
18. Ribeiro A, Lindmarker P, Johnsson H, et al. Pulmonary embolism: one-year follow-up with echocardiography Doppler and five-year survival analysis. Circulation 1999; 99:1325–1330.
19. Wolf M, Boyer-Neumann C, Parent F, et al. Thrombotic risk factors in pulmonary hypertension. Eur Resp J 2000; 15:395–399.
20. Colorio CC, Martinuzzo ME, Forastiero RR, et al. Thrombophilic factors in chronic thromboembolic pulmonary hypertension. Blood Coagul Fibrinolysis 2001; 12:427–432.
21. Bonderman D, Turecek PL, Jakowitsch J, et al. High prevalence of elevated clotting Factor VIII in chronic thromboembolic pulmonary hypertension. Thromb Haemost 2003; 90: 372–376.
22. Bonderman D, Jakowitsch J, Adlbrecht C, et al. Medical conditions increasing the risk of chronic thromboembolic pulmonary hypertension. Thromb Haemost 2005; 93:512–516.
23. Rosenhek R, Korschineck I, Gharehbaghi-Schnell E, et al. Fibrinolytic imbalance of the arterial wall: pulmonary artery displays increased fibrinolytic potential compared with the aorta. Lab Invest 2003; 83:871–876.
24. Lang IM, Marsh JJ, Olman MA, et al. Parallel analysis of tissue-type plasminogen activator and type 1 plasminogen activator inhibitor in plasma and endothelial cells derived from patients with chronic pulmonary thromboemboli. Circulation 1994; 90:716–712.
25. Morris TA, Marsh JJ, Giles PG, et al. Fibrin derived from patients with chronic thromboembolic pulmonary hypertension is resistant to lysis. Am J Resp Crit Care Med 2006; 173:1270–1275.
26. Moser KM, Bloor CM. Pulmonary vascular lesions occurring in patients with chronic major vessel thromboembolic pulmonary hypertension. Chest 1993; 103:685–692.
27. Ryan KL, Fedullo PF, Davis GB, et al. Perfusion scan findings understate the severity of angiographic and hemodynamic compromise in chronic thromboembolic pulmonary hypertension. Chest 1988; 93:1180–1185.
28. Azarian R, Wartski M, Collignon MA, et al. Lung perfusion scans and hemodynamics in acute and chronic pulmonary embolism. J Nucl Med 1997; 38:980–983.
29. Du L, Sullivan CC, Chu D, et al. Signaling molecules in nonfamilial pulmonary hypertension. N Engl J Med 2003; 348(6):500–509.
30. Kim H, Yung GL, Marsh JJ, et al. Endothelin mediates pulmonary vascular remodeling in a canine model of chronic thromboembolic pulmonary hypertension. Eur Resp J 2000; 15(4): 640–648.

31. Bauer M, Wilkens H, Langer F, et al. Selective upregulation of endothelin B receptor gene expression in severe pulmonary hypertension. Circulation 2002; 105(9):1034–1036.

32. Thistlethwaite PA, Lee SH, Du L, et al. Human angiopoietin gene expression is a marker of pulmonary hypertension in patients undergoing pulmonary thromboendarterectomy. J Thorac Cardiovasc Surg 2001; 122:65–73.

33. Yao W, Firth AL, Sacks RS, et al. Identification of putative endothelial progenitor cells in Endarterectomized tissue of patients with chronic thromboembolic pulmonary hypertension. Am J Physiol Lung Cell Mol Physiol 2009 Mar 13 [Epub].

34. Simonneau G, Azarian R, Brenot F, et al. Surgical management of unresolved pulmonary embolism: a personal series of 72 patients. Chest 1995; 107:52S–55S.

35. Fedullo PF, Auger WR, Kerr KM, et al. Chronic thromboembolic pulmonary hypertension. N Engl J Med 2001; 345:1465–1472.

36. Auger WR, Moser KM. Pulmonary flow murmurs: a distinctive physical sign found in chronic pulmonary thromboembolic disease. Clin Res 1989; 37:145A.

37. Woodruff WW III, Hoeck BE, Chitwood WR Jr., et al. Radiographic findings in pulmonary hypertension from unresolved embolism. Am J Roentgenol 1985; 144:681–686.

38. Morris TA, Auger WR, Ysrael MZ, et al. Parenchymal scarring is associated with restrictive spirometric defects in patients with chronic thromboembolic pulmonary hypertension. Chest 1996; 110:399–403.

39. Steenhuis LH, Groen HJM, Koeter GH, et al. Diffusion capacity and haemodynamcs in primary and chronic thromboembolic pulmonary hypertension. Eur Respir J 2000; 16:276–281.

40. Kapitan KS, Buchbinder M, Wagner PD, et al. Mechanisms of hypoxemia in chronic thromboembolic pulmonary hypertension. Am Rev Respir Dis 1989; 139:1149–1154.

41. Blanchard DG, Malouf PJ, Gurudevan SV, et al. Utility of right ventricular Tei index in the noninvasive evaluation of chronic thromboembolic pulmonary hypertension before and after pulmonary thromboendarterectomy. JACC Cardiovasc Imaging 2009; 2:143–149.

42. Dittrich HC, McCann HA, Blanchard DG. Cardiac structure and function in chronic thromboembolic pulmonary hypertension. Am J Card Imaging 1994; 8:18–27.

43. Mahmud E, Raisinghani A, Hassankhani A, et al. Correlation of left ventricular diastolic filling characteristics with right ventricular overload and pulmonary artery pressure in chronic thromboembolic pulmonary hypertension. J Am Coll Cardiol 2002; 40:318–324.

44. Lisbona R, Kreisman H, Novales-Diaz J, et al. Perfusion lung scanning: differentiation of primary from thromboembolic pulmonary hypertension. Am J Roentgenol 1985; 144:27–30.

45. Powe JE, Palevsky HI, McCarthy KE, et al. Pulmonary arterial hypertension: value of perfusion scintigraphy. Radiology 1987; 164:727–730.

46. Bailey CL, Channick RN, Auger WR, et al. "High probability" perfusion lung scans in pulmonary venoocclusive disease. Am J Respir Crit Care Med 2000; 162:1974–1978.

47. Rush C, Langleben D, Schlesinger RD, et al. Lung scintigraphy in pulmonary capillary hemangiomatosis: a rare disorder causing primary pulmonary hypertension. Clin Nucl Med 1991; 16:913–917.

48. Kerr KM. Pulmonary artery sarcoma masquerading as chronic thromboembolic pulmonary hypertension. Nat Clin Pract Cardiovasc Med 2005; 2:108–112.

49. Kerr KM, Auger WR, Fedullo PF, et al. Large vessel pulmonary arteritis mimicking chronic thromboembolic disease. Am J Respir Crit Care Med 1995; 152:367–373.

50. Berry PF, Buccigrossi D, Peabody J, et al. Pulmonary vascular occlusion and fibrosing mediastinitis. Chest 1986; 89:296–301.

51. King MA, Bergin CJ, Yeung D, et al. Chronic pulmonary thromboembolism: detection of regional hypoperfusion with CT. Radiology 1994; 191:359–363.

52. Schwickert HC, Schweden F, Schild HH, et al. Pulmonary arteries and lung parenchyma in chronic pulmonary embolism: preoperative and postoperative CT findings. Radiology 1994; 191:351–357.

53. Tunariu N, Gibbs SJR, Win Z, et al. Ventilation-perfusion scintigraphy is more sensitive than multidetector CTPA in detecting chronic thromboembolic pulmonary disease as a treatable cause of pulmonary hypertension. J Nucl Med 2007; 48:680–684.
54. Moser KM, Fedullo PF, Finkbeiner WE, et al. Do patients with primary pulmonary hypertension develop extensive central thrombi? Circulation 1995; 91:741745.
55. Silversides CK, Granton JT, Konen E, et al. Pulmonary thrombosis in adults with Eisenmenger syndrome. J Am Coll Cardiol 2003; 42:1982–1987.
56. Russo A, De Luca M, Vigna C, et al. Central pulmonary artery lesions in chronic obstructive pulmonary disease. A transesophageal echocardiography study. Circulation 1999; 100:1808–1815.
57. Kim HS, Fesler P, Channick RN, et al. Preoperative partitioning of pulmonary vascular resistance correlates with early outcome after thromboendarterectomy for chronic thromboembolic pulmonary hypertension. Circulation 2004; 109:18–22.
58. Pitton MB, Duber C, Mayer E, et al. Hemodynamic effects of nonionic contrast bolus injection and oxygen inhalation during pulmonary angiography in patients with chronic major-vessel thromboembolic pulmonary hypertension. Circulation 1996; 94:2485–2491.
59. Auger WR, Fedullo PF, Moser KM, et al. Chronic major-vessel chronic thromboembolic pulmonary artery obstruction: Appearance at angiography. Radiology 1992; 183:393–398.
60. Kreitner K-F, Kunz RP, Ley S, et al. Chronic thromboembolic pulmonary hypertension-assessment by magnetic resonance imaging. Eur Radiol 2007; 17:11–21.
61. Krietner K-F, Ley S, Kauczor H-U, et al. Chronic thromboembolic pulmonary hypertension: pre- and postoperative assessment with breath-hold magnetic resonance techniques. Radiology 2004; 232:535–543.
62. Nikolaou K, Schoenberg SO, Attenberger U, et al. Pulmonary arterial hypertension: diagnosis with fast perfusion imaging and high-spatial-resolution MR angiography—preliminary experience. Radiology 2005; 236:694–703.
63. Alfakih K, Reid S, Jones T, et al. Assessment of ventricular function and mass by cardiac magnetic resonance imaging. Eur Radiol 2004; 14:1813–1822.
64. Beygui F, Furber A, Delepine S, et al. Routine breath-hold gradient echo MRI-derived right ventricular mass, volumes and function: accuracy, reproducibility and coherence study. Int J Cardiovasc Imaging 2004; 20:509–516.
65. Miller FNAC, Coulden RA, Sonnex E, et al. The use of MR flow mapping in the assessment of pulmonary artery blood flow following pulmonary thrombo-endarterectomy. Radiol RSNA Proc 2003; 462P.
66. Jamieson SW, Kapelanski DW, Sakakibara N, et al. Pulmonary endarterectomy: experience and lessons learned in 1,500 cases. Ann Thoracic Surg 2003; 76:1457–1462.
67. Riedel M, Stanek V, Widimsky J, et al. Long-term follow-up of patients with pulmonary thromboembolism: late prognosis and evolution of hemodynamic and respiratory data. Chest 1982; 81:151–158.
68. Lewczuk J, Piszko P, Jagas J, et al. Prognostic factors in medically treated patients with chronic pulmonary embolism. Chest 2001; 119:818–823.
69. Dartevelle P, Fadel E, Mussot S, et al. Chronic thromboembolic pulmonary hypertension. Eur Resp J 2004; 23:637–648.
70. Thistlethwaite P, Kemp A, Lingling D, et al. Outcomes of pulmonary thromboendarterectomy for treatment of extreme thromboembolic pulmonary hypertension. J Thorac Cardiovasc Surg 2006; 131:307–313.
71. Nakajima N, Masuda M, Mogi K. The surgical treatment for chronic pulmonary thromboembolism: our experience and current review of the literature. Ann Thorac Cardiovasc Surg 1997; 3:15–21.
72. Mayer E, Kramm T, Dahm M, et al. Early results of pulmonary thromboendarterectomy in chronic thromboembolic pulmonary hypertension. Z Kardiol 1997; 86:920–927.

73. Gilbert TB, Gaine SP, Rubin LJ, et al. Short-term outcome and predictors of adverse events following pulmonary thromboendarterectomy. World J Surg 1998; 22:1029–1032.
74. Dartevelle P, Fadel E, Chapelier A, et al. Angioscopic video-assisted pulmonary endarterectomy for post-embolic pulmonary hypertension. Eur J Cardiothorac Surg 1999; 16:38–43.
75. Ando M, Okita Y, Tagusari O, et al. Surgical treatment for chronic thromboembolic pulmonary hypertension under profound hypothermia and circulatory arrest in 24 patients. J Card Surg 1999; 14:377–385.
76. Rubens FD, Bourke M, Hynes M, et al. Surgery for chronic thromboembolic pulmonary hypertension—inclusive experience from a national referral center. Ann Thorac Surg 2007; 83:1075–1081.
77. Mares P, Gilbert TB, Tschernko EM, et al. Pulmonary artery thromboendarterectomy: a comparison of two different postoperative treatment strategies. Anesth Analg 2000; 90:267–273.
78. D'Armini AM, Cattadori B, Monterosso C, et al. Pulmonary thromboendarterectomy in patients with chronic thromboembolic pulmonary hypertension: hemodynamic characteristics and changes. Eur J Cardiothorac Surg 2000; 18:696–702.
79. Tscholl D, Langer F, Wendler O, et al. Pulmonary thromboendarterectomy: risk factors for early survival and hemodynamic improvement. Eur J Cardiothorac Surg 2001; 19:771–776.
80. Masuda M, Nakajima N. Our experience of surgical treatment for chronic pulmonary thromboembolism. Ann Thorac Cardiovasc Surg 2001; 7:261–265.
81. Piovella F, D'Armini AM, Barone M, et al. Chronic thromboembolic pulmonary hypertension. Semin Thromb Hemost 2006; 32:848–855.
82. Mellemkjaer S, Ilkjaer LB, Klaaborg KE, et al. Pulmonary endarterectomy for chronic thromboembolic pulmonary hypertension. Ten years experience in Denmark. Scand Cardiovasc J 2006; 40:49–53.
83. Madani M, Jamieson SW. Technical advances of pulmonary endarterectomy for chronic thromboembolic pulmonary hypertension. Semin Thorac Cardiovasc Med 2006; 18:243–250.
84. Mayer E, Klepetko W. Techniques and outcome of pulmonary endarterectomy for chronic thromboembolic pulmonary hypertension. Proc Am Thorac Soc 2006; 3:589–593.
85. Zund G, Pretre R, Niederhauser U, et al. Improved exposure of the pulmonary arteries for thromboendarterectomy. Ann Thorac Surg 1998; 66:1821–1823.
86. Hagl C, Khaladj N, Peters T, et al. Technical advances of pulmonary thromboendarterectomy for chronic thromboembolic pulmonary hypertension. Eur J Cardiothorac Surg 2003; 23:776–781.
87. Thomson B, Tsui SSL, Dunning J, et al. Pulmonary endarterectomy is possible and effective without the use of complete circulatory arrest—the UK experience in over 150 patients. Eur J Cardiothorac Surg 2008; 33:157—163.
88. Mikus PM, Mikus E, Martin-Suarez S, et al. Pulmonary endarterectomy: an alternative to circulatory arrest and deep hypothermia: mid-term results. Eur J Cardiothorac Surg 2008; 34:159–163.
89. Menzel T, Wagner S, Mohr-Kahaly S, et al. Reversibility of changes in left and right ventricular geometry and hemodynamics in pulmonary hypertension. Echocardiographic characteristics before and after pulmonary thromboendarterectomy. Z Kardiol 1997; 86:928–935.
90. Mayer E, Dahm M, Hake U, et al. Mid-term results of pulmonary thromboendarterectomy for chronic thromboembolic pulmonary hypertension. Ann Thorac Surg 1996; 61:1788–1792.
91. Corsico AG, D'Armini AM, Cerveri I, et al. Long-term outcome after pulmonary thromboendarterectomy. Am J Resp Crit Care Med 2008; 178:419–424.
92. Archibald CJ, Auger WR, Fedullo PF, et al. Long-term outcome after pulmonary thromboendarterectomy. Am J Respir Crit Care Med 1999; 160:523–528.

93. Zoia MC, D'Armini AM, Beccaria M, et al., Pavia Thromboendarterectomy Group. Mid term effects of pulmonary thromboendarterectomy on clinical and cardiopulmonary functional status. Thorax 2002; 57:608–612.
94. Tanabe N, Okada O, Nakagawa Y, et al. The efficacy of pulmonary thromboendarterectomy on long-term gas exchange. Eur Respir J 1997; 10:2066–2072.
95. Auger WR, Kim NH, Kerr KM, et al. Chronic thromboembolic pulmonary hypertension. Clin Chest Med 2007; 28:255–269.
96. Hartz RS, Byme JG, Levitsky S, et al. Predictors of mortality in pulmonary thromboendarterectomy. Ann Thorac Surg 1996; 62:1255–1260.
97. Manecke GR, Kotzyr A, Atkins G, et al. Massive pulmonary hemorrhage after pulmonary thromboendarterectomy. Anesth Analg 2004; 99:672–675.
98. Levinson R, Shure D, Moser KM. Reperfusion pulmonary edema after pulmonary artery thromboendarterectomy. Am Rev Resp Dis 1986; 134:1241–1245.
99. Miller WT, Osiason AW, Langlotz CP, et al. Reperfusion edema after thromboendarterectomy: radiographic patterns of disease. J Thorac Imaging 1998; 13:178–183.
100. Bresser P, Pepke-Zaba J, Jais X, et al. Medical therapies for chronic thromboembolic pulmonary hypertension. Proc Am Thorac Soc 2006; 3:594–600.
101. Jensen KW, Kerr KM, Fedullo PF, et al. Prevalence of medical therapy for pulmonary arterial hypertension (PAH) in chronic thromboembolic pulmonary hypertension (CTEPH) prior to referral for pulmonary thromboendarterectomy (PTE). Am J Resp Crit Care Med 2008; 177:A181.
102. Suntharalingam J, Treacy CM, Doughty NJ, et al. Long-term use of sildenafil in inoperable chronic thromboembolic pulmonary hypertension. Chest 2008; 134:229–236.
103. Reichenberger F, Voswinckel R, Enke B, et al. Long-term treatment with sildenafil in chronic thromboembolic pulmonary hypertension. Eur Resp J 2007; 30:922–927.
104. Ulrich S, Speich R, Domenighetti G, et al. Bosentan therapy for chronic thromboembolic pulmonary hypertension (BOCTEPH STUDY). Swiss Med Wkly 2007; 137:573–580.
105. Hughes RJ, Jais X, Bonderman D, et al. Bosentan in inoperable chronic thromboembolic pulmonary hypertension: efficacy at 1 year. Eur Resp J 2006; 28:138–143.
106. Jais X, D'Armini AM, Jansa P, et al. Bosentan for treatment of inoperable chronic thromboembolic pulmonary hypertension: BENEFiT (Bosentan Effects in iNopErable Forms of chronic Thromboembolic pulmonary hypertension), a randomized, placebo-controlled trial. J Am Coll Cardiol 2008; 52:2127–2134.
107. Cabrol S, Souza R, Jais X, et al. Intravenous epoprostenol in inoperable thromboembolic pulmonary hypertension. J Heart Lung Transplant 2007; 26:357–362.
108. Skoro-Sajer N, Bonderman D, Wiesbauer F, et al. Treprostinil for severe inoperable chronic thromboembolic pulmonary hypertension. J Thromb Haemost 2007; 5:483–489.

22
Pulmonary Arterial Hypertension: Conventional Therapy

OLIVIER SITBON
Université Paris Sud 11, Service de Pneumologie et Réanimation Respiratoire, Hôpital Antoine Béclère, Assistance Publique Hôpitaux de Paris, Clamart, France

I. Introduction

The definition of "conventional therapy" for pulmonary arterial hypertension (PAH) is sometimes unclear for clinicians. What is "conventional" to one may be considered differently by another, depending on a disease's awareness, availability of therapies, and a clinician's habits. Indeed, it would be better to consider conventional therapy as the combination of general measures (first of all, not to harm) and supportive therapies (anticoagulants, diuretics, supplemental oxygen, etc.). Historically, treatment with calcium channel blockers (CCBs) was also considered as conventional therapy as it was the only vasodilator that has demonstrated clinical efficacy (in a small subset of patients with idiopathic PAH) before availability of treatments targeting endothelial dysfunction [prostanoids, endothelin receptor antagonists (ERAs), phosphodiesterase inhibitors, etc.]. No randomized controlled study has been performed to evaluate conventional therapy in patients with PAH, and the rationale for using it is based on the results of uncontrolled observational studies only (1). In addition, these studies were performed mostly in patients with idiopathic PAH, and extension of their conclusions to PAH associated with other diseases and conditions has to be done with caution. In the national North American Registry of 194 patients with PAH, most received conventional therapy including oral anticoagulants, diuretics, supplemental oxygen, cardiac glycosides, and CCBs (2). At that time, the median survival was 2.8 years (2). Medical advances over the last twenty years have resulted in significant improvement in the prognosis of this condition. Today, conventional therapy has to be considered in combination with disease-specific targeted PAH treatments in patients with PAH.

In this chapter, we will cover general measures to prevent clinical deterioration (limitation of physical activity, birth control, avoidance of hypoxia, etc.), supportive therapies (anticoagulants, diuretics, oxygen, etc.) and vasodilator therapy with CCBs.

II. General Measures

Although there is no evidence-based guidance regarding physical activity, patients with PAH require sensible advice about general activities of daily living and need to adapt to the uncertainty associated with a serious chronic life-threatening disease. An important general measure for patients with PAH is the avoidance of circumstances and substances that may aggravate the disease. PAH patients have a restricted pulmonary circulation, and peripheral vasodilatation or increased cardiac demand can precipitate worsening of pulmonary hypertension (PH) and put patients with PAH at risk of acute right-heart failure and syncope (3–5).

A. Physical Activity and Lifestyle

Exercise can aggravate or trigger symptoms of PH including dyspnea, fatigue, chest pain, presyncope, or syncope. Also, physicians traditionally advise patients against physical activity. They are taught to stay active while adapting effort according to their symptoms. Nevertheless, the appropriate level of physical activity is difficult to define as too much rest also has its attendant risks, physical deconditioning, and muscular involution, leading to functional limitation and worsened symptoms. A compromise should be found to encourage patients to have a moderate exercise activity while avoiding heavy physical activity that would be potentially dangerous (5,6). To date, only one study has evaluated the effect of cardiorespiratory training in 30 patients with PAH and chronic thromboembolic PH (7). The program involved 3 weeks of inpatient rehabilitation followed by 12 weeks of training at home with phone call supervision. No modification on cardiac hemodynamic was observed on echocardiography, but six-minute walk distance and quality of life were improved (7). In addition, rehabilitation has been found to be safe in these patients. More data are however needed to recommend cardiopulmonary rehabilitation in patients with PAH, and studies are ongoing.

In addition to limitation of heavy physical activity, hot baths should be avoided and patients are advised to be cautious on hot days because induced cutaneous vasodilation may significantly decrease right ventricular preload and cardiac output (6).

B. Altitude and Travel

As hypoxic vasoconstriction is an aggravating factor in PAH, stays at altitudes of >800 to 1000 m and air flight in unpressurized cabin must be proscribed. In these circumstances, supplemental oxygen therapy may be indicated for symptomatic purposes as well as to avoid PAH deterioration (3,4). In flight oxygen administration should be considered for patients in functional classes III and IV and those with an oxygen saturation <92%. A flow rate of 2 L/min will raise inspired PO_2 to values found at sea level. Nevertheless, the usefulness of this supplemental oxygen therapy is debatable. Finally, patients should be advised to travel with written information about their disease and be advised how to contact local PH clinics in close proximity to where they are traveling.

C. Pregnancy, Birth Control, and Hormonal Therapy

Pregnancy is associated with 30% to 50% mortality in patients with PAH (8). As a consequence, PAH is a formal contraindication of pregnancy. The hemodynamic and hormonal changes occurring during pregnancy and peripartum period can lead to severe, and sometimes fatal, right-heart failure (8,9). Consequently, a safe and effective method of contraception is always recommended in PAH women of childbearing age (8,9). Barrier contraceptive methods are safe but with an unpredictable effect. Mechanical contraception (intrauterine device) or surgical sterilization is typically recommended. Combined estrogen-progesterone oral contraceptive is theoretically contraindicated as their prothrombotic activity would worsen PH (10). Progesterone-only preparations are effective approaches to contraception for PAH women without history of venous thromboembolism or documented thrombophilia and receiving effective oral anticoagulation. They avoid potential issues of estrogens (11). It should be remembered that ERAs may reduce the efficacy of oral contraceptive agents. A combination of two methods may also be indicated. The patient who becomes pregnant should be informed of the high risk of pregnancy, and termination of pregnancy should be discussed. Patients who chose to continue pregnancy should be treated with disease-targeted therapies, planned elective delivery, and effective close collaboration between obstetricians and the PAH team (8,12).

Finally, it is not clear if the use of hormonal therapy in postmenopausal women with PAH is advisable or not. It may be considered in cases of intolerable menopausal symptoms in conjunction with oral anticoagulation.

D. Infection Prevention

Patients with PAH are susceptible to developing pulmonary infections, which may aggravate PH and be the cause of death in about 7% of cases. While there are no controlled trials, it is recommended to consider routine immunizations against influenza and pneumococcal infection in patients with PAH.

E. Anesthesia and Surgery

Elective surgery is expected to have an increased risk in patients with PAH. Hypotension is a common side effect seen with the use of sedative and anesthetic drugs. This is generally poorly tolerated by PAH patients, to the extent of being potentially life threatening. If hemodynamic instability occurs, it will be more difficult to manage in such patients and can rapidly be out of control. Consequently, it is recommended in general in PAH patients to avoid the use of sedatives as much as possible and to conduct any necessary surgery at centers specialized in the treatment of PAH, to coordinate surgical and medical interventions (5).

F. Proscribed Drugs

Sympathomimetic drugs, often used in medication to relieve nasal congestion, are vasoconstrictors and should therefore be avoided in patients with PAH. β-Blockers, often used for cardiac comorbidities or esophageal variceal prevention, counteract chronotropic response (13). This has been shown to be deleterious to PAH patients because it is a very important adaptative physiological response that allows preservation of adequate cardiac output. To discontinue such a drug in a PAH patient may lead, by itself, to important clinical and hemodynamic improvement (13). Of course, this intervention should be discussed with a cardiologist or hepatologist.

G. Psychosocial Support

Patients with PAH often feel isolated by their diagnosis. Many of them develop anxiety and depression leading to impairment in quality of life. Timely referral to a psychiatrist or psychologist should be made when appropriate. Information on the severity of the disease is available from many nonprofessional sources, and an important role of the PAH multidisciplinary team is to support patients with accurate and up-to-date information. Patient support groups may also play an important role in this area. Encouraging patients and their family members to join patient support groups can have positive effects on coping, confidence, and outlook.

III. Supportive Therapy

A. Anticoagulation

There is a strong rationale for the use of anticoagulant therapy in patients with PAH. This is based on the observation, reported in large pathological series, of pulmonary arteriopathy with thrombotic lesions defined by the presence of eccentric intimal fibrosis and recanalized thrombi (14,15). Endothelial dysfunction that predisposes patients to pulmonary arteriopathy also promotes intravascular thrombosis (16). Abnormalities in coagulation and fibrinolytic pathways have also been reported (17–19). Moreover, the presence of right-heart failure and immobility are risk factors for acute venous thromboembolism, and in patients with PAH who die suddenly, fresh intrapulmonary clots may be found at autopsy (15,20). In addition, the presence of an indwelling central venous catheter in patients treated with continuous intravenous prostacyclin infusion may also be considered as a risk factor for venous thromboembolism.

Although there is no controlled trial examining the effect of anticoagulation in PAH, three open-label studies suggested that oral anticoagulant therapy may be beneficial in patients with PAH (20–22). In a retrospective study performed in 120 patients with idiopathic PAH, Fuster et al. showed a significant beneficial effect of anticoagulant therapy on overall survival (Fig. 1) (20). In this study, the three-year survival was 49% in patients treated with oral anticoagulants and 21% in the others (20). In a small prospective study, Rich et al. have shown that patients who did not respond to CCBs and who were treated with warfarin had improved survival as compared with those who did not receive anticoagulation (Fig. 2) (21). However, this beneficial effect of anticoagulants was not observed in "responders" to CCBs (21). In the most recent retrospective study, Frank et al. examined the effect of anticoagulant therapy with warfarin on the long-term prognosis in 173 patients with idiopathic and aminorex-induced PAH (22). In both groups, the use of oral warfarin was associated with a better survival, particularly in patients with aminorex-associated PAH (mean survival time of 8.3 years in anticoagulated aminorex-treated patients compared with 6.1 years in non-anticoagulated aminorex-treated patients). In addition, an improvement of symptoms like dyspnea on exertion was seen in 44.8% of the anticoagulated aminorex-treated patients, while deterioration was evident in 72.2% of the nonanticoagulated aminorex-treated patients (22).

Although all these three studies suggest a survival benefit with oral anticoagulants in patients with PAH, evidence in favor of oral anticoagulation is confined to patients

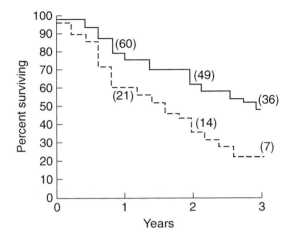

Figure 1 Effect of oral anticoagulant therapy on PAH survival (retrospective observational analysis from Mayo Clinic performed before availability of "modern" PAH-specific therapies). Patients treated with warfarin (*n* = 78; *solid line*) had a better survival than those treated without oral anticoagulants (*n* = 37; *dashed line*). *Abbreviation*: PAH, pulmonary arterial hypertension. *Source*: From Ref. 20.

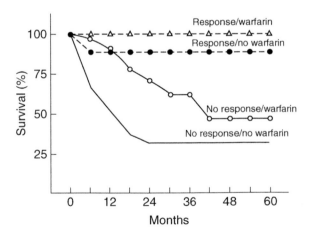

Figure 2 Survival in patients with idiopathic pulmonary arterial hypertension according to the response to calcium channel blockers therapy and to the use of concurrent anticoagulation. *Source*: From Ref. 21.

with idiopathic or anorexigen-associated PAH. The potential risks of oral anti-coagulation should be weighed against the risks for patients with other forms of PAH especially when there is an increased risk of bleeding such as congenital heart diseases (increased risk of hemoptysis), portopulmonary hypertension, or human immunodeficiency virus (HIV)-associated PAH with severe thrombocytopenia. In addition, none of these studies were conducted during the current era of targeted PAH therapies [prostanoids, ERAs, phosphodiesterase-5 (PDE-5) inhibitors]. Whether anticoagulation further improves survival in patients receiving these "modern" therapies remains uncertain.

Despite the absence of randomized controlled trials, international guidelines recommend the use of oral anticoagulants in patients with idiopathic, heritable, or anorexigen-associated PAH (23). The use of anticoagulants in other forms of PAH, that is, those that are associated with a concomitant disease, is more questionable.

Oral warfarin is the most widely used anticoagulant therapy in patients with PAH. Advice regarding the target international normalized ratio (INR) in patients with idiopathic PAH varies from 1.5 to 2.5 in most centers of North America and 2.0 to 3.0 in European centers. Generally, patients with PAH receiving therapy with long-term intravenous prostaglandins are anticoagulated in the absence of contraindications due, in part, to the additional risk of catheter-associated thrombosis.

In some cases, curative doses of low molecular weight heparin or unfractionated heparin can be used. However, the use of these anticoagulant drugs has not been studied.

B. Oxygen Therapy

Although oxygen administration has been demonstrated to reduce the pulmonary vascular resistance (PVR) in some patients with PAH, there are no robust data to suggest that long-term oxygen therapy is beneficial in PAH. Most patients with PAH except those with right-to-left shunt (patients with congenital heart diseases or having *patent foramen ovale*) have minor degrees of arterial hypoxemia at rest (mean PaO_2 was 71 mmHg in the NIH Registry of patients with PAH) (24). In PAH, mild hypoxemia is at least in part the consequence of impaired cardiac output, resulting in low mixed venous pulmonary saturation (SvO_2) and only minimally altered ventilation-perfusion matching (25). A minority of patients with PAH have severe hypoxemia caused by right-to-left shunt through a *patent foramen ovale*. In this case, shunt-induced hypoxemia is refractory to increased oxygen fraction. Theoretically, hypoxemia may aggravate PH by increasing pulmonary vasoconstriction, and supplemental oxygen therapy should be considered in patients with severe hypoxemia at rest (<55 mmHg). Although improvement in PH with supplemental oxygen has been reported in some patients, this has not been confirmed by controlled study. In PAH patients with severe hypoxia, oxygen therapy can improve quality of life by improving dyspnea and exercise capacity. On the other hand, oxygen equipment can limit mobility and can be a major constraint, leading to worsened functional impairment, so indication for supplemental oxygen therapy should be discussed case by case taking in consideration the patient's motivation and behavior (6). Ambulatory oxygen supplementation may be considered for PAH patients when there is evidence of symptomatic benefit and correctable desaturation on exercise.

C. Diuretics

Right ventricular overload is part of PAH clinical presentation and has been identified as a negative prognostic factor (2,26). Although there are no randomized controlled trials of diuretics in PAH, clinical experience shows clear symptomatic benefit in fluid-overloaded patients treated with this therapy. Diuretics and sodium-restricted diet (<2400 mg/day) relieve hypervolemia and associated symptoms such as hepatic congestion and peripheral edema. Whether this strategy improves prognosis is unknown. Furthermore, careful dosage adjustment is needed, on the basis of clinical, echocardiographic, and hemodynamic findings, because hypovolemia can lead to a reduction in the right ventricular preload and decrease in cardiac output (6). Furosemide and/or spironolactone may be prescribed and increased as needed. Large doses of furosemide, up to 500 mg/day, may be sometimes necessary (5,9). It is also important to monitor renal function and blood biochemistry in patients to avoid hypokalemia and the effects of decreased intravascular volume leading to prerenal failure.

Cardiac Glycosides

Digoxin has been shown to improve cardiac output acutely in patients with idiopathic PAH (27). Its long-term effectiveness is, however, unknown. Furthermore, digitalis toxicity may be enhanced if hypoxemia and diuretic-induced hypokalemia are also present. Therefore, digoxin is now reserved for patients with PAH who have atrial fibrillation secondary to atrial dilatation (27).

IV. Calcium Channel Blockers

Vasoconstriction has traditionally been assumed to be a preponderant mechanism in the pathogenesis of PAH (3). This is supported by pathological examination, which had shown medial hypertrophy and hyperplasia of the media of muscular pulmonary arteries in PAH patients (14,15). Also, Raynaud's phenomenon is found in 10% to 14% of patients with idiopathic PAH (24,28), suggesting abnormal underlying vasospastic response of systemic and pulmonary vessels (29). Finally, acute vasodilatation challenge with pulmonary vasodilators such as inhaled nitric oxide (NO) may reduce substantially both pulmonary pressures and PVR in a subset of patients with PAH.

Historically, many vasodilator treatments were proposed in PAH with debatable results. Early publications in small series of patients reported beneficial effects of chronic oral administration of phentolamine, diazoxide, hydralazine, isoproterenol, or angiotensin-converting enzyme (ACE) inhibitors (30–33). By contrast others reported mainly deleterious effects with these drugs (34,35). Among all vasodilators tested, only CCBs have been proven effective in long term in rare carefully selected patients (21,36,37). Unfortunately, no clinical or hemodynamical parameter can predict acute and/or chronic response to CCBs in patients with PAH (21,37,38). It is generally accepted that the initial response to acute pulmonary vasodilator testing accurately identifies patients with PAH who are likely to respond to chronic treatment with oral vasodilators including CCBs (32). The rationale for acute vasodilator testing in the evaluation of PAH patients is to select those who are more likely to have a sustained beneficial response to CCBs and a better prognosis. This test must be performed in all patients during initial right-heart catheterization in experts PH centers. The most widely used drugs for vasoreactivity testing include intravenous prostacyclin (39), adenosine

Table 1 Short-Acting Agents Used for Acute Vasodilator Testing in Pulmonary Arterial Hypertension

	Route of administration	Dose range	Side effects
Nitric oxide	Inhaled	10–20 ppm	None
Epoprostenol	Intravenous	2–10 ng/kg/min	Headache, nausea, hypotension
Adenosine	Intravenous	50–250 µg/kg/min	Chest pain, dyspnea, atrioventricular block

(40,41), or inhaled NO (37,38,42,43) (Table 1). Recent data suggest that inhaled iloprost may be more effective than NO to decrease PVR although it is not currently known whether such response is predictable of the outcome with oral CCBs therapy (44). NO has the advantages to be the most selective agent for the pulmonary vascular bed, to have an easy route of administration, good safety, and low cost.

At the beginning of the 1990s, Rich et al. showed in an open prospective study that high dose of CCBs (nifedipine 90–240 mg/day or diltiazem 360–900 mg/day) significantly improved outcome in PAH patients, with a positive response to acute vasodilatation testing with CCBs (Fig. 2) (21). In this study, the rate of "responders" to CCBs was lower (26.6%) than that reported by Weir et al. in the NIH Registry (55%) (45). Subsequently, Sitbon et al. (37) showed that only 70 out of the 557 patients (12.6%) evaluated in the French Reference Center for Pulmonary Arterial Hypertension could be treated by CCBs according to criteria established by Rich et al. (21). More importantly, only 38 out of the 70 acute responders (6.8% of the total idiopathic PAH study population) maintained long-term improvement with CCBs, defined as New York Heart Association (NYHA) functional class I or II at one year with near normalization in pulmonary hemodynamics without the need for another specific PAH treatment (Fig. 3) (37). Based largely on the data from this series, the 3rd World Congress on Pulmonary Arterial Hypertension Task Force (46), the European Society of Cardiology (23), and the American College of Chest Physicians (47) guidelines proposed that an acute response to acute vasodilator testing be defined as a drop in mean pulmonary arterial pressure (mPAP) by at least 10 mmHg to reach an absolute level of <40 mmHg, with a stable or increased cardiac output (Figs. 4 and 5). Patients with idiopathic PAH who meet the criteria for a positive vasodilator response and are treated with CCBs should be followed closely for both safety and efficacy with an initial reassessment after three to four months of therapy including hemodynamic evaluation in all cases (Fig. 5). In other forms of PAH (BMPR2 mutation carriers, patients with PAH associated with connective tissue diseases, HIV infection, portal hypertension, or congenital cardiac shunts), the rate of acute responders is even rarer, and long-term response to CCBs is exceptional in these patients (37).

CCBs, which are given at high dosages in PAH, must be avoided in the absence of proven significant vasoreactivity because of the risk of significantly reduced cardiac output and systemic blood pressure without reduction in PVR (37). In addition, acute titration with CCBs, as proposed by Rich et al. (21), has been progressively abandoned for a progressive up-titration of the dose over a few weeks (48). The doses of CCBs that have shown efficacy in idiopathic PAH are relatively high: 120 to 240 mg/day for nifedipine (21), 240 to 720 mg/day for diltiazem, and up to 20 mg/day for amlodipine (49). The long-term effects of lower dosages have, however, never been evaluated. The

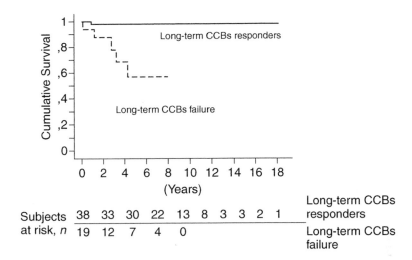

Figure 3 Outcome of long-term CCBs responders (i.e., patients who are in New York Heart Association classes I and II with near-normal pulmonary hemodynamics after one year onward on CCBs; *solid line*) compared with patients who failed on CCBs (*dashed line*); $p = 0.0007$ (Cox-Mantel log-rank test). *Abbreviation*: CCBs, calcium channel blockers. *Source*: From Ref. 37.

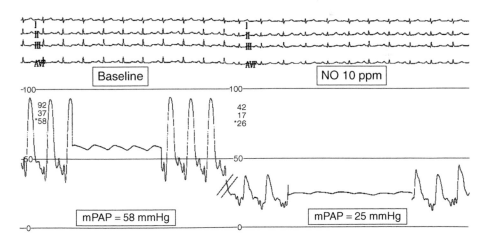

Figure 4 Acute vasodilator testing with inhaled NO in a 45-year-old male with idiopathic PAH. mPAP dropped from 58 mmHg to 25 mmHg during inhalation of 10 ppm NO. This patient was subsequently treated with diltiazem (360 mg/day). Seven years later, he is still alive without any PAH-related symptom and a normal resting pulmonary hemodynamics on diltiazem therapy. *Abbreviations*: PAH, pulmonary arterial hypertension; NO, nitric oxide; mPAP, mean pulmonary arterial pressure.

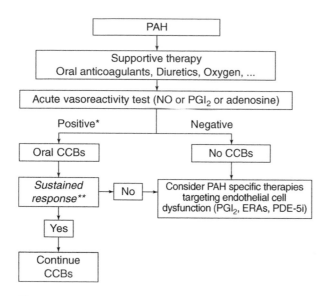

Figure 5 Treatment algorithm for "conventional" therapy. (*) A positive response to acute vasodilator testing is defined as a decrease in mPAP by at least 10 mmHg to reach an absolute level of <40 mmHg without a decrease in cardiac output. (**) Patients with a sustained benefit from CCBs are defined as those in New York Heart Association functional class I or II who have near normal hemodynamic values after at least one year of follow-up. *Abbreviations*: CCBs, calcium channel blockers; ERAs, endothelin receptor antagonists; NO, nitric oxide; PAH, pulmonary arterial hypertension; PDE-5i, phosphodiesterase-5 inhibitor; PGI_2, prostacyclin.

choice between nifedipine and diltiazem is guided by heart rate at rest: diltiazem is given to patients with a heart rate >80/min (21). Verapamil is not recommended because of negative inotropic effects (50). The side effects most frequently observed with CCBs are systemic hypotension and edema of the lower limbs (38). Association with low dose of diuretics and elastic stockings will help to reverse these side effects.

V. Conclusion

Conventional therapy mostly includes general measures, supplemental oxygen, diuretics, and oral anticoagulants. Treatment with high-dose CCBs should be restricted to rare patients with idiopathic PAH who demonstrate acute vasodilator response during right-heart catheterization. Beside the subset of vasoreactive patients who have an excellent prognosis, mean survival for PAH patients remains low while they are on conventional therapy alone. Today, conventional therapy may be considered as adjunctive therapy in combination with effective targeted therapies available (prostanoids, ERAs, and PDE-5 inhibitors for most PAH patients and CCBs for acute responders). However, in the absence of randomized controlled trials with these conventional therapies, their indication is mostly based on an expert's opinion and experience.

References

1. Channick RN. Conventional therapy in pulmonary arterial hypertension. In: Barst RJ, ed. Pulmonary Arterial Hypertension Diagnosis and Evidence-Based Treatment. Chicester, UK: John Wiley & Sons, 2008:47–60.
2. D'Alonzo GE, Barst RJ, Ayres SM, et al. Survival in patients with primary pulmonary hypertension. Results from a national prospective study. Ann Intern Med 1991; 115:343–549.
3. Rubin LJ. Primary pulmonary hypertension. N Engl J Med 1997; 336:111–117.
4. Gaine SP, Rubin LJ. Primary pulmonary hypertension. Lancet 1998; 352:719–725.
5. Humbert M, Sitbon O, Simonneau G. Treatment of pulmonary arterial hypertension. N Engl J Med 2004; 351:1425–1436.
6. Naeije R, Vachiery JL. Medical therapy of pulmonary hypertension. Conventional therapies. Clin Chest Med 2001; 22:517–527.
7. Mereles D, Ehlken N, Kreuscher S, et al. Exercise and respiratory training improve exercise capacity and quality of life in patients with severe chronic pulmonary hypertension. Circulation 2006; 114:1482–1489.
8. Bonnin M, Mercier FJ, Sitbon O, et al. Severe pulmonary hypertension during pregnancy: mode of delivery and anesthetic management of 15 consecutive cases. Anesthesiology 2005; 102:1133–1137.
9. Sitbon O, Humbert M, Simonneau G. Primary pulmonary hypertension: current therapy. Prog Cardiovasc Dis 2002; 45:115–128.
10. Kleiger RE, Boxer M, Ingham RE, et al. Pulmonary hypertension in patients using oral contraceptives. Chest 1976; 69:143–147.
11. Thorne S, Nelson-Piercy C, MacGregor A, et al. Pregnancy and contraception in heart disease and pulmonary arterial hypertension. J Fam Plann Reprod Health Care 2006; 32:75–81.
12. Bendayan D, Hod M, Oron G, et al. Pregnancy outcome in patients with pulmonary arterial hypertension receiving prostacyclin therapy. Obstet Gynecol 2005; 106:1206–1210.
13. Provencher S, Herve P, Jais X, et al. Deleterious effects of beta-blockers on exercise capacity and hemodynamics in patients with portopulmonary hypertension. Gastroenterology 2006; 130:120–126.
14. Bjornsson J, Edwards WD. Primary pulmonary hypertension: a histopathological study of 80 cases. Mayo Clin Proc 1985; 60:16–25.
15. Palevsky HI, Schloo BL, Pietra GG, et al. Primary pulmonary hypertension. Vascular structure, morphometry and responsiveness to vasodilators agents. Circulation 1989; 80: 1207–1221.
16. Christman BW, McPherson CD, Newman JH, et al. An imbalance between the excretion of thromboxane and prostacyclin metabolites in pulmonary hypertension. N Engl J Med 1992; 327:70–75.
17. Huber K, Beckmann R, Frank H, et al. Fibrinogen, t-PA, and PAI-1 plasma levels in patients with pulmonary hypertension. Am J Respir Crit Care Med 1994; 150:929–933.
18. Hoeper MM, Sosada M, Fabel H. Plasma coagulation profiles in patients with severe primary pulmonary hypertension. Eur Respir J 1998; 12:1446–1449.
19. Herve P, Humbert M, Sitbon O, et al. Pathobiology of pulmonary hypertension. The role of platelets and thrombosis. Clin Chest Med 2001; 22:451–458.
20. Fuster V, Steele PM, Edwards WD, et al. Primary pulmonary hypertension: natural history and the importance of thrombosis. Circulation 1984; 70:580–587.
21. Rich S, Kaufmann E, Levy PS. The effect of high doses of calcium-channel blockers on survival in primary pulmonary hypertension. N Engl J Med 1992; 327:76–81.
22. Frank H, Mlczoch J, Huber K, et al. The effect of anticoagulant therapy in primary and anorectic drug-induced pulmonary hypertension. Chest 1997; 112:714–721.

23. Galie N, Torbicki A, Barst R, et al. Guidelines on diagnosis and treatment of pulmonary arterial hypertension. The task force on diagnosis and treatment of pulmonary arterial hypertension of the European Society of Cardiology. Eur Heart J 2004; 25:2243–2278.

24. Rich S, Dantzker DR, Ayres SM, et al. Primary pulmonary hypertension: a national prospective study. Ann Intern Med 1987; 107:216–223.

25. Dantzker DR, Bower JS. Mechanisms of gas exchange abnormality in patients with chronic obliterative pulmonary vascular disease. J Clin Invest 1979; 64:1050.

26. Sitbon O, Humbert M, Nunes H, et al. Long-term intravenous epoprostenol infusion in primary pulmonary hypertension. Prognostic factors and survival. J Am Coll Cardiol 2002; 40:780–788.

27. Rich S, Seidlitz M, Dodin E, et al. The short-term effects of digoxin in patients with right ventricular dysfunction from pulmonary hypertension. Chest 1998; 114:787–792.

28. Brenot F. Primary pulmonary hypertension: case series from France. Chest 1994; 105: 33S–36S.

29. Fahey PJ, Utell MJ, Condemi JJ, et al. Raynaud's phenomenon of the lung. Am J Med 1984; 76:263–269.

30. Rubin LJ, Peter RH. Oral hydralazine therapy for primary pulmonary hypertension. N Engl J Med 1980; 302:69–73.

31. Packer M. Vasodilator therapy for primary pulmonary hypertension. Ann Intern Med 1985; 103:258–270.

32. Reeves JT, Groves BM, Turkevich D. The case for treatment of selected patients with primary pulmonary hypertension. Am Rev Respir Dis 1986; 134:342–346.

33. Hughes JD, Rubin LJ. Primary pulmonary hypertension. An analysis of 28 cases and a review of the literature. Medicine (Baltimore) 1986; 65:56–72.

34. Packer M, Greenberg B, Massie B, et al. Deleterious effects of hydralazine in patients with pulmonary hypertension. N Engl J Med 1982; 306:1326–1331.

35. McGoon MD, Vlietstra RE. Vasodilator therapy for primary pulmonary hypertension. Mayo Clin Proc 1984; 59:672–677.

36. Packer M. Therapeutic application of calcium-channel antagonists for pulmonary hypertension. Am J Cardiol 1985; 55:196B–201B.

37. Sitbon O, Humbert M, Jais X, et al. Long-term response to calcium channel blockers in idiopathic pulmonary arterial hypertension. Circulation 2005; 111:3105–3111.

38. Sitbon O, Humbert M, Jagot JL, et al. Inhaled nitric oxide as a screening agent for safely identifying responders to oral calcium-channel blockers in primary pulmonary hypertension. Eur Respir J 1998; 12:265–270.

39. Rubin LJ, Groves BM, Reeves JT, et al. Prostacyclin-induced acute pulmonary vasodilation in primary pulmonary hypertension. Circulation 1982; 66:334–338.

40. Schrader BJ, Inbar S, Kaufmann L, et al. Comparison of the effects of adenosine and nifedipine in pulmonary hypertension. J Am Coll Cardiol 1992; 19:1060–1064.

41. Nootens M, Schrader B, Kaufmann E, et al. Comparative acute effects of adenosine and prostacyclin in primary pulmonary hypertension. Chest 1995; 107:54–57.

42. Sitbon O, Brenot F, Denjean A, et al. Inhaled nitric oxide as a screening vasodilator agent in primary pulmonary hypertension. A dose-response study and comparison with prostacyclin. Am J Respir Crit Care Med 1995; 151:384–389.

43. Cockrill BA, Kacmarek RM, Fifer MA, et al. Comparison of the effects of nitric oxide, nitroprusside, and nifedipine on hemodynamics and right ventricular contractility in patients with chronic pulmonary hypertension. Chest 2001; 119:128–136.

44. Hoeper MM, Olschewski H, Ghofrani HA, et al. A comparison of the acute hemodynamic effects of inhaled nitric oxide and aerosolized iloprost in primary pulmonary hypertension. German PPH study group. J Am Coll Cardiol 2000; 35:176–182.

45. Weir EK, Rubin LJ, Ayres SM, et al. The acute administration of vasodilators in primary pulmonary hypertension. Experience from the National Institutes of Health Registry on primary pulmonary hypertension. Am Rev Respir Dis 1989; 140:1623–1630.

46. Barst RJ, McGoon M, Torbicki A, et al. Diagnosis and differential assessment of pulmonary arterial hypertension. J Am Coll Cardiol 2004; 43:40S–47S.

47. Badesch DB, Abman SH, Ahearn GS, et al. Medical therapy for pulmonary arterial hypertension: ACCP evidence-based clinical practice guidelines. Chest 2004; 126:35S–62S.

48. Gaine S. Pulmonary hypertension. JAMA 2000; 284:3160–3168.

49. Woodmansey PA, O'Toole L, Channer KS, et al. Acute pulmonary vasodilatory properties of amlodipine in humans with pulmonary hypertension. Heart 1996; 75:171–173.

50. Packer M, Medina N, Yushak M, et al. Detrimental effects of verapamil in patients with primary pulmonary hypertension. Br Heart J 1984; 52:106–111.

23
Medical Treatment of PAH: Prostacyclins

PAUL R. FORFIA
University of Pennsylvania, Philadelphia, Pennsylvania, U.S.A.
VALLERIE V. MCLAUGHLIN
University of Michigan Health System, Ann Arbor, Michigan, U.S.A.

I. Introduction

Initially described by Moncada and Vane in 1976, prostacyclin (epoprostenol, PGI_2) is a member of the prostacylin family produced by the vascular endothelial cells (1,2). PGI_2 is a major metabolite of arachidonic acid formed via the cyclooxygenase pathway, and is a potent vasodilator of both the pulmonary and systemic vascular beds, as well as an inhibitor of platelet aggregation (1,2). Chronically, PGI_2 has antiproliferative effects and has been shown in vitro to inhibit smooth muscle cell growth (3). PGI_2 may also have positive inotropic effects, although this is controversial. Interest in the use of PGI_2 as a treatment for pulmonary arterial hypertension (PAH) commenced in the early 1980s, even before the recognition of the relative imbalance between vasodilating and vaso-constricting prostacyclin metabolites in this population (4,5). Several smaller observations during the 1980s paved the way for the landmark trials that established the role of prostanoids for PAH.

II. Intravenous Epoprostenol

In 1982, Rubin et al. studied the hemodynamic effects of escalating doses of intravenous (IV) epoprostenol (2–12 ng/kg/min) in seven patients with idiopathic pulmonary arterial hypertension (IPAH) and severe hemodynamic compromise (6). At a mean dose of 5.7 ng/kg/min, epoprostenol reduced total pulmonary resistance by approximately 43% while cardiac output increased by 56%. Longer-term infusions (1–25 months) led to hemodynamic improvement, clinical stabilization, and improved exercise capacity in patients with severe IPAH who were refractory to oral vasodilators, digoxin, and diuretic therapy (7). These early observational studies led to the first randomized trial with epoprostenol in 1990 (8). Patients with IPAH ($n = 23$) were randomized to epoprostenol (mean dose 7.1 ng/kg/min) or placebo, and functional classification, six-minute walk distance (6MWD), and cardiopulmonary hemodynamics were compared at baseline and two months after therapy. All 10 patients treated with epoprostenol improved by at least one functional class, and on average increased their 6MWD from 246 to 378 m. Total pulmonary resistance fell from 21.6 to 13.9 mmHg/L/min, and cardiac output rose from

3.3 to 3.9 L/min. In contrast, the majority of placebo-treated patients did not symptomatically improve, had a lesser increase in walk distance, with no significant changes in hemdoynamics. Of note, three patients in the placebo arm died over the eight-week study period versus one subject treated with epoprostenol. Nine patients were treated with epoprostenol for an additional 6 to 18 months and enjoyed sustained symptomatic and hemodynamic effects. These findings also provided the impetus for a multicenter open-label trial, which randomized 81 IPAH patients, functional class III or IV, to epoprostenol plus conventional therapy versus conventional therapy alone (9). At 12 weeks, the epoprostenol-treated group (mean dose 9.2 ng/kg/min) had improved quality of life scores, improved functional class, and increased their median 6MWD (+31 m vs. −29 m in conventional therapy group) versus conventional therapy alone. Pulmonary vascular resistance (PVR) fell by approximately 25% (placebo increased 9%) and cardiac index rose by 15%, while mean systemic arterial pressure fell by only 5%. Patients with the greatest hemodynamic improvements over the study period tended to have the largest improvements in 6MWD. Eight patients died during the 12-week study period; all eight deaths occurred in the conventional therapy group. Importantly, the hemodynamic and clinical improvements seen in the epoprostenol-treated patients were not predicted by short-term hemodynamic responsiveness to epoprostenol prior to randomization, confirming previous observations that the long-term effects of epoprostenol are not well predicted by short-term acute vasodilator responsiveness. The results of this study led to FDA approval of epoprostenol in 1995 for patients with idiopathic PAH.

Epoprostenol has also been studied specifically in population with PAH related to the scleroderma spectrum of diseases. Badesch et al. studied epoprostenol in 111 such patients in a randomized, open-label trial conducted over a 12-week period (10). In relative terms, patients in the epoprostenol treatment group were quite ill at baseline, with a mean 6MWD of only 272 m, right atrial pressure of 13 mmHg, and cardiac index of 1.9 L/min/m^2. In response to epoprostenol (mean dose 11.2 ng/kg/min), PVR declined by 32% and cardiac index increased 0.5 L/min/m^2, while 6MWD increased (270–316 m). In patients treated with conventional therapy the 6MWD declined (240–192 m), for an impressive net 6MWD difference of +108 m. There were no survival differences detected (4 deaths in epoprostenol group, 5 deaths in conventional treatment group) over this relatively short follow-up period, but neither study was powered to detect a survival benefit.

Longer-term observational studies have demonstrated improved outcomes in IPAH patients treated with epoprostenol. In 2002, McLaughlin et al. reported on the long-term clinical outcomes of 162 patients with IPAH treated with epoprostenol (median follow-up 36 months) (11). The observed survival rates at one, two, three, and five years were 88%, 76%, 63%, and 47%, respectively; these rates were significantly greater than the expected one-, two-, and three-year survival rates of 59%, 46%, and 35%, respectively as predicted by the NIH survival. Baseline predictors of survival included exercise capacity, right atrial pressure, and vasodilator responsiveness in response to adenosine. On follow-up, subjects who remained functional class I to II fared far better (3- and 5-year survival rates of 89% and 73%, respectively) than those who were class III (3- and 5-year survival rates of 62% and 35%, respectively); patients who remained class IV did especially poorly (survival rates 42% at 2 years, 0% at 3 years). A total of 70 episodes of sepsis were reported, 4 of which were fatal; 1 patient died due to interruption of epoprostenol therapy. Similarly, Sitbon et al. reported overall survival rates of 85%, 70%, 63%, and 55%, respectively at one, two, three, and five years in 178 patients with IPAH treated with continuous IV epoprostenol (12). After three months on therapy, a history of right-heart failure, persistence of class III or IV functional status, and a <30% fall in total pulmonary resistance were associated with poor survival. These findings provide the basis for the recommendation of referral for lung transplantation in PAH patients who remain class III or IV despite prostacyclin therapy. Observational series have also demonstrated beneficial effects of epoprostenol in associated forms of PAH including congenital heart disease (CHD), human immunodeficiency virus (HIV), and portopulmonary hypertension, in addition to sarcoid-related and chronic thromboembolic pulmonary hypertension (CTEPH).

A. Practical Considerations

Epoprostenol sodium is the IV formulation of PGI_2, with a half-life of about six minutes. The two major pharmacologic actions of epoprostenol are inhibition of platelet aggregation and potent vasodilation of systemic and pulmonary vascular beds, both of which are mediated via stimulation of adenylate cyclase and increased production of cyclic adenosine monophosphate (cAMP). Patients are generally hospitalized for initiation of epoprostenol. The initial dose of epoprostenol is 2 ng/kg/min and can be uptitrated by 2 ng/kg/min at varying time intervals over the first few days of the hospitalization, with the rate of increase being dictated by the severity of the PAH and patient's tolerability to its side effects. Side effects commonly include jaw pain, flushing, nausea, headache, diarrhea, and systemic hypotension. Blood stream infections can be life-threatening. Given its potent hemodynamic effects and rapid offset of action, sudden interruption of epoprostenol therapy can lead to rebound pulmonary vasoconstriction, acute right ventricular (RV) failure, and death. Thus, although infusion may be initiated via a peripheral line or peripherally inserted central catheter (PICC) line, a more durable form of IV access, typically a tunneled, cuffed central venous catheter is required prior to hospital discharge.

Continuous epoprostenol is a complex therapy that requires daily reconstitution and self-administration of medication, operation of a continuous infusion pump, and central venous access care. Due to its instability at room temperature, the medication must be kept cold within the infusion pump using ice packs. Patients must have a backup pump available in the rare event of infusion pump malfunction. Therefore, extensive patient education is required prior to hospital discharge. Patients should have appropriate support systems. The patient must be educable and demonstrate proficiency with this therapy before being discharged; inappropriate patient selection for epoprostenol infusion can lead to potentially catastrophic outcomes related to inadvertent interruption of therapy or line-related sepsis.

In the outpatient setting, the epoprostenol infusion is generally uptitrated by 2 ng/kg/min once or twice per week until a desired clinical effect, balanced by patient tolerance to side effects. Patients should be monitored frequently in the office during the first 6 to 12 months of therapy. While there is considerable patient variability, the optimal dose of epoprostenol is likely between 25 and 40 ng/kg/min. Epoprostenol overdose can occur, typically manifesting clinically with stereotypical, but excessive prostanoid side effects (diarrhea, flushing) and a high cardiac output state by right-heart catheterization (13).

III. Treprostinil

Developed with the hopes of obviating the need for IV infusion, the stable prostacyclin analogue treprostinil was initially tested in a series of three pilot studies in patients with IPAH (14). In the first study, the acute hemodynamic effects of IV treprostinil were demonstrated to be similar to IV epoprostenol. Importantly, the acute hemodynamic effects of subcutaneously delivered treprostinil were also similar to IV epoprostenol. Lastly, a randomized trial in 26 patients with IPAH demonstrated that continuous subcutaneous (SC) treprostinil infusion led to significant increases in 6MWD (+37 m) versus placebo group (−6 m) over an eight-week follow-up period. These findings led to a large scale, placebo-controlled randomized international trial of SC treprostinil infusion in 470 patients with PAH with class II to IV symptoms over a 12-week period (15). The study included patients with IPAH (58%), PAH associated with connective tissue disease (CTD) (19%), and PAH associated with systemic to pulmonary shunts (23%). The primary endpoint was a median change in 6MWD. Treprostinil was started at 1.25 ng/kg/min and titrated progressively over the 12-week period to a maximal dose of 22.5 ng/kg/min. Typical prostanoid side effects occurred, including jaw pain, diarrhea, and flushing; 18 (8%) patients discontinued therapy due to intolerable site pain. At 12 weeks, there was a modest median difference of 16 m in the 6MWD between the treprostinil versus placebo groups. Importantly, the final dose achieved was only 9.3 ng/kg/min; the subgroup of patients who were treated with doses >13.8 ng/kg/min improved their 6MWD 36 m. The dose limitation was largely related to pain at the site of the SC infusion, which occurred in 85% of subjects. Also, the 6MWD treatment effect was only 2 m in the 53 patients who were functional class II at baseline, versus 17 and 54 m for the subjects who were class III and IV at baseline, respectively. Taken together, these findings suggested that relative underdosing of treprostinil and inclusion of a diverse, and overall less impaired PAH cohort may have led to the relatively modest improvements in 6MWD. In clinical practice, target treprostinil doses are routinely two to four times higher than epoprostenol doses.

Rubenfire et al. randomized 22 PAH patients, stable on IV epoprostenol, to either SC treprostinil or placebo. The transition was made in a closely monitored setting given the concern for clinical deterioration (16). Over the eight-week trial, 7 of 8 patients randomized to placebo deteriorated, while 1 of 14 patients randomized to treprostinil deteriorated ($p = 0.00023$), suggesting that patients on epoprostenol could be safely transitioned to SC treprostinil. At the end of the eight-week trial, the dose of treprostinil was 153% of the epoprostenol dose in those who were transitioned.

Longer-term observation studies have suggested improved outcomes with treprostinil. Barst et al. reported an observational, uncontrolled series of 860 patients with PAH of varying etiology [IPAH (48%), CHD-PAH (21%), CTD-PAH (18%), porto-pulmonary (5%), CTEPH (6%)] treated with SC treprostinil (17). The average dose was 42 ng/kg/min at four years; 23% of patients discontinued therapy due to adverse events, primarily site pain/reaction, 16% died, and 11% switched to an alternative prostanoid. Survival at one and four years in the overall cohort was 87% and 68%, and 91% and 72% for the IPAH subgroup. Similar observations were found in another multicenter retrospective study of SC treprostinil in 99 patients with PAH and 23 patients with CTEPH (18). Taken together, these findings suggest that long-term SC treprostinil is a viable alternative to IV epoprostenol in the treatment of PAH in selected patients.

Given the limitation of site pain/reaction from SC infusion, and that SC and IV treprostinil have virtually the same bioavailability and hemodynamic effects, long-term IV treprostinil has also been studied in PAH (19). Tapson et al. reported on 16 patients with PAH (8 IPAH, 6 CTD-PAH, 2 CHD-PAH) treated with IV treprostinil as their initial therapy in an open-label, uncontrolled series (20). Over 12 weeks, the primary endpoint, 6MWD, improved from 319 to 400 m. In an open-label uncontrolled trial, Gomberg-Maitland transitioned 31 patients with PAH on IV epoprostenol to IV treprostinil (21). Four patients were transitioned back to epoprostenol over the 12-week study. Among those 27 who remained on IV treprostinil, the 6MWD was unchanged, although the mean PAP was slightly higher, and the cardiac output was slightly lower than baseline. At week 12, the mean dose of treprostinil was more than twice the dose of epoprostenol.

A. Practical Considerations

Treprostinil is a tricyclic benzidene analogue of prostacyclin that has similar antiplatelet and cardiopulmonary hemodynamic effects as epoprostenol. Unlike epoprostenol, treprostinil is stable at room temperature at a neutral pH, and has an elimination half-life of 4.6 hours. Treprostinil can be delivered by either SC or IV routes.

Patients are generally hospitalized for initiation of IV treprostinil; however SC treprostinil can be initiated in the hospital, the office, or at home if the patient has demonstrated proficiency during the education process. The recommended initial dose of treprostinil is 1.25 ng/kg/min and is typically increased by 1.25 ng/kg/min per week for the first four weeks and then by 2.5 ng/kg/min per week until the desired clinical effect is achieved in balance with patient tolerability to its side effects. In practice, the starting dose is often 2.5 ng/kg/min and will be uptitrated to approximately 15 to 20 ng/kg/min by the first month as per patient tolerance. Similar to epoprostenol, side effects commonly include jaw pain, flushing, diarrhea, and headache. Studies have consistently reported site pain in 80% to 85% of patients receiving SC treprostinil; however, the proportion of patients who eventually discontinue therapy on account of site pain varies widely from study to study, and center to center. Site pain should be aggressively and preemptively managed with topical analgesics (i.e., PLO gel with 5% lidocaine, ketoprofen), local or systemic neuropathic modulating agents (i.e., gabapentin), and hot/cold packs particularly for the two- to five-day period following site change. Patients often report that certain sites are less painful than others; thus, patients should be encouraged to change their injection site less frequently once they find a site that is less painful. Due its longer half-life, interruption of therapy is an urgent but not emergent matter, typically allowing the patient time to seek medical attention before the biologic effects of therapy have worn off. For long-term IV administration, a tunneled, cuffed central venous catheter is recommended.

Treprostinil comes in premixed 20 mL vials containing either 1, 2.5, 5, or 10 mg/mL concentrations, and does not require daily reconstitution with diluent when used subcutaneously. Due to its stability at room temperature, ice packs are not needed. For SC administration, the medication cartridge must be changed every 72 hours and for IV administration every 48 hours. Patients must have a backup pump available in the rare event of infusion pump malfunction. While blood stream infection is a concern with IV agents, a concern for an increased risk of gram-negative infections has been raised with IV treprostinil (22). Oral and inhaled forms of treprostinil are currently being studied in clinical trials.

IV. Iloprost

Iloprost is a stable synthetic prostacyclin analogue with a half-life of 20 to 30 minutes delivered via aerosolized inhalation. This inhaled formulation was developed as an alternative to epoprostenol with hopes of greater pulmonary vascular selectivity, less systemic vasodilatory effects, and a less invasive and potentially safer delivery mechanism. The pivotal randomized, placebo-controlled trial with iloprost was a 12-week study that assessed the combined clinical endpoint of (*i*) improvement by at least one functional class, (*ii*) a >10% improvement in 6MWD, and (*iii*) no death or deterioration (23). The study enrolled 203 patients with PAH or CTEPH, all of whom were functional class III or IV. The combined clinical endpoint was met by 16.8% of the patients randomized to iloprost and 4.9% in those randomized to placebo ($p = 0.007$). Cough, headache, and syncope were more common in the iloprost group.

Longer-term observations with iloprost have demonstrated conflicting results. While Hoeper's observation of 24 patients followed over one year suggested improvements in exercise endurance and hemodynamics, Opitz's description of long-term event-free survival with iloprost in 76 patients was less impressive (24,25). Iloprost has also been studied in two trials as add-on therapy in patients who remain symptomatic while on bosentan. One, which was designed as a safety study, randomized 65 such PAH patients to inhaled iloprost or placebo (26). The combination appeared to be safe, and there were also improvements in efficacy endpoints including 6MWD, functional class, time to clinical worsening, and postinhalation hemodynamics. The other was aborted after enrollment of 40 patients, as a futility analysis predicted failure with respect to the predetermined sample size (27).

A. Practical Considerations

Inhaled iloprost is delivered via aerosolized inhalation with a specific device (I-Neb, Pro-dose), and therapy is generally instituted in the home with close observation after requisite patient education. Best results are achieved with slow deep inspiration and faster expiration. The initial dose is 2.5 µg every two to three hours while awake. Treatments are prescribed six to nine times per day, although in our experience, the average frequency is five times per day. If the low dose is tolerated, the dose is generally increased to 5 µg. Care should be taken in those with low blood pressure, and inhaled iloprost should not be initiated if the systolic blood pressure is <85 mmHg. The most common side effects include flushing, cough, and headache.

V. Beraprost

Beraprost sodium is an orally active prostacylin analogue with a stable structure due to its cyclopentabenzofuranyl skeleton (28). It is rapidly absorbed and has an elimination

TABLE 1 Selected Prospective Clinical Trials with prostanoids in PAH

Study	Study Name	Duration (wks)	Patients (N)	Baseline 6MWD (m)	Functional Class %	Etiology %	Comparison	Outcomes
Epoprostenol–IPAH(8)	none	8	24	246 (A) 205 (C)	II–8 III–63 IV–29	IPAH– 100	Randomized, unblinded i.v. epo + conventional therapy vs conventional therapy alone	Compared to control: • 6MWD increased 45 m • mPAP decreased 9 mmHg • PVR decreased 8 U • 1 death compared to 3 in control group
Epoprostenol–IPAH(9)	none	12	81	316 (A) 272 (C)	II–0 III–74 IV–26	IPAH– 100	Randomized, unblinded i.v. epo + conventional therapy vs conventional therapy alone	Compared to control: • 6MWD increased 47 m • mPAP decreased 6.7 mmHg • PVR decreased 4.9 U • No deaths compared to 8 in control group
Epoprostenol–CTD–(10)	none	12	111	271 (A) 240 (C)	II–5 III–78 IV–17	CTD– 100	Randomized, unblinded i.v. epo + conventional therapy vs conventional therapy alone	Compared to control: • 6MWD increased 108 m • mPAP decreased 6 mmHg • PVR decreased 5.5 U • 21 improved functional class compared to none in control group • No difference in 12-week survival
Treprostinil (15)	none	12	470	326 (A) 327 (C)	II–12 III–81 IV–7	IPAH– 58 CTD–19 CHD–24	Randomized, double-blind s.c. treprostinil vs s.c. placebo	Compared to placebo: • 6MWD increased 10 m • mPAP decreased 3 mmHg • PVR decreased 4.7 U • No difference in survival 85% had infusion site pain vs 27% in placebo group

Drug (ref)	Trial	Weeks	N	6MWD (m)	NYHA	Etiology	Study design	Results
Treprostinil (20)	none	12	16	319	III–88 IV–4	IPAH-50 CTD-38 CHD-13	Open label IV treprostinil	Compared to baseline 6MWD increased 82 m mPAP decreased 4.2 mmHg PVR decreased 9.4 U
Treprostinil (21)	none	12	31	438	II–77 III–23	IPAH-68 CTD-19 CHD-13	Open label transition from IV epoprostenol to IV treprostinil	6MWD unchanged mPAP increased by 4 mmHg PVRI increased by 3 U-m2 4 patients transitioned back to IV epoprostenol
Treprostinil (16)	none	8	22	437 (A) 424 (C)	I–4 II–55 III41	IPAH-73 CTD-14 CHD-4 PoP-9	Randomized, double-blind transition from IV epoprostenol to sc treprostinil	7/8 patients transitioned to placebo deteriorated, 1/14 patients transition to sc treprostinil deteriorated, $p = 0.00023$ Maximum treprostinil dose 152% of baseline epoprostenol dose
Iloprost(23)	AIR	12	203	332 (A) 315 (C)	III–59 IV–41	IPAH-54 CTD-17 CTEPH –28	Randomized, double-blind inhaled iloprost vs inhaled placebo	Compared to placebo: • 6MWD increased 36.4 m • mPAP decreased 4.4 mmHg (after inhalation; no difference before inhalation) • PVR decreased 4 U (after inhalation; 1.2 U before inhalation) • NYHA class improved in 24.8% compared to 12. 7% of placebo
Iloprost(26)	STEP	12	67	335	II–1.5 III–94 IV–4.5	IPAH-55 APAH-45	Randomize, double-blind, inhaled iloprost vs inhaled placebo in patient on bosentan	Compared to placebo: • 6MWD increased 26 m • mPAP decreased 8 mmHg (after inhalation; no difference before inhalation)

(Continued)

TABLE 1 Selected Prospective Clinical Trials with prostanoids in PAH (*Continued*)

Study	Study Name	Duration (wks)	Patients (N)	Baseline 6MWD (m)	Functional Class %	Etiology %	Comparison	Outcomes
Iloprost(27)	COMBI	12	40	317 (A) 296 (C)	III–100	IPAH–100	Randomize, double-blind, inhaled iloprost vs inhaled placebo in patient on bosentan	• PVR decreased 3.2 U (after inhalation • NYHA class improved in 34% compared to 6% of placebo • Terminated early due to futility analysis. 6MWD +1 m in placebo and −9 m in iloprost
Beraprost(31)	none	52	116	433 (A) 445 (C)	II–53% III–47%	IPAH– 74% CTD– 10% CHD– 16%	Randomized, double-blind max tolerated oral dose of beraprost vs placebo	• Compared to placebo • 6MWD was 23 m further (NS) at 52 weeks (and unchanged from baseline) • Hemodynamics unchanged • No difference in disease progression at 52 weeks
Beraprost(30)	ALPHABET	12	130	362 (A) 383 (C)	II–49 III–51	IPAH– 48 CTD–10 CHD–18 PoPH–17 HIV–7	Randomize, double-blind max tolerated oral dose of beraprost vs placebo	• Compared to placebo • 6MWD increased 23 m • Hemodynamics unchanged • Functional class unchanged

half-life of 35 to 40 minutes when administered in the fasting state but 3 to 3.5 hours when administered with a meal. Like other prostanoids, the main physiologic effects include vasodilatation, inhibition of platelet aggregation, and in vitro inhibition of smooth muscle cell proliferation (3,29). Several small observational studies that suggested improvements in exercise endurance and hemodynamics with beraprost led to its evaluation in two randomized controlled trials.

In a prospective, double-blind placebo-controlled randomized study of beraprost, Galie and colleagues studied 130 patients with PAH for 12 weeks (30). The primary endpoint of 6MWD improved by 25 m ($p = 0.036$). However, a year long, double-blind placebo-controlled trial of 116 PAH patients led by Barst et al. did not demonstrate sustained improvements with beraprost (31). Benefits noted in 6MWD and disease progression at 3 and 6 months were not sustained at 9 and 12 months.

A. Practical Considerations

Beraprost is an oral prostacyclin analogue that is generally administered in doses up to 80 μg four times per day. Most common side effects include headache, flushing, jaw pain, diarrhea, and leg pain.

VI. Conclusions

There is excellent rationale for the use of prostacyclin analogues in PAH based on the basic mechanisms of the disease, and indeed, clinical trials have demonstrated the benefit of this class of therapy in PAH patients. Table 1 summarizes selected prospective clinical trials with prostacylin analogues. In the most critically ill patients, IV epoprostenol is the drug of choice, as the most rapid acting, reliable, and potent prostanoid for which there is a wealth of evidence. Parenteral (IV and SC) prostanoids are complicated therapies and are most appropriately managed by practices with considerable experience in their use. Investigational trials of additional prostacyclin analogues and prostacyclin receptor agonists are under way.

References

1. Moncada S, Gryglewski R, Bunting S, et al. An enzyme isolated from arteries transforms prostaglandin endoperoxides to an unstable substance that inhibits platelet aggregation. Nature 1976; 263:663–665.
2. Moncada S, Vane JR. Arachidonic acid metabolites and the interactions between platelets and blood-vessel walls. N Engl J Med 1979; 300:1142–1147.
3. Clapp LH, Finney P, Turcato S, et al. Differential effects of stable prostacyclin analogs on smooth muscle proliferation and cyclic AMP generation in human pulmonary artery. Am J Respir Cell Mol Biol 2002; 26:194–201.
4. Christman BW, McPherson CD, Newman JH, et al. An imbalance between the excretion of thromboxane and prostacyclin metabolites in pulmonary hypertension. N Engl J Med 1992; 327:70–75.
5. Tuder RM, Cool CD, Geraci MW, et al. Prostacyclin synthase expression is decreased in lungs from patients with severe pulmonary hypertension. Am J Respir Crit Care Med 1999; 159:1925–1932.

6. Rubin LJ, Groves BM, Reeves JT, et al. Prostacyclin-induced acute pulmonary vasodilation in primary pulmonary hypertension. Circulation 1982; 66:334–338.

7. Higenbottam T, Wheeldon D, Wells F, et al. Long-term treatment of primary pulmonary hypertension with continuous intravenous epoprostenol (prostacyclin). Lancet 1984; 1:1046–1047.

8. Rubin LJ, Mendoza J, Hood M, et al. Treatment of primary pulmonary hypertension with continuous intravenous prostacyclin (epoprostenol). Results of a randomized trial. Ann Intern Med 1990; 112:485–491.

9. Barst RJ, Rubin LJ, Long WA, et al. A comparison of continuous intravenous epoprostenol (prostacyclin) with conventional therapy for primary pulmonary hypertension. N Engl J Med 1996; 334:296–301.

10. Badesch DB, Tapson VF, McGoon MD, et al. Continuous intravenous epoprostenol for pulmonary hypertension due to the scleroderma spectrum of disease. Ann Intern Med 2000; 132:425–434.

11. McLaughlin VV, Shillington A, Rich S. Survival in primary pulmonary hypertension: the impact of epoprostenol therapy. Circulation 2002; 106:1477–1482.

12. Sitbon O, Humbert M, Nunes H, et al. Long-term intravenous epoprostenol infusion in primary pulmonary hypertension: prognostic factors and survival. J Am Coll Cardiol 2002; 40:780–788.

13. Rich S, McLaughlin VV. The effects of chronic prostacyclin therapy on cardiac output and symptoms in primary pulmonary hypertension. J Am Coll Cardiol 1999; 34:1184–1187.

14. McLaughlin VV, Gaine SP, Barst RJ, et al. Efficacy and safety of treprostinil: an epoprostenol analogue for primary pulmonary hypertension. J Cardiovasc Pharmacol 2003; 41:293–299.

15. Simonneau G, Barst RJ, Galie N, et al. Continuous subcutaneous infusion of treprostinil, a prostacyclin analogue, in patients with pulmonary arterial hypertension. Am J Respir Crit Care Med 2002; 165:800–804.

16. Rubenfire M, McLaughlin VV, Allen RP, et al. Transition from IV epoprostenol to subcutaneous treprostinil in pulmonary arterial hypertension: a controlled trial. Chest 2007; 132:757–763.

17. Barst R, Galie N, Naeije R, et al. Long-term outcome in pulmonary arterial hypertension patients treated with subcutaneous treprostinil. Eur Respir J 2006; 47:2049–2056.

18. Lang I, Gomez-Sanchez M, Kneussl M, et al. Efficacy of long-term subcutaneous treprostinil sodium therapy in pulmonary hypertension. Chest 2006; 129:1636–1643.

19. McSwain CS, Benza R, Shapiro S, et al. Dose proportionality of treprostinil sodium administered by continuous subcutaneous and intravenous infusion. J Clin Pharmacol 2008; 48:19–25.

20. Tapson VF, Gomberg-Maitland M, McLaughlin VV, et al. Safety and efficacy of IV treprostinil for pulmonary arterial hypertension: a prospective, multicenter, open-label, 12-week trial. Chest 2006; 129:683–688.

21. Gomberg-Maitland M, Tapson VF, Benza RL, et al. Transition from intravenous epoprostenol to intravenous treprostinil in pulmonary hypertension. Am J Respir Crit Care Med 2005; 172:1586–1589.

22. Kallen AJ, Lederman E, Balaji A, et al. Bloodstream infections in patients given treatment with intravenous prostanoids. Infect Control Hosp Epidemiol 2008; 29:342–349.

23. Olschewski H, Simonneau G, Galie N, et al. Inhaled iloprost for severe pulmonary hypertension. N Engl J Med 2002; 347:322–329.

24. Hoeper MM, Schwarze M, Ehlerding S, et al. Long-term treatment of primary pulmonary hypertension with aerosolized iloprost, a prostacyclin analogue. N Engl J Med 2000; 342:1866–1870.

25. Opitz CF, Wensel R, Winkler J, et al. Clinical efficacy and survival with first-line inhaled iloprost therapy in patients with idiopathic pulmonary arterial hypertension. Eur Heart J 2005; 26:1895–1902.

26. McLaughlin VV, Oudiz RJ, Adaani F, et al. Randomized study of adding inhaled iloprost to existing bosentan in pulmonary arterial hypertension. Am J Respir Crit Care Med 2006; 174:1257–1263.

27. Hoeper MM, Leuchte H, Halank M, et al. Combining inhaled iloprost with bosentan in patients with idiopathic pulmonary arterial hypertension. Eur Respir J 2006; 28:691–694.

28. Sim AK, McCraw AP, Cleland ME, et al. Effect of a stable prostacyclin analogue on platelet function and experimentally-induced thrombosis in the microcirculation. Arzneimittelforschung 1985; 35:1816–1818.

29. Murata T, Murai T, Kanai T, et al. General pharmacology of beraprost sodium. 2nd communication: effect on the autonomic, cardiovascular and gastrointestinal systems, and other effects. Arzneimittelforschung 1989; 39:867–876.

30. Galie N, Humbert M, Vachiery J, et al. Effects of beraprost sodium, an oral prostacyclin analogue, in patients with pulmonary arterial hypertension: a randomized, double-blind, placebo-controlled trial. J Am Coll Cardiol 2002; 39:1496–1502.

31. Barst RJ, McGoon MD, McLaughlin VV, et al. Beraprost therapy for pulmonary arterial hypertension. J Am Coll Cardiol 2003; 41:2119–2125.

24
Phosphodiesterase Type 5 Inhibitors

NAZZARENO GALIÈ
University of Bologna, Bologna, Italy

I. Introduction

Pulmonary arterial hypertension (PAH) is associated with impaired release of nitric oxide (1) due, at least in part, to reduced expression of nitric oxide synthase in the vascular endothelium of pulmonary arteries (2). Although inhaled nitric oxide is used for testing acute vasoreactivity (3), its chronic administration is cumbersome and requires a complex delivery system (4).

Downstream activation of soluble guanylate cyclase is thus reduced in patients with PAH with less cellular synthesis of cyclic guanosine monophosphate (cGMP), the second messenger of nitric oxide. Phosphodiesterase type 5 (PDE-5) inactivates cGMP in the pulmonary vasculature, and it appears to be upregulated in pulmonary hypertension (5,6). Inhibition of PDE-5 increases cGMP levels, which may mediate the antiproliferative (7) and vasodilating (8) effects of endogenous nitric oxide. These data represent the rationale for the development of PDE-5 inhibitors to treat PAH. All three PDE-5 inhibitors approved for the treatment of erectile dysfunction, sildenafil, tadalafil, and vardenafil, cause significant pulmonary vasodilation with maximum effects observed after 60, 75 to 90, and 40 to 45 minutes, respectively (9). The upregulation of PDE-5 in the lung vasculature of patients with PAH may exert (theoretically) a preferential effect of the PDE-5 inhibitors on these vessels (5,6).

II. Sildenafil

Sildenafil is an orally active, potent, and selective inhibitor of PDE-5. In a study on human pulmonary artery smooth muscle cells treated with the platelet-derived growth factor (PDGF), sildenafil exerted an antiproliferative effect (7).

Animal studies in the classical model of monocrotalin-induced pulmonary hypertension in rats have shown favorable effects of sildenafil on pulmonary arterial pressure, right ventricular hypertrophy, and survival (10,11). In particular sildenafil prevented myocardial remodeling in pulmonary hypertension through an indirect action via right ventricular unloading (11).

A number of uncontrolled studies have reported favorable effects of sildenafil in patients with idiopathic PAH, PAH associated with connective tissue diseases (CTDs), congenital heart diseases, and chronic thromboembolic pulmonary hypertension

(CTEPH) (12–14). Five randomized controlled studies of sildenafil in the treatment of PAH patients cited improvement in exercise capacity, hemodynamic parameters, and clinical status (15–19).

The Sildenafil Use in Pulmonary artERial hypertension (SUPER) trial of 278 PAH patients treated with sildenafil 20, 40, or 80 mg three times daily, compared with placebo, confirmed favorable results on exercise capacity, symptoms, and hemodynamics (16). The durability of the effect over time was shown only for the dose of 80 mg TID (16).

A post hoc analysis of 84 patients with CTD-associated PAH receiving sildenafil in the SUPER-1 trial revealed improved exercise capacity, hemodynamics, and functional class at 12 weeks when compared with placebo (20).

In a small randomized controlled study in PAH patients [Sildenafil vs. Endothelin Receptor Antagonist for Pulmonary Hypertension (SERAPH) study], the effects of sildenafil on functional capacity were comparable to those of bosentan; only sildenafil reduced the right ventricular muscle mass as assessed by cardiac magnetic resonance (18).

In a randomized controlled study with crossover design in patients with idiopathic PAH or PAH associated with congenital heart diseases, sildenafil improved the symptomatic status, exercise capacity, New York Heart Association (NYHA) class, and hemodynamic parameters (17).

The Pulmonary Arterial Hypertension Combination Study of Epoprostenol and Sildenafil (PACES) trial addressed the effects of adding sildenafil 80 mg TID compared with placebo in 267 PAH patients chronically treated with intravenous epoprostenol (19). The addition of sildenafil improved exercise capacity, hemodynamic measurements, time to clinical worsening, and quality of life in this severe patient population. Of note, seven deaths occurred in this trial, all in the placebo group.

Most side effects of sildenafil are mild to moderate and mainly related to vasodilation (headache, flushing, epistaxis).

Sildenafil plasma levels are reduced and bosentan plasma levels are increased if the two drugs are coadministered due to a pharmacokinetic interaction mediated by the cytochrome P450 3A4 (21). Even if the clinical relevance of this interaction is unknown, higher doses of sildenafil might theoretically be needed in patients with bosentan background therapy, and specific trials may be required to clarify this issue. Sildenafil coadministration with nitrates is contraindicated due to a synergistic effect on the induction of hypotension.

The approved dose of sildenafil is 20 mg TID, but the durability of effect up to one year has been demonstrated only with the dose of 80 mg TID (16,19). In clinical practice, uptitration beyond 20 mg TID (mainly 40–80 mg TID) may be needed.

III. Tadalafil

Tadalafil, an orally administered, once-daily dosing, selective inhibitor of PDE-5, is currently approved for the treatment of erectile dysfunction (22). Preliminary data on tadalafil for the treatment of PAH are limited to a single-dose hemodynamic evaluation (9), anecdotal clinical use (23), and a trial on Eisenmenger syndrome patients (24). In this last study, tadalafil was well tolerated, with an improvement in functional class, six-minute walk distance, and hemodynamics. None of the patients had a fall in systemic arterial pressure, worsening of oxygen saturation, or any adverse reactions to the drug.

The Pulmonary arterial Hypertension and ReSponse to Tadalafil (PHIRST) study on 406 PAH patients (about 50% on background bosentan therapy) treated with tadalafil 5, 10, 20, or 40 mg once daily demonstrated favorable results on exercise capacity, symptoms, hemodynamics, and time to clinical worsening at the largest dose (25). In addition, favorable results were observed in patients on background bosentan therapy but to a lesser extent. The reasons for this observation are not clear, but may be related to a pharmacokinetic interaction between tadalafil and bosentan mediated by the cytochrome P450 3A4 and leading to reduced tadalafil plasma levels (reducing the pharmacodynamic effects) and increased bosentan plasma levels (26). Higher doses of tadalafil might theoretically be needed in patients with bosentan background therapy, and specific trials may be required to clarify this issue. Tadalafil coadministration with nitrates is contraindicated due to a synergistic effect on the induction of hypotension. The most common treatment-related adverse events reported with tadalafil were headache, myalgias, and flushing.

IV. Vardenafil

Vardenafil is an orally administered, once-daily dosed, selective inhibitor of PDE-5, which is currently approved for the treatment of erectile dysfunction. Preliminary data on the efficacy of vardenafil to treat PAH are limited to a single-dose hemodynamic evaluation (9) and a small study on five patients with different types of pulmonary hypertension (27) In this study, the maintenance dose of vardenafil was 10 to 15 mg daily.

Vardenafil coadministration with nitrates is contraindicated due to a synergistic effect on the induction of hypotension.

Reference

1. Archer SL, Djaballah K, Humbert M, et al. Nitric oxide deficiency in fenfluramine- and dexfenfluramine-induced pulmonary hypertension. Am J Respir Crit Care Med 1998; 158(4): 1061–1067.
2. Giaid A, Saleh D. Reduced expression of endothelial nitric oxide synthase in the lungs of patients with pulmonary hypertension. N Engl J Med 1995; 333(4):214–221.
3. Task FM, Galie N, Torbicki A, et al. Guidelines on diagnosis and treatment of pulmonary arterial hypertension: the task force on diagnosis and treatment of pulmonary arterial hypertension of the European Society of Cardiology. Eur Heart J 2004; 25(24):2243–2278.
4. Channick RN, Newhart JW, Johnson FW, et al. Pulsed delivery of inhaled nitric oxide to patients with primary pulmonary hypertension: an ambulatory delivery system and initial clinical tests. Chest 1996; 109(6):1545–1549.
5. Wharton J, Strange JW, Moller GMO, et al. Antiproliferative effects of phosphodiesterase type 5 inhibition in human pulmonary artery cells. Am J Respir Crit Care Med 2005; 172(1): 105–113.
6. Corbin JD, Beasley A, Blount MA, et al. High lung PDE5: a strong basis for treating pulmonary hypertension with PDE5 inhibitors. Biochem Biophys Res Commun 2005; 334(3):930–938.
7. Tantini B, Manes A, Fiumana E, et al. Antiproliferative effect of sildenafil on human pulmonary artery smooth muscle cells. Basic Res Cardiol 2005; 100(2):131–138.

8. Michelakis E, Tymchak W, Lien D, et al. Oral sildenafil is an effective and specific pulmonary vasodilator in patients with pulmonary arterial hypertension: comparison with inhaled nitric oxide. Circulation 2002;105(20):2398–2403.
9. Ghofrani HA, Voswinckel R, Reichenberger F, et al. Differences in hemodynamic and oxygenation responses to three different phosphodiesterase-5 inhibitors in patients with pulmonary arterial hypertension: a randomized prospective study. J Am Coll Cardiol 2004; 44(7):1488–1496.
10. Schermuly RT, Kreisselmeier KP, Ghofrani HA, et al. Chronic sildenafil treatment inhibits monocrotaline-induced pulmonary hypertension in rats. Am J Respir Crit Care Med 2004; 169(1): 39–45.
11. Schafer S, Ellinghaus P, Janssen W, et al. Chronic inhibition of phosphodiesterase 5 does not prevent pressure-overload-induced right-ventricular remodelling. Cardiovasc Res 2009; cvp002.
12. Bhatia S, Frantz RP, Severson CJ, et al. Immediate and long-term hemodynamic and clinical effects of sildenafil in patients with pulmonary arterial hypertension receiving vasodilator therapy. Mayo Clin Proc 2003; 78(10):1207–1213.
13. Michelakis ED, Tymchak W, Noga M, et al. Long-term treatment with oral sildenafil is safe and improves functional capacity and hemodynamics in patients with pulmonary arterial hypertension. Circulation 2003; 108(17):2066–1069.
14. Ghofrani HA, Schermuly RT, Rose F, et al. Sildenafil for long-term treatment of nonoperable chronic thromboembolic pulmonary hypertension. Am J Respir Crit Care Med 2003; 167(8): 1139–1141.
15. Sastry BKS, Narasimhan C, Reddy NK, et al. Clinical efficacy of sildenafil in primary pulmonary hypertension: a randomized, placebo-controlled, double-blind, crossover study. J Am Coll Cardiol 2004; 43(7):1149–1153.
16. Galie N, Ghofrani HA, Torbicki A, et al., the Sildenafil Use in Pulmonary Arterial Hypertension (SUPER) Study Group. Sildenafil citrate therapy for pulmonary arterial hypertension. N Engl J Med 2005; 353(20):2148–2157.
17. Singh T, Rohit M, Grover A, et al. A randomized, placebo-controlled, double-blind, crossover study to evaluate the efficacy of oral sildenafil therapy in severe pulmonary artery hypertension. Am Heart J 2006; 151(4):851.e1–851.e5.
18. Wilkins MR, Paul GA, Strange JW, et al. Sildenafil versus Endothelin Receptor Antagonist for Pulmonary Hypertension (SERAPH) Study. Am J Respir Crit Care Med 2005; 171(11): 1292–1297.
19. Simonneau G, Rubin L, Galie N, et al., For the Pulmonary Arterial Hypertension Combination Study of Epoprostenol and Sildenafil (PACES) Study Group. Addition of sildenafil to long-term intravenous epoprostenol therapy in patients with pulmonary arterial hypertension. Ann Intern Med 2008; 149:521–530.
20. Badesch DB, Hill NS, Burgess G, et al. Sildenafil for pulmonary arterial hypertension associated with connective tissue disease. J Rheumatol 2007; 34(12):2417–2422.
21. Burgess G, Hoogkamer H, Collings L, et al. Mutual pharmacokinetic interactions between steady-state bosentan and sildenafil. Eur J Clin Pharmacol 2008; 64:43–50.
22. Cialis (tadalafil) Product Label. Food and Drugs Administration Website 2008 February 1. Available at: http://www.fda.gov/cder/drug/infopage/cialis/default.htm. Accessed February 1, 2008.
23. Palmieri EA, Affuso F, Fazio S, et al. Tadalafil in primary pulmonary arterial hypertension. Ann Intern Med 2004; 141(9):743–744.
24. Mukhopadhyay S, Sharma M, Ramakrishnan S, et al. Phosphodiesterase-5 inhibitor in Eisenmenger syndrome: A preliminary observational study. Circulation 2006; 114(17):1807–1810.

25. Galiè N, Brundage B, Ghofrani A, et al. Tadalafil therapy in pulmonary arterial hypertension: results of a randomized, double-blind, placebo-controlled, phase III study. Eur Heart J 2008; 29(abstr suppl):519.
26. Wrishko RE, Dingemanse J, Yu A, et al. Pharmacokinetic interaction between tadalafil and bosentan in healthy male subjects. J Clin Pharmacol 2008; 48:610–618.
27. Aizawa K, Hanaoka T, Kasai H, et al. Long-term vardenafil therapy improves hemodynamics in patients with pulmonary hypertension. Hypertens Res 2006; 29(2):123–128.

25

Medical Treatment of Pulmonary Arterial Hypertension: Endothelin Receptor Antagonists

KRISTINA KEMP and MARC HUMBERT
Université Paris Sud 11, Service de Pneumologie et Réanimation Respiratoire, Hôpital Antoine Béclère, Assistance Publique Hôpitaux de Paris, Clamart, France

I. Introduction

Pulmonary arterial hypertension (PAH) is a disease of the small pulmonary arteries, characterized by vascular proliferation and remodeling (1,2). It leads to progressive increase in pulmonary vascular resistance (PVR), ultimately causing right ventricular failure and death. Despite recent major improvements, no current treatments of PAH are curative for this devastating condition. However, in less than 20 years, treatment for patients with PAH has evolved from a state of no hope to one in which prolonged survival and improvements in quality of life can be achieved (1).

Three factors are thought to cause the increased PVR that characterizes PAH: vasoconstriction, remodeling of the pulmonary vessel wall, and thrombosis in situ (2). A substantial list of molecules have been implicated as putative candidates in the pathogenesis of PAH (2). Advances in the understanding of the molecular mechanisms involved in PAH suggest that endothelial dysfunction plays a key role in this condition (2). Chronically impaired production of vasoactive mediators such as nitric oxide and prostacyclin, along with prolonged overexpression of vasoconstrictors such as endothelin (ET)-1, not only affects vascular tone but also promotes vascular remodeling. Thus, these substances represent logical pharmacological targets (2).

II. Endothelin-1

ET-1 is a vasoconstrictor produced by vascular endothelial cells (2,3). It is a 21–amino acid peptide that was first characterized in 1988 (3). Big ET, the 38–amino acid precursor, is activated when hydrolyzed by ET-converting enzymes present within the lungs (4,5). Once activated, ET acts in an autocrine/paracrine role (6,7). Not only is ET-1 one of the most potent vasoconstrictors, it also has proliferative effects and is involved in inflammation and fibrosis (7–10) (Fig. 1). A variety of factors can stimulate the biosynthesis of ET, including hypoxia, ischemia, angiotensin II, vasopressin, catecholamines, cytokines, growth factors, and thrombin (7).

ET-1 has been implicated in the pathophysiology of PAH. Patients with PAH have been shown to have increased synthesis and expression of this important molecule,

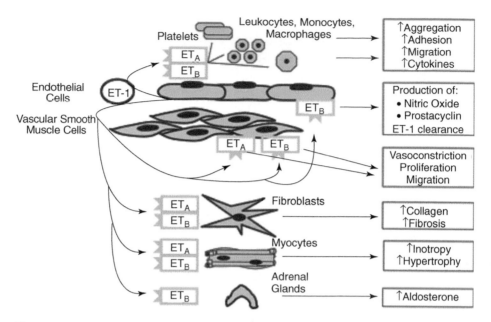

Figure 1 Schematic representation of ET-1 effects in different cell types. *Abbreviations*: ET-1, endothelin-1; ETA, endothelin-1 receptor A; ETB, endothelin-1 receptor B. *Source*: From Ref. 7.

particularly within the pulmonary microvasculature (11). ET-1 plasma concentrations correlate with indices of disease severity as assessed by exercise capacity and hemodynamic parameters (12) (Fig. 2). Therefore, there has been interest in modulating the actions of ET-1 for treatment of PAH via receptor antagonism.

III. Endothelin Receptors

ET-1 binds within the lung by one of two receptors known as endothelin receptor A (ETA) and endothelin receptor B (ETB), both of which belong to the G protein–coupled receptors (13). ETA and ETB are expressed on smooth muscle cells and cardiac myocytes, however, only ETB receptors are expressed on endothelial cells (14).

Activation of ETA and ETB receptors causes sustained vasoconstriction and proliferation of vascular smooth muscular cells within the pulmonary arteries. ETB receptors also mediate pulmonary ET clearance and induce endothelial cell production of local mediators of vascular tone, including nitric oxide and prostacyclin (15).

IV. Endothelin Receptor Antagonists

Presently, there are several ET receptor antagonists available for treatment of PAH. They are differentiated by their affinities for ETA and ETB blockade. Bosentan was the first available ET receptor antagonist and is a dual or nonselective blocker, with an

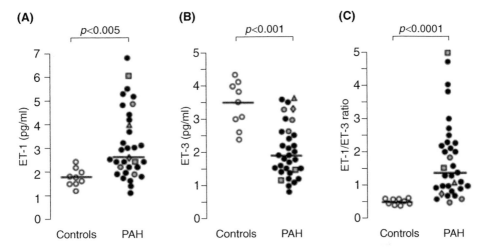

Figure 2 ET-1 and ET-3 plasma concentrations and ET-1/ET-3 ratio in control subjects and patients with PAH. (**A**) ET-1 plasma concentrations were measured in control subjects ($n = 9$) and in patients with PAH ($n = 26$). In patients with PAH, ET-1 plasma concentrations were increased in comparison with control subjects ($p < 0.005$, Mann-Whitney U test). (**B**) ET-3 plasma concentrations were measured in control subjects ($n = 9$) and in subjects with PAH ($n = 26$). In patients with PAH, ET-3 plasma concentrations were decreased in comparison with control subjects ($p < 0.001$, Mann-Whitney U test). (**C**) ET-1/ET-3 ratio was defined as the ratio of ET-1 plasma concentrations to ET-3 plasma concentrations. ET-1/ET-3 ratio was calculated in control subjects ($n = 9$) and in patients with PAH ($n = 26$). In patients with PAH, ET-1/ET-3 ratio was increased in comparison with control subjects ($p < 0.0001$, Mann-Whitney U test). Measurements in control subjects (*open circles*). Measurements in subjects with idiopathic, familial, or appetite suppressant–associated PAH (*black circles*). Measurements in PAH associated with other conditions (*gray shapes*) [PAH associated with scleroderma (*square*), portopulmonary hypertension (*circle*), HIV-associated PAH (*triangle*), and veno-occlusive disease (*diamond*)]. *Abbreviation*: ET, endothelin. *Source*: From Ref. 12.

ETA/ETB affinity ratio of approximately 40:1 (16). Sitaxsentan is considered an ETA selective antagonist with ETA/ETB affinity ratio of approximately 6000:1 (17). Ambrisentan is another ETA selective antagonist with ETA/ETB affinity ratio of 77:1 (18). All three of these agents have been evaluated with randomized clinical trials and are presented below.

V. Bosentan

Bosentan is a dual ETA and ETB receptor antagonist. An initial clinical study with bosentan showed favorable hemodynamic effects with decreased PVR (19). The phase II trial was a randomized, double-blind, placebo-controlled, multicenter study (study 351), which evaluated the effects of bosentan on exercise capacity and hemodynamics in 32 patients with severe idiopathic PAH or PAH associated with scleroderma (20).

Enrolled patients were in New York Heart Association (NYHA) functional class III and were treated for 12 weeks with oral bosentan 62.5 mg b.i.d. for four weeks, followed by 125 mg b.i.d. Results showed that the six-minute walk distance (6MWD) significantly improved by 70 m in the bosentan arm, whereas no improvement was seen with placebo (20). The difference between treatment arms in the mean change in the 6MWD was 76 ± 31 m (mean $\pm$ SEM) in favor of bosentan. Bosentan also improved hemodynamic parameters as the cardiac index improved, with the mean difference at week 12 between treatment groups of 1.0 ± 0.2 L/min/m^2 (mean $\pm$ SEM) in favor of bosentan (20). Bosentan decreased PVR by 223 dyne.sec/cm^5, whereas it increased with placebo by 191 dyne.sec/cm^5. Bosentan also decreased the mean pulmonary artery pressure and the mean right atrial pressure, and both variables increased in the placebo group. The functional class improved in patients treated with bosentan. The medication was tolerated, however, there were asymptomatic increases in hepatic aminotransferases observed in two bosentan-treated patients, but these normalized without discontinuation or change of dose (20).

Subsequently, BREATHE-1, a phase III clinical trial, was performed (21). This double-blind, placebo-controlled study evaluated bosentan in 213 patients with PAH (idiopathic or associated with connective tissue disease), who were randomized to placebo, bosentan 125 or 250 mg b.i.d. (following 62.5 mg b.i.d. for four weeks), for a minimum of 16 weeks at target dose. End points were change in 6MWD, changes in Borg dyspnea index, NYHA functional class, and time to clinical worsening. Patients had symptomatic, severe PAH (NYHA functional class III–IV) despite treatment with anticoagulants and/or vasodilators, diuretics, cardiac glycosides, or supplemental oxygen and had a 6MWD between 150 and 450 m. The majority of patients enrolled (195 out of 213) were in NYHA functional class III. At week 16, patients treated with bosentan improved the 6MWD by 36 m, whereas deterioration (-8 m) was seen with placebo, giving a significant mean 6MWD difference between treatment groups of 44 m in favor of bosentan (21) (Fig. 3). In subgroup analysis, patients with idiopathic PAH improved their walk distance with bosentan treatment, however, in scleroderma patients, bosentan prevented deterioration as compared with placebo. No dose-response relation for efficacy could be ascertained. Bosentan significantly increased the time to clinical worsening as compared with placebo.

Abnormal hepatic function, as indicated by elevated levels of alanine aminotransferase (ALT) and/or aspartate aminotransferase (AST), occurred more frequently in the bosentan group. Abnormal hepatic function $>3 \times$ the upper limit of normal values was dose dependent, reported more frequently in the 250 mg b.i.d. bosentan group over the 125 mg b.i.d. dosage group (14% vs. 4%, respectively) (21). Two patients (3%) in the 125 mg b.i.d. group and five (7%) in the 250 mg b.i.d. group experienced hepatic transferase elevations of over eight times the upper limit of normal. The most frequent hepatic function abnormalities were transient except in three patients who were in the high-dosage bosentan group. These patients were withdrawn prematurely from the study. There were three patient deaths during the course of the study; two in the placebo group and one in the 125 mg bosentan group. Given the results of this study, bosentan 125 mg b.i.d. was given approval.

More long-term observational data are available for the 169 patients enrolled in study 351 and BREATHE-1 receiving bosentan treatment (22). After 12 and 24 months of treatment with bosentan as first-line therapy, with transition or addition of alternative

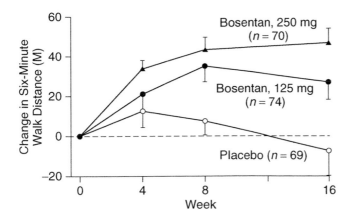

Figure 3 Mean (±SE) change in six-minute walk distance from baseline to week 16 in the placebo and bosentan groups. $p < 0.01$ for the comparison between the 125-mg dose of bosentan and placebo, and $p < 0.001$ for the comparison between the 250-mg dose and placebo by the Mann-Whitney U test. There was no significant difference between the two bosentan groups ($p = 0.18$ by the Mann-Whitney U test). *Source*: From Ref. 21.

therapies as required, 96% and 89% of patients remained alive, respectively. Another study compared survival in patients with class III idiopathic PAH treated with first-line bosentan with that in a historical cohort of patients started on epoprostenol (23). Survival estimates after one and two years were 97% and 91%, respectively, in the 139 patients in the bosentan-treated cohort and 91% and 84% in the 346 patients in the epoprostenol cohort. Baseline characteristics suggested that the epoprostenol cohort had more severe disease, and no evidence was found to suggest that initial treatment with bosentan, followed by or with the addition of other treatment, if needed, adversely affected the long-term outcome when compared with initial epoprostenol therapy (23).

As BREATHE-1 evaluated patients with more advanced PAH as noted by the NYHA functional classes III and IV, the EARLY study was performed to evaluate the effects of bosentan with milder disease (24). This double-blind, placebo-controlled study evaluated bosentan in 185 patients with NYHA functional class II PAH due to idiopathic, familial, anorexigen, human immunodeficiency virus (HIV), connective tissue/autoimmune, congenital heart defects. Patients were required to have a 6MWD of <500 m or <80% of their normal predicted value. The coprimary end points were PVR and 6MWD. The results indicated that at six months, the mean PVR was 83.2% of the baseline value in the bosentan group and 107.5% in the placebo group, giving a statistically significant treatment effect of −22.6% (24). The 6MWD did not show a statistically significant improvement, however, the placebo group did show a decline. Regarding secondary outcomes, NYHA functional class and time to clinical worsening remained stable in the bosentan group but deteriorated in the placebo group. There were also statistically significant reductions in plasma concentrations of N terminal (NT)-pro-BNP (brain natriuretic peptide) and improvement in SF-36 health transition index in bosentan-treated patients as compared with patients receiving placebo (24). Patients received concomitant sildenafil in 15% and 14% for each of the bosentan and placebo groups, respectively. Despite treatment with sildenafil, the benefit of bosentan on the pulmonary hemodynamics was maintained (24). The study was not adequately powered to evaluate monotherapy effectiveness in comparison with dual therapy with bosentan and sildenafil. The safety profile of bosentan showed elevation in aminotransferases of >3 × the upper limit of normal in 12 patients (13%) of bosentan-treated patients. These increases returned to normal in all patients, without intervention, after dose reduction, or with discontinuation of bosentan treatment. There were two deaths during the study, one in each arm.

As hepatic side effects had been observed with administration of bosentan therapy, European authorities required the introduction of a post-marketing surveillance system to obtain further data on its safety profile (25). After bosentan received approval for treatment of PAH in the European Union, a prospective, internet-based post-marketing surveillance system was developed to evaluate further safety data (25). Within 30 months, 4994 patients were included, representing 79% of patients receiving bosentan in Europe. A total of 4623 patients were naïve to treatment, and 352 had elevated aminotransferases. This corresponds to an annualized rate of 10.1% (25). Bosentan was discontinued in 150 bosentan-naïve patients (3.2%) because of elevated aminotransferases. Reversal of aminotransferase elevation occurred in all cases. Monthly liver function tests are recommended while on bosentan therapy.

Bosentan therapy has been evaluated in children (26). In an open-label study, 19 pediatric patients with idiopathic PAH or PAH related to congenital heart defects were treated with bosentan therapy adjusted according to weight (26). No patients had Eisenmenger syndrome, and approximately half of the patients were on stable doses of epoprostenol. Patients were predominantly NYHA functional class II (15/19). Results showed that pulmonary hemodynamics significantly improved when compared with baseline after 12 weeks of treatment, as mean pulmonary artery pressure fell by 8.0 mmHg and PVR index fell by 300 dyne.sec/cm^5/m^2. A retrospective trial evaluating the long-term effects of bosentan included 86 children with IPAH or PAH associated with congenital heart disease or connective tissue disease who received bosentan treatment (27). Patients were permitted stable doses of concomitant intravenous epoprostenol or subcutaneous treprostinil. The median exposure to bosentan was 14 months, and at the cutoff date, 79% of patients were still treated with bosentan. In 90% of the patients, NYHA functional class improved (46%) or was unchanged (44%) with bosentan treatment. Mean pulmonary artery pressure and PVR decreased, and Kaplan-Meier survival estimates at one and two years were 98% and 91%, respectively.

BREATHE-5 evaluated bosentan therapy in a multicenter, double-blind, randomized, and placebo-controlled study in patients with NYHA functional class III Eisenmenger syndrome (28). Fifty-four patients were randomized 2:1 to bosentan versus placebo for 16 weeks. Results indicate that, when compared with placebo, bosentan did not worsen oxygen saturation (+1%), reduced PVR (−472 dyne.sec/cm^5/m^2), decreased mean pulmonary arterial pressure (−5.5 mmHg), and increased exercise capacity (+32 m). Four patients discontinued because of adverse events, two (5%) in the bosentan arm and two (12%) in the placebo arm.

BREATHE-4 was an open multicenter study of bosentan therapy in 16 patients with HIV-associated PAH (29). Results indicate improvements in exercise capacity, NYHA functional class, quality of life, and cardiopulmonary hemodynamics (29). There appeared to be no significant impact on the control of HIV infection, and the safety profile was within the range of previous studies with bosentan therapy.

BENEFIT evaluated bosentan in a double-blind, randomized, placebo-controlled study in chronic thromboembolic pulmonary hypertension (CTEPH) (30). Patients were enrolled if they had CTEPH considered either inoperable or persistent/recurrent pulmonary hypertension >6 months after pulmonary endarterectomy (PEA). The study enrolled 157 patients, 80 in the placebo arm and 77 in the bosentan arm. Just over one quarter of patients had previous PEA at entry. After 16 weeks, a statistically significant mean treatment effect was noted in the PVR between bosentan and placebo (−24.1%) (30). Mean change in exercise capacity was not significantly changed between groups (+2.2 m). The secondary end points of total pulmonary resistance and cardiac index significantly improved, however, the NYHA functional class and time to clinical worsening were not significantly affected by treatment. The results do not explain why the hemodynamic improvements did not translate into a favorable effect on exercise capacity, and the authors conclude that a greater understanding of the disease is required (30).

VI. Sitaxsentan

Sitaxsentan is a selective ETA receptor antagonist. An open-label pilot study showed beneficial effects of sitaxsentan on 6MWD exercise capacity and hemodynamics (31). However, an important safety signal of acute hepatitis was identified, with one fatality, which was thought to represent nonlinear pharmacokinetics of sitaxsentan at higher doses.

STRIDE-1 was a randomized, double-blind, placebo-controlled trial where 178 NYHA functional class II, III, and IV patients with idiopathic PAH, PAH related to connective tissue disease, or PAH related to congenital systemic to pulmonary shunts were equally randomized to receive placebo, sitaxsentan 100 mg, or sitaxsentan 300 mg po once daily (32). In this study, sitaxsentan failed to improve VO_2 (primary end point), while it significantly improved secondary end points such as 6MWD and NYHA functional class after 12 weeks of treatment in both the 100-mg and 300-mg groups. The 6MWD treatment effect in the sitaxsentan group was +35 m for the 100-mg dose and +33 m for the 300-mg dose. PVR significantly decreased with sitaxsentan treatment (mean ± SD for 100-mg group, 1025 ± 694 to 805 ± 553 dyne.sec/cm⁵; and for 300-mg group, 946 ± 484 to 753 ± 524 dyne.sec/cm⁵) and increased with placebo (911 ± 484 to 960 ± 535 dyne.sec/cm⁵). Cardiac index did not change after 12 weeks of placebo but increased with sitaxsentan treatment (100 mg, 2.4 ± 0.8 to 2.7 ± 0.8 L/min/m²; and 300 mg, 2.3 ± 0.7 to 2.7 ⊥ 0.9 L/min/m²). NYHA functional class improved in 16 out of 55 (29%) patients in the 100-mg group and in 19 out of 63 (30%) patients in the 300-mg group, but only 9 out of 60 (15%) patients in the placebo group.

The most frequently reported clinical adverse events with sitaxsentan treatment, experienced more frequently by the treatment group than by the placebo group, were headache, peripheral edema, nausea, nasal congestion, and dizziness. The most frequently reported laboratory adverse event was increased international normalized ratio (INR) or prothrombin time (PT), related to sitaxsentan's inhibitory effect on the CYP2C9 P450 enzyme, the principal hepatic enzyme involved in the metabolism of warfarin. The incidence was higher in the 300-mg group. This drug interaction necessitates a dose reduction of warfarin and careful follow-up of the INR. The incidence of

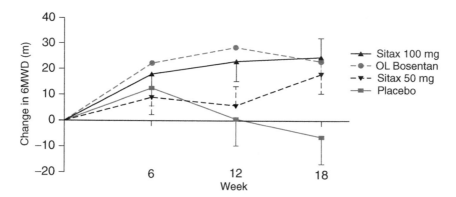

Figure 4 Mean (±SE) change in 6MWD from baseline to week 18 in the placebo, 50 mg sitaxsentan, 100 mg sitaxsentan, and OL bosentan groups. $p = 0.03$ (95% confidence interval 5.37, 57.44) for comparison between the 100-mg dose of sitaxsentan and placebo; $p = 0.05$ for OL bosentan versus placebo; and $p = 0.07$ for 50 mg sitaxsentan versus placebo. *Abbreviations*: 6MWD, six-minute walk distance; OL, open-label. *Source*: From Ref. 33.

elevated aminotransferase values of $>3 \times$ the upper limit of normal was 3% for the placebo group, 0% for the 100-mg group, and 10% for the 300-mg group.

  STRIDE-2 was a second randomized, double-blind, placebo-controlled trial that evaluated 247 patients (245 patients treated) with blinded sitaxsentan 50 mg or 100 mg, open-label bosentan, or blinded placebo (33). Included patients carried a diagnosis of idiopathic PAH, PAH associated with connective tissue disease, or congenital heart disease, and were in NYHA functional class II, III and IV. After 18 weeks, patients treated with sitaxsentan 100 mg had a significantly increased 6MWD (31.4 m) compared with the placebo group, and improved functional class. The placebo-subtracted treatment effect for sitaxsentan 50 mg was 24.2 m and for open-label bosentan was 29.5 m (Fig. 4) (33). Time to clinical worsening was not significantly improved with sitaxsentan. The incidence of elevated hepatic transaminases ($>3 \times$ the upper limit of normal) was 6% for placebo, 5% for sitaxsentan 50 mg, 3% for sitaxsentan 100 mg, and 11% for bosentan.

  STRIDE-2X is a one-year, prospective, open-label observation of outcomes and survival as an extension of STRIDE-2 (34): 229 patients were enrolled, and patients initially receiving sitaxsentan 50 mg were excluded from the analysis. Of the 92 patients receiving sitaxsentan 100 mg, overall one-year survival was 96%, and there was a 34% risk of a clinical-worsening event by one year. There was a 6% risk of elevated aminotransferases $>3 \times$ the upper limit of normal with a 3% cumulative risk of discontinuation at one year due to elevated aminotransferases. There was an overall 15% risk of discontinuation due to adverse events in the 100 mg sitaxsentan group.

VII. Ambrisentan

Ambrisentan is another selective ETA receptor antagonist. In contrast to sitaxsentan, ambrisentan is propanoic acid based. A phase II, double-blind, dose-ranging study evaluated the efficacy and safety of four doses of ambrisentan (1, 2.5, 5, or 10 mg) once daily for 12 weeks in patients with PAH (35). Sixty-four patients with idiopathic PAH or PAH associated with connective tissue disease, anorexigen use, or HIV infection were included. The 6MWD significantly improved with ambrisentan (+36.1 m), with similar increases for each dose group (range +33.9 to +38.1 m). Other parameters, including the Borg dyspnea index, NYHA functional class, subject global assessment, mean pulmonary arterial pressure, and cardiac index, also improved. Adverse events were mild and unrelated to dose, including the incidence of elevated serum aminotransferase concentrations >3 times the upper limit of normal (incidence of 3.1%).

ARIES-1 and ARIES-2 were concurrent phase III randomized, double-blind, placebo-controlled studies evaluating ambrisentan in PAH (idiopathic or associated with connective tissue disease, HIV infection, or anorexigen use) (36). ARIES-1 enrolled 202 patients who were allocated to placebo, ambrisentan 5 or 10 mg po daily, while ARIES-2 enrolled 192 patients who were allocated to placebo, ambrisentan 2.5 or 5 mg po daily. After 12 weeks, the 6MWD significantly increased in all ambrisentan groups; mean placebo-corrected treatment effects were 31 m and 51 m for the 5- and 10 mg ambrisentan groups, respectively, in ARIES-1, while 6MWD significantly increased to 32 m and 59 m for the 2.5 and 5 mg ambrisentan groups, respectively, in ARIES-2 (36) (Fig. 5). Improvements in time to clinical worsening (ARIES-2), NYHA functional class (ARIES-1), SF-36 (ARIES-2), Borg dyspnea score (both studies), and B-type natriuretic peptide (both studies) were observed (36). None of the patients who received ambrisentan therapy developed aminotransferase levels >3 times the upper limit of normal. The long-term treatment effect was evaluated in an open-label extension of the ARIES-1 and ARIES-2 trials (36): 280 patients completed 48 weeks of treatment with ambrisentan monotherapy. From baseline, the 6MWD increased 39 m from baseline in this group.

VIII.   Safety

ET receptor antagonists are generally well tolerated. The effect on increasing hepatic aminotransferases is recognized as a class effect and requires monthly monitoring of these markers. This effect appears less frequent with ambrisentan, although real-life data are still missing. As hemoglobin can fall with treatment, as a class effect, it is recommended that this is checked after one and three months of treatment. Sitaxsentan does have a drug interaction with warfarin, and therefore, a dose reduction in warfarin is recommended with this treatment. ET receptor antagonists may interact with other medications, and with combination therapy, there is a possible interaction between bosentan and sildenafil. However, hundreds of patients are currently treated with a combination of bosentan and sildenafil, and no safety signal has been detected in recent post-marketing studies (25).

ET receptor antagonists are potentially teratogenic. ET-1 receptor antagonists, as a class, have consistently produced teratogenic effects in animals. Pregnancy must be excluded before initiation of treatment and prevented thereafter by use of at least two reliable methods of contraception unless patients have had a tubal sterilization or copper T 380A intrauterine device (IUD) or LNg-20 IUD inserted. Because of drug-to-drug interaction, oral contraceptives are likely to be ineffective in patients receiving bosentan or sitaxsentan.

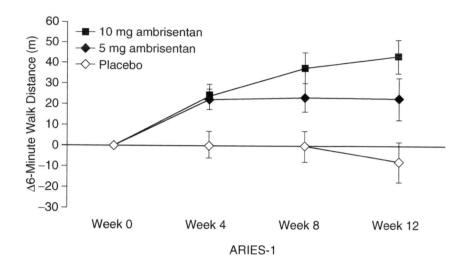

ARIES-1

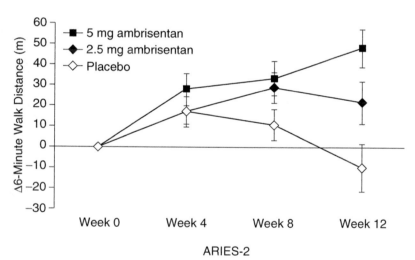

ARIES-2

Figure 5 Mean (±SE) changes from baseline in the six-minute walk distance at week 12 in the placebo and ambrisentan groups of ARIES-1 and ARIES-2. Comparisons of individual ambrisentan dose groups with placebo for change in six-minute walk distance were analyzed by use of a Wilcoxon test with stratification by cause. For ARIES-1, $p = 0.008$, 5-mg ambrisentan once daily versus placebo; $p < 0.001$, 10-mg ambrisentan once daily versus placebo. For ARIES-2, $p = 0.022$, 2.5-mg ambrisentan once daily versus placebo; $p < 0.001$, 5-mg ambrisentan once daily versus placebo. A total of 201 patients in ARIES-1 and 192 patients in ARIES-2 were included in these intention-to-treat analyses. *Source*: From Ref. 36.

IX. Conclusion

In conclusion, bosentan, sitaxsentan, and ambrisentan have all undergone randomized controlled trials, indicating benefit in the management of PAH. These agents have variable approval worldwide. There are also other agents in current development, which have not been discussed in the present chapter. The question of superiority between these therapies is debated but unknown as no good-quality long-term studies comparing agents are available. The issue of ETA/ETB selectivity also remains a much-discussed point concerning choice of treatment. The choice of ET receptor antagonist treatment at the present time appears to surround safety and side effect profiles. As clinical experience continues to expand and also with the advent of high-quality long-term studies, treatment decisions will hopefully be more clearly defined.

References

1. Humbert M, Sitbon O, Simonneau G. Treatment of pulmonary arterial hypertension. N Engl J Med 2004; 351:1425–1436.
2. Humbert M, Morrell NW, Archer SL, et al. Cellular and molecular pathobiology of pulmonary arterial hypertension. J Am Coll Cardiol 2004; 43:13S–24S.
3. Yanagisawa M, Kurihara H, Kimura S, et al. A novel potent vasoconstrictor peptide produced by vascular endothelial cells. Nature 1998; 332:411–415.
4. Takahashi M, Matshushita Y, Iijima Y, et al. Purification and characterization of endothelin-converting enzyme from rat lung. J Biol Chem 1993; 268:21394–21398.
5. Inoue A, Yanagisawa M, Kimura S, et al. The human endothelin family: three structurally and pharmacologically distinct isopeptides predicted by three separate genes. Proc Natl Acad Sci U S A 1989; 86:2863–2867.
6. Eguchi S, Hirata Y, Imai T, et al. Endothelin-1 as an autocrine growth factor for endothelial cells. J Cardiovasc Pharmacol 1995; 26:S279–S283.
7. Galiè N, Manes A, Branzi A. The endothelin system in pulmonary arterial hypertension. Cardiovasc Res 2004; 61:227–237.
8. Davie N, Hallen SJ, Upton PD, et al. ETA and ETB receptors modulate the proliferation of human smooth muscle cells. Am J Respir Crit Care Med 2002; 165:398–405.
9. Shi-Wen X, Chen Y, Denton CP, et al. Endothelin-1 promotes myofibroblast induction through the ETA receptor via a rac/phosphoinositide 3-kinase/Akt-dependent pathway and is essential for the enhanced contractile phenotype of fibrotic fibroblasts. Mol Biol Cell 2004; 15:2707–2719.
10. Préfontaine A, Calderone A, Dupuis J. Role of endothelin receptors on basal and endothelin-1-stimulated lung myofibroblast proliferation. Can J Physiol Pharmacol 2008; 86:337–342.
11. Giaid A, Yanagisawa M, Langleben D, et al. Expression of endothelin-1 in the lungs of patients with pulmonary hypertension. N Engl J Med 1993; 328:1732–1739.
12. Montani D, Souza R, Binkert C, et al. Endothelin-1/endothelin-3 ratio: a potential prognostic factor of pulmonary arterial hypertension. Chest 2007; 131:101–108.
13. Masuda Y, Miyazaki H, Kondoh M, et al. Two different forms of endothelin receptors in rat lungs. FEBS Lett 1989; 257:208–210.
14. Eguchi S, Kozuka M, Hirose S, et al. Identification of G protein-coupled endothelin receptors in cultured bovine endothelial cells. Biochem Biophys Res Commun 1991; 174:1343–1346.
15. Humbert M, Simonneau G. Drug Insight: endothelin-receptor antagonists for pulmonary arterial hypertension in systemic rheumatic diseases. Nat Clin Pract Rheumatol 2005; 1:93–101.
16. Clozel M. Effects of bosentan on cellular processes involved in pulmonary arterial hypertension: do they explain the long-term benefit? Ann Med 2003; 35:605–613.

17. Wu C, Chan MF, Stavros F, et al. Discovery of TBC11251, a potent, long acting, orally active endothelin receptor-A selective antagonist. J Med Chem 1997; 40:1690–1697.

18. Vatter H, Zimmermann M, Jung C, et al. Effect of the novel endothelin (A) receptor antagonist LU 208075 on contraction and relaxation of isolated rat basilar artery. Clin Sci (Lond) 2002; 103:408S–413S.

19. Williamson DJ, Wallman LL, Jones R, et al. Hemodynamic effects of bosentan, an endothelin receptor antagonist, in patients with pulmonary hypertension. Circulation 2000; 102:411–418.

20. Channick RN, Simonneau G, Sitbon O, et al. Effects of the dual endothelin-receptor antagonist bosentan in patients with pulmonary hypertension: a randomised placebo-controlled study. Lancet 2001; 358:1119–1123.

21. Rubin LJ, Badesch DB, Barst RJ, et al. Bosentan therapy for pulmonary arterial hypertension. N Engl J Med 2002; 346:896–903.

22. McLaughlin VV, Sitbon O, Badesch DB, et al. Survival with first-line bosentan in patients with primary pulmonary hypertension. Eur Respir J 2005; 25:244–249.

23. Sitbon O, McLaughlin VV, Badesch DB, et al. Survival in patients with class III idiopathic pulmonary arterial hypertension treated with first line oral bosentan compared with an historical cohort of patients started on intravenous epoprostenol. Thorax 2005; 60:1025–1030.

24. Galiè N, Rubin LJ, Hoeper MM, et al. Treatment of patients with mildly symptomatic pulmonary arterial hypertension with bosentan (EARLY study): a double-blind, randomised controlled trial. Lancet 2008; 371:2093–2100.

25. Humbert M, Segal ES, Kiely DG, et al. Results of European post-marketing surveillance of bosentan in pulmonary hypertension. Eur Resp J 2007; 30:338–343.

26. Barst RJ, Dunbar D, Dingemanse J, et al. Pharmacokinetics, safety, and efficacy of bosentan in pediatric patients with pulmonary arterial hypertension. Clin Pharmacol Ther 2003; 73:372–382.

27. Rosenzweig EB, Ivy DD, Widlitz A, et al. Effects of long-term bosentan in children with pulmonary arterial hypertension. J Am Coll Cardiol 2005; 46:697–704.

28. Galiè N, Beghetti M, Gatzoulis MA, et al. Bosentan therapy in patients with Eisenmenger syndrome: a multicenter, double-blind, randomized, placebo-controlled study. Circulation 2006; 114:48–54.

29. Sitbon O, Gressin V, Speich R, et al. Bosentan for the treatment of human immunodeficiency virus-associated pulmonary arterial hypertension. Am J Respir Crit Care Med 2004; 170:1212–1217.

30. Jais X, D'Armini AM, Jansa P, et al. Bosentan for Treatment of inoperable chronic thromboembolic pulmonary hypertension (BENEFiT), a randomized, placebo-controlled trial. J Am Coll Cardiol 2008; 52:2127–2134.

31. Barst RJ, Rich S, Widlitz A, et al. Clinical efficacy of sitaxsentan, an endothelin-A receptor antagonist, in patients with pulmonary arterial hypertension: open-label pilot study. Chest 2002; 121:1860–1868.

32. Barst RJ, Langleben D, Frost A, et al. Sitaxsentan therapy for pulmonary arterial hypertension. Am J Respir Crit Care Med 2004; 169:441–447.

33. Barst RJ, Langleben D, Badesch D, et al. Treatment of pulmonary arterial hypertension with the selective endothelin-A receptor antagonist sitaxsentan. J Am Coll Cardiol 2006; 47:2049–2056.

34. Benza RL, Barst RJ, Galiè N, et al. Sitaxsentan for the treatment of pulmonary arterial hypertension: a 1-year, prospective, open-label observation of outcome and survival. Chest 2008; 134:775–782.

35. Galiè N, Badesch D, Oudiz R, et al. Ambrisentan therapy for pulmonary arterial hypertension. J Am Coll Cardiol 2005; 46:529–535.

36. Galiè N, Olschewski H, Oudiz RJ, et al. Ambrisentan for the treatment of pulmonary arterial hypertension: results of the ambrisentan in pulmonary arterial hypertension, randomized, double-blind, placebo-controlled, multicenter, efficacy (ARIES) study 1 and 2. Circulation 2008; 117:3010–3019.

26
Medical Treatment of PAH: Combination Therapy, Novel Agents, Future Directions, and Current Recommendations

LEWIS J. RUBIN
University of California, San Diego School of Medicine, La Jolla, California, U.S.A.

SEAN P. GAINE
Mater Misericordiae University Hospital, University College Dublin, Dublin, Ireland

I. Introduction

Despite the remarkable advances in the development of targeted therapies for pulmonary arterial hypertension (PAH) over the past decade, a substantial number of patients either manifest an incomplete response to monotherapy or fail to respond altogether. This is not particularly surprising, given the likelihood that multiple pathogenic pathways are operative in PAH (1). As in other complex medical conditions in which multiple interfacing pathways play pathogenic roles, such as HIV infection, cancer, and congestive heart failure, a treatment strategy that targets several pathways has appeal in PAH; although only a handful of clinical trials using combination strategies have been completed to date and critical questions remain unanswered, combination therapy is widely used in clinical practice. In this chapter we will review current recommendations, explore the role of combination therapy and discuss future targets for drug development in PAH.

II. Combination Therapy

To date, most clinical trials focused on combination therapy have implemented an add-on strategy: There have been three small and two large placebo-controlled combination therapy trials. The first trial addressing combination therapy (BREATHE-2), and the only one thus far implementing a de novo combination strategy, evaluated functional class III or IV patients with either idiopathic pulmonary arterial hypertension (IPAH) or PAH related to connective tissue diseases starting on intravenous epoprostenol and randomized them to also receive bosentan or placebo (2). This small underpowered study failed to demonstrate significant improvement in exercise capacity, although more patients receiving the combination achieved a >30% reduction in total pulmonary resistance compared with the epoprostenol alone group. More recently, the STEP study, a U.S. multicenter randomized, placebo-controlled double-blind study, evaluated the addition of inhaled iloprost to bosentan in persistently symptomatic patients (NYHA functional class III or IV) (3). After 12 weeks, the 6-minute walk distance improved by 30 m in the iloprost group and 4 m in the placebo group, a treatment effect that achieved borderline statistical significance. There were, however, significant improvements in NYHA functional class, time to clinical worsening, and postinhalation mean pulmonary artery pressure and pulmonary vascular resistance with add-on iloprost. Subsequently, a European study with a similar design was terminated early due to lack of effect (4). Two small uncontrolled trials evaluating the effects of inhaled treprostinil added to background therapy with bosentan in patients with persistent functional class III symptoms demonstrated improved hemodynamics and exercise capacity (5,6), and preliminary results of a large multicenter placebo-controlled trial of add-on inhaled treprostinil to background oral therapy with either bosentan or sildenafil demonstrated modest but statistically significant improvement in six-minute walk distance and reduction in N-terminal pro-BNP levels. The largest trial evaluating combination therapy performed to date is the PACES trial in which sildenafil or placebo was added to background intravenous epoprostenol (7). The addition of sildenafil resulted in improved exercise capacity, hemodynamics, clinical worsening, and survival. Interestingly, a post hoc analysis revealed that the subgroup in which the benefit in exercise capacity, but not survival, was observed was the least impaired (baseline 6-min walk > 325 m), while the survival benefit, but not exercise capacity benefit, was observed in the most impaired (baseline 6-min walk < 325 m). Of note, the dose of sildenafil used in this trial was 80 mg three times daily, which is not the approved dose for the treatment of PAH. Whether the impressive findings in this study are applicable to the use of approved doses of sildenafil is unknown.

The optimal timing of combination therapy remains unclear, but Hoeper and colleagues have developed an algorithm that utilizes assessment of parameters known to have prognostic significance to select the proper timing for additional therapy (Fig. 1) (8). These parameters include exercise capacity (both 6-min walk test and measurement of maximal oxygen consumption during cardiopulmonary exercise testing), systolic blood pressure, and assessment of functional class. Applying this algorithm to their decision making led to improved survival compared with matched historical controls from their center.

A number of unanswered questions remain concerning combination therapy for PAH that should be addressed in the future.

1. Which of the current targets of therapy are the most important to address as part of a combination strategy?
2. Is the initiation of a combination therapy strategy at the onset more effective than starting with monotherapy, and is this more important in patients with either certain forms of PAH or degrees of severity?
3. What are the most robust and meaningful endpoints for clinical trials assessing efficacy of combination therapies?

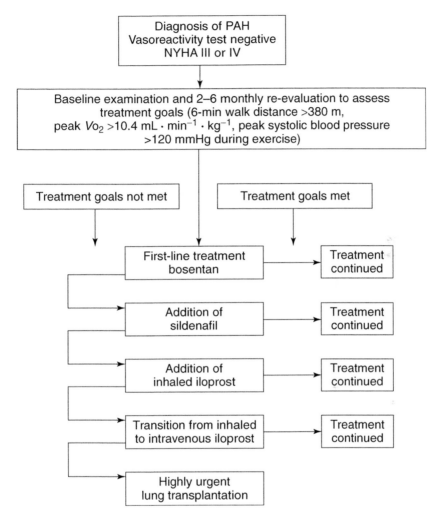

Figure 1 Goal-oriented treatment strategy for patients not initially requiring parenteral prostanoid therapy. *Source:* From Ref. 8.

III. Future Therapies

Future studies targeting newly identified alterations in endothelial and smooth muscle cell function may provide novel treatments. Several of the most promising targets are discussed below:

A. Serotonin Receptor and Transporter Function

Serotonin (5-hydroxytryptamine, 5-HT) is a potent vasoconstrictor and mitogen that has long been suspected to play a pathogenic role in PAH (9). Recent work suggests that

5-HT receptors may be upregulated in PAH, providing a novel therapeutic target since antagonists to these receptors have been developed (10). Others have shown that the serotonin transporter (SERT), a molecule that facilitates transmembrane transport of serotonin into the cell, is upregulated in PAH (11); additionally, the fenfluramine anorexigens, which are known to increase the risk of developing PAH, produce an upregulation of the SERT in vitro, supporting a pathogenic mechanism for this system in PAH (12). Drugs that downregulate the SERT, such as the selective serotonin reuptake inhibitors (SSRIs) that are used to treat depression, may be worth exploring as treatment options in the future.

B. Vasoactive Intestinal Polypeptide

Vasoactive intestinal polypeptide (VIP) is a neuropeptide that is produced by a variety of cells that has both potent vasodilating properties and cellular antiproliferative effects (13). VIP receptors appear to be upregulated in PAH, suggesting that this may be a compensatory mechanism in this disease. In a preliminary case series, eight patients with IPAH who were treated with inhaled VIP at doses of 200 μg four times daily showed marked clinical and hemodynamic improvement (14). Further studies confirming these encouraging preliminary findings and clarifying optimal dosing and long-term safety are being undertaken presently.

C. Rho Kinase Inhibitors

Rho kinase is part of a family of enzymes that is involved in the processes of cellular growth and regulation of smooth muscle tone (15). Studies in animal models of pulmonary hypertension suggest that fasudil, and inhibitor of Rho kinase, may ameliorate the hemodynamic and pathologic severity of pulmonary vascular injury (16), and provide a rationale for clinical development of this agent in PAH.

D. Inhibitors of Growth Factor Synthesis

PAH is characterized pathologically by uncontrolled angiogenesis, a process that is reminiscent of malignant transformation (17). In support of this concept, monoclonal expansion has been demonstrated in the plexiform lesion of IPAH (18). Imatinib, a tyrosine kinase inhibitor that is approved for the treatment of hematopoietic malignancies, produced improvement in a handful of PAH patients refractory of other available treatments (19), suggesting that this novel approach may be of benefit in PAH.

Adrenomedullin is a peptide that causes vasodilation and inhibits proliferation of pulmonary vascular smooth muscle cells (20). Both intravenous and inhaled adrenomedullin lower pulmonary vascular resistance in patients with IPAH (21,22). Long-term data are not available, but this substance also has potential as a future treatment for PAH.

E. Guanylate Cyclase Activators

Nitric oxide induces the synthesis of cyclic guanosine monophosphate (cGMP) by activating the soluble guanylate cyclase. Soluble guanylate cyclase stimulators have been shown to produce pulmonary vasodilation and augment the response to nitric oxide in experimental pulmonary hypertension (23), and a preliminary acute clinical study with BAY 63-2521 (riociguat) demonstrated improved pulmonary hemodynamic parameters (24) that warrant further investigation in larger studies.

F. Cell-Based Therapy

Several recent studies have demonstrated that infusions of endothelial progenitor cells in animal models of pulmonary hypertension attenuate the injury, particularly when these cells are transfected with nitric oxide synthase, the enzyme responsible for the generation of nitric oxide from L-arginine (25,26). Thus, while cell-based therapies have yet to fulfill their promise in other conditions, particularly in cardiovascular diseases, pilot safety and efficacy trials are now under way with progenitor cell infusions in patients with severe PAH refractory to medical therapy.

Drugs currently used to treat other conditions may have effects that are beneficial in PAH as well. For example, the hydroxymethylglutaryl coenzyme-A reductase inhibitors (statins) manifest pleiotropic effects that have been suggested to be responsible for a component of their benefit in atherosclerotic disease (27), and these agents attenuate the pulmonary arteriopathy induced by the administration of monocrotaline to experimental animals (28,29). A small clinical trial evaluating a statin for PAH is ongoing. Similarly, currently available platelet inhibitors (i.e., aspirin) and newer antithrombotic agents may have a role in the treatment of PAH, in light of the beneficial effects (and inherent risks) of anticoagulation with warfarin in idiopathic PAH.

IV. General Recommendations

With the advent of targeted therapies, the management of PAH has become more complex and challenging. Clinicians must choose the appropriate agents for initiation of therapy and identify the appropriate timing and selection of additional or alternative therapies. Several multidisciplinary evidence-based guidelines for the management of PAH have been published recently that assist the physician in formulating a management plan for patients with PAH of varying degrees of severity (30,31).

V. General Measures

General measures for patients with PAH include avoidance of environments and medications that can aggravate the condition, physical activity and rehabilitation, supplemental oxygen when hypoxemia is present, and the use of diuretics for peripheral edema or other signs of right heart failure. The role of anticoagulation remains controversial, particularly in forms of PAH other than IPAH, due to limited evidence from clinical studies; however most experts advocate the use of vitamin K antagonists, unless contraindicated, with a target INR of 2.0 to 2.5.

VI. Acute Vasodilator Testing

The rationale for vasodilator testing in PAH patients is based on the premise that acute responders are more likely to have a sustained beneficial response to oral calcium channel blockers (CCBs) than nonresponders and could, accordingly, be treated with these inexpensive drugs (31).

A. Agents for Acute Vasodilator Testing

Acute vasodilator testing is usually performed during the same procedure as the diagnostic catheterization. The ideal vasodilator agent for PAH is selective for the pulmonary circulation and has rapid onset and offset of effect. Acute vasodilator testing can be performed using inhaled nitric oxide (iNO), or intravenous prostacylin (prostaglandin I_2, epoprostenol) or adenosine (31). The choice of vasodilator remains one of physician preferences; however, one should not use nonselective and nontitratable agents such as CCBs or nitrates for acute vasodilator testing.

B. Definition of Responders to Acute Vasodilator Testing in PAH

Based largely on the findings of Sitbon et al. (32), the European Society of Cardiology and the American College of Chest Physicians guidelines define an acute response to acute vasodilator testing as: A decrease in mean pulmonary artery pressure of at least 10 mmHg to an absolute level of less than 40 mmHg *without* a decrease in cardiac output. Patients with PAH due to conditions other than IPAH have a very low rate of long-term responsiveness to oral CCB therapy. Accordingly, the value of acute testing in such patients is less clear and should be individualized. While these criteria do not identify all patients who may be responsive to long-term CCB therapy, they are sufficiently specific to identify patients who are unlikely to benefit from this form of therapy and for whom other treatments are indicated.

VII. Evidence-Based Treatment Algorithm

The primary goals of treatment in PAH patients are to improve symptoms and pulmonary hemodynamic derangements, to prevent disease progression, and, ideally, to improve survival.

A. Calcium Channel Blockers

The rationale for CCBs in PAH is based on the premise that vasoconstriction is a significant factor in the pathogenesis of pulmonary hypertension and that systemic vasodilator agents can exert similar effects on the pulmonary arteries. Early studies in a highly selected population of IPAH patients demonstrated a five-year survival of 95% in responders to CCBs (33); However, recent experience has shown that only approximately 5% to 10% of IPAH patients, and even fewer patients with other forms of PAH, are long-term responders to therapy with CCBs (32). Patients who meet the criteria for an "acute responder" to acute vasodilator testing may be treated initially with CCBs, but they should be followed closely since many patients lose responsiveness over time.

B. Prostanoids

Prostacyclin synthase is reduced in PAH patients, resulting in the inadequate production of prostacyclin I_2, a vasodilator with both antiplatelet and antiproliferative effects (34). Prostacyclin replacement therapy has been a mainstay of PAH therapy for over a decade. The three commercially available prostacyclin analogues, epoprostenol, treprostinil, and iloprost, are described in greater detail elsewhere in this book.

Epoprostenol

Epoprostenol is indicated for patients with functional class IV symptoms or those with functional class III symptoms that are refractory to nonparenteral therapy. Given its considerable complexity, epoprostenol use should be limited to centers experienced with its administration.

Treprostinil

Treprostinil is a stable prostacyclin analogue with a half-life of four hours that is approved for use either by intravenous or by subcutaneous continuous infusion in functional class II, III, and IV PAH, although it is almost never used in class II patients.

Iloprost

Iloprost is a prostacyclin analogue that can be delivered by nebulization and is indicated for functional class III and IV PAH that is refractory of background oral therapy.

C. Endothelin Receptor Antagonists

Endothelin-1 is a vasoconstrictor and a smooth muscle mitogen that is overproduced by the injured pulmonary vascular endothelium and therefore appears to contribute to the development of PAH. Three endothelin receptor antagonists (ERAs) are commercially available: one (bosentan) that is a dual ET_A and ET_B receptor antagonist, while the other two (sitaxsentan and ambrisentan) are more selective antagonists of the ET_A receptor. While there are no head-to-head studies comparing the efficacy or safety of these agents against each other, the general impression is that they are equally effective, but each has unique advantages and disadvantages. Accordingly, the choice of ERA to use is largely an individual one, based on interpretation of the evidence and clinical experience.

Hepatic toxicity is the most serious adverse effect of ERAs and, while its frequency varies from one drug to another, all patients receiving any ERA should undergo monthly blood tests of liver function to monitor for incipient drug-induced hepatic injury.

D. Phosphodiesterase Inhibitors

Nitric oxide (NO) is an endothelial-derived vasodilator and antiproliferative molecule whose pulmonary endothelial synthesis is diminished in PAH. The NO-mediated effects are due to activation of guanylate cyclase, which increases cGMP production. Cyclic GMP is rapidly degraded by phosphodiesterases. Phosphodiesterase inhibitors (PDEi), particularly those that inhibit phosphodiesterase type 5 (PDE-5), the primary PDE in pulmonary vascular smooth muscle, such as sildenafil and tadalafil, have been demonstrated to produce sustained benefit in PAH. Sildenafil, and more recently tadalafil, are approved as PAH therapy. Sildenafil has been shown to be effective both as a monotherapy and in combination with epoprostenol. There are no comparison studies of initial therapy using ERA or PDE5; accordingly, the choice of initial oral therapy-ERA or PDE5- is based on individual preference, cost, availability, and other individual clinical features.

References

1. Yuan JXJ, Rubin LJ. Pathogenesis of pulmonary artery hypertension: need for multiple hits. Circulation 2005; 111:534–538.
2. Humbert M, Barst RJ, Robbins IM, et al. Combination of bosentan with epoprostenol in pulmonary arterial hypertension: BREATHE-2. Eur Respir J 2004; 24:1–7.
3. McLaughlin VV, Oudiz RJ, Frost A, et al. Randomized study of adding to existing bosentan in pulmonary arterial hypertension. Am J Respir Crit Care Med 2006; 174:1257–1263.
4. Hoeper MM, Leuchte H, Halank M, et al. Combining inhaled iloprost with bosentan in patients with idiopathic pulmonary arterial hypertension. Eur Respir J 2006; 28:691–694.
5. Channick RN, Olschewski H, Seeger W, et al. Safety and efficacy of inhaled treprostinil as add-on therapy to bosentan in pulmonary arterial hypertension. J Am Coll Cardiol 2006; 48:1433–1437.
6. Voswinckel R, Enke B, Reichenberger F, et al. Favorable effects of inhaled treprostinil in severe pulmonary hypertension: results from randomized controlled pilot studies. J Am Coll Cardiol 2006; 48:1672–1681.
7. Simonneau G, Rubin LJ, Galiè N, et al. Safety and efficacy of the addition of sildenafil to long-term intravenous epoprostenol therapy in patients With pulmonary arterial hypertension: a randomized clinical trial. Ann Intern Med 2008; 149(8):521–530.
8. Hoeper MM, Markevych I, Spiekerkoetter E, et al. Goal-oriented treatment and combination therapy for pulmonary arterial hypertension. Eur Respir J 2005; 26:858–863.
9. Fanburg BL, Lee SL. A new role for an old molecule: serotonin as a mitogen. Am J Physiol 1997; 272:L795–L806.
10. MacLean MR, Herve P, Eddahibi S, et al. 5-hydroxytryptamine and the pulmonary circulation: receptors, transporters and relevance to pulmonary arterial hypertension. Br J Pharmacol 2000; 13:161–168.
11. Dempsie Y, Morecroft I, Welsh DJ, et al. Converging evidence in support of the serotonin hypothesis of dexfenfluramine-induced pulmonary hypertension with novel transgenic mice. Circulation 2008; 117:2928–2937.

12. Eddhaibi S, Humbert M, Fadel E, et al. Serotonin transporter overexpression is responsible for pulmonary artery smooth muscle hyperplasia in primary pulmonary hypertension. J Clin Invest 2001; 108:1141–1150.

13. Said SI. Mediators and modulators of pulmonary arterial hypertension. Am J Physiol Lung Cell Mol Physiol 2006; 291:547–558.

14. Petkov V, Mosgeoller W, Ziesche, R. et al. Vasoactive intestinal polypeptide as a new drug for treatment of primary pulmonary hypertension. J Clin Invest 2003; 111:1339–1146.

15. Oka M, Homma N, Taraseviciene-Stewart L, et al. Rho kinase-mediated vasoconstriction is important in severe occlusive pulmonary arterial hypertension in rats. Circ Res 2007; 100(6): 923–929.

16. Abe K, Shimokawa H, Morikawa K, et al. Long-term treatment with a Rho-kinase inhibitor improves monocrotaline-induced fatal pulmonary hypertension in rats. Circ Res 2004; 94(3): 385–393.

17. Schermuly RT, Dony E, Ghofrani HA, et al. Reversal of experimental pulmonary hypertension by PDGF inhibition. J Clin Invest 2005; 115:2811–2821.

18. Lee SD, Shroyer KR, Markham NE, et al. Monoclonal endothelial cell proliferation is present in primary but not secondary pulmonary hypertension. J Clin Invest 1998; 101(5):927–934.

19. Ghofrani HA, Seeger W, Grimminger F. Imatinib for the treatment of pulmonary arterial hypertension. N Engl J Med 2005; 353:1412–1413.

20. Nagaya N, Kangawa K. Adrenomedullin in the treatment of pulmonary hypertension. Peptides 2004; 25(11):2013–2018.

21. von der Hardt K, Kandler MA, Chada M, et al. Brief adrenomedullin inhalation leads to sustained reduction of pulmonary artery pressure. Eur Respir J 2004; 24(4):615–623.

22. Nagaya N, Nishikimi T, Uematsua M, et al. Haemodynamic and hormonal effects of adrenomedullin in patients with pulmonary hypertension. Heart 2000; 84:653–658.

23. Evgenov OV, Ichinose F, Evgenov NV, et al. Soluble guanylate cyclase activator reverses acute pulmonary hypertension and augments the pulmonary vasodilator response to inhaled nitric oxide in awake lambs. Circulation 2004; 110:2253–2259.

24. Grimminger F, Weimann G, Frey R, et al. First acute hemodynamic study of soluble guanylate cyclase stimulator riociguat in pulmonary hypertension. Eur Respir J 2009; 33(4):785–792.

25. Zhao YD, Courtman DW, Deng Y, et al. Rescue of monocrotaline-induced pulmonary arterial hypertension using bone marrow-derived endothelial-like progenitor cells: efficacy of combined cell and eNOS gene therapy in established disease. Circ Res 2005; 96(4):442–450.

26. Wang XX, Zhang FR, Shang YP, et al. Transplantation of autologous endothelial progenitor cells may be beneficial in patients with idiopathic pulmonary arterial hypertension: a pilot randomized controlled trial. J Am Coll Cardiol 2007; 49(14):1566–1571.

27. Indolfi C, Cioppa A, Stabile E, et al. Effects of hydroxymethylglutaryl coenzyme-A reductase inhibitor simvastatin on smooth muscle cell proliferation in vitro and neointimal formation in vivo after vascular injury. J Am Coll Cardiol 2000; 35:214–221.

28. Nishimura T, Faul JL, Berry GJ, et al. Simvastatin attenuates smooth muscle neointimal proliferation and pulmonary hypertension in rats. Am J Respir Crit Care Med 2002; 166: 1403–1408.

29. Nishimura T, Vaszar LT, Faul JL, et al. Simvastatin rescues rats from fatal pulmonary hypertension by inducing apoptosis in neointimal smooth muscle. Circulation 2003; 108: 1640–1645.

30. Galié N, Torbicki A, Barst R, et al. European Society of Cardiology Guidelines On Diagnosis and Treatment of Pulmonary Artery Hypertension. Eur J Cardiol 2004; 25:2243–2278.

31. Badesch DB, Abman SH, Simonneau G, et al. Medical therapy for pulmonary arterial hypertension: Updated ACCP evidence-based clinical practice guidelines. Chest 2007; 131(6):1917–1928.

32. Sitbon O, Humbert M, Jais X, et al. Long-term response to calcium channel blockers in idiopathic pulmonary arterial hypertension. Circulation 2005; 111:3105–3111.
33. Rich S, Kaufmann E, Levy PS. The effect of high doses of calcium-channel blockers on survival in primary pulmonary hypertension. N Engl J Med 1992; 327:76–81.
34. Tuder RM, Cool CD, Geraci MW, et al. Prostacyclin synthase expression is decreased in lungs from patients with severe pulmonary hypertension. Am J Respir Crit Care Med 1999; 159:1925–1932.

27

Goal-Oriented Therapy in Pulmonary Arterial Hypertension

MARIUS M. HOEPER
Hannover Medical School, Hannover, Germany

I. Introduction

The term goal-oriented therapy describes a relatively new therapeutic concept in the field of pulmonary arterial hypertension (PAH), which focuses on the question when a response to therapy can be considered sufficient and when not. This question is of fundamental importance in guiding therapeutic decisions, that is, when to maintain a therapy, when to switch from one medication to another, and when to combine several medications. The goal of modern PAH therapy is not simply to achieve a certain degree of clinical improvement but to achieve disease control, which means to ascertain an acceptable clinical status and to keep the patient stable for as long as possible.

The clinical problem that has led to the concept of goal-oriented therapy can be exemplified by a hypothetical but realistic case scenario: a 30-year-old woman is diagnosed with idiopathic PAH. She presents in WHO functional class III with a six-minute walk distance of 350 m. Disease-targeted treatment is started, for instance, with an endothelin receptor antagonist or a phosphodiesterase 5 (PDE-5) inhibitor. Three months later, she reports better exercise tolerance, but she is still not capable of climbing two flights of stairs without pausing. Thus, despite improvement, she remains in functional class III. Her six-minute walk test (6MWT) is now 420 m. This is a typical clinical situation in which physicians have to decide whether this treatment result is satisfying, which would mean that treatment would be continued, or whether the treatment result is not sufficient, which would trigger an adjustment of the medical therapy, most likely the addition of another drug. The evolving concept of goal-oriented therapy has been introduced to guide these treatment decisions.

A. Definition of Patient Status

According to the recent guidelines on pulmonary hypertension published jointly by the European Society of Cardiology and the European Respiratory Society, the clinical condition of a patient can be defined as stable and satisfactory, stable but not satisfactory, or unstable and deteriorating.

Stable and satisfactory: These patients meet the criteria listed in the "green zone" of Table 1. The most important features are absence of clinical signs of right ventricular (RV)

Table 1 Risk Determinants in Pulmonary Arterial Hypertension

Low risk	Determinants of risk	High risk
No	Clinical evidence of RV failure	Yes
Gradual	Progression	Rapid
II, III	WHO class	IV
Longer (>400–500 m)	6-min walk distance	Shorter (<300 m)
VO_2max > 14.5 mL/min/kg	Cardiopulmonary exercise testing	VO_2max < 12 mL/min/kg
Minimally elevated and stable	BNP/NT-pro-BNP	Very elevated and/or rising
$PaCO_2$ > 34 mmHg	Blood gases	$PaCO_2$ < 32 mmHg
Minimal RV dysfunction TAPSE > 2.0 cm	Echocardiographic findings	Pericardial effusion RV dysfunction TAPSE < 1.5 cm
Normal/near-normal RAP and CI	Hemodynamics	High RAP and low CI

The values shown in the "green zone" on the left side are associated with a good prognosis, whereas the values in the "red zone" signal clinical instability.

Abbreviations: RV, right ventricular; VO_2max, maximum oxygen uptake; BNP, brain natriuretic peptide; NT-pro-BNP, N-terminal fragment of pro–brain natriuretic peptide; TAPSE, tricuspid annular plane systolic excursion; RAP, right atrial pressure; CI, cardiac index.

failure, stable WHO functional class I or II, absence of syncope, a six-minute walk distance >400 to 500 m depending on the individual patient, a peak oxygen uptake >15 mL/min/kg, normal or near-normal brain natriuretic peptide (BNP) or the N-terminal fragment of pro–brain natriuretic peptide (NT-pro-BNP) plasma levels, no pericardial effusion, tricuspid annular plane systolic excursion (TAPSE) determined by echocardiography >2,0 cm, and right-heart catheterization showing a right atrial pressure <8 mmHg and a cardiac index >2.5 L/min/m^2.

Stable but not satisfactory: These patients are not deteriorating but have not achieved the status that the patient and treating physician would consider desirable. Some of the limits described above for a stable and satisfactory condition and included in the green zone of Table 1 are not fulfilled. These patients require reevaluation and consideration for additional or different treatment.

Unstable and deteriorating: These patients meet some or all of the criteria listed in the "red zone" of Table 1. In particular, these patients present with RV failure, progression of symptoms and signs, worsening in functional class, a six-minute walk distance <300 to 400 m, a peak oxygen uptake <12 mL/min/kg, rising BNP/NT-pro-BNP plasma levels, evidence of pericardial effusion, TAPSE <1.5 cm, a right atrial pressure >15 mmHg and rising, and a cardiac index below 2.0 L/min/m^2. Clinical warning signs are increasing edema and the need to escalate diuretic therapy, new onset, or increasing frequency of angina. Another important warning sign is syncope, which requires immediate attention as it is a common manifestation of a low cardiac output.

The goal of therapy is to bring and maintain the patient in the first category, that is, stable and satisfactory. A comprehensive prognostic evaluation is required to ascertain that the patient meets this goal.

II. Comprehensive Prognostic Evaluation and Treatment Goals

Several groups of parameters can help determine clinical status and stability. These can be categorized into three different groups: (*i*) clinical signs and exercise performance, (*ii*) biomarkers, and (*iii*) RV function and hemodynamics.

A. Clinical Signs and Exercise Performance

Clinical assessment often provides the most important information on a patient's status. Signs of right-heart failure should be absent. In this context, it is helpful to keep in mind that edema is not always a sign of right-heart failure but may also occur as a side effect of PAH-targeted therapy. Exercise capacity should be normal or only mildly impaired, and ideally, patients should be in WHO functional class I or II.

The most widely used tool to measure exercise capacity is the 6MWT. Improvement in six-minute walk distance has been the primary end point in most of the pivotal trials that have been performed in the field of PAH (1–4). It was demonstrated some years ago, however, that it is not the extent of improvement in six-minute walk distance achieved with medical therapy that is of prognostic importance but the overall walking distance a patient is able to cover (5,6). In a study of patients suffering from idiopathic PAH treated with epoprostenol, Sitbon et al. showed that a six-minute walk distance >380 m, three months after institution of therapy, was associated with a three-year survival rate of 81% compared with 56% in patients who walked <380 m (5). Similar data were later reported for patients treated with bosentan (6). Thus, a six-minute walk distance >380 m was originally proposed as an important treatment goal for PAH patients (7). Meanwhile, however, it has become clear that especially younger patients are often capable of walking >400 m despite the presence of severe pulmonary hypertension. For this reason, the 6MWT treatment goal is now set between 400 and 500 m depending on the patient's age, height, physical condition, and comorbidities.

Cardiopulmonary exercise testing is also used by many PH centers to assess the functional status of their patients (8). Cardiopulmonary exercise testing can be performed safely in almost all disease stages, but this tool is most useful in patients with mild to moderate symptoms and six-minute walk distances above 400 m. In these patients, cardiopulmonary exercise testing often provides invaluable information as it may uncover patients who seem to have an acceptable functional status based on self-reporting and 6MWT but who still have severely impaired RV function and, therefore, a questionable prognosis. Several parameters obtained during cardiopulmonary exercise testing are of prognostic importance, the most widely used being the peak oxygen uptake. It has been shown that a peak oxygen uptake <10.4 mL/min/kg is associated with a poor prognosis (9). Patients in functional class II usually have a peak oxygen uptake of 15.0 mL/min/kg or higher (8). Thus, another treatment goal is to achieve a peak oxygen uptake >15.0 mL/min/kg. Other parameters of prognostic importance include the peak systolic blood pressure during exercise and the ventilatory efficacy (9).

B. Biomarkers

Biomarkers are increasingly being used to assess the status of patients with PAH. Plasma levels of BNP or NT-pro-BNP are most widely used as they correlate with RV function and provide prognostic information (10,11). Cutoff levels associated with either a good or a poor outcome have not yet been sufficiently validated; however, markedly elevated BNP/NT-pro-BNP values that further increase despite targeted therapy are an indicator of a poor prognosis, whereas normal or near-normal BNP and NT-pro-BNP values are usually associated with a well-preserved RV function and a good outcome.

Other biomarkers might also be useful: Troponin is an indicator of myocardial injury, and PAH patients with elevated troponin levels have a high risk of death (12).

A low arterial $PaCO_2$ is a marker of disease severity in PAH as these patients with PAH tend to hyperventilate, which means that their $PaCO_2$ is often lower than normal. The extent of hyperventilation worsens as cardiac output deteriorates, and $PaCO_2$ values <32 mmHg indicate a poor prognosis (13). $PaCO_2$ levels <32 mmHg in patients who seemingly do well must be interpreted as a warning sign and should trigger a further assessment of the RV function.

C. Right Ventricular Function and Hemodynamics

Regular assessment of RV function and hemodynamics is critical in the management of PAH patients. The most widely used tools are echocardiography and right-heart catheterization.

Echocardiography is frequently used as follow-up tool in PAH, although it has not been well standardized for this purpose. One of the main problems is the interpretation of the pulmonary arterial pressure during the course of the disease. Physicians tend to interpret changes in the pulmonary arterial pressure as indicators of worsening or improvements of the disease. This interpretation, however, can be fundamentally wrong. There is virtually no correlation between the pulmonary arterial pressure and the severity of the disease. This is due to the fact that the magnitude of pulmonary arterial pressure elevation reflects not only the extent of pulmonary vascular obstruction but also the performance of the right ventricle. Both factors tend to change the pulmonary arterial pressure in opposite directions. Thus, a fall in the pulmonary arterial pressure can be a result of effective therapy as well as declining RV function. It is for these reasons that the pulmonary arterial pressure is not a useful marker of disease severity (5,14). Currently, the pulmonary arterial pressure is not included in goal-oriented therapeutic concepts.

Echocardiographic parameters that are more useful to assess RV function include the right atrial area, TEI index, TAPSE, and presence or absence of a pericardial effusion (see chap. 8 by Drs. Torbicki and Fijalkowska for more details) (15–18). TAPSE has become one of the most widely used echocardiography indicators of RV function and a value >2.0 cm has been suggested as treatment goal (18).

Right-heart catheterization is an invasive procedure but remains the gold standard in the assessment of pulmonary hypertension and RV function. The main rule for interpreting right-heart catheterization data during follow-up of PAH patients is the same as that for echocardiography: The pulmonary arterial pressure is a poor determinant of disease severity and prognosis (5,14). The most important reason to conduct invasive reassessments during the course of the disease is to make sure that the determinants of RV function, that is, right atrial pressure, cardiac output, and mixed venous oxygen saturation, are in the normal range.

III. Criteria for the Initial Therapy of PAH

Goal-oriented therapy usually starts as monotherapy; combination therapy is reserved for advanced disease or when the response to the initial therapy is not sufficient. Several factors influence the choice of the initial therapy of PAH patients: the severity of the disease, underlying condition and concomitant diseases, availability of drugs, local reimbursement regulations, physicians' and patients' preferences, and many more.

A. Patients Presenting in Functional Class II

The initial clinical trials in PAH included mostly patients in functional classes III and IV, and it was unclear if patients in functional class II would also derive benefit from medical therapy. Meanwhile, however, it has been shown that the PDE-5 inhibitor sildenafil as well as the endothelin receptor antagonist ambrisentan improve exercise capacity in patients presenting in functional class II (2,3). More importantly, the Endothelin antagonist trial in mildly symptomatic PAH patients (EARLY) study has demonstrated that the endothelin receptor antagonist bosentan slows disease progression in patients presenting with mild symptoms, that is, in functional class II (19).

On the basis of these data, endothelin receptor antagonists and PDE-5 inhibitors are recommended as first-choice therapy for PAH patients presenting in functional class II. However, as no head-to-head comparison studies are available, it is unknown if any of these agents is more efficacious than the other.

B. Patients Presenting in Functional Class III

For patients presenting in functional class III, a variety of agents have been approved, including the endothelin receptor antagonists bosentan, sitaxentan, and ambrisentan, the PDE-5 inhibitors sildenafil and tadalafil, intravenous epoprostenol, treprostinil and iloprost, inhaled iloprost, inhaled treprostinil, and subcutaneous treprostinil. Again, as there are no head-to-head comparisons between any of these treatments, the selection of the first-choice treatment remains difficult. Endothelin receptor antagonists and PDE-5 inhibitors are the most frequently used compounds in patients presenting in class III. These drugs are more convenient than prostanoids as they can be administered orally and have few side effects. In addition, they are efficacious in terms of improving exercise capacity and hemodynamics, and there is an increasing amount of data showing that these drugs slow disease progression. Some experts keep arguing that intravenous epoprostenol should remain the treatment of choice for patients in functional class III as this remains the only therapy for which a survival benefit has been proven (20,21). The survival advantage with epoprostenol treatment, however, has been shown only in patients with a baseline six-minute walk distance <150 m, that is, only in patients presenting in functional class IV (20). In fact, earlier studies by the Cambridge group found no survival benefit in PAH patients treated with intravenous prostanoids when the baseline mixed venous oxygen saturation was >60%, that is, when these patients had a normal or near-normal cardiac output (22,23). In addition, a study from France has provided data suggesting that the survival of patients in functional class III with first-line bosentan therapy is the same as that with first-line epoprostenol therapy (6).

C.   Patients Presenting in Functional Class IV

Current treatment guidelines recommend intravenous prostacyclin derivative, such as epoprostenol, treprostinil, or iloprost, as first-line treatment for patients presenting in functional class IV. Some centers also use subcutaneous treprostinil in these patients. In treatment-naive patients who are hemodynamically stable, a treatment trial with PDE-5 inhibitors and/or endothelin receptor antagonists may be justified, but these patients need to be monitored closely, and parenteral prostanoid therapy should be started once they do not improve rapidly and substantially. Patients presenting with overt right-heart failure should be treated with parenteral prostanoids as soon as possible. After stabilization, some of these patients may eventually be transitioned to less invasive therapies, but this needs to be done with great caution. Some centers use up-front combination therapy with two or three classes of substances in this patient population, although there is a shortage of data to support this approach.

IV.   When to Switch and When to Combine?

In the vast majority of PAH patients, disease-targeted treatment is started as monotherapy with an endothelin receptor antagonist, a PDE-5 inhibitor, or a prostanoid. If a patient responds well to his or her current medication or, in other words, when treatment goals are met, therapy will be continued (7). The situation is less clear when treatment goals are not met, that is, when patients fail to improve sufficiently, when they show no improvement at all, or when they even deteriorate while receiving active therapy. The EARLY trial, as mentioned above, has shown that active therapy can slow the progression of the disease even if patients have no improvement in their exercise capacity (19). Therefore, it is probably useful to continue a disease-targeted therapy even if it is not having a direct impact on the patient's performance. Thus, most experts tend to add new treatments to previous ones when treatment goals are not met with monotherapy and consider withdrawing PAH-targeted therapy in situations where a patient would not tolerate a medication.

As outlined in detail in chapter 26, there is growing evidence that various combinations improve hemodynamics, exercise capacity, and outcome in patients with PAH (7,24–27). The optimal time to institute combination therapy, however, is unknown, and the same is true for the best choice of drugs. In view of the progressive nature and the poor prognosis of PAH, it seems reasonable to start combination therapy up front, that is, once the diagnosis has been made. This strategy has not yet been studied. For the present time, the standard of care is a sequential approach starting with monotherapy and moving on to combination therapy once a treatment is not found to be sufficiently active (7). To decide whether or not combination therapy is necessary, the patient's status must be reassessed on a regular basis and treatment goals need to be defined for individual patients to guide treatment decisions.

A. Timing of Follow-Up Evaluations

It is usually recommended to reassess PAH every 3 months, although this interval can vary from a few days in unstable patients to 6 to 12 months in patients who have been stable for several years. Assessment of the disease status should not be based on a single variable alone. At least, one objective parameter of exercise capacity should be measured at every visit, ideally together with at least one biomarker and either echocardiography or right-heart catheterization to determine RV function.

There are no generally accepted rules regarding when and how often right-heart catheterization should be repeated in PAH patients. Individual decisions are probably the best approach outside scientific programs. Follow-up right-heart catheterizations should be considered when changes in the therapeutic strategy are to be expected. Some centers find it useful to perform a right-heart catheter whenever they consider changing the PAH medication, especially prior to starting combination therapy. However, in many cases, the decision to change or adapt therapy can be based on the clinical presentation together with the abovementioned noninvasive assessments. Thus, other centers are more conservative and perform follow-up catheters mostly when the clinical presentation and the noninvasive findings are not concordant or when major treatment decisions such as the introduction of intravenous prostacyclin therapy or listing for lung transplantation are being discussed. There are no data to show that the outcome of patients treated in centers who perform right-heart catheterizations on a regular basis is different from the outcome of patients treated in centers where right-heart catheterizations are performed less frequently.

V. Goal-Oriented Therapy

Currently, most PAH centers use a goal-directed treatment strategy (7). As treatment goals have not been prospectively and comparatively assessed, they vary from center to center and from patient to patient. Table 1 shows several risk determinants and thresholds for which there are data in the medical literature that allow linking these values to either a good or a poor outcome. These parameters have been discussed in some detail in the previous section of this chapter.

According to the concept of goal-oriented therapy, all prognostically relevant parameters should be in the green zone (Table 1). As long as this is the case, it is reasonable to continue the current therapeutic strategy. If treatment goals are not met and if the comprehensive assessment shows that this is due to the severity of pulmonary hypertension and not due to concomitant diseases, treatment is usually intensified, which, in the vast majority of the cases, means that new treatments are added to the existing regimen. The order of drugs and the choices of combination partners are currently left up to the discretion of the physician and the preferences of the patient as there are no data comparing long-term safety and efficacy of various combination strategies.

The first study that addressed the concept of goal-oriented therapy in patients with PAH was started in 2002 at Hannover Medical School, Hannover, Germany, and defined three treatment goals for the reasons described above: (*i*) a six-minute walk distance >380 m, (*ii*) a peak oxygen uptake >10.4 mL/min/kg, and (*iii*) a peak systolic blood pressure during exercise >120 mmHg (7). Right-heart catheterization was not used on a

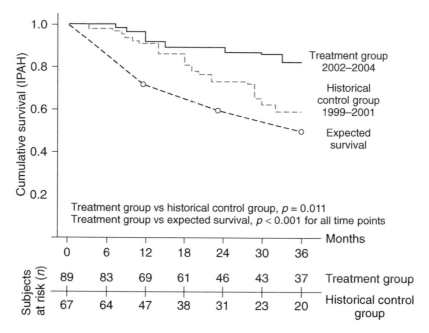

Figure 1 (*See color insert*) Survival of patients with idiopathic pulmonary arterial hypertension with goal-oriented therapy compared with a historical group, and the expected survival as calculated from the National Institutes of Health Registry equation. *Abbreviation*: IPAH, idiopathic pulmonary arterial hypertension.

routine basis but only when the clinical picture was not clear. Treatment was started with bosentan, and this treatment was continued as monotherapy as long as the treatment goals were met. If this was not or no longer the case, sildenafil was added to bosentan and again, treatment was continued as long as the treatment goals were met. If the treatment goals were not met with oral combination therapy, inhaled iloprost was added. The next step was the transition from inhaled to intravenous iloprost, while the oral drugs were continued. If triple combination therapy was not successful, patients were considered for lung or heart-lung transplantation. With this concept, >50% of the patients eventually needed combination therapy during a three-year observation period, but <10% of all patients required intravenous prostacyclin therapy. The three-year survival with this therapeutic concept was 83% in patients with idiopathic PAH, which was not only significantly better than the expected survival rate based on the National Institutes of Health (NIH) Registry equation (28) but also significantly better than the survival rate of a historical control group that was treated in the same center with a conventional approach that included oral beraprost, inhaled and intravenous iloprost, and lung transplantation (Fig. 1).

Meanwhile, the treatment goals and the therapeutic regimen have been modified (Fig. 2): The target six-minute walk distance now ranges from 400 to 500 m depending on the individual patients. The peak oxygen uptake should exceed 15.0 mL/kg/min, and other parameters such as NT-pro-BNP levels are also being taken into consideration. Right-heart

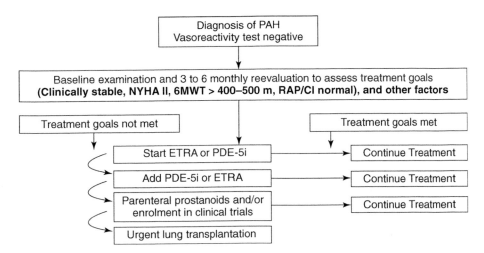

Figure 2 (*See color insert*) Proposal for a goal-oriented approach to PAH as it is currently (2008) used at Hannover Medical School, Hannover, Germany. *Abbreviations*: PAH, pulmonary arterial hypertension; NYHA, New York Heart Association; 6MWT, six-minute walk test; RAP, right atrial pressure; CI, cardiac index; ETRA, endothelin receptor antagonists; PDE-5i, phosphodiesterase-5 inhibitor.

catheterization is still not used on a regular basis but more frequently than before to make sure that right atrial pressure and cardiac index are within the normal range with medical therapy. Treatment is usually started with an oral drug, either an endothelin receptor antagonist or a PDE-5 inhibitor. In patients with advanced disease, a combination of these compounds is often used up front. Inhaled iloprost is no longer used as it is deemed not sufficiently effective in patients deteriorating despite oral combination therapy. In patients not reaching treatment goals with oral combination therapy, addition of parenteral prostanoids should be considered. If these patients are stable, enrollment into clinical trials is an alternative option, especially as several ongoing and future trials assess the safety and efficacy of novel drugs on top of established therapies.

    Taken together, goal-oriented combination therapy is constantly evolving and has become more ambitious than ever. As a consequence, combination therapy is used more frequently and earlier in the course of the disease than before. It is likely that these adjustments will result in further improvements in the quality of life and the survival of patients with PAH, but many questions still need to be addressed in clinical trials.

References

1. Rubin LJ, Badesch DB, Barst RJ, et al. Bosentan therapy for pulmonary arterial hypertension. N Engl J Med 2002; 346:896–903.
2. Galie N, Ghofrani HA, Torbicki A, et al. Sildenafil citrate therapy for pulmonary arterial hypertension. N Engl J Med 2005; 353:2148–2157.
3. Galie N, Olschewski H, Oudiz RJ, et al. Ambrisentan for the treatment of pulmonary arterial hypertension: results of the ambrisentan in pulmonary arterial hypertension, randomized, double-blind, placebo-controlled, multicenter, efficacy (ARIES) study 1 and 2. Circulation 2008; 117:3010–3019.

4. Barst RJ, Langleben D, Badesch D, et al. Treatment of pulmonary arterial hypertension with the selective endothelin-A receptor antagonist sitaxsentan. J Am Coll Cardiol 2006; 47:2049–2056.
5. Sitbon O, Humbert M, Nunes H, et al. Long-term intravenous epoprostenol infusion in primary pulmonary hypertension: prognostic factors and survival. J Am Coll Cardiol 2002; 40:780–788.
6. Provencher S, Sitbon O, Humbert M, et al. Long-term outcome with first-line bosentan therapy in idiopathic pulmonary arterial hypertension. Eur Heart J 2006; 27:589–595.
7. Hoeper MM, Markevych I, Spiekerkoetter E, et al. Goal-oriented treatment and combination therapy for pulmonary arterial hypertension. Eur Respir J 2005; 26:858–863.
8. Sun XG, Hansen JE, Oudiz RJ, et al. Exercise pathophysiology in patients with primary pulmonary hypertension. Circulation 2001; 104:429–435.
9. Wensel R, Opitz CF, Anker SD, et al. Assessment of survival in patients with primary pulmonary hypertension: importance of cardiopulmonary exercise testing. Circulation 2002; 106:319–324.
10. Nagaya N, Nishikimi T, Uematsu M, et al. Plasma brain natriuretic peptide as a prognostic indicator in patients with primary pulmonary hypertension. Circulation 2000; 102:865–870.
11. Fijalkowska A, Kurzyna M, Torbicki A, et al. Serum N-terminal brain natriuretic peptide as a prognostic parameter in patients with pulmonary hypertension. Chest 2006; 129:1313–1321.
12. Torbicki A, Kurzyna M, Kuca P, et al. Detectable serum cardiac troponin T as a marker of poor prognosis among patients with chronic precapillary pulmonary hypertension. Circulation 2003; 108:844–848.
13. Hoeper MM, Pletz MW, Golpon H, et al. Prognostic value of blood gas analyses in patients with idiopathic pulmonary arterial hypertension. Eur Respir J 2007; 29:944–950.
14. McLaughlin VV, Sitbon O, Badesch DB, et al. Survival with first-line bosentan in patients with primary pulmonary hypertension. Eur Respir J 2005; 25:244–249.
15. Hinderliter AL, Willis PW IV, Long W, et al. Frequency and prognostic significance of pericardial effusion in primary pulmonary hypertension. PPH Study Group. Primary pulmonary hypertension. Am J Cardiol 1999; 84:481–484, A10.
16. Raymond RJ, Hinderliter AL, Willis PW, et al. Echocardiographic predictors of adverse outcomes in primary pulmonary hypertension. J Am Coll Cardiol 2002; 39:1214–1219.
17. Yeo TC, Dujardin KS, Tei C, et al. Value of a Doppler-derived index combining systolic and diastolic time intervals in predicting outcome in primary pulmonary hypertension. Am J Cardiol 1998; 81:1157–1161.
18. Forfia PR, Fisher MR, Mathai SC, et al. Tricuspid annular displacement predicts survival in pulmonary hypertension. Am J Respir Crit Care Med 2006; 174:1034–1041.
19. Galie N, Rubin L, Hoeper M, et al. Treatment of patients with mildly symptomatic pulmonary arterial hypertension with bosentan (EARLY study): a double-blind, randomised controlled trial. Lancet 2008; 371:2093–2100.
20. Barst RJ, Rubin LJ, Long WA, et al. A comparison of continuous intravenous epoprostenol (prostacyclin) with conventional therapy for primary pulmonary hypertension. The Primary Pulmonary Hypertension Study Group. N Engl J Med 1996; 334:296–302.
21. Rich S. The current treatment of pulmonary arterial hypertension: time to redefine success. Chest 2006; 130:1198–1202.
22. Higenbottam T, Butt AY, McMahon A, et al. Long-term intravenous prostaglandin (epoprostenol or iloprost) for treatment of severe pulmonary hypertension. Heart 1998; 80:151–155.
23. Higenbottam TW, Butt AY, Dinh-Xaun AT, et al. Treatment of pulmonary hypertension with the continuous infusion of a prostacyclin analogue, iloprost. Heart 1998; 79:175–179.
24. Ghofrani HA, Rose F, Schermuly RT, et al. Oral sildenafil as long-term adjunct therapy to inhaled iloprost in severe pulmonary arterial hypertension. J Am Coll Cardiol 2003; 42:158–164.
25. Mathai SC, Girgis RE, Fisher MR, et al. Addition of sildenafil to bosentan monotherapy in pulmonary arterial hypertension. Eur Respir J 2007; 29:469–475.

26. Hoeper MM, Faulenbach C, Golpon H, et al. Combination therapy with bosentan and sildenafil in idiopathic pulmonary arterial hypertension. Eur Respir J 2004; 24:1007–1010.
27. Hoeper MM, Taha N, Bekjarova A, et al. Bosentan treatment in patients with primary pulmonary hypertension receiving nonparenteral prostanoids. Eur Respir J 2003; 22:330–334.
28. D'Alonzo GE, Barst RJ, Ayres SM, et al. Survival in patients with primary pulmonary hypertension. Results from a national prospective registry. Ann Intern Med 1991; 115:343–349.

28
Atrial Septostomy for the Treatment of Severe Pulmonary Hypertension

JULIO SANDOVAL, JORGE GASPAR, and TOMÁS PULIDO
Instituto Nacional de Cardiologia, Ignacio Chavez, Mexico

I. Introduction

Survival in pulmonary arterial hypertension (PAH) is highly dependent on the functional status of the right ventricle. Hemodynamic variables that reflect right ventricular (RV) dysfunction, such as a low cardiac output (CO) and, in particular, elevated mean right-atrial pressures (mRAPs) are associated with poor prognosis (1). The main objectives of the contemporary management of PAH are (*i*) to alleviate pulmonary microvascular obstruction as the primary objective and (*ii*) to alleviate right ventricular failure (RVF) as a secondary goal. Medical treatments for PAH are reviewed in other chapters of this book. There is no question that pharmacological interventions such as long-term intravenous infusion of prostacyclin and, more recently, other prostacyclin analogues, endothelin-receptor antagonists, and phosphodiesterase-5 inhibitors have improved the quality of life and survival of patients with PAH (2,3). Despite all these interventions, however, RVF may progress or reoccur in some patients (4). This chapter reviews the role of atrial septostomy (AS), an intervention specifically oriented to the relief of RVF, in the treatment scheme of PAH.

II. Background

The notion that right to left shunting might be beneficial in PAH was first suggested by Austen et al. (5). These authors showed that the surgical creation of an atrial septal defect in the setting of a canine model of chronic RV hypertension produced beneficial hemodynamic effects, particularly during exercise, as well as a favorable effect on the survival of the animals. In 1966 Rashkind and Miller described the catheter-balloon technique for the creation of an atrial defect without thoracotomy (6). This technique, indicated to increase pulmonary blood flow (PBF) in children with transposition of the great vessels or with mitral and pulmonary atresia, was subsequently replaced by blade septostomy, a procedure introduced by Park et al. (7). Blade balloon atrial septostomy (BBAS) as a palliative therapy for refractory PAH was first reported by Rich and Lam in 1983 (8). Subsequent studies (9,10) demonstrated that BBAS could be successfully performed in patients with advanced PAH and result in significant clinical and hemo-dynamic improvement. Graded balloon dilation atrial septostomy (BDAS), a variant of

BBAS introduced by Hausknecht et al. (11) and Rothman et al. (12), is the technique most used in recent series (13–26) and has produced similar results.

III. Rationale

The use of AS in patients with idiopathic PAH is supported by the fact that in these patients RV failure and recurrent syncope are associated with poor short-term prognosis (1). Apart from the experimental support of the animal studies reported by Austen et al. (5) (see previous section), several clinical observations have also suggested that an interatrial defect might be of benefit in severe pulmonary hypertension. Rozkovec et al. (27) showed that patients with idiopathic PAH who had a patent foramen ovale lived longer than those without intracardiac shunting. Similarly, patients with Eisenmenger syndrome live longer and have heart failure less frequently than patients with idiopathic PAH (28,29). Taken together, these studies have suggested that deterioration in symptoms, RVF, and death in idiopathic PAH are associated with obstruction to systemic flow and failure of the right ventricle. An atrial septal defect in this setting would allow right to left shunting to increase systemic output that, in spite of the fall in systemic arterial oxygen saturation, will produce an increase in systemic oxygen transport (9,10,30). Furthermore, the shunt at the atrial level would allow decompression of the right atrium and right ventricle, alleviating signs and symptoms of right-heart failure.

IV. Atrial Septostomy in PAH

The precise role of AS in the treatment of PAH remains uncertain because most of the knowledge regarding its use comes from small series or case reports. The limitations of these studies include the noncontrolled nature of the studies, a different etiology and/or different indication for the procedure, and, in particular, the fact that the medical treatment has changed over the past two decades (31). Despite these limitations, AS appears to have a place as a therapeutic modality for advanced PAH.

The indications for AS in the setting of PAH, the potential benefits, and the recommendations to reduce the risk for procedure-related mortality were addressed in a review derived from a collective analysis of 64 cases from the literature (30) and have been reviewed and expanded in most recent guidelines (32,33). The knowledge has now expanded with the report of new cases in the last few years (25,26,34–39). The authors have reviewed the updated literature regarding the results of this intervention in the setting of pulmonary hypertension. Important issues derived from the analysis of the collective worldwide experience were discussed and debated at the world symposium— Pulmonary Hypertension 2008 in Dana Point, California, United States (40). Most information derived from this analysis is presented in this chapter.

V. Patients

The literature holds 223 reported cases (mean age 27 ± 17 years) (40). Most of them (70%) are women and severe idiopathic PAH has been the etiological indication for the procedure in 81.4%. Other etiologies have included PAH associated to surgically cor-rected congenital heart disease (8.3%), PAH associated to collagen vascular disease (4.6%), peripheral (distal) chronic thromboembolic pulmonary hypertension not ame-nable to surgical treatment (2.8%), and miscellaneous etiologies (2.8%). In some of the patients, the procedure was performed on emergency basis; in others it was performed electively for severe pulmonary hypertension and functional limitation. Congestive heart failure (42.5%), syncope (38%), or both (19.4%) have been the main symptomatic indications for the procedure. The mean NYHA functional class for the group, before septostomy, was 3.56 ± 0.4. In 96 of these patients, the procedure was performed after the failure of maximal medical treatment, including long-term intravenous prostacyclin infusion ($n = 57$), bosentan ($n = 18$), sildenafil ($n = 8$), beraprost ($n = 6$), subcutaneous treprostinil ($n = 4$), and inhaled Iloprost ($n = 3$). In 10 of these patients, different combinations of these drugs were used. The simultaneous use of these drugs and AS in the reports, as well as the evidence for the safe administration of intravenous epo-prostenol or oral bosentan in the setting of PAH associated with congenital heart disease (41,42) is in support for the nondeleterious nature of this potential combination therapy.

VI. Procedures

Two types of atrial septostomy, BBAS (31.8%) and BDAS (68.2%), have been used in the treatment of PAH. The basic difference between the two procedures is that, in contrast to BBAS, in BDAS, the Park blade septostomy catheter is not used and the interatrial orifice is created by puncture with a Brockenbrough needle and use of pro-gressively larger balloon catheters in a step-by-step fashion (Fig. 1). In BDAS, a 10%

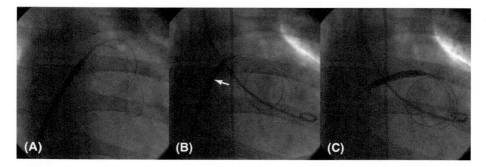

Figure 1 Balloon dilation atrial septostomy. The procedure involves a standard right- and left-heart catheterization. Transseptal puncture is performed with the Mullins introducer and Brock-enbrough needle using standard techniques. Once the correct and stable position of the Mullins introducer in the left atrium is confirmed, the needle is withdrawn and a Inoue circular-end guidewire is passed to the left atrium. Over this guidewire, septostomy dilatation is done, in a graded step-by-step approach, beginning at 4 mm diameter with the Inoue septostomy dilator (**A**) and completed using peripheral balloons of successive diameters (**B, C**). Inflation of the balloon with contrast media is increased just enough to eliminate balloon waist (*arrow*) and is repeated at least twice to counter elastic recoil.

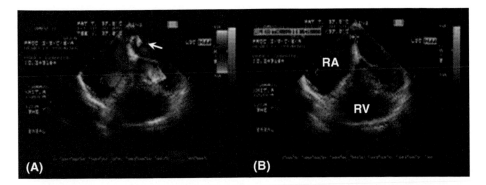

Figure 2   (*See color insert*) Transesophageal echocardiography to confirm (**A**) and measure the diameter (**B**) of the created interatrial defect. Note the right to-left shunt at the level of atrial septum (*arrow*). *Abbreviations*: RA, right atrium; RV, right ventricle.

decrease in $SaO_2\%$ and an increase in left ventricular end-diastolic pressure approaching 18 mmHg preclude further dilatation (43).

Following the procedure, the patients are monitored in an intensive care setting during the first 48 hours after the procedure in a $30°–45°$ upright position, with continuous supplementary oxygen administration. For the management of severe hypoxemia after septostomy, the use of inhaled Iloprost has been recently suggested (25). Echocardiography is useful to monitor for evidence of LV volume overload and is also useful in determining the baseline interatrial orifice diameter, which should be approximately 20% smaller than the maximal balloon diameter used due to tissue recoil (Fig. 2).

A prospective evaluation of potential differences between the two procedures in regard to hemodynamic results and risk of complications has not been done. The election to perform BBAS or BDAS should be a decision taken at each center based on institutional expertise. Regardless of the technique employed, several issues regarding patient selection and preparation for the procedure, monitoring of variables during the procedure, and management after the intervention have been described. These issues are summarized as recommendations to minimize the risk of death during the procedure in Table 1 (30). The procedures should be performed only in centers experienced in both atrial septostomy and pulmonary hypertension (30,44).

VII.   Immediate Outcome After Atrial Septostomy

In most of the reported series, the septostomy has been performed in the setting of severe PAH and RVF. Accordingly, there is an inherent risk of complications and death during the procedure. Since recommendations to minimize this risk have been established, procedure-related mortality appears to be decreasing. In the analysis of the current worldwide experience, there are 16 immediate (24 hours) procedure-related deaths (7.1%), and one-month mortality has occurred in 33 patients (14.8%). For the BDAS technique these figures

Table 1 Recommendations to Minimize the Risk of Procedure-Related Mortality of Atrial Septostomy

---

1. Atrial septostomy should be attempted only by those institutions with an established track record in the treatment of advanced pulmonary hypertension where atrial septostomy is performed with low morbidity.

2. Atrial septostomy should not be performed in the patient with impending death and severe right ventricular failure on maximal cardiorespiratory support. An mRAP > 20 mmHg, a PVRI > 55 U/m^2, and a predicted 1-year survival $<40\%$ are all significant predictors of procedure-related death.

3. Before cardiac catheterization, it is important to confirm an acceptable baseline systemic oxygen saturation ($>90\%$ in room air) as well as to optimize cardiac function (adequate right-heart filling pressure, additional inotropic support if needed).

4. During cardiac catheterization is mandatory:

    a. Supplemental oxygen if needed
    b. Mild and appropriate sedation to prevent anxiety
    c. Careful monitoring of variables (LAP, SaO$_2$%, and mRAP)
    d. To attempt a step-by-step procedure.

5. After atrial septostomy, it is important to optimize oxygen delivery. Transfusion of packed red blood cells or erythropoietin (prior to and following the procedure if needed) may be necessary to increase oxygen content.

Abbreviations: MRAP, mean right-atrial pressure; PVRI, pulmonary vascular resistance index; LAP, left atrial pressure; SaO$_2$%, arterial oxygen saturation.
Source: From Ref. 30.

are 4.2% and 10.3%, respectively (Table 2). Causes of immediate death in the 33 cases reported were refractory hypoxemia ($n = 20$), progressive right-heart failure ($n = 6$), procedure complications ($n = 4$), multiple organ failure ($n = 1$), hemoptysis ($n = 1$), and unrelated (voluntary dialysis withdrawal 1 case).

Variables associated with periprocedural death (at 1 month) in the current worldwide experience are shown in Table 3. As in the previous analysis of the world-wide experience (30), an mRAP > 20 mmHg remains as the most significant risk factor for procedure-related death (risk rate $= 30.5; p < 0.001$). Higher NYHA functional class and congestive heart failure also tended to be associated with an increased risk of death, whereas syncope, as an indication for AS, had a protective effect against such a risk. Finally, a higher SaO$_2$ after the procedure had also a protective effect against the risk of death at one month.

On the other hand, symptoms and signs of RVF are improved immediately after AS in the majority of surviving patients (i.e., syncope and systemic venous congestion either disappear or decrease in frequency or intensity) (30). From a total of 186 surviving patients in whom an immediate follow-up outcome was reported in the current world-wide experience, 163 patients (87.6%) were reported as improved and 23 (12.4%) as not improved (40). NYHA functional class of the surviving patients decreased from 3.49 ± 0.58 to 2.1 ± 0.67 ($p < 0.001$). Exercise endurance, as assessed by the six-minute walk, was also improved in most of the patients after septostomy in the three studies

Table 2 Procedure-Related Mortality in Balloon Dilation Atrial Septostomy for Pulmonary Hypertension

Author	Procedures (number of patients)	Deaths 24 hr	Deaths 1 mo
Hayden et al. (24)	6 (6)	0	2
Sandoval et al. (13)	22 (15)	1	1
Thanopoulos et al. (18)	6 (6)	0	0
Rothman et al. (14)	13 (12)	0	2
Reichenberger et al. (15)	20 (17)	3	5
Kothari et al. (19)	11 (11)	2	3
Vachiery et al. (16)	18 (16)	1	2
Moscussi et al. (17)	1 (1)	0	0
Allcock et al. (20)	12 (9)	0	0
Kurzyna et al. (21)	3 (3)	0	1
Chau et al. (22)	1 (1)	0	0
Micheletti et al. (23)	22 (20)	0	0
Kurzyna et al. (25)	14 (11)	0	1
Ciarka et al. (26)	11(11)	0	0
Wawrzynska et al. (35)	1 (1)	0	0
Rogan et al. (36)	1 (1)	0	0
Fraisse et al. (37)	1 (1)	0	0
Prieto et al. (38)	1 (1)	0	0
O'Loughlin et al. (39)	1 (1)	0	0
Total	165 (144)	7 (42%)	17 (10.3%)

Table 3 Baseline Variables Associated with Procedure-Related Mortality (One Month)

Variable	HR (95% CI)	p
Age (yr)	0.99 (0.96–1.03)	<0.966
Age > 18 yr old	1.12 (0.29–4.34)	<0.865
Gender, female	0.73 (0.18–2.8)	<0.635
NYHA functional class	8.53 (0.89–81.2)	<0.062
Diagnosis of CVD	3.18 (0.67–14.9)	<0.143
Syncope	0.14 (0.03–0.66)	<0.013
RHF	5.97 (0.75–47.2)	<0.089
Septostomy type, blade	1.19 (0.30–4.6)	<0.800
Mean RAP (mmHg)	1.19 (1.1–1.29)	<0.000
RAP > 20 mmHg	30.5 (3.8–244)	<0.001
Mean PAP (mmHg)	1.01(0.98–1.05)	<0.321
Mean LAP (mmHg)	1.11(0.86–1.43)	<0.420
Baseline CI (L/min/m^2)	0.38 (0.09–1.6)	<0.189
Baseline PVRI (U/m^2)	1.04 (0.98–1.09)	<0.148
Baseline SaO$_2$%	0.97 (0.83–1.14)	<0.773
SaO$_2$% after procedure	0.90 (0.84–0.96)	<0.001
Mean SAP (mmHg)	0.96 (0.92–1.01)	<0.148

Abbreviations: CVD, collagen vascular disease; RHF, right-heart failure; RAP, right atrial pressure; PAP, pulmonary artery pressure; LAP, left atrial pressure; CI, cardiac index; PVRI, pulmonary vascular resistance index; SaO$_2$%, arterial oxygen saturation; SAP, systemic artery pressure.
Source: From Ref. 40.

evaluating this parameter (13,16,20). Thirty-one out of the 186 surviving patients (16.6%) were transplanted.

VIII. Immediate Hemodynamic Effects

Hemodynamics before and after septostomy have been described in only 117 of the reported cases. Analyzed as a group, there was a significant ($p < 0.001$) decrease in mean RAP (from 14.6 ± 8 to 11.6 ± 6.3 mmHg) and SaO_2% (from 93.3 ± 4.1 to 83 ± 8.5 %); this was accompanied by an also significant ($p < 0.001$) increase in mLAP (from 5.7 ± 3.3 to 8.10 ± 3.98 mmHg) and CI (from 2.04 ± 0.69 to 2.62 ± 0.84 L/min/m^2). Pulmonary and systemic pressure did not change after septostomy.

The magnitude of hemodynamic improvement is not the same for all patients and depends on baseline mean RAP (30,43). Changes after AS are progressively more important where the mRAP is higher (Table 4) (40). In patients with an RAP < 10 mmHg, the decrease in RAP was not significant (10.6% from already low baseline reading) yet there was a 22.5% increase in CI. In patients with an RAP more than 20 mmHg (where procedural mortality is highest), RAP and SaO_2% decreased 25% and 14.5%, respectively, and CI increased 38% from baseline. Patients with a baseline RAP between 11 and 20 mmHg had an intermediate response, but a better risk benefit ratio. It has to be stressed that all these measurements represent only the resting state and are likely to be different at exercise as shown in dogs with RV hypertension (5) where an increase in cardiac output in the face of minimal elevation of RV end-diastolic pressure occurred only in dogs with an atrial septal defect. Hemodynamics during exercise in humans after septostomy have not been established.

Regarding the effect of AS on other hemodynamic variables such as PBF and, therefore, on pulmonary vascular resistance are difficult to assess as in most of the studies reported so far, a direct measurement of PBF has not been done. In a recent work by Kurzyna and coworkers (25), a significant increase in PVR was seen in some of the patients correlating with the level of mixed venous pO_2 after the procedure, and it was though to be responsible, in part, for refractory hypoxemia following septostomy. This was successfully managed with inhaled Iloprost. This most interesting finding deserves future investigation.

Mechanisms for hemodynamic and clinical benefit include decompression of the RV at rest, prevention of further RV dilation and dysfunction during exercise, and an increase in CO and systemic oxygen transport (SOT) at rest and during exercise (via right to left shunt). A recent study of patients with PAH (45) showed a decrease in the levels of brain-type natriuretic peptide after septostomy, a finding in support of the decompression phenomenon. The increase in SOT and delivery might also produce beneficial effects on peripheral oxygen utilization and be responsible for the improvement in exercise capacity.

Other mechanisms for improvement after septostomy are also likely. It has been shown that PAH patients have an increase in sympathetic nervous activity (46), which may, in fact, be one of the pathophysiological mechanisms leading to RVF (43,47). In a recent study, Ciarka et al. (26) demonstrated a significant decrease in sympathetic overactivity, as assessed by a decrease in muscle sympathetic nerve activity, after septostomy in patients with PAH. By decreasing sympathetic overdrive, septostomy may also improve RV function.

Table 4 Hemodynamic Effects of Atrial Septostomy According to Baseline Mean Right Atrial Pressure

Variable	RAP < 10 mmHg (n = 42)			RAP = 11–20 mmHg (n = 49)			RAP > 20 mmHg (n = 26)		
	Before	After	p	Before	After	p	Before	After	p
mRAP (mmHg)	6.6 ± 2.4	5.9 ± 3.2	<0.214	14.8 ± 2.8	11.9 ± 3.5	<0.001	26.6 ± 4.4	19.9 ± 3.8	<0.001
mPAP (mmHg)	62 ± 16	64 ± 19	<0.329	66.4 ± 17	66.4 ± 16	<1.000	63.4 ± 20	67.5 ± 20	<0.102
mLAP (mmHg)	5.0 ± 2.7	6.8 ± 2.4	<0.005	5.3 ± 3.6	7.8 ± 4.5	<0.001	7.9 ± 3.0	10.9 ± 4.0	<0.029
SaO$_2$%	93.8 ± 4	85.8 ± 7	<0.001	93.0 ± 4.0	82.8 ± 7.2	<0.001	93.1 ± 4.3	78.6 ± 10.3	<0.001
CI (L/min/m^2)	2.36 ± 0.58	2.89 ± 0.72	<0.001	2.04 ± 0.71	2.65 ± 0.96	<0.001	1.55 ± 0.49	2.14 ± 0.56	<0.001
MSAP (mmHg)	83 ± 15	83 ± 13	<0.931	84.5 ± 14	88.8 ± 15	<0.065	78 ± 20	81 ± 18	<0.254
NYHA class	3.25 ± 0.64	2.00 ± 0.65	<0.001	3.63 ± 0.49	2.21 ± 0.78	<0.001	3.71 ± 0.49	2.00 ± 0.0	<0.001

Abbreviations: mRAP, mean right-atrial pressure; PAP, mean pulmonary artery pressure; mLAP, mean left atrial pressure; SaO$_2$, arterial oxygen saturation; CI, cardiac index; mSAP, mean systemic arterial pressure; NYHA, New York Heart Association.

Source: From Ref. 40.

IX. Long-Term Effects

Two studies have evaluated the long-term hemodynamic effects of AS (10,34). Both studies found an improvement in RV function (higher CI and lower RAP) over time in patients who had repeat catheterization after a mean of about two years. AS may also exert beneficial effects on right-heart structure and function. Echocardiography studies performed before and six months after septostomy in patients with PAH showed a decrease in right atrial and RV systolic and diastolic areas as a reflection of less right-heart dilation after the procedure (48). This simple decompression effect (decrease in radius) reduces wall stress and may improve RV performance via the Laplace relationship (43,47).

X. Spontaneous Closure of Atrial Septostomy

In most of the reported series, subsequent closure of the defect has been a relatively frequent and undesirable outcome of BDAS. In the worldwide experience, 27 out of the 223 cases reported (12.1%) spontaneous closure of the septostomy occurred. The reason for this remains unknown. In our experience, there have not been significant differences in age, hemodynamic profile, or septostomy size between patients with spontaneous closure and those in whom the septostomy remained open. To solve the problem of closure, we have elected to repeat septostomy as many times as necessary and achieved this without complications (13,49).

Recently, however, this problem has been approached differently by other investigators. Micheletti et al. (23) placed a custom-made fenestrated atrial septal device at the end of the procedure to maintain the septostomy open. By doing this in 7 out of 20 children, the spontaneous closure of the defect was successfully avoided. This approach has been followed by other investigators (37–39). These additional interventions may help in reducing the risk of the subsequent closure of the defect. At present, however, it is difficult to anticipate the long-term risk/benefit of this approach. There is always the chance of paradoxical embolus if the patient is not adequately anticoagulated. The benefit is also questionable. In a recent communication, Lammers et al. (50) reported the occlusion of the fenestration in four out of nine patients, after a follow-up of 10 months, despite the concomitant use of aspirin or warfarin.

XI. Effect of Atrial Septostomy on Long-Term Survival

Although most reported series have suggested a beneficial effect (9,10,13,34,49), the impact of septostomy on survival of patients with PAH has not been established in prospective and controlled studies. From these reports, it is also clear that long-term survival is limited by late deaths, primarily as a result of progression of the pulmonary vascular disease. From the current worldwide experience (40), we have analyzed the survival characteristics of 106 patients in whom follow-up and outcome after septostomy (that is excluding procedural deaths) was available. The mean survival time was 63 months (95%CI, 50–76 months). Mortality after septostomy in these patients was associated with increasing age (HR 1.04; $p < 0.001$), scleroderma diagnosis (HR 8.32; $p < 0.004$), NYHA class after septostomy (HR 4.71; $p < 0.000$), and NYHA functional

Table 5 Real Versus Predicted Survival for Patients with Pulmonary Hypertension Surviving Atrial Septostomy

Author	1-Yr survival		2-Yr survival		3-Yr survival	
	Predicted (%)[a]	Real (%)	Predicted (%)[a]	Real (%)	Predicted (%)[a]	Real (%)
Kerstein (10) ($n = 13$)	62	80	48	73	39	65
Law (34) ($n = 33$)	68	84	55	77	46	69
Sandoval (49) ($n = 33$)	65	90	52	81	43	77

[a]Predicted by the equation developed from the National Institutes of Health PPH registry data.
Source: From Ref. 1.

class 3 and 4 after septostomy (HR 6.24; $p < 0.009$). CI after septostomy (HR 0.179; $p < 0.002$), left atrial pressure after septostomy (HR 0.737; $p < 0.005$), and SOT after septostomy (HR 0.99; $p < 0.002$) all had a protective effect against the risk of death.

At our center we have recently analyzed our experience with 50 septostomy procedures performed in 34 patients (age 35 ± 10 years) (49). Only one procedure-related death occurred (2%). Septostomy was repeated in 10 patients due to spontaneous closure of the defect. In 21 patients, AS was the only form of treatment while 11 received additional PAH-specific pharmacotherapy after AS. During follow-up (mean 58.5 ± 38 months) 21 patients died; median survival of the group was 60 months (95% CI, 43–77), which is better than their predicted survival. Median survival for patients on pharmacotherapy additional to AS was 83 months (95% CI, 57–109), which is better than that for patients with AS alone [53 months (95% CI, 39–67); log rank, 6.52; $p = 0.010$]. The potential benefit of an early combination of AS and PAH-specific drug therapies suggested by these results is appealing and, in our opinion, worthwhile to be further evaluated.

Although there are limitations in regard to the studied populations, the impact of AS on the survival of patients with severe pulmonary hypertension and right-heart failure appears beneficial and at least comparable to that of other current pharmacological therapeutic interventions. Three relatively large series have demonstrated this survival benefit to a similar extent (10,34,49) (Table 5). Given the fact that a significant proportion of patients in these series were receiving some of the current medications and in many cases they continue to receive them after the procedure, it is difficult to separate the potential beneficial effect that these medications could have had on the survival of these patients.

XII. Summary

Current practice in the management of PAH is to consider AS for treatment only after maximal medical (pharmacological) therapy has failed. The advanced stage of PAH and RVF of the patients undergoing the procedure in the analysis of the current worldwide experience is in support of this. Despite the lack of a prospective and controlled study, AS stands as an additional, promising strategy in the treatment of RVF from severe PAH. Experience with this procedure is limited in part due to the relative availability and success of the new forms of pharmacological interventions. Uptake may also be related to a lack of training pathway. However, based on analyses of the worldwide experience, several general conclusions can be made: (*i*) AS can be performed successfully in selected patients with advanced pulmonary vascular disease. (*ii*) In patients with PAH who have undergone successful AS, the procedure has resulted in a significant clinical improvement, beneficial and long-lasting hemodynamic effects at rest, and a trend toward improved survival. (*iii*) The procedure-related mortality is still high but appears to be decreasing. Operator experience and adherence to WHO recommendations account for a low fatality rate. (*iv*) Because the disease process in PAH is unaffected by the procedure itself (late deaths), the long-term effects of an AS must be considered to be palliative. (*iv*) Procedure-related mortality is clearly associated with the advanced stage of the disease. Accordingly, we should attempt AS in an earlier stage of the disease. Likewise, the potential benefit of an early combination of AS and PAH-specific drug therapies is appealing and, in our opinion, worthwhile to be further evaluated.

Justification for the use of AS stands on the deleterious impact of RVF on survival of patients, the unpredictable response to medical treatment, the limited access to lung transplantation, and finally the disparity in the availability of these treatments throughout the world. Indications for the procedure include the following: (*i*) Failure of maximal medical therapy (including oral calcium channel blockers (CCB), prostacyclin analogues, bosentan, and phosphodiesterase-5 inhibitors, alone or combined) with persisting RV failure and/or recurrent syncope. (*ii*) As a bridge to transplantation. (*iii*) When no other therapeutic options exist, as is the case in health care systems without PAH-specific drug access.

References

1. D'Alonso GE, Barst RJ, Ayres SM, et al. Survival in patients with primary pulmonary hypertension. Results of a national prospective study. Ann Intern Med 1991; 115:343–349.
2. Badesch DB, Abman SH, Ahearn GS, et al. Medical therapy for pulmonary arterial hypertension. ACCP Evidence-Based Clinical Practice Guidelines. Chest 2004; 126:35S–62S.
3. Galie N, Seeger W, Naeije R, et al. Comparative analysis of clinical trials and evidence-based treatment algorithm in pulmonary arterial hypertension. J Am Coll Cardiol 2004; 43:81S–88S.
4. McLaughlin VV, Shillington A, Rich S. Survival in primary pulmonary hypertension: the impact of epoprostenol therapy. Circulation 2002; 106:1477–1482.
5. Austen WG, Morrow AG, Berry WB. Experimental studies of the surgical treatment of primary pulmonary hypertension. J Thorac Cardiovasc Surg 1964; 48:448–455.
6. Rashkind WJ, Miller WW. Creation of an atrial septal defect without thoracotomy. A palliative approach to complete transposition of the great arteries. JAMA 1966; 196:991–992.
7. Park SC, Neches WH, Zuberbuhler JR, et al. Clinical use of blade atrial septostomy. Circulation 1978; 58:600–606.
8. Rich S, Lam W. Atrial septostomy as palliative therapy for refractory primary pulmonary hypertension. Am J Cardiol 1983; 51:1560–1561.
9. Nihill MR, O'Laughlin MP, Mullins CE. Effects of atrial septostomy in patients with terminal cor pulmonale due to pulmonary vascular disease. Catheter Cardiovasc Diagn 1991; 24:166–172.
10. Kerstein D, Levy PS, Hsu DT, et al. Blade balloon atrial septostomy in patients with severe primary pulmonary hypertension. Circulation 1995; 91:2028–2035.
11. Hausknecht MJ, Sims RE, Nihill MR, et al. Successful palliation of primary pulmonary hypertension by atrial septostomy. Am J Cardiol 1990; 65:1045–1046.

12. Rothman A, Beltran D, Kriett JM, et al. Graded balloon dilation atrial septostomy as a bridge to transplantation in primary pulmonary hypertension. Am Heart J 1993; 125:1763–1766.
13. Sandoval J, Gaspar J, Pulido T, et al. Graded balloon dilation atrial septostomy in severe primary pulmonary hypertension. A therapeutic alternative for patients non-responsive to vasodilator treatment. J Am Coll Cardiol 1998; 32:297–304.
14. Rothman A, Slansky MS, Lucas VW, et al. Atrial septostomy as a bridge to lung transplantation in patients with severe pulmonary hypertension. Am J Cardiol 1999; 84:682–686.
15. Reichenberger F, Pepke-Zaba J, McNeil K, et al. Atrial septostomy in the treatment of severe pulmonary arterial hypertension. Thorax 2003; 58:797–800.
16. Vachiery JL, Stoupel E, Boonstra A, et al. Balloon atrial septostomy for pulmonary hypertension in the prostacyclin era. Am J Respir Crit Care Med 2003; 167:A692.
17. Moscussi M, Dairywala IT, Chetcuti S, et al. Balloon atrial septostomy in end-stage pulmonary hypertension guided a novel intracardiac echocardiographic transducer. Catheter Cardiovasc Interv 2001; 52: 530–534.
18. Thanopoulos BD, Georgakopoulos D, Tsaousis GS, et al. Percutaneous balloon dilation of the atrial septum: immediate and midterm results. Heart 1996; 76:502–506.
19. Kothari SS, Yusuf A, Juneja R, et al. Graded balloon atrial septostomy in severe pulmonary hypertension. Indian Heart J 2002; 54:164–169.
20. Allcock RJ, O'Sullivan JJ, Corris PA. Atrial septostomy for pulmonary hypertension. Heart 2003; 89:1344–1347.
21. Kurzyna M, Dabrowsky M, Torbicki A, et al. Atrial septostomy for severe primary pulmonary hypertension. Report of two cases. Kardiol Pol 2003; 58:27–33.
22. Chau EMC, Fan KYY, Chow WH. Combined atrial septostomy and oral sildenafil for severe right ventricular failure due to primary pulmonary hypertension. Hong Kong Med J 2004; 10:281–284.
23. Micheletti A, Hislop A, Lammers A, et al. Role of atrial septostomy in the treatment of children with pulmonary arterial hypertension. Heart 2006; 92:969–972.
24. Hayden AM. Balloon atrial septostomy increases cardiac index and may reduce mortality among pulmonary hypertension patients awaiting lung transplantation. J Transpl Coord 1997; 7:131–133.
25. Kurzyna M, Dabrowski M, Bielecki D, et al. Atrial septostomy in treatment of end-stage right heart failure in patients with pulmonary hypertension. Chest 2007; 131:947–948.
26. Ciarka A, Vachiery JL, Houssiere A, et al. Atrial septostomy decreases sympathetic overactivity in pulmonary arterial hypertension. Chest 2007; 131:1831–1837.
27. Rozkovec A, Montanes P, Oakley CM. Factors that influence the outcome of primary pulmonary hypertension. Br Heart J 1986; 55:449–458.
28. Hopkins WE, Ochoa LL, Richardson GW, et al. Comparison of the hemodynamics and survival of adults with severe primary pulmonary hypertension or Eisenmenger syndrome. J Heart Lung Transplant 1996; 15:100–105.
29. Hopkins WE. The remarkable right ventricle of patients with Eisenmenger syndrome. Coronary Artery Disease 2005; 16:19–25.
30. Sandoval J, Rothman A, Pulido T. Atrial septostomy for pulmonary hypertension. Clin Chest Med 2001; 22:547–560.
31. Barst RJ. Role of atrial septostomy in the treatment of pulmonary vascular disease. Thorax 2000; 55:95–96.
32. Doyle RL, McCrory D, Channick RN, et al. Surgical treatments/interventions for pulmonary arterial hypertension. ACCP Evidence-Based Clinical Practice Guidelines. Chest 2004; 126:63S–71S.
33. Klepetko W, Mayer E, Sandoval J, et al. Interventional and surgical modalities of treatment for pulmonary arterial hypertension. J Am Coll Cardiol 2004; 43:73S–80S.

34. Law MA, Grifka RG, Mullins CE, et al. Atrial septostomy improves survival in select patients with pulmonary hypertension. Am Heart J 2007; 153:779–784.
35. Wawrzynska L, Remiszewski P, Kurzyna M, et al. A case of a patient with idiopathic pulmonary arterial hypertension treated with lung transplantation: a bumpy road to success. Pol Arch Med Wewn 2006; 115:565–571
36. Rogan MP, Walsh KP, Gaine SP. Migraine with aura following atrial septostomy for pulmonary arterial hypertension. Nat Clin Pract Cardiovasc Med 2007; 4:55–58.
37. Fraisse A, Chetaille P, Amin Z, et al. Use of Amplatzer fenestrated atrial septal defect device in a child with familial pulmonary hypertension. Pediatr Cardiol 2006; 27:759–762.
38. Prieto LR, Latson LA, Jennings C. Atrial septostomy using a butterfly stent in a patient with severe pulmonary arterial hypertension. Catheter Cardiovasc Interv 2006; 68:642–647.
39. O'loughlin AJ, Keogh A, Muller DW. Insertion of a fenestrated Amplatzer atrial septostomy device for severe pulmonary hypertension. Heart Lung Circ 2006; 15:275–277.
40. Keogh A, Mayer E, Benza R, et al. Interventional and surgical modalities of treatment in PAH (in press).
41. Rosenzweig EB, Kerstein D, Barst RJ. Long-term prostacyclin for pulmonary hypertension with associated congenital heart defects. Circulation 1999; 99:1858–1865.
42. Galie N, Beghetti M, Gatzoulis MA, et al. Bosentan therapy in patients with Eisenmenger syndrome: a multicenter, double-blind, randomized, placebo-controlled study. Circulation 2006; 114:48–54.
43. Sandoval J, Gaspar J. Atrial septostomy. In: Peacock AJ, Rubin LJ, eds. Pulmonary Circulation. 2nd ed. London, UK: Edward Arnold Publishers Ltd., 2004:319–333.
44. Rich S, Dodin E, McLaughlin VV. Usefulness of atrial septostomy as a treatment for primary pulmonary hypertension and guidelines for its application. Am J Cardiol 1997; 80:369–371.
45. O'Byrne ML, Berman-Rosenzweig ES, Barst RJ. The effect of atrial septostomy on the concentration of brain-type natriuretic peptide in patients with idiopathic pulmonary arterial hypertension. Cardiol Young 2007; 17:557–559.
46. Velez Roa S, Ciarka A, Najem B, et al. Increased sympathetic nerve activity in pulmonary artery hypertension. Circulation 2004; 110:1308–1312.
47. Bristow MR, Zisman LS, Lances BD, et al. The pressure-overloaded right ventricle in pulmonary hypertension. Chest 1998; 114(suppl):101S–106S.
48. Espínola-Zavaleta N, Vargas-Barrón J, Tazar JI, et al. Echocardiographic evaluation of patients with pulmonary hypertension before and after atrial septostomy. Echocardiography 1999; 16:625.
49. Sandoval J, Gaspar J, Peña H, et al. Effect of atrial septostomy on the survival of patients with severe pulmonary arterial hypertension. The benefit of combining strategies (editorial review).
50. Lammers AE, Derrick G, Haworth SG, et al. Efficacy and long-term patency of fenestrated amplatzer devices in children. Catheter Cardiovasc Interv 2007; 70:578–584.

29
Surgical Management of Pulmonary Hypertension

**PHILIPPE G. DARTEVELLE, ELIE FADEL, SACHA MUSSOT,
DOMINIQUE FABRE and OLAF MERCIER**
Marie Lannelongue Hospital, Université Paris Sud 11, Le Plessis Robinson, France

MARC HUMBERT and GÉRALD SIMONNEAU
Université Paris Sud 11, Service de Pneumologie et Réanimation Respiratoire, Hôpital Antoine
Béclère, Assistance Publique Hôpitaux de Paris, Clamart, France

I. Introduction

Pulmonary hypertension (PH) is a severe condition that has been ignored for a long time. Over the past 20 years, there has been increased interest from respirologists, cardiologists, and thoracic surgeons due to the development of new therapies that have improved the outcome of PH patients' life.

Among these new therapeutic options, surgery has a major role and consists of either lung transplantation (LT) for PH failing medical therapy or curative surgical procedures when PH is caused by an obstruction of the pulmonary arteries by fibrotic tissue resulting from pulmonary embolism, tumors (particularly angiosarcomas), ecchinococcal cysts, etc. Potts procedure may sometimes be performed in children with suprasystemic pulmonary arterial hypertension (PAH).

II. Lung Transplantations

LT is indicated for end-stage pulmonary vascular diseases not curable by any medical therapy or conservative procedure, provided that no specific contraindications to LT exist (discussed in detail in chap. 30) (1).

The number of lung transplants performed is much lower than that of liver, kidney, or heart transplants. In contrast to other solid organ transplants, the lungs are in contact with the external milieu through the tracheobronchial tree and are at risk of pneumonia during donor resuscitation (Fig. 1) (2).

Recipient selection criteria currently include age less than 60 to 65 years, the absence of mechanical respiratory insufficency due to scoliosis, absence of phrenic nerve paralysis, absence of recent neoplastic disease, or other potentially life-threatening diseases.

LT for PAH is indicated for patients with a life expectancy of less than one year, consistent with a functional status of NYHA stage III or IV. Recent worsening of dyspnea and hemodynamic parameters such as a right atrial pressure of greater than

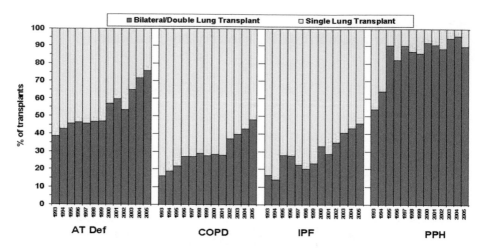

Figure 1 (*See color insert*) Adult lung transplantation: procedure type within indication, by year from 1993 to 2005. *Source*: From Ref. 2, with permission from Elsevier.

12 mmHg, pulmonary arterial pressure greater than 60 mmHg, cardiac index less than 2.2 L/min/m^2, or indexed pulmonary resistance greater than 30 UI are indications for LT. Selection criteria and timing of listing for LT are discussed in detail in chapter 30.

Bilateral sequential lung transplantation (BSLT) and heart-lung transplantation (HLT) are the usual procedures performed in PAH because of the frequent V/Q mismatch observed after single LT for this indication. Transplantation in pulmonary vascular diseases requires a higher organ donor quality than other indications because the perioperative management is more difficult in PAH. In PH, LT are performed under cardiopulmonary (CP) bypass and the heart function is often altered.

A. Types of Transplantation

All three types of LT procedures can reduce or normalize the pulmonary vascular resistance (PVR) in patients with PH, but each procedure has advantages and disadvantages in terms of allocation facilities, complications, length and difficulty of the postoperative course, airway complications, and long-term results.

Heart-Lung Transplantation

This transplantation has an advantage as the operation is relatively simple for the following reasons: (*i*) a standard median sternotomy is performed, (*ii*) the donor heart is normal (avoiding postoperative left-heart dysfunction), (*iii*) the airway receives blood supply from the coronary arteries, thereby preventing airway ischemic complications, (*iv*) two lungs are transplanted in one step (Fig. 2).

After institution of CP bypass between both vena cavae and the ascending aorta, the heart is removed, as for a heart transplantation, leaving in place the posterior part of the left atrium and ostia of the pulmonary veins and a large part of the right atrium. After right pleural aperture, the right lung is removed by stapling the lung hilum, except the

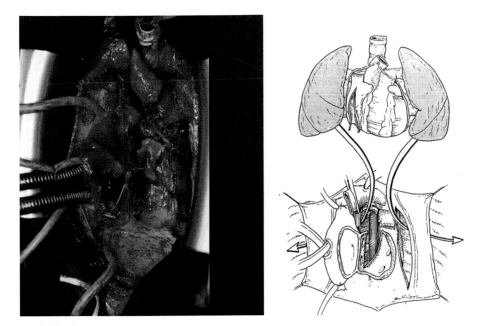

Figure 2 (*See color insert*) Photo and schematic drawing showing the principle of "en bloc" heart-lung transplantation.

main bronchus, which is cautiously dissected with ligation of all surrounding tissue and particularly bronchial arteries that are well developed in obstructive PH or Eisenmenger syndromes. The azygos vein arch is also divided to facilitate implantation of the heart-lung block. The left lung is then removed separately with care to avoid injury to the phrenic and recurrent laryngeal nerves. The next step consists of dissecting free and removing the tracheobronchial bifurcation. Again all the bronchial arteries have to be secured by numerous ligatures to avoid postoperative bleeding from the posterior mediastinum that is difficult to approach after heart-lung block reimplantation. Reimplantation of the heart-lung block requires one tracheal anastomosis, one right atrial anastomosis between the donor right atrium opened from the inferior vena cava (IVC) to the appendage and the recipient right atrium, and finally an end-to-end aortic anastomosis at the level of the ascending aorta.

Single-Lung Transplantation

This is a less desirable procedure in PH even though only one lung is needed. Technically, single-lung transplantation (SLT) is a relatively simple procedure performed via a posterolateral thoracotomy. Three successive anastomoses are required; one on the main bronchus, another on the right atrium, and the last on the pulmonary artery (PA). In SLT recipients, the postoperative course is usually difficult in PAH owing to severe ventilation-perfusion (V/Q) mismatch at every postoperative event (e.g., reperfusion edema, infection, rejection, etc.). Compared with BSLT or HLT, survival rate, maximum workload, and quality of life are worse with SLT.

Bilateral Sequential Lung Transplantation

BSLT is performed sequentially without airway revascularization. Compared with HLT, the native heart of the recipient is preserved, and the donor's heart is allocated to another recipient. BSLT must be performed under CP bypass or extracorporeal membrane oxygenation (ECMO). We believe that the optimal surgical approach is a bilateral anterolateral thoracotomy without sternal division. This contrasts with the clamshell incision that dramatically impairs respiratory mechanics. BSLT consists of successively performing two SLT with a total of six anastomoses. Major complications related to impaired cardiac function in patients with PAH may be averted by cautious intra-operative management. Unfortunately, among patients with severe muscular hypertro-phy of the right ventricle (RV), administration of inotropic agents may obstruct the RV outflow tract, impeding ejection. Further, an overflow ejected by the RV into the low-resistance vascular bed may cause pulmonary edema because the dysfunctional left heart is no longer capable of dealing with a high cardiac output.

B.   Late Complications and Survival

Irrespective of the type of transplant operation, early mortality rate following LT for PAH is higher than other end-stage pulmonary diseases. Additional complications fol-lowing LT include the need for life-long immunosuppression, heightened susceptibility to infections, posttransplant lymphoproliferative disease (PTLD), malignant neoplasms, complications of prolonged immunosuppression (e.g., renal failure, hypertension, hypercholesterolemia, diabetes mellitus, etc.), and (most worrisome) chronic allograft rejection leading to bronchiolitis obliterans syndrome (BOS) and respiratory failure.

Finally, the postoperative mortality in lung and heart-lung transplant recipients is about 20%; overall 5- and 10-year survival rates are 49% and 36%, respectively. In the Paris-Sud University series of 207 LTs for PAH, survival was better for HLT compared to DLT (Fig. 3).

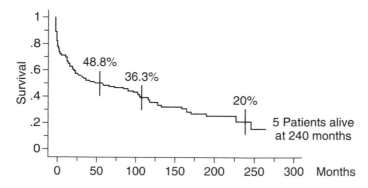

Figure 3   (*See color insert*) Overall survival in transplantation for PAH from 1986 to 2008 concerning 207 transplantations from Paris-Sud University series. *Abbreviation*: PAH, pulmonary arterial hypertension.

III. Potts Procedure

This procedure consists of performing a direct anastomosis between the left PA and the descending thoracic aorta without any prosthetic interposition (3) (Fig. 4). It permits discharge of the pulmonary circulation into the lower part of the body, which consequently is less oxygen saturated than the upper body. The principle of this procedure relies on the fact that PAH in Eisenmenger syndrome is much better tolerated than idiopathic PAH, and survival may be prolonged.

This operation has to be performed through a left thoracotomy without CP bypass; it is associated with a 20% mortality rate and excellent long-term results in terms of function, quality of life, and survival. Potts anastomoses might be an appropriate alternative to LT in children with suprasystemic PAH.

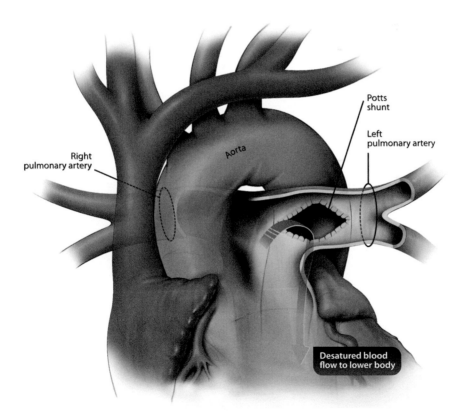

Figure 4 (*See color insert*) Potts procedure consists of performing a direct anastomosis between the left pulmonary artery and the descending thoracic aorta without any prosthetic interposition.

IV. Pulmonary Endarterectomy in Chronic Thromboembolic Pulmonary Diseases

Chronic thromboembolic pulmonary arterial disease is the only cause of PH that is totally curable by a surgical procedure that consists of restoring the pulmonary arterial tree by removing endoluminal and fibrotic material resulting from pulmonary emboli (4–8) (Fig. 5).

Chronic thromboembolic pulmonary hypertension (CTEPH) is caused by obstruction of large pulmonary arteries by acute and recurrent pulmonary emboli and organization of these blood clots. This disease, initially considered to be rare, is diagnosed more and more frequently, likely because of the availability of successful medical and surgical treatment. The development of centers specialized in the diagnosis and treatment of PAH and more consistent follow-up of patients presenting with acute pulmonary emboli also contribute to the ongoing increase in the number of patients diagnosed and treated for CTEPH.

This surgical procedure is an endarterectomy of the entire vascular bed starting at the origin of each PA and extending into all the segmental and subsegmental arteries up to 2 cm from the pleura. Since a major systemic vascularization has developed to supply the obstructed territories, the pulmonary endarterectomy (PEA) requires a circulatory arrest that permits the surgeon to perform this procedure without major back-bleeding originating from the systemic circulation. As a circulatory arrest is always mandatory, the first step of the procedure after CP bypass institution is to cool the patient down to 20°C.

Because clinically evident acute pulmonary embolism episodes are absent in approximately half of the patients with CTEPH, the diagnosis can be difficult. Lung scinti-nuclear scan showing segmental unmatched perfusion defects is the best diagnostic tool to suspect chronic thromboembolic disease. Accessibility to endarterectomy can be assessed only in reference centers for PH after evaluation by pulmonologists, radiologists, and thoracic surgeons with extensive experience in the surgical treatment of

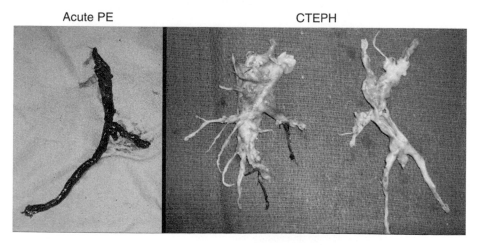

Figure 5   (*See color insert*) Material removed by endarterectomy from the right pulmonary artery (R) and the left one (L) compared with thrombus from acute pulmonary embolism.

this disease. Pulmonary angiography and multislice angio CT scan confirm the diagnosis and determine the feasibility of endarterectomy according to the location of the disease, proximal versus distal. The lesions must start at the level of the PA trunk or at the level of the lobar arteries to find a plan for the endarterectomy.

When the hemodynamic gravity corresponds to the degree of obliteration, PEA can be performed with minimal perioperative mortality, providing definitive excellent functional results in almost all cases. Currently in experienced centers, the mortality rate of PEA is lower than 3%, and more than 85% of the patients are definitively cured by surgery.

A. Technique of Pulmonary Endarterectomy

PEA is performed during circulatory arrest. Obstructive material is removed from each PA and all lobar and segmental branches (in total 20 to 30 branches); this is the only way to reduce the PVR by at least 50%. The intraluminal material is at this stage composed of fibrous tissue inseparable from the intima, and therefore inaccessible to thrombectomy or dilatation. Thus, a true endarterectomy is required, starting at the level of right and left pulmonary arteries inside the pericardium and progressively extending distally into each of the branches of the pulmonary arterial tree.

Patients suffering from chronic thromboembolic disease may develop systemic hypervascular neovascularization from bronchial and intercostal arteries via residual adhesions between the chest wall and the visceral pleura due to previous emboli. The development of a systemic to PA circulation at the precapillary level results in significant back-bleeding from the PA at the time of endarterectomy. The only way to stop this bleeding, which continuously fills the PA and obstructs the surgical field, is to suspend the systemic circulation under conditions of deep hypothermia between 18°C and 20°C. To limit the time of circulatory arrest, CP bypass is stopped only after identification of the correct plane for endarterectomy. After completion of endarterectomy on the first side, the extracorporeal circulation is resumed for about 15 minutes before the contralateral endarterectomy is performed. This sequential technique with intermediate reperfusion limits the cumulated period of circulatory arrest to less than 55 minutes.

The operation is entirely performed through a median sternotomy and through the pericardium without having to open the pleura or dissect the PA outside the pericardium. This approach avoids the dissection of highly vascularized tissue surrounding blood vessels and pleural adhesions.

PEA is truly an *endovascular procedure* that can benefit from video technology. The angioscope illuminates the lumen of the PA, and the video camera allows the distal arterial divisions to be better seen, displayed on screen for the surgeon and surgical assistants.

Briefly, the operation is divided into four stages:

1. The first stage is to perform a median extrapleural sternotomy, a vertical pericardiotomy, to initiate CP bypass between the superior and inferior vena cavae and aorta. Profound cooling is immediately started and as the patient's temperature falls, the superior vena cava is completely dissected to access the right PA. A vent is inserted through the right superior pulmonary vein into the left ventricle; decompression of the left heart is essential because of the

significant venous return from the hypervascularized bronchial arteries through the pulmonary veins. Once the body temperature reaches 20°C, the ascending aorta is clamped and retrograde crystalloid cardioplegia is injected into the aortic root. A longitudinal arteriotomy is performed along the anterior aspect of the right PA in the segment between the aorta and the superior vena cava. The endarterectomy is started by identifying the correct plane in the media of the posterior surface of the PA. This plane is developed circumferentially in the mediastinal artery and its branches and then in the intermediary arterial trunk and its branches. CP bypass is then stopped to work in bloodless vessels and the endarterectomy plane is pursued into the lobar and segmental branches distally to the subsegmental branches of the basilar segments.

2. As the arteriotomy is closed, the patient is reperfused with CP bypass for approximately 15 minutes, the time necessary to close the arteriotomy with a back-and-forth running suture of 6-0 polypropylene. Cardioplegia is repeated at this stage.

3. An arciform arteriotomy is made on the left PA and the endarterectomy is performed according to the same principles as the right side.

4. The patient is reperfused during closure of the left arteriotomy, the cardiac chambers are deaired, the aorta is unclamped, and the patient is slowly rewarmed to 37°C.

The postoperative course may be complicated by postreperfusion pulmonary edema causing hypoxemia and occasionally requiring prolonged mechanical ventilation. Other complications include right-heart failure secondary to persistently high PA pressure, arteriotomy rupture during a spike of pulmonary hypertension, nosocomial pneumonia, hemoptysis (easily treated by embolization), or phrenic nerve palsy, which can prolong dependence on mechanical ventilation. Rethrombosis of an endarterectomized area can rarely occur particularly in unilateral obstruction and warrants anticoagulation as soon as possible after surgery. The patients often continue to improve hemodynamically and functionally for several months after the operation.

The mortality rate of this surgery is approximately 2% in experienced centers; this low mortality reflects refinement in techniques to properly assess indications, high-quality imaging, surgical expertise, and improved postoperative care; intra- and post-operative improvements including maintaining low cardiac output to avoid reperfusion pulmonary edema; the possible use of ECMO to treat hemodynamic instability; and bronchial artery embolization to control postoperative hemoptysis.

Long-term outcome of patients undergoing PEA is excellent with normalization of hemodynamics in most cases. In patients with incomplete immediate results the hemodynamics may deteriorate after several months or years even in the absence of new embolic events and adequate anticoagulation.

B. Indications, Contraindications, and Limits of PEA

Indications for this operation are directly related to the technical feasibility of PEA and the experience of the surgical team (9–11) (Fig. 6). The lesions must start at the level of the PA trunks or at the level of the lobar arteries to find a suitable

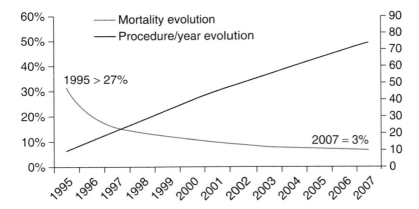

Figure 6 (*See color insert*) Experience and mortality correlated from Paris-Sud University series.

endarterectomy plane. Good results are achieved in almost all cases where the hemodynamic compromise corresponds to the degree of vascular obliteration. In contrast, in severe, long-standing cases where resistances are disproportionately high compared with the degree of anatomic lesions seen on angiography, pulmonary arteritis is usually present in the nonobstructed territories (12,13). These patients should be selected for endarterectomy only if one predicts that the surgical procedure can reduce the PVR by 50%.

The most difficult aspect of patient selection is differentiating secondary obstruction due to macroscopic pulmonary emboli and PAH with upstream thrombosis in the distal part of the segmental arteries. In this situation, submillimeter CT slices with high-quality reconstruction is very helpful (14). Pulmonary hypertension by micro-emboli secondary to intravenous catheters appears similar to the latter. In conclusion, patients presenting with chronic thromboembolic disease should undergo surgery as soon as the diagnosis is made, before the development of an arteritis in the non-obstructed territories and severe PAH. The risk of surgery is low at this early stage of the disease and the future development of arteritis is avoided.

V.   Special Procedures in Obstructive PH

CTEPH is by far the most common cause of obstructive PH. Other causes of pulmonary arterial obstruction, be it extrinsic, endoluminal, or parietal, must however be excluded.

A.   Endarterectomy for Angiosarcomas

Among cases of obstructive PH, approximately 3% are due to angiosarcomas within the main PA trunks (Fig. 7). This primary malignancy of the PA usually has its origin in the pulmonary arterial trunk, surrounds the pulmonary valve, and progressively extends toward branches of the PA, most often bilaterally. The diagnosis is suggested by slowly

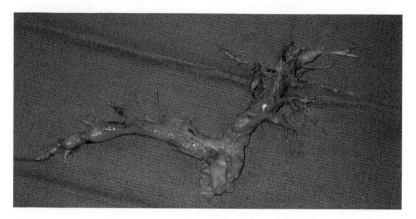

Figure 7 (*See color insert*) Specimen of angiosarcoma resected by endarterectomy.

progressive symptoms without acute episodes or previous thromboembolic disease and the presence of a large quantity of endoluminal material proximally in the main PA on CT scan. The diagnosis is confirmed by a preoperative endovascular biopsy or during surgery.

Treating this type of malignant obstructive PH lies on the same principles as a postembolic PH because the tumor rarely develops outside of the arterial wall. Consequently, a true PEA can be performed with satisfactory tumor removal and major postoperative hemodynamic improvement.

Chemotherapy and lung metastasectomies usually portend a poor long-term prognosis due to frequent tumor recurrence, but in our series of 20 cases, 20% of patients have survived more than five years.

B. Tumor Emboli into the Pulmonary Artery

A variety of carcinomas (particularly renal, testicular, and uterine) may release emboli to the pulmonary arteries that become obstructed either by embolization or by direct extension of the tumor through the vena cava and right-heart chambers. Uterine leiomyomatosis, a benign tumor with vascular tropism, can invade the IVC and obstruct the pulmonary arteries. Similarly, testicular tumors may continue to grow as teratomas in the IVC and in the pulmonary arteries after response to chemotherapy and normalization of tumoral markers.

C. Hydatic Emboli

Hydatic cysts of the liver can migrate spontaneously or during hepatic surgery into the IVC and the pulmonary arteries causing downstream thrombosis and obstruction of a large part of the pulmonary vascular bed. The diagnosis of this form of PH is aided by the clinical context and positive serology. This type of PH may also be treated by PEA when the distal bed is obliterated, or by resection of the intraluminal hydatic cyst when the distal bed is free of thrombus.

References

1. McCurry KR, Shearon TH, Edwards LB, et al. Lung transplantation in the United States, 1998–2007. Am J Transplant 2009; 9(4 pt 2):942–958.
2. Trulock EP, Christie JD, Edwards LB, et al. Registry of the International Society for Heart and Lung Transplantation: twenty-fourth official adult lung and heart-lung transplantation report-2007. J Heart Lung Transplant 2007; 26(8):782–795.
3. Blanc J, Vouhe P, Bonnet D. Potts shunt in patients with pulmonary hypertension. N Engl J Med 2004; 350(6):623.
4. Dartevelle P, Fadel E, Chapelier A, et al. [Surgical treatment of post-embolism pulmonary hypertension]. Rev Pneumol Clin 2004; 60(2):124–134.
5. Dartevelle P, Fadel E, Mussot S, et al. [Surgical treatment of chronic thromboembolic pulmonary hypertension]. Presse Med 2005; 34(19 pt 2):1475–1486.
6. Dartevelle P, Fadel E, Mussot S, et al. Chronic thromboembolic pulmonary hypertension. Eur Respir J 2004; 23(4):637–648.
7. Klepetko W, Mayer E, Sandoval J, et al. Interventional and surgical modalities of treatment for pulmonary arterial hypertension. J Am Coll Cardiol 2004; 43(12 suppl S):73S–80S.
8. Madani MM, Jamieson SW. Technical advances of pulmonary endarterectomy for chronic thromboembolic pulmonary hypertension. Semin Thorac Cardiovasc Surg 2006; 18(3):243–249.
9. Galie N, Torbicki A, Barst R, et al. Guidelines on diagnosis and treatment of pulmonary arterial hypertension. The Task Force on Diagnosis and Treatment of Pulmonary Arterial Hypertension of the European Society of Cardiology. Eu Heart J 2004; 25(24):2243–2278.
10. Jais X, Dartevelle P, Parent F, et al. [Postembolic pulmonary hypertension]. Rev Mal Respir 2007; 24(4 pt 1):497–508.
11. Manecke GR Jr., Wilson WC, Auger WR, et al. Chronic thromboembolic pulmonary hypertension and pulmonary thromboendarterectomy. Semin Cardiothorac Vasc Anesth 2005; 9(3):189–204.
12. Thistlethwaite PA, Kemp A, Du L, et al. Outcomes of pulmonary endarterectomy for treatment of extreme thromboembolic pulmonary hypertension. J Thorac Cardiovasc Surg 2006; 131(2): 307–313.
13. Cabrol S, Souza R, Jais X, et al. Intravenous epoprostenol in inoperable chronic thromboembolic pulmonary hypertension. J Heart Lung Transplant 2007; 26(4):357–362.
14. Paul JF, Khallil A, Sigal-Cinqualbre A, et al. Findings on submillimeter MDCT are predictive of operability in chronic thromboembolic pulmonary hypertension. AJR Am J Roentgenol 2007; 188(4):1059–1062.

30
The Selection and Timing of Transplantation for Patients with Pulmonary Arterial Hypertension

PAUL A. CORRIS
Institute of Cellular Medicine, Newcastle University and Freeman Hospital,
Newcastle upon Tyne, U.K.

I. Introduction

Lung transplantation is now a generally accepted therapy for the management of a wide range of severe lung disorders, with evidence supporting improved quality of life and survival benefit for lung transplant recipients (1). However, the number of donor organs available remains far fewer than the number of patients with end-stage lung disease who might potentially benefit from the procedure. It is of primary importance, therefore, to optimize the use of this resource, such that the selection of patients who receive a transplant represents those with realistic prospects of favorable long-term outcomes. There is a clear ethical responsibility to respect these altruistic gifts from all donor families and to balance the medical resource requirements of one potential recipient against those of others in their society. These concepts apply equally to listing a candidate with the intention of transplant and potentially delisting (perhaps only temporarily) a candidate whose health condition changes such that a successful outcome is no longer predicted.

In addition to considering absolute and relative contraindications to lung transplantation, this chapter discusses specific factors that may be used in deciding when a patient with pulmonary arterial hypertension (PAH) should be referred to a transplant center and when transplantation should be considered.

II. Patient Selection—General

A. Indications

Lung transplantation is indicated for patients with PAH or associated medical conditions such as pulmonary capillary hemangiomatosis (PCH) who fail maximal medical therapy or for whom no effective medical therapy exists. Potential candidates should be well informed and demonstrate adequate health behavior and willingness to adhere to guidelines from health care professionals.

The primary goal of lung transplantation is to provide a survival benefit. Several studies have demonstrated that lung transplantation confers such benefit, particularly in patients with advanced cystic fibrosis, idiopathic pulmonary fibrosis, and idiopathic pulmonary hypertension (2–5). Reports for emphysema patients are conflicted (6), and two studies including patients with Eisenmenger syndrome did not find a survival benefit (2,3). Uncertainties regarding the methodology and the validity of several assumptions used in the analysis together with improved posttransplant survival rates over time affect conclusions drawn from these studies.

How to weigh expected survival benefit with gains in quality of life is a topic of considerable discussion in the transplant community. Lung transplantation for most patients is a palliative rather than curative treatment, and improvements in quality of life in addition to survival should be used to assess the effectiveness of the procedure (7,8), a view shared by patients themselves (9). Thus, the patient's quality of life should be taken into account when the need for a lung transplant is assessed, but owing to the storage of donor organs, it is not currently possible to support transplantation solely for quality-of-life purposes.

B. General Contraindications

Lung transplantation remains a complex therapy with a significant risk of perioperative morbidity and mortality; therefore, it is important to consider the overall sum of contraindications and comorbidities. The following lists are not intended to include all possible clinical scenarios, but rather to highlight common areas of concern.

Absolute Contraindications

- Malignancy in the last two years, with the exception of cutaneous squamous and basal cell tumors. In general, a five-year disease-free interval is prudent. The role of lung transplantation for localized bronchoalveolar cell carcinoma remains controversial.
- Untreatable advanced dysfunction of another major organ system (e.g., heart, liver, or kidney). Coronary artery disease not amenable to percutaneous intervention or bypass grafting, or associated with significant impairment or left ventricular function, is an absolute contraindication to lung transplantation, but heart-lung transplantation (HLT) could be considered in highly selected cases.
- Noncurable chronic extrapulmonary infection including chronic active viral hepatitis B, hepatitis C, and human immunodeficiency virus.
- Significant chest wall/spinal deformity.
- Documented nonadherence or inability to follow through with medical therapy or office follow-up, or both.
- Untreatable psychiatric or psychological condition associated with the inability to cooperate or comply with medical therapy.
- Absence of a consistent or reliable social support system.
- Substance addiction (e.g. alcohol, tobacco, or narcotics), either active or within the last six months.

Relative Contraindications

- Age older than 65 years. Older patients have less optimal survival (1), likely due to comorbidities, and therefore, recipient age should be a factor in candidate selection. Although there cannot be endorsement of an upper age limit as an absolute contraindication (recognizing that advancing age alone in an otherwise acceptable candidate with few comorbidities does not necessarily compromise successful transplant outcomes), the presence of several relative contraindications can combine to increase the risks of transplantation above a safe threshold.

- Critical or unstable clinical condition (e.g., shock, mechanical ventilation, or extracorporeal membrane oxygenation).
- Severely limited functional status with poor rehabilitation potential.
- Colonization with highly resistant or highly virulent bacteria, fungi, or mycobacteria.
- Severe obesity defined as a body mass index (BMI) exceeding 30 mg/m^2 (3,10).
- Severe or symptomatic osteoporosis.
- Mechanical ventilation, carefully selected candidates on mechanical ventilation without other acute or chronic organ dysfunction, who are able to actively participate in a meaningful rehabilitation program, may be successfully transplanted.
- Other medical conditions that have not resulted in end-stage organ damage, such as diabetes mellitus, systemic hypertension, peptic ulcer disease, or gastroesophageal reflux should be optimally treated before transplantation.

C. Timing of Referral

In general, referral for transplantation assessment is advisable when patients have a less than 50%, two- to three-year predicted survival or New York Heart Association (NYHA) class III or IV level of function, or both. The chance of surviving the waiting period will depend on the waiting time, underlying disease, and the existing system for allocation of donor organs. Waiting time tends to be variable and is based on many factors such as height and blood group. It tends to be longer for small women compared with taller patients and for recipients with blood groups other than AB. Patients who have idiopathic pulmonary fibrosis, cystic fibrosis, or idiopathic pulmonary hypertension experience lower survival rates while awaiting lung transplantation compared with patients who have emphysema or Eisenmenger syndrome (2).

III. Patient Selection—PAH

A. Introduction

Because of new and efficacious medical therapies in PAH, patients are registered on waiting lists later than before, after failing medical therapy, and consequently they are in a more end-stage disease, often with major distension of the heart, ascites, edema, and renal insufficiency. Their survival after waiting list registration is consequently very short; many patients are transplanted emergently, in very severe condition, and because of that, they may not have optimal donors.

Development of these medical therapies has taught teams in charge of PAH to better recognize pulmonary veno-occlusive disease (PVOD) and PCH, which usually do not respond to medical therapy and worsen under epoprostenol due to the development of pulmonary edema. These patients must be registered very urgently on the waiting list, in view of the absence of a medical alternative to lung transplantation.

In PAH related to congenital cardiac abnormalities, criteria for registration remain very difficult to define, considering the length of their evolution. On the basis of the better tolerance of Eisenmenger syndrome compared with PAH, the concept of Pott's anastomosis in idiopathic PAH in children has been developed and seems to considerably increase the quality of life of these patients and their survival.

Transplantation in congenital cardiac abnormalities, which is always performed after a long evolution of disease, is still associated with high mortality, due to liver and kidney dysfunction and bleeding during surgery.

It is important to mention that transplantation for vascular disease is currently performed in patients on intravenous prostaglandin and combination therapy or even circulatory support (ECMO), and consequently finding heart-lung and lung donors is a high priority.

In contrast with the trend for using increasingly marginal donors, lung transplantation for PAH needs optimal donors, because the newly transplanted lungs are facing a different circulation, both from the right ventricle, which has increased its output, and the left chamber cavities that have difficulty in dealing with the increased flow.

B. Specific Characteristics

The advent of disease-targeted therapy for severe PAH has reduced patient referral for lung transplant programs. The long-term outcomes of medically treated patients remains uncertain, and transplantation will remain an important mode of therapy for those who fail on such therapies. Studies indicate that up to 25% of patients with IPAH may fail to improve on disease-targeted therapy, and the prognosis of patients who remain in WHO functional class III or IV remains poor (11,12). International guidelines to aid referral and listing have been published by the International Society for Heart and Lung Transplantation (ISHLT) (13).

The prognosis of PAH varies according to the etiology, and PAH associated with connective tissue disease (CTD) has a worse prognosis than IPAH even when treated with prostanoids, while patients with PAH associated with congenital heart disease (CHD) have a better survival. The worst prognosis is seen in patients with PVOD and PCH because of the lack of effective medical treatments, and these patients should be listed for transplantation at the time of diagnosis. Patients with features identifying a worse prognosis profile including clinical, functional, and hemodynamic parameters (see later in the chapter) despite maximal medical therapy should be referred for transplant listing. Both heart-lung and isolated double-lung transplantation have been performed for PAH though the threshold of unrecoverable right ventricular (RV) dysfunction is unknown. As a consequence, most patients are considered for double-lung transplantation. While afterload is immediately reduced after surgery, RV function does not improve immediately, and hemodynamic instability is a common problem in the early postoperative period following isolated lung transplantation. Both single and bilateral procedures have been performed with apparent similar survival, any complication occurring in the allograft following single-lung transplantation (SLT) is associated with severe hypoxemia. Currently the vast majority of patients receive bilateral lungs as evidenced by the ISHLT Registry figures.

Patients with PAH related to complex CHD should be considered for HLT, while patients with Eisenmenger syndrome due to simple shunts have been treated by isolated lung transplantation and repair of the cardiac defect; patients with ventricular septal defect (VSD) have a better outcome with combined HLT.

C. Choice of Transplant Operation

There are three operative procedures currently used in patients with PAH, and each procedure has its own advocates, including single-lung (14–18), bilateral lung (19,20), and heart-lung (21–23) transplantation.

Proponents of SLT have argued that it is technically an easier procedure to perform, has less morbidity and mortality when compared with bilateral lung transplant (BLT) and HLT and allows more patients to receive lung transplants. Opponents have argued that patients transplanted with a single lung are more at risk not only for developing severe postoperative pulmonary edema (14,24) but also for severe ventilation/perfusion mismatches in case of acute or chronic rejection (25,26), both adversely affecting early and late survival and functional outcome. Any dysfunction that changes the compliance in the allograft can lead to rapid and sometimes marked hypoxemia in the recipient due to further shifting of ventilation from the allograft to the native lung. Early graft dysfunction due to reperfusion injury may be extremely difficult to manage, leading to severe hypoxemia and hemodynamic instability. Diffuse alveolar damage may result and is often associated with infection (14). SLT is a very satisfactory procedure in patients with PAH secondary to pulmonary parenchymal diseases, with no differences in outcome when compared with a same group of patients without PAH (27).

Proponents of BLT have argued that this procedure results in fewer ventilation/ perfusion mismatches, and as a result, patients are easier to look after in the immediate postoperative period. Moreover, this allows more marginal donor lungs to be utilized and hence makes best of the rare resource of donor lungs. Patients also have better pulmonary function and better long-term survival. According to a recent survey, this type of transplant procedure was preferred by 83% of responding centers (4). Interestingly, 100% of the North American centers respond that double-lung transplantation was their preferred type of procedure compared with only 29% in Europe and Israel where HLT remains the first choice.

HLT historically was the first and only procedure in these patients (1). Advocates of this procedure argue that the operation is not only technically more straightforward and thus associated with fewer postoperative complications, but also that obliterative bronchiolitis responsible for late death seems to occur less frequently with this type of procedure (21). Opponents of this procedure argue that isolated lung transplantation alone will result in immediate and long-term normalization of pulmonary vascular resistance (PVR) and RV ejection fraction (16,17,28,29). The donor heart can be used for isolated cardiac transplantation. Patients subjected to HLT are also at risk for accelerated graft coronary disease, although the incidence in the series from Stanford University was only 8% at five years following the transplant (21). For all these reasons, many authors have pointed out that HLT should be reserved for special indications such as patients with Eisenmenger syndrome caused by complex CHD (20,30,31) or children.

D. Comparative Studies

No prospective randomized studies are available to relieve the uncertainty as to the best lung transplant procedure for patients with PAH.

Four single centers have reported the outcomes between different transplant types for both primary and secondary hypertension. Chapelier and his colleagues reported on the results of HLT, BLT, and SLT for PAH from the Paris-Sud University Lung Transplant Group (32). There was a similar improvement in early and late right-sided hemodynamic function, pulmonary function, and two-year and four-year survival between HLT and BLT recipients. The sole patient who received a single lung developed severe pulmonary edema, left ventricular failure, persistent desaturation, and an important ventilation/perfusion mismatch. They concluded that HLT and BLT are equally effective, but SLT should be avoided.

The Pittsburgh group reported on their experience in two studies. In the first study published in 1994 by Bando et al. (33), pulmonary artery (PA) pressures decreased in all three allograft groups but remained higher in the single-lung recipients, compared with the two other groups. A significant ventilation/perfusion mismatch occurred in the SLT recipients but not in the others because of preferential blood flow to the allograft. Graft-related mortality was significantly higher and the overall functional recovery was significantly lower at one year in the SLT compared with BLT and HLT recipients. The authors concluded that BLT is a more satisfactory option for patients with pulmonary hypertension and that HLT should be preserved for recipients with complex CHDs or left ventricular dysfunction. In the second study from this group reported by Gammie et al. in 1998, SLT was compared with BLT with primary or secondary pulmonary hypertension (34). There was no difference in median duration of intubation; length of stay in the intensive care unit; hospital stay; one-month, one-year, and four-year survival; and late functional status between both groups. During this study period, 58 patients with PAH died awaiting transplantation. The authors concluded that SLT could be preferentially applied for patients on the waiting list. The group from Ann Arbor compared the outcome of SLT and simultaneous intracardiac repair versus HLT for patients with pulmonary hypertension secondary to congenital cardiac anomalies (30). One SLT recipient died perioperatively. Three of the four remaining patients surviving the first year died during the second year. The two HLT recipients were doing well 15 and 18 months after the operation. The authors concluded that SLT and simultaneous repair of intracardiac defects may have good early results, but long-term results are considerably less favorable.

Finally, the group at Johns Hopkins Hospital in Baltimore recently reported their results in 57 recipients with primary and secondary pulmonary hypertension (35). The survival of up to four years in patients with primary pulmonary hypertension was superior in BLT compared with SLT recipients (100% vs. 67%; $p = 0.02$). There was no clear advantage to SLT versus BLT for secondary pulmonary hypertension, although four-year survival was better in single-lung recipients if PA pressure was ≤ 40 mmHg (91% vs. 75%; $p = 0.11$), and it was better in bilateral lung recipients if this value was ≥ 40 mmHg (88% vs. 62%; $p = 0.19$). The authors concluded that BLT is the procedure of choice for patients with primary pulmonary hypertension and also with secondary hypertension with PA pressures ≥ 40 mmHg.

No true consensus exists for the optimal lung transplant procedure for pulmonary hypertension and likely never will. The choice will largely depend on the local situation regarding organ donors and experience of the transplant team, although the majority favor BLT.

E. Timing of Transplantation in PAH

There has been considerable change in the approach to the assessment and listing of patients with severe PAH since the development of prostanoid therapy. Until the 1990s, medical treatment had focused on chronic vasodilator therapy based on calcium channel blockade, anticoagulation, and use of diuretics, digoxin, and oxygen. In the National Institutes of Health (NIH) Registry of 1991 (36), the median survival was 2.8 years and hence patients were generally referred for consideration of transplantation when they had reached NYHA class III or class IV. A better comprehension of the pathogenesis of PAH has changed the focus of medical treatments to evaluate drugs that may reverse the vasoproliferative effects resulting in pulmonary vascular remodeling. The first drug shown to be effective was epoprostenol (PGI_2) given by a continuous intravenous infusion. In a pivotal study by Barst and colleagues (37), 81 patients were randomized to receive epoprostenol or conventional therapy. The survival was significantly improved at five years from 27% to 54% in the epoprostenol-treated group. More recent studies suggest that median survival may be approaching six years and exercise performance and quality of life are also significantly improved. Moreover, the advent of oral therapy in combination with prostenoids is now in routine practice, although the impact of such combination therapy on long-term outcomes is unknown. This has clearly impacted greatly on the timing of transplant listing, and, moreover, two studies have now demonstrated that 60% to 70% of patients who had previously been listed for transplantation on pre-epoprostenol criteria can be delisted because of clinical improvement (38,39). Survival data from the ISHLT Registry suggests a five-year survival of approximately 40% to 50% following HLT or BLT; however, PAH is one of the major risk factors for both early and late mortality with an odds ratio of 1.52 (40).

It is in this setting that pulmonary hypertension and transplant centers must decide whom to refer for listing and the timing of such a referral. One study (41) has surveyed current practices in a wide variety of transplant centers throughout North America, Europe, and Australia. Forty percent of centers felt all NYHA class III patients should be referred to transplant centers. By contrast, 57% of centers limited referral to those NYHA class III and IV patients who had failed to show benefit after an average of three months of epoprostenol therapy. A recent single-center report has demonstrated the value of assessment after three months of epoprostenol therapy. An improvement in NYHA to class II and a decrease in PVR of 30% or more is associated with a survival of 90% at five years.

Only 40% of centers use one or more hemodynamic criteria for listing. These include a mean right atrial pressure of more than 15 mmHg, PVR of 4 to 15 Wood units, a mixed venous oxygen saturation of less than 63%, and a cardiac index of less than 2 L/min (42,43). The vast majority of centers use some form of exercise testing and echocardiography to help determine functional status referral and listing (44). No single measurement on echocardiogram has emerged as most useful. The evidence suggests, however, that exercise testing can be more helpful. A six-minute walking test of more than 332 m is associated with a good prognosis, and this simple exercise test is both reproducible and correlated reasonably well with hemodynamics. It is also very sensitive in the detection of improvements related to therapy. A more formal exercise test with measurement of metabolic gas exchange is utilized by approximately 25% of centers with a mean oxygen consumption of less than 10 mL/kg/min used as an indicator for listing.

Overall, the results show that major pulmonary hypertension and transplant centers vary considerably regarding patterns of referral, listing, and transplantation of patients, and it is only with continued carefully collected registry data that guidelines for best practice will be refined. One important issue relates to the potential delay, for a NYHA class IV patient who fails to respond to intravenous epoprostenol over three months, in listing for transplantation and the effect this has on his or her overall chances of receiving a graft.

Patients who remain in a stable clinical state at NYHA class III will also prove a potentially difficult group, and it is suggested that careful note is taken of the patients' informed views in this situation.

Patients who are experiencing problems with exertional syncope but who otherwise seem to have a good quality of life should be considered for atrial septostomy in addition to receiving prostenoid therapy.

Finally, potentially life-threatening hemoptysis should also be considered an indication for listing for transplant patients.

References

1. Trulock EP, Edwards LB, Taylor DO, et al. Registry of the International Society for Heart and Lung Transplantation (twenty-second official adult lung and heart-lung transplant report—2005). J Heart Lung Transplant 2005; 24:956–967.
2. Charman SC, Sharples LD, McNeil KD, et al. Assessment of survival benefit after lung transplantation by patient diagnosis. J Heart Lung Transplant 2002; 21:226–232.
3. Demeester J, Smits J, Persijn GG, et al. Listing for lung transplantation (life expectancy and transplant effect, stratified by type of end-stage lung disease, the Eurotransplant Experience). J Heart Lung Transplant 2001; 29:518–524.
4. Thabut G, Mal H, Castier Y, et al. Survival benefit of lung transplantation for patients with idiopathic pulmonary fibrosis. J Thorac Cardiovasc Surg 2003; 126:469–475.
5. Geertsma A, ten Vergert EM, Bonsel GJ, et al. Does lung transplantation prolong life? A comparison of survival with and without transplantation. J Heart Lung Transplant 1998; 17:511–516.
6. Hosenpud JD, Bennett LE, Keck BM, et al. Effect of diagnosis on survival benefit of lung transplantation for end-stage lung disease. Lancet 1998; 351:24–27.
7. Gerbase MW, Spiliopoulos A, Rochat T, et al. Health-related quality of life following single or bilateral lung transplantation (a 7-year comparison to functional outcome). Chest 2005; 128:1371–1378.
8. Gross C, Savik K, Bolman M, et al. Long-term health status and quality-of-life outcomes of lung transplant recipients. Chest 1995; 108:1587–1593.
9. Maish AB. Priorities for lung transplantation among patients with cystic fibrosis. JAMA 2002; 287:1524–1525.
10. Kanasky WF, Anton SD, Rodrigue JR, et al. Impact of body weight on long-term survival after lung transplantation. Chest 2002; 121:401–406.
11. Sitbon O, Humbert M, Nunes H, et al. Long-term intravenous epoprostenol infusion in primary pulmonary hypertension: prognostic factors and survival. J Am Coll Cardiol 2002; 40(4):780–788.

12. McLaughlin VV, Shillington A, Rich S. Survival in primary pulmonary hypertension: the impact of epoprostenol therapy. Circulation 2002; 106(12):1477–1482.
13. Orens JB, Estenne M, Arcasoy S, et al. International guidelines for the selection of lung transplant candidates: 2006 update—a consensus report from the pulmonary scientific council of the International Society of Heart and Lung Transplantation. J Heart Lung Transplant 2006; 25:745–755.
14. Bando K, Keenan RJ, Paradis IL, et al. Impact of pulmonary hypertension on outcome after single lung transplantation. Ann Thorac Surg 1994; 58:1336–1342.
15. McCarthy PM, Rosenkranz ER, White RD, et al. Single lung transplantation with atrial septal defect repair for Eisenmenger's syndrome. Ann Thorac Surg 1991; 52:300–303.
16. Pasque MK, Trulock EP, Kaiser LR, et al. Single lung transplantation for pulmonary hypertension: three month haemodynamic follow up. Circulation 1991; 84:2275–2279.
17. Pasque MK, Trulock EP, Cooper JD, et al. Single lung transplantation for pulmonary hypertension: single institution experience in 34 patients. Circulation 1995; 92:2252–2258.
18. Starnes VA, Stinson EB, Oyer PE, et al. Single lung transplantation: a new therapeutic option for patients with pulmonary hypertension. Transplant Proc 1991; 23:1209–1210.
19. Ueno T, Smith JA, Snell GI, et al. Bilateral sequential single lung transplantation for pulmonary hypertension and Eisenmenger's syndrome. Ann Thorac Surg 2000; 69:381–387.
20. Birsan T, Zuckermann Z, Artemiou O, et al. Bilateral lung transplantation for pulmonary hypertension. Transplant Proc 1997; 29:2892–2894.
21. White RI, Robbins RC, Altinger J, et al. Heart-lung transplantation for primary pulmonary hypertension. Ann Thorac Surg 1999; 67:937–942.
22. Mikhail G, Al-Kattan K, Banner N, et al. Long-term results of heart lung transplantation for pulmonary hypertension. Transplant Proc 1997; 29:633.
23. Stoica SC, McNeil KD, Perreas K, et al. Heart lung transplantation for Eisenmenger syndrome: early and long term results. Ann Thorac Surg 2001; 72:1887–1891.
24. Boujoukos AJ, Martich GD, Vega JD, et al. Reperfusion injury in single lung transplant recipients with pulmonary hypertension and emphysema. J Heart Lung Transplant 1997; 16:440–448.
25. Kramer MR, Marshall SE, McDougall IR, et al. The distribution of ventilation and perfusion after single lung transplantation in patients with pulmonary fibrosis and pulmonary hypertension. Transplant Proc 1991; 23:1215–1216.
26. Levine SM, Jenkinson SG, Bryan CL, et al. Ventilation-perfusion inequalities during graft rejection in patients undergoing single lung transplantation for primary pulmonary hypertension. Chest 1992; 101:401–405.
27. Huerd SS, Hodges TN, Grover FL, et al. Secondary pulmonary hypertension does not adversely affect outcome after single lung transplantation. J Thorac Cardiovasc Surg 2000; 119:458–465.
28. Kramer MR, Valantine HA, Marshall SE, et al. Recovery of the right ventricle after single lung transplantation. Am J Cardiol 1994; 73:494–500.
29. Shulman LR, Leibowitz DW, Anadarangam T, et al. Variability of right ventricular functional recovery after lung transplantation. Transplantation 1996; 62:622–625.
30. Lupinetti FM, Bolling SF, Bove EL, et al. Selective lung or heart lung transplantation for pulmonary hypertension associated with congenital cardiac anomalies. Ann Thorac Surg 1994; 57:1545–1549.
31. Waddell TK, Bennett LW, Kennedy R, et al. Lung or heart lung transplantation for Eisenmenger's syndrome: analysis of the ISHLT/UNOS joint thoracic registry (abstract). J Heart Lung Transplant 2000; 19:57.
32. Chapelier A, Vouhe P, Macchiarini P, et al. Comparative outcome of heart lung and lung transplantation for pulmonary hypertension. J Thorac Cardiovac Surg 1993; 106:299–307.

33. Bando K, Armitage JM, Paradis IL, et al. Indications for, and results of, single, bilateral and heart lung transplantation for pulmonary hypertension. J Thorac Cardiovasc Surg 1994; 108:1056–1065.
34. Gammie JS, Keenan RJ, Pham SM, et al. Single versus double lung transplantation for pulmonary hypertension. J Thorac Cardiovasc Surg 1998; 115:397–403.
35. Conte JV, Borja MJ, Patel CB, et al. Lung transplantation for primary and secondary pulmonary hypertension. Ann Thorac Surg 2001; 72:1673–1680.
36. D'Alonzo GE, Barst RJ, Ayers SM, et al. Survival in patients with primary pulmonary hypertension. Ann Intern Med 1991; 115:343–349.
37. Barst RJ, Rubin LJ, Long WA, et al. A comparison of continuous intravenous epoprostenol (prostacyclin) with conventional therapy for primary pulmonary hypertension. N Engl J Med 1996; 334:296–301.
38. Robbins IM, Christman BW, Newman JH, et al. A survey of diagnostic practices and the use of epoprostenol in patients with primary pulmonary hypertension. Chest 1998; 114:1269–1275.
39. Conte JV, Gaine SP, Orens JB, et al. The influence of continuous intravenous prostacyclin therapy for primary pulmonary hypertension on the timing and outcome of transplantation. J Heart Lung Transplant 1998; 17:679–685.
40. Hosenpud JD, Bennett LE, Keck BM, et al. The registry of the International Society for Heart and Lung Transplantation: seventeenth official report. J Heart Lung Transplant 2000; 19:909–931.
41. Pielsticker EJ, Martinex FJ, Rubenfire M. Lung and heart lung transplant practice patterns in pulmonary hypertension centres. J Heart Lung Transplant 2001; 20:1297–1304.
42. Rich S, Levy PS. Characteristics of surviving and non-surviving patients with primary pulmonary hypertension. Am J Med 1984; 76:573–578.
43. Glanville AR, Burke CM, Theodore J, et al. Primary pulmonary hypertension: length of survival of patients referred for heart and lung transplantation. Chest 1987; 91:675–681.
44. Eysmann SB, Palevsky HI, Reichek N, et al. Two dimensional echocardiography and cardiac catheterisation correlates of survival in primary pulmonary hypertension. Circulation 1989; 79:353–360.

31
Pulmonary Arterial Hypertension and Pregnancy

XAVIER JAÏS, LAURA CLAIRE PRICE, FLORENCE PARENT, and MARC HUMBERT
Université Paris Sud 11, Service de Pneumologie et Réanimation Respiratoire, Hôpital Antoine Béclère, Assistance Publique Hôpitaux de Paris, Clamart, France

I. Introduction

Pulmonary arterial hypertension (PAH) is defined as a mean pulmonary artery pressure (mPAP) greater than 25 mmHg in the setting of normal or reduced cardiac output (CO) and normal pulmonary capillary wedge pressure (PCWP) ($\leq$15 mmHg) (1). PAH is a disease of the small pulmonary arteries characterized by vascular proliferation and remodeling (2). It results in a progressive increase in pulmonary vascular resistance (PVR), right ventricular failure, and ultimately death. PAH can be characterized as idiopathic (IPAH) or familial, or may be associated with other conditions including collagen vascular disease, congenital heart disease (CHD), portal hypertension, HIV infection, and the use of certain drugs (3). PAH most commonly occurs in women of childbearing age (4). During the last decade, new advanced therapies for the treatment of PAH have evolved, improving the quality of life and outcomes of PAH patients. However, despite these recent therapeutic advances, no treatment can cure this devastating condition (5).

Pregnancy in women with PAH including IPAH or PAH associated with CHD or other conditions is reported to be associated with a high maternal mortality, historically estimated between 30% and 56% (6). Indeed, the major hemodynamic changes that occur during pregnancy are poorly tolerated in these patients. Therefore, clinical practice guidelines strongly discouraged pregnancy and recommended an effective method of contraception in women of childbearing age (7). Over recent years, new advanced therapies have been shown to improve outcome and have resulted in more women of childbearing age considering pregnancy (5). In addition, several reports of successful pregnancies in patients treated with advanced PAH therapies have been published (8–19) and may suggest that advances in the multidisciplinary approach have decreased the high mortality rate previously reported (6). This chapter will focus on the management of PAH during pregnancy in the current era and its impact on the maternal outcome.

II. Physiological Considerations

A. Hemodynamic Changes in Normal Pregnancy

Important changes occur as early as 5 to 8 weeks into the pregnancy and gradually return to normal 2 to 12 weeks postpartum. These changes follow the estrogen- and prostaglandin-induced relaxation of vascular smooth muscle, leading to an increase in the venous capacitance and a reduction in the systemic vascular resistance (SVR) (20).

Total blood volume rises above the prepregnancy level by 10%, 30%, and 45% over the first, second, and third trimesters, respectively. This increases the end-diastolic volume and heart rate by 10–20 beats/ minute while CO increases by 30% to 50% by the second trimester mostly due to an increase in stroke volume (21). There is a remarkable fluctuation in resting CO with changes in position; the compression of the inferior vena cava by the enlarged gravid uterus in the supine position results in decreased venous return and a concomitant significant decrease in CO. The CO usually exceeds the nonpregnant level by 50% at week 20 to 24. During the final trimester it can remain at this level, increase further, or even decrease (22).

In contrast, there is no change in central venous pressure (CVP) or PCWP, as both SVR and PVR are reduced. The 20% to 30% fall in SVR is a fundamental physiological change in pregnancy and is a consequence of systemic vasodilatation and the development of the low-resistance uteroplacental circulation. Lastly, pulmonary pressures remain normal due to a similar decrease in PVR to accommodate the increased CO (21). Table 1 summarizes the main hemodynamic changes during a normal pregnancy.

Other significant cardiovascular changes occur at the time of labor, delivery, and in the postpartum period. CO increases even further during labor, up to 15% in the first stage and 50% in the second stage, especially during contractions, when oxygen consumption is greatly increased, but also between contractions. The sympathetic response to pain and anxiety further elevate heart rate and blood pressure. Uterine contractions lead to an autotransfusion of a total of 300 to 500 mL of blood back into the circulation, and following delivery of the baby, up to 1 L of placental blood may be returned to the circulation following aortocaval decompression and contraction of the uterus. Intrathoracic blood volume rises, and CO increases up to 80% of preterm values. This is followed by a rapid reduction in heart rate, SVR, and CO within hours of delivery. Postpartum, all these changes revert quite rapidly during the first week postpartum, and more slowly over the following six weeks (23,24).

Table 1 Hemodynamic Changes in Normal Pregnancy

Parameter	Effect of normal pregnancy
Heart rate (32 wk)	Elevated 10–20 beats/min
SVR	20–30% lower
PVR	20–30% lower
Cardiac output (25 wk)	30–50% higher
Blood volume	Elevated 40%
Plasma volume	Elevated 45–50%
Red cell mass	Elevated 20–30%
PCWP	No change
CVP	No change

B. Physiological Consequences of Gestational Hemodynamic Changes in PAH

The increased blood volume and CO throughout pregnancy, and especially the fluid shifts following delivery, will be an extreme maternal challenge in PAH patients, with their high and fixed resistance to pulmonary vascular flow. In normal subjects, the low-resistance pulmonary vascular bed usually copes easily with the large increase in blood flow seen in pregnancy (as with exercise) through vasodilatation and recruitment of pulmonary capillaries. This allows large changes in pulmonary blood flow to be tolerated with little change in PAP. In PAH, obliteration of pulmonary vessels reduces the total area of the pulmonary vascular bed, and remodeled pulmonary vessels are less able to vasodilate; hence this ability for pulmonary vascular recruitment is diminished. The resulting excessive afterload on the right ventricle (RV) will be poorly tolerated, and with increasing right ventricular pressure overload, a downward spiral of RV failure will follow (25).

III. Epidemiology and Prognosis

Some data regarding the overall incidence of PAH in pregnancy are available from a large health survey. A 2002 to 2004 U.S.-wide analysis reported 182 patients with IPAH out of 11.2 million deliveries (26).

Outcome data are mostly limited to retrospective review of cases. Two major series reviewed all published reports of pregnancies in women with PAH to evaluate their characteristics, management, and outcome (6,27). The first one analyzed all cases published between 1978 and 1996 and included 125 patients undergoing PAH pregnancies beyond 22 weeks, of which 73 patients had Eisenmenger syndrome, 27 had IPAH, and 25 had what was then termed "secondary pulmonary hypertension" (anorexigen-induced PAH, connective tissue disease–PAH, sickle cell disease PAH, and portopulmonary hypertension), and chronic thromboembolic pulmonary hypertension (CTEPH) (6). Maternal mortality was found to be 36% in mothers with Eisenmenger syndrome, 30% in "primary PH" (now termed IPAH), and 56% in secondary PH. Except for three prepartal deaths due to Eisenmenger syndrome, all fatalities occurred within 35 days after delivery. Late diagnosis of PAH and timing of hospital admission (risk increasing by 9% with each week of pregnancy) were independent risk factors of maternal mortality. Moreover, operative delivery, severity of pulmonary hypertension (PH), and number of previous pregnancies and deliveries were contributing factors. Lastly, neonatal survival ranging from 87% to 89% was similar in the three groups and was significantly influenced by maternal outcome. During the last decade, new advanced therapies for the treatment of PAH have emerged, and the management of high-risk pregnancies has improved. Therefore, a recent study examined whether the contemporary approach to pregnancy and PAH (since 1997) has had an impact on maternal outcome (27). In this study, the authors performed a systematic review of all cases published in the past decade (1997–2007), representing 73 parturients with IPAH, CHD-associated PAH (CHD-PAH), or PAH of other etiology (connective tissue disease–associated PAH, CTEPH, HIV infection–associated PAH, medication-induced PAH). Outcome data observed in this study were then compared with relevant data published between 1978 and 1996 by Weiss and colleagues (6,27). Overall, maternal mortality for parturients with PAH was lower in the last decade compared with previous area ($p = 0.047$). Mortality decreased substantially in all three subgroups (from 30% to 17% in IPAH, 36% to 28% in CHD-PAH, and 56% to 33% in PAH of other etiology), although not reaching statistical significance. The majority of deaths occurred during the post-partum period, mainly within the first month after delivery. Patients receiving general anesthesia (GA) were four times more likely to die, compared with those receiving regional anesthesia (RA). Primigravidae were at higher mortality risk compared with parturients with previous pregnancies (27).

IV. Clinical Presentation

Deterioration of PH during pregnancy has been reported to occur between the 20th and 24th weeks of gestation, when pregnancy-related hemodynamic changes are the most important (17). Fatigue, worsening of dyspnea, syncope, and chest pain are the most frequently observed symptoms (8). Patients are likely to be admitted antenatally mainly because of clinical deterioration as it is indicated in the U.S. series where IPAH led to a fivefold increase in antenatal hospitalizations (26). More patients with CHD-PAH (76–81%) have a preexisting diagnosis of PAH prior to pregnancy, compared to IPAH (26–45%), which are relatively more likely to present with de novo PAH (6,27). In this setting, dyspnea, excessive peripheral edema and weight gain, for example, may be considered as normal during pregnancy, and diagnosis of PAH can easily be delayed.

V. Investigations

A. Echocardiography and Right-Heart Catheterization

As in the nonpregnancy setting, echocardiography is a very useful screening technique to detect patients with suspected PH. A study of 11 critically ill obstetric patients, where echocardiography and right-heart catheterization (RHC) were performed simulta-neously, showed a good correlation between the two techniques in the estimation of cardiac index, intracardiac pressures, or pulmonary artery systolic pressure (28). A more recent study evaluated the correlation of estimated PAPs by echocardiography with RHC measurements in pregnant women (29). Here again, the results showed a good corre-lation between right ventricular systolic pressure (estimated by echo) and PAP measured by RHC. However, in 30% of cases, RHC eliminated the diagnosis of PH when echo-cardiography suspected the presence of PH. Lastly, a study was undertaken to compare the accuracy of echocardiography versus RHC to estimate PAPs in pregnant women with suspected PH (30). Of the 20 patients evaluated in the study, PAP was significantly greater when estimated by echocardiography than when measured by catheterization (59.6 vs. 54.8 mmHg; $p < 0.004$). In addition, 32% of the patients had PH when estimated by echocardiography but had normal PAPs on subsequent catheterization. Therefore, RHC remains the gold standard to confirm the presence of PAH, to assess the severity of the disease, and to guide treatment decisions such as pregnancy interruption or preterm delivery. Roberts and Keast have been able to provide some prognostic data on pregnant patients with PAH, using RHC values demonstrating an improvement in survival, with a cardiac index of >4 L/min, right atrial pressure <10 mmHg, and PVR <1000 dyne.sec/cm^5 (31).

VI. Management of Pregnant Women with PAH

Mortality rates among pregnant women with PAH remain prohibitively high, although they seem to have decreased in the last decade (27). Therefore, pregnancy should continue to be contraindicated in patients with PAH and an effective method of contraception is strongly recommended in women of childbearing age (5,27). Barrier contraceptive methods are safe but with an unpredictable effect. Oral contraception with progesterone only preparation such as medroxyprogesterone acetate and etonogestrel is an effective approach to contraception and avoids potential issues of estrogens. It should be remembered that endothelin receptor antagonist (ERA) bosentan may reduce the efficacy of oral contraceptive agents. Levonorgestrel-releasing intrauterine device (Mirena coil) is also effective but rarely leads to a vasovagal reaction when inserted, and this may be poorly tolerated in the setting of severe PAH. A combination of two methods may also be utilized (32). If pregnancy occurs in a patient with known PAH and/or if PAH is detected early in pregnancy, termination should be considered and performed as soon as the decision has been made, preferably in the first trimester and in any case before 22 weeks. Suction curettage under local anesthesia is the preferred method (27,33). Indeed, there are no data regarding medical abortion with oral antiprogesterones. For patients with PAH who continue with the pregnancy, a multidisciplinary approach including obstetricians, anesthetists, PAH specialists, and close monitoring at a referral PAH center is recommended. Pregnant women with PAH should be seen at least monthly and, in addition to full clinical evaluation, echocardiography should be performed (34). Moreover, repeated ultrasonography should be recommended to assess for intrauterine growth retardation that has been reported to occur in 33% of cases of PH, especially in patients with antiphospholipid antibodies and lupus-associated PAH (14,35).

A. General Measures and Conventional Medical Therapy

Given their preexisting cardiopulmonary limitations, women are advised to minimize additional cardiac demands by limiting their physical activity. Periods of bed rest in the lateral position are recommended to avoid inferior vena cava compression by the fetus and reduced venous return to the heart. Although diuretics are usually avoided during pregnancy, many patients with PAH who develop right-heart failure require diuretics under careful supervision to reduce volume overload (34). Furosemide may be the loop diuretic of choice, and the dose may be escalated as required. Supplemental oxygen may be needed when patients are hypoxemic in an effort to avoid further increases in PVR.

Lifelong anticoagulation is recommended in patients with IPAH to reduce the risk of in situ thrombosis and thromboembolism. These patients generally receive vitamin K antagonists (VKAs). However, VKAs are contraindicated during pregnancy. Therefore, anticoagulation with full-dose subcutaneous low molecular weight heparin (LMWH) is recommended throughout the pregnancy, although there are no clear guidelines on the use of prophylactic versus full dosage (17,34,36). Antepartum anticoagulation is debated in Eisenmenger patients with thrombotic and bleeding diathesis and needs to be discussed for each patient by the multidisciplinary team (36).

B. PAH-Specific Therapy

Although the treatment of PAH in pregnancy is not well documented, case reports, which provide a low level of evidence, have described the successful use of targeted pulmonary antiproliferative and/or vasodilator therapy in this patient population (8–19). In addition, some studies have demonstrated that an increased mortality was associated with both severe PH and late diagnosis (6). Therefore, early treatment is indicated.

Calcium Channel Blockers

In the patients who have evidence of a positive response to inhaled nitric oxide (iNO) during acute vasoreactivity testing, high-dose calcium channel blockers (CCBs) are indicated (37), and both nifedipine and diltiazem are safe to use during pregnancy (33,38). Sometimes, in those "responders" to iNO, high-dose CCB may produce near-normalization of pulmonary arterial pressure and right ventricular function after long-term use (37). Those patients, with near-normal hemodynamics, may represent the only subgroup of PAH patients for whom pregnancy could be allowed (17,38).

Prostanoids

Prostacyclin induces relaxation of vascular smooth muscle and inhibits the growth of smooth muscle cells. In addition, it is a powerful inhibitor of platelet aggregation. Intravenous prostacyclin (IV epoprostenol) was the first prostacyclin used to treat PAH in the 1980s and remains today the first-line therapy for the most severe patients (5). Reproductive studies in rats and rabbits have shown no impaired fertility or fetal harm at 2.5 to 4.8 times the recommended human dose (36). At least 12 case reports have described the use of IV epoprostenol in pregnant patients with PAH, including those with severe disease (8,9,11–14,17,38). In these case reports, epoprostenol was initiated for most patients several weeks before or near the time of delivery. There have been at least two reported maternal deaths despite treatment with epoprostenol: one with a late diagnosis made of severe right ventricular failure due to PAH presenting in pregnancy (38) and another with severe PH when prostanoids were not started until after cesarean section (8). Conversely, no adverse fetal outcome was recorded.

Iloprost, a stable prostacyclin analogue that can be delivered by inhalation to patients, has been also used during pregnancy (8,15,16). At least five cases of pregnant patients in NYHA functional class II or III who received nebulized iloprost for PAH have been published. Iloprost was started during the second and third trimester of pregnancy for the majority of patients. All infants were free from congenital abnormalities, and there was no postpartum maternal or infant mortality.

Phosphodiesterase Type 5 Inhibitors

Sildenafil is effective in PAH through a reduction in cyclic GMP breakdown, thus increasing the sensitivity of pulmonary vascular smooth muscle to nitric oxide. In addition, sildenafil causes uterine artery vasodilatation and has been shown to have beneficial effects on myometrial thickness. There have been at least two reports of its successful use in pregnancy (18,19). Neither case reported adverse fetal outcomes.

Endothelin Receptor Antagonists

Bosentan, sitaxsentan, and ambrisentan are potent teratogens and are, therefore, contraindicated in pregnancy (39,40). Pregnancy is thus excluded prior to starting treatment with antagonist receptor antagonist.

Nitric Oxide

Nitric oxide is mostly used to assess pulmonary vasoreactivity (5), but has also been used as treatment during pregnancy and the peripartum period in many cases (10,17).

Recommendations

IV epoprostenol should be the preferred treatment for patients in NYHA functional class III or IV and should be started as early as possible (14,17,36). Nebulized iloprost (15,16) or oral sildenafil (18,19) may be an option for patients in NYHA functional class II with more stable PAH.

An algorithm for the management of pregnant women with PAH is proposed in Figure 1.

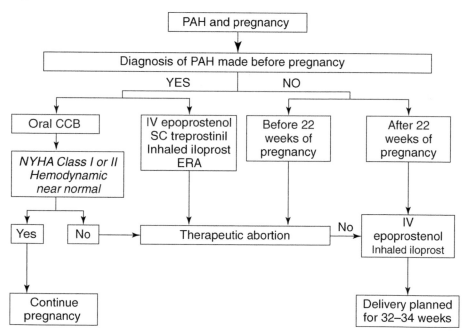

Figure 1 Algorithm for the management of pregnant women with PAH. *Abbreviations*: CCB, calcium channel blocker; ERA, endothelin receptor antagonist; PDE-5 I, phosphodiesterase type-5 inhibitors.

C. Mode of Delivery and Anesthetic Management

Multidisciplinary care and good planning is central to the overall care of these patients, and ideally their peripartum management should be managed in a center with suitable facilities and expertise (17,27,34). The goal for management of delivery includes avoiding increases in PVR and maintenance of right ventricular preload. The timing and optimum mode of delivery (vaginal vs. caesarean section) remains debated (6,17,27,34,41). A recent study in mothers with congenital heart disease including CHD-PAH patients showed no influence of the delivery method on maternal cardiac event rate (42). Vaginal delivery is associated with less blood loss and thromboembolic risk, although the latter is reduced with thromboprophylaxis, and a lower risk of infection (43). There are also less abrupt hemodynamic changes during vaginal delivery, particularly when assisted by effective analgesia and a short second stage of labor. However, prolonged, difficult, and painful labors can have detrimental pulmonary vascular effects. Caesarean section (CS) may become necessary in cases of maternal hemodynamic deterioration or fetal distress requiring urgent delivery (27). Moreover, the proportion of premature deliveries is reported to be high (59–85%) in several studies (17,27,35). Therefore, lack of predictable delivery time where the team can be fully prepared makes a case for the planned induction of labor. Scheduled caesarean delivery is now frequently used and seems to be a safe procedure (8,15,17,44–48). In the 2002 to 2004 U.S. report, 105 out of 182 (57.9%) IPAH cases were delivered under caesarean compared with 31.1% in controls ($p < 0.05$) (26). Scheduled caesarean delivery has the advantage of taking place during the day and avoiding the risk of an urgent caesarean delivery during labor with the hemodynamic instability that could occur under such conditions. The timing is usually 32 to 34 weeks for planned deliveries to allow sufficient fetal maturity while avoiding unplanned emergency deliveries. The hemodynamic principles of anesthetic management in these women are the maintenance of oxygenation, normovolemia and normotension. They also involve minimizing increases in catecholamine surges with adequate analgesia, and reducing ventricular preload in the immediate postpartum period. Successful deliveries by CS under GA have been reported (17,44). However, other authors have described increased pulmonary arterial pressure during laryngoscopy and tracheal intubation; moreover, adverse effects of positive-pressure ventilation on venous return may ultimately lead to cardiac failure (49). In addition, in their systematic review of all cases of parturient women with PAH published between 1997 and 2007, Bédard and colleagues found that parturient women who received GA were at higher risk of death (27). Therefore, there is an increasing body of evidence suggesting that CS under RA is preferable. Nonetheless, the dense and extended block needed to prevent pain during cesarean delivery may have significant hemodynamic consequences. Specifically, single-shot spinal anesthesia is considered contraindicated in these patients. Therefore, incremental epidural anesthesia is thought to be the ideal anesthetic technique (45,46). However, for a better sensory block, some authors preferred using combined spinal-epidural anesthesia (17,46,47). For patients on anticoagulation, even at prophylactic doses, care needs to be taken during RA to minimize the risk of neuraxial hematoma. The potential additional bleeding risk due to the antiplatelet effects of prostacyclin has been considered; however, as far as we are aware, there have been no reported cases of this potential complication when heparinization is temporarily discontinued (14,17).

Intraoperative monitoring at delivery is always advocated with ECG, pulse oximetry, and invasive arterial blood pressure monitoring (8,17,38,45,46). In contrast, the use of the pulmonary arterial catheter is debated owing to associated complications such as pulmonary artery perforation and the lack of evidence that it improves outcomes in parturient with PAH (6,17,27). In a single-center series, standard vascular access included a radial artery catheter, a central venous line, and a large bore catheter for rapid fluid infusion (17).

Oxytocic drugs such as oxytocin, which improve uterine contraction, may also have major hemodynamic effects. Continuous infusion of oxytocin, at the lowest effective rate, in low-volume fluid, has minimal cardiovascular effects and avoids the circulatory overload (17,33,49).

D. Postpartum Management

The postpartum period is the most critical time for acute PH exacerbations (8,17,27). The possible risk of a PH crisis and/or severe right ventricular (RV) failure should be anticipated by the multidisciplinary team and ideally a management plan preconceived. Current recommendations are to continue close maternal monitoring for at least 72-hour postpartum in an intensive care unit (17,25,33,44). The onset of severe hypoxemia and/ or hypotension may suggest worsening RV failure, which may relate to placental autotransfusion, excessive PVR due to any cause or to adverse hemodynamic effects of oxytocin. The principles of management of RV failure include minimization of RV afterload, maintenance of appropriate RV preload with sufficient SVR, and off-loading of the RV, as appropriate (17,25). In the setting of a PH crisis, with equalization of systemic and pulmonary vascular pressures, the minimization of RV afterload is absolutely crucial. Therapies for postpartum PH crises have included iNO (8,17), epoprostenol (8,9,14,17), or inhaled iloprost (8,15,16). Systemic vasopressors and inotropes may also be needed in case of unstable hemodynamic status, with dobutamine being a good choice of inotrope as it increases contractility but not PVR/SVR ratio. In terms of vasopressors, norepinephrine is often used (17,49). Anticoagulation is widely indicated in the postpartum period. LMWH can usually be restarted 12 hours after delivery in the absence of persistent bleeding (50).

VII. Conclusion

Despite recent advances in the management of pregnant women with PAH, maternal mortality still remains high. Therefore, pregnancy should continue to be strongly discouraged in patients with PAH. Patients who become pregnant should be informed of the high risk of pregnancy and early termination, when it is possible, should be discussed. The patients who choose to continue pregnancy should be treated early with PAH-targeted therapies including IV epoprostenol and/or sildenafil. In addition, the treatment and care of the pregnant woman with PAH can be challenging and is best undertaken at PAH referral centers that can manage this unique state with a multidisciplinary team approach. This allows formulation of an agreed and documented management strategy for planned delivery and postpartum monitoring.

References

1. Barst RJ, McGoon MD, Torbicki A, et al. Diagnosis and differential assessment of pulmonary arterial hypertension. J Am Coll Cardiol 2004; 43:40S–47S.
2. Rubin LJ. Primary pulmonary hypertension. N Engl J Med 1997; 336:111–117.
3. Simonneau G, Galie N, Rubin LJ, et al. Clinical classification of pulmonary hypertension. J Am Coll Cardiol 2004; 43:5S–12S.
4. Rich S, Dantzker DR, Ayres SM, et al. Primary pulmonary hypertension: a national prospective study. Ann Intern Med 1987; 107:216–223.
5. Humbert M, Sitbon O, Simonneau G. Treatment of pulmonary arterial hypertension. N Engl J Med 2004; 351:1425–1436.
6. Weiss BM, Zemp L, Seifert B, et al. Outcome of pulmonary vascular disease in pregnancy: a systematic overview from 1978 through 1996. J Am Coll Cardiol 1998; 31:1650–1657.
7. Badesh DB, Abman SH, Aheam GS, et al. Medical therapy for pulmonary arterial hypertension. ACCP evidence-based clinical practice guidelines. Chest 2004; 126:35S–62S.
8. Monnery L, Nanson J, Charlton G. Primary pulmonary hypertension in pregnancy; a role for novel vasodilators. Br J Anaesth 2001; 87:295–298.
9. Stewart R, Tuazon D, Olson G, et al. Pregnancy and primary pulmonary hypertension: successful outcome with epoprostenol therapy. Chest 2001; 119:973–975.
10. Lam GK, Stanford RE, Thorp J, et al. Inhaled nitric oxide for primary pulmonary hypertension in pregnancy. Obstet Gynecol 2001; 98:895–898.
11. Geohas C, McLaughlin VV. Successful management of pregnancy in a patient with eisenmenger syndrome with epoprostenol. Chest 2003; 124:1170–1173.
12. Bildirici I, Shumway JB. Intravenous and inhaled epoprostenol for primary pulmonary hypertension during pregnancy and delivery. Obstet Gynecol 2004; 103:1102–1105.
13. Avdalovic M, Sandrock C, Hoso A, et al. Epoprostenol in pregnant patients with secondary pulmonary hypertension: two case reports and a review of the literature. Treat Respir Med 2004; 3:29–34.
14. Bendayan D, Hod M, Oron G, et al. Pregnancy outcome in patients with pulmonary arterial hypertension receiving prostacyclin therapy. Obstet Gynecol 2005; 106:1206–1210.
15. Wong PS, Constantinides S, Kennedy CR, et al. Primary pulmonary hypertension in pregnancy. J R Soc Med 2001; 94:523–526.
16. Elliot CA, Stewart P, Webster VJ, et al. The use of iloprost in early pregnancy in patients with pulmonary arterial hypertension. Eur Respir J 2005; 26:168–173.
17. Bonnin M, Mercier FJ, Sitbon O, et al. Severe pulmonary hypertension during pregnancy: mode of delivery and anesthetic management of 15 consecutive cases. Anesthesiology 2005; 102:1133–1137.
18. Lacassie HJ, Germain AM, Valdés G, et al. Management of Eisenmenger syndrome in pregnancy with sildenafil and L-arginine. Obstet Gynecol 2004; 103:1118–1120.
19. Molelekwa V, Akhter P, Mc Kenna P, et al. Eisenmenger's syndrome in a 27 week pregnancy–management with bosentan and sildenafil. Ir Med J 2005; 98:87–88.
20. Capeless EL, Clapp JF. Cardiovascular changes in early phase of pregnancy. Am J Obstet Gynecol 1989; 161:1449–1453.
21. Ueland K. Pregnancy and cardiovascular disease. Med Clin North Am 1977; 61:17–41.
22. Van Oppen A, Van der Tweel I, Alsbach GP, et al. A longitudinal study of maternal hemodynamics during normal pregnancy. Obstet Gynecol 1996; 13:135–146.
23. Duvekot JJ, Peeters LLH. Maternal cardiovascular hemodynamic adaptation to pregnancy. Obstet Gynecol Surv 1994; 49:S1–S14.
24. Clapp JF III, Capeless E. Cardiovascular function before, during, and after the first and subsequent pregnancies. Am J Cardiol 1997; 80:1469–1473.

25. Budev MM, Arroliga AC, Emery S. Exacerbation of underlying pulmonary disease in pregnancy. Crit Care Med 2005; 33:S313–S318.
26. Chakravarty EF, Khanna D, Chung L. Pregnancy outcomes in systemic sclerosis, primary pulmonary hypertension, and sickle cell disease. Obstet Gynecol 2008; 111:927–934.
27. Bédard E, Dimopoulos K, Gatzoulis MA. Has there been any progress made on pregnancy outcomes among women with pulmonary arterial hypertension? Eur Heart J 2009; 30: 256–265.
28. Belfort MA, Rokey R, Saade GR, et al. Rapid echographic assessment of left and right heart hemodynamics in critically ill obstetric patients. Am J Obstet Gynecol 1994; 171: 884–892.
29. Wylie BJ, Epps KC, Gaddipati S, et al. Correlation of transthoracic echocardiography and right heart catheterization in pregnancy. J Perinat Med 2007; 35(6):497–502.
30. Penning S, Robinson KD, Major CA, et al. A comparison of echocardiography and pulmonary artery catheterization for evaluation of pulmonary artery pressures in pregnant patients with suspected pulmonary hypertension. Am J Obstet Gynecol 2001; 184(7):1568–1570.
31. Roberts NV, Keast PJ. Pulmonary hypertension and pregnancy: a lethal combination. Anaesth Intensive Care 1990; 18:366–374.
32. Thorne S, Nelson-Piercy C, MacGregor A, et al. Pregnancy and contraception in heart disease and pulmonary arterial hypertension. J Fam Plann Reprod Health Care 2006; 32:75–81.
33. Chamaidi A, Gatzoulis MA. Heart disease and pregnancy. Hellenic J Cardiol 2006; 47:275–291.
34. Madden BP. Pulmonary hypertension and pregnancy. Int J Obstet Anesth 2009; 18(2): 156–164 (Epub February 14, 2009).
35. McMillan E, Martin WL, Waugh J, et al. Management of pregnancy in women with pulmonary hypertension secondary to SLE and anti-phospholipid syndrome. Lupus 2002; 11:392–398.
36. Huang S, DeSantis ER. Treatment of pulmonary arterial hypertension in pregnancy. Am J Health Syst Pharm 2007; 64:1922–1926.
37. Sitbon O, Humbert M, Jais X, et al. Long-term response to calcium channel blockers in idiopathic pulmonary arterial hypertension. Circulation 2005; 111:3105–3111.
38. Easterling TR, Ralph DD, Schmucker BC. Pulmonary hypertension in pregnancy: treatment with pulmonary vasodilators. Obstet Gynecol 1999; 93:494–498.
39. Clouthier D, Williams S, Hammer R, et al. Cell-autonomous and nonautonomous actions of endothelin-A receptor signalling in craniofacial and cardiovascular development. Dev Biol 2003; 261:506–519.
40. Kurihara Y, Kurihara H, Suzuki H, et al. Elevated blood pressure and craniofacial abnormalities in mice deficient in endothelin 1. Nature 1994; 368:703–710.
41. Siu SC, Sermer M, Colman JM, et al. Prospective multicenter study of pregnancy outcomes in women with heart disease. Circulation 2001; 104:515–521.
42. Song YB, Park SW, Kim JH, et al. Outcomes of pregnancy in women with congenital heart disease: a single center experience in Korea. J Korean Med Sci 2008; 23:808–813.
43. Uebing A, Steer PJ, Yentis SM, et al. Pregnancy and congenital heart disease. Br Med J 2006; 332:401–406.
44. O'Hare R, McLoughlin C, Milligan K, et al. Anaesthesia for caesarean section in the presence of severe primary pulmonary hypertension. Br J Anaesth 1998; 81:790–792.
45. Weiss BM, Maggiorini M, Jenni R, et al. Pregnant patient with primary pulmonary hypertension: inhaled pulmonary vasodilators and epidural anesthesia for cesarean delivery. Anesthesiology 2000; 92:1191–1194.
46. Olofsson C, Bremme K, Forsell G, et al. Cesarean section under epidural ropivacaine 0,75% in a parturient with severe pulmonary hypertension. Acta Anaesthesiol Scand 2001; 45: 258–260.

47. Duggan AB, Katz SG. Combined spinal and epidural anaesthesia for caesarean section in a parturient with severe primary pulmonary hypertension. Anaesth Intensive Care 2003; 31: 565–569.
48. Parneix M, Fanou L, Morau E, et al. Low-dose combined spinal-epidural anaesthesia for caesarean section in a patient with Eisenmenger's syndrome. Int J Obstet Anesth 2009; 18: 81–84.
49. Price LC, Forrest P, Sodhi V, et al. Use of vasopressin after caesarean section in idiopathic pulmonary arterial hypertension. Br J Anaesth 2007; 99:552–555.
50. Duhl AJ, Paidas MJ, Ural SH, et al. Antithrombotic therapy and pregnancy: consensus report and recommendations for prevention and treatment of venous thromboembolism and adverse pregnancy outcomes. Am J Obstet Gynecol 2007; 197:457.e1–457.e21.

32
Pediatric Pulmonary Hypertension

CECILE TISSOT and MAURICE BEGHETTI
University Children's Hospital, Geneva, Switzerland

I. Introduction

Prior to the current treatment era, the prognosis of pulmonary arterial hypertension (PAH) was extremely poor with a high mortality rate (1,2) and less than one-year survival in untreated children (2–4); prognosis has improved markedly in recent years. This has coincided with improvements in diagnosis and general management, as well as the off-label application of adult PAH-specific therapies to children (5–8). The prognosis of PAH has changed dramatically with a 97% five-year survival in children with severe PAH responding to acute vasodilator testing treated with calcium channel blockade and a 92% five-year survival in nonresponders treated with intravenous (IV) prostacyclin (9,10). Nevertheless, PAH has no cure, and the aim of the treatment is to improve quality of life, symptoms, hemodynamics, and exercise capacity and to prolong survival. This chapter reviews the current understanding of pediatric pulmonary hypertension, classification, diagnostic evaluation, and available treatment with description of targeted pharmacological therapy and new treatments in children.

II. Clinical Presentation and Diagnosis of PAH in Children

PAH is defined as a mean pulmonary artery pressure (mPAP) $\geq$25 mmHg at rest or $\geq$30 mmHg during exercise, with a normal pulmonary capillary wedge pressure ($\leq$15 mmHg) and increased pulmonary vascular resistance (PVR) index ($\geq$3 Wood units $\times$ m^2) (11,12), a definition that applies to all but the youngest patients.

Symptoms of PAH in children are frequently misleading and the diagnosis may be unrecognized for some time. PAH should be suspected in any child with excessive fatigue, shortness of breath, or unexplained syncopal episode(s). The physical signs of PAH include a left parasternal right ventricular (RV) lift and an accentuated pulmonary component of the second heart sound. A diastolic murmur of pulmonary insufficiency and a holosystolic murmur of tricuspid regurgitation may be audible. In case of heart failure, cool extremities related to poor cardiac output may be found. The resting systemic arterial oxygen saturation should be normal in the absence of any intracardiac shunt.

Chest X ray, electrocardiogram, and echocardiography are integral to the initial evaluation of PAH. Chest X ray demonstrates enlarged central pulmonary arteries and diminished peripheral pulmonary vascular markings. The electrocardiogram shows signs of RV hypertrophy and strain, right atrial enlargement, and right axis deviation. Transthoracic echocardiography allows estimation of the RV systolic pressure (RVSP) from the tricuspid regurgitant flow velocity (13,14) and of the end-diastolic and mPAP from the end-diastolic and maximal pulmonary regurgitant flow velocity, respectively (15,16). Echocardiography may reveal dilation of the right-heart chambers and RV hypertrophy with bowing of the interventricular septum to the left, compressing the left ventricle, estimated by the left ventricular eccentricity index (EI) (17). RV function can be estimated by the fractional area change (FAC), which is considered abnormal in adults if ≤40% (18). Tricuspid annular plane systolic excursion (TAPSE), defined as the total displacement of the tricuspid annulus in centimeters from end diastole to end systole, is a useful echocardiographic-derived measure of RV function and correlates with survival in adults with PAH (19). In children aged six years or more, exercise capacity can be assessed with a six-minute walk test (6MWT). Cardiopulmonary exercise testing to determine maximum oxygen capacity (max VO_2) and anaerobic threshold may be useful. Ventilation/perfusion (V/Q) scan, pulmonary function tests, chest computed tomographic (CT) scan and abdominal ultrasonography should be performed to define potential etiologies. Similarly, serological studies and blood screening for connective tissue diseases, human immunodeficiency virus (HIV) testing, and coagulation studies may detect potential causes of PAH (20) (Table 1). When pulmonary veno-occlusive disease (PVOD), pulmonary capillary hemangiomatosis (PCH), or alveolar hypoplasia/dysplasia is suspected, a lung biopsy may be indicated. Brain natriuretic peptide (BNP) and N-terminal pro–brain natriuretic peptide (NT-pro-BNP) may be useful to assess the progression of the disease. BNP appears to correlate positively with functional status in children with PAH (21), and change in BNP measurements over time correlates with the change in the hemodynamic and echocardiographic parameters of children with PAH (BNP value > 180 pg/mL predicts decreased survival) (22). NT-pro-BNP also correlates with outcome in children with PAH (23). After initiation of treatment, NT-pro-BNP appears to decrease, which correlates with an increase in exercise capacity as documented by the 6MWT (23).

Table 1 Suggested Diagnostic Evaluation of Children with Pulmonary Hypertension

Chest radiograph	• Cardiomegaly • Enlarged central pulmonary arteries • Peripheral pulmonary hypoperfusion
Electrocardiogram	• Right ventricular hypertrophy and dilation • Right atrial hypertrophy • Right axis deviation • ST segment changes
Echocardiogram	• Right ventricular hypertrophy and dilation • Decreased right ventricular function (FAC, TAPSE) • TR jet velocity >2.5 m/sec • Flattening of the interventricular septum (EI) • Pericardial effusion

Table 1   Suggested Diagnostic Evaluation of Children with Pulmonary Hypertension (*Continued*)

Cardiac catheterization with acute vasodilator testing	• Cardiac output • Pulmonary artery pressure • Pulmonary vascular resistance • Pulmonary vasoreactivity testing • Right atrial pressure • Aortopulmonary collaterals
Liver evaluation	• Liver function tests with γGT • Abdominal ultrasound (portopulmonary hypertension) • Hepatitis profile
Complete blood count (CBC)	• Anemia • Erythrocytosis • Abnormal red blood cells • Thrombopenia
Urinalysis	• Proteinuria
Hypercoagulable evaluation	• Disseminated intravscular coagulation (DIC) screen • Factor V Leiden • Antithrombin III • Prothrombin mutation 22010 • Protein C • Protein S • Anticardiolipin IgM and IgG
Collagen vascular disease workup	• Antinuclear antibody (ANA) with profile (DNA, Smith, RNP, SSA, SSB, centromere, SCL-70) • Rheumatoid factor • Erythrocyte sedimentation rate • Complement
Lung evaluation	• Pulmonary function tests with DLCO and bronchodilator • Sleep study and pulse oxymetry • Chest CT scan • Ventilation/perfusion scan • Lung biopsy[a]
Six-minute walk test, cardiopulmonary exercise test	• VO_2 max • Work rate • Anaerobic threshold
HIV tests	• HIV-1 IgG test (EIA) • p24, gp41, gp120 antigens
Thyroid function tests	• TSH, thyroxin
BNP, NT-pro-BNP	• Increase in BNP and NT-pro-BNP
Toxicology screen	• Cocaine • Methamphetamine

[a]May be of interest in very young patients with unclear etiology.
Abbreviations: FAC, fractional area change; TAPSE, tricuspid annular plane systolic excursion; EI, eccentricity index; BNP, brain natriuretic peptide.

Finally, PAH must be confirmed by cardiac catheterization, and pulmonary vasoreactivity testing must be performed during this study. The acute testing should be performed preferably with inhaled nitric oxide (iNO), but inhaled iloprost, IV epoprostenol, or IV adenosine may be used. According to the new definition for adults, acute responders should show a decrease of ≥ 10 mmHg in mPAP with a mPAP of ≤ 40 mmHg, and an unchanged or increased cardiac output (24,25). It is still a matter of debate if this should be applied also for children. The percentage of responders in children is somewhere between 6% and 40% (4,9,26).

III. Etiology of PAH in Children

Understanding the epidemiology and natural history of pediatric PAH is essential to guide management decisions. Nevertheless, data on pediatric epidemiology are sparse. Registries can provide valuable information with respect to epidemiology, diagnosis, most appropriate end-point assessments, treatment, and outcomes. While there are many registries of adult patients with PAH, registries of children with PAH are less well established and less well powered. It has been possible to gain some data on PAH etiology in children from clinical trials or postmarketing surveillance studies of medical therapy, but these populations may be preselected with respect to inclusion criteria. In a two-center, U.S. clinical trial of bosentan in 86 pediatric patients with PAH (7), the predominant diagnoses were PAH associated with congenital heart disease (CHD, 56%) and idiopathic PAH (42%). A similar trend was observed in a European, prospective, Internet-based, postmarketing surveillance database (27).

There are established national registries in the United Kingdom, Switzerland, and France (8,28), but several other countries are currently establishing similar registries. The U.K. national registry was established in 2001, and analyses of treatment patterns and survival over the ensuing five years in 216 children with PAH were published recently (29). PAH associated with CHD was the most common form of PAH (48%), followed by idiopathic PAH (28%), consistent with previous studies.

The diagnostic classification of PAH in children follows that adopted for adults (30) because there is no current classification system that is specific for children. However, the sparse data collected to date already show a different pattern of diagnoses and etiologies for PAH in children compared with adults. The predominant diagnoses in children are idiopathic PAH and PAH related to CHD, which probably account for about 90% of children with PAH encountered in clinical practice. So far very few patients with other forms of PAH have been reported, but we need to know if this is due to the lack of diagnosis, lack of reporting, or a true absence of these forms of PAH in children. It is possible that PAH associated with lung developmental anomalies or bronchopulmonary dysplasia is currently underreported (31). It is not uncommon to encounter children with combination of etiologies and/or rare syndromes.

To address the paucity of registry data for pediatric patients with PAH, the first international registry in pediatric PAH was recently established: the Tracking Outcomes and Practice in Pediatric PAH (TOPP) registry (32). Up to 450 children aged ≥ 3 months and ≤ 18 years with previously or newly diagnosed PAH (two-thirds and one-third of the registry population, respectively), confirmed by right-heart catheterization will be enrolled and followed for ≥ 3 years at 39 specialist centers in 22 countries (Australia,

Austria, Belgium, Brazil, Canada, China, Denmark, France, Germany, Greece, Hungary, Italy, Japan, Mexico, Netherlands, Norway, Poland, Portugal, Switzerland, Turkey, United Kingdom, and United States), covering four continents. The main aims of the registry are to describe the demographic and clinical characteristics of PAH in children, to determine medical treatment and disease-management patterns in clinical practice, and to describe risk factors for and the clinical course of disease progression. From these data it is hoped that diagnosis and treatment guidelines will be formulated and long-term patient care improved.

IV. Pathophysiology of PAH in Children

The pathophysiology of PAH shows some similarities in adults and children but there are specificities for children. The role of endothelial dysfunction and the abnormal balance of antimitotic and promitotic substances and of vasodilators and vaso-constrictors is also true for the pediatric population. Increased thromboxane, endothelin, and serotonin and decreased prostacyclin and nitric oxide (NO) have been described (33–39). PAH is a process driven not only by pulmonary vasoconstriction but by pro-liferation and remodeling of the pulmonary vascular bed (40–42). In young children, there is suggestion of failure of the pulmonary vasculature to relax in addition to a reduction in arterial number/surface area (43). In older children, intimal hyperplasia and occlusive change as well as plexiform lesions are found in the pulmonary arterioles (44). In contrast to adults, children with IPAH are thought to have more pulmonary vascular medial hypertrophy, less intimal fibrosis, and fewer plexiform lesions (45,46). This suggests that vasoconstriction, leading to medial hypertrophy, may occur early in the course of the disease and may precede the development of plexiform lesions and other fixed pulmonary vascular changes. This may explain why severe acute pulmonary hypertensive crisis occur more often in young than in older children or adults in response to pulmonary vasoconstrictor triggers.

However, PAH appears to be a disease of "predisposed" individuals in whom various stimuli may initiate the pulmonary vascular disease process. A genetic mutation of bone morphogenetic protein receptor type 2 (BMPR2) on chromosome 2q33 (the PPH1 gene), a gene encoding a transforming growth factor β (TGF-β) receptor, has been recognized in some patients with familial PAH (>50% of the patients), idiopathic PAH (∼20–25%) (47), and in some sporadic cases of PAH (26%) (48). Genetics in the pediatric population is still not completely clear, but BMPR2 seems to be also involved in some patients (49,50) whereas some data suggest that children may have a different genetic background than adults (51). The familial form of PAH accounts for about 6% of all cases and shows genetic anticipation, presentation occurring at younger age in successive generations (52).

V. Treatment of Children with PAH

A. Treatment Algorithms

There are no evidence-based treatment recommendations for children with PAH, pri-marily because of the lack of randomized clinical trials in pediatric patients. The aim of medical treatment is to dilate and reverse the abnormal remodeling of the pulmonary vascular bed, to restore the endothelial function, and to allow growth of the peripheral pulmonary arteries, by acting on the prostacyclin, endothelin, and NO pathways. No drug therapy is approved for use in children with PAH, and off-label therapy has been the pragmatic norm in this population. In practice, the therapeutic algorithm developed for PAH in adults (12,24) appears to guide treatment of children with PAH (20). Nevertheless, there are some difficulties in applying adult criteria and dosage regimens to children; standard end points to evaluate the response to treatment [e.g., the WHO (World Health Organization) classification and exercise capacity] may not be applicable or reliable in small children. Moreover, children with PAH should be referred to centers specialized for PAH so that optimal care is given, follow-up studies can be made, compliance can be addressed, and transition to adult care is considered when necessary.

Children who respond acutely to vasodilator testing should initially be treated with calcium channel blockers (CCBs) whereas nonresponders to *acute* vasoreactivity testing should be treated with other forms of therapy (9). In "nonresponders" with right-heart failure, first-line treatment is continuous IV epoprostenol (10). In the absence of right-heart failure, other agents may be tried first (Fig. 1). Endothelin receptor antagonists (bosentan, sitaxentan, ambrisentan), prostanoids (trepostinil, iloprost), and phosphodiesterase 5 (PDE-5) inhibitors (sildenafil) have been approved for the treatment of adult PAH, but none have been approved for the pediatric population. Combination therapy may be considered but has not been well studied.

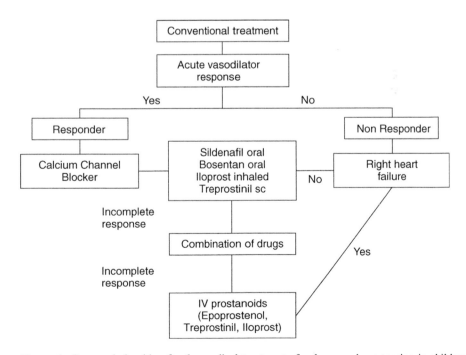

Figure 1 Proposed algorithm for the medical treatment of pulmonary hypertension in children.

B. General Measures

Since children are thought to have a more reactive pulmonary vascular bed than adults, even if this is still highly controversial, any respiratory tract infection resulting in V/Q mismatch can result in exacerbation of PAH. Therefore, aggressive therapy of PAH with iNO may be necessary during the acute phase of a respiratory viral illness. Standard immunization schedule is recommended as well as annual influenza and pneumococcal vaccinations unless there are contraindications. Very young children may benefit from respiratory syncytial virus prophylaxis. Fever should be treated aggressively to minimize the consequences of increased metabolic demand. Valsalva maneuvers, by decreasing the systemic venous return to the right side of the heart, may precipitate syncopal episodes and should be avoided.

C. Conventional Therapy

Conventional therapy for PAH in children may include, beyond the neonatal period, digitalis, diuretics, anticoagulation, and supplemental oxygen when required.

Diuretic therapy should be initiated cautiously since children with PAH may be preload dependent to maintain an optimal cardiac output. In the presence of overt right-heart failure, diuretics are often needed and some patients may need relatively high doses of diuretics. Although the use of digitalis in PAH is still highly controversial, children with frank right-heart failure may benefit from digoxin therapy (53). However, similar to adult trials, digoxin therapy has not shown a clear benefit in children with PAH. Consideration of anticoagulation in children with PAH is based on studies in adults (54,55). Thrombotic lesions within the pulmonary arteries have been well demonstrated in histopathological examination of adult patients with IPAH, and laboratory data are consistent with a hypercoagulable state in some patients. Moreover, small pulmonary emboli can be life threatening in patients with a pulmonary vascular bed unable to vasodilate or recruit additional vessels. In addition, postmortem examination of patients presenting with sudden death often demonstrates fresh clots in the pulmonary vascular bed. The use of anticoagulation in PAH is controversial but may be beneficial in patients with low cardiac output in whom sluggish blood flow through the pulmonary arteries may predispose to the formation of thrombi in situ. Clinical data supporting the use of chronic anticoagulation are limited. Warfarin has been associated with improved survival in adult patients with PAH (54–56), while the use of chronic anticoagulation has not been widely studied in children. Whenever beneficial, anticoagulation should be dosed to achieve an international normalized ratio (INR) of 1.5 to 2.0. A safe approach is to anticoagulate children with hypercoagulable state and eventually those in right-heart failure, as they are the most at risk of thrombosis in situ. Risks of anticoagulation, particularly in small children, must be weighed against benefits. For patients with contraindication to warfarin therapy, heparin is a reasonable alternative, either intravenous heparin or low molecular weight heparin, with a targeted partial thromboplastin time (aPTT) of 1.5 times that of control. Antiaggregation therapy with acetylsalicylic acid is widely used in children but there are no data showing efficacy.

Some children, while fully saturated during the day, demonstrate arterial desaturation during sleep, related to mild hypoventilation, which can exacerbate PAH. This can be avoided using nocturnal supplemental oxygen. Some children with PAH should have oxygen available at home in case of emergency. They should receive supplemental oxygen during any respiratory tract infection associated with desaturation as well as during air travel. In children with Eisenmenger syndrome or with a right to left intra-cardiac shunt, oxygen supplementation does not usually improve oxygen saturation, and the benefit of systematic oxygen supplementation on survival is controversial (57).

D. Nitric Oxide

NO is a potent vasodilator with selective effect on pulmonary circulation. It activates guanylate cyclase in the pulmonary smooth muscle cells, which increases cyclic gua-nosine monophosphate (GMP) and decreases intracellular calcium concentration, lead-ing to smooth muscle relaxation and vasodilation (58–60). iNO is useful in all forms of PAH, comprising acute PAH exacerbation and in perioperative and postoperative PAH following cardiac surgery. Nevertheless, the role of chronic administration of iNO has yet to be determined (61,62). Chronic home administration of iNO can be achieved using a novel pulsed nasal delivery system that appears to be as effective as the con-tinuous delivery system (63), but difficulties in chronic administration of iNO may preclude its use.

E. Calcium Channel Blockers

CCBs inhibit calcium influx through slow channels into cardiac and smooth muscle cells, causing pulmonary vasodilation. Acute pulmonary vasoreactivity testing during right-heart catheterization is the initial step in determining the suitability of long-term CCB therapy for children with severe PAH. As mentioned earlier, the prevalence of acute vasoreactivity is higher in children than in adults, allowing a higher proportion of children to be treated effectively with CCB therapy (9). In children with idiopathic PAH, Barst et al. (9) showed that five-year survival rates improved significantly in acute vasoreactive responders treated with CCB compared with that in nonresponders ($n = 31$ and $n = 43$, respectively; $p = 0.0002$). Longer-term follow-up revealed a 10-year survival rate of 81% among the responders, but careful follow-up is essential as some acute responders may become nonresponders with time and require additional treatment (6,25).

Relatively high dose of CCB are used and the optimal dose for children is uncertain. Most commonly used CCB are long-acting nifedipine 120 to 240 mg daily or amlodipine 20 to 40 mg daily, less commonly diltiazem 60 to 180 mg three times a day. Side effects are systemic hypotension, pulmonary edema, and RV failure.

F. Intravenous Prostanoids

Prostacyclin is a metabolite of arachidonic acid, which is endogenously produced by the vascular endothelium. It is a potent vasodilator in both the systemic and pulmonary circulation and has antiplatelet activity. Prostacyclin has been used for almost two decades and was approved for the treatment of severe PAH in adults in 1995. Long-term IV epoprostenol was shown to be effective in children with idiopathic PAH in 1999 (9). Survival was significantly improved in children treated with long-term IV epoprostenol ($n = 31$) compared with those in whom it was indicated but not administered ($n = 28$, $p = 0.002$): the four-year survival rates for treated and untreated patients were 94% and

38%, respectively. Longer-term follow-up in 35 patients treated with IV epoprostenol revealed a 10-year survival rate (including transplantation as a censoring event) of 61%, while 10-year treatment success rate (defined as freedom from death, transplantation, or atrial septostomy) was 37% for this group (6). The optimal dose of IV epoprostenol is unclear with significant patient variability, requiring incremental titration with the most rapid increase during the first months of treatment. The development of a tolerance is possible, and some children need periodic dose escalation. Maintenance doses of IV epoprostenol per kilogram of body weight appear to be higher in children than adults (12): in adults, the mean dose is 20 to 40 ng/kg/min compared with a mean dose of 50 to 80 ng/kg/min in young children. Adverse effects are inhibition of platelet aggregation, systemic vasodilation, and hepatic enzymes alteration. Common side effects include diarrhea and jaw pain. Epoprostenol is chemically unstable at neutral pH and at room temperature and has a short half-life (1–2 minutes) rendering a continuous intravenous system necessary. A permanent central venous access is required, and complications like line sepsis, local infection, and catheter dislodgement are not unusual (64). In addition, pump malfunction can be a life-threatening event as sudden interruption of the medication can lead to severe rebound pulmonary hypertension (43). There has been little or no published experience with other prostacyclins, such as trepostinil, iloprost, or beraprost in children (12). Pain at the site of administration frequently associated with subcutaneous (SC) trepostinil (65) generally precludes its administration in children (12,26).

G. Inhaled Iloprost

Inhaled iloprost has been investigated as an alternative to parenteral prostacyclins, owing to the inherent problems associated with parenteral medication. Administration by inhalation also enables direct delivery of the drug to the lungs, thus reducing systemic side effects and improving gas exchange in case of V/Q mismatch. The effects of inhaled iloprost as add-on therapy were investigated in 22 children (median age 11.5 years) with PAH (66). The majority of the children were severely ill; 10 of the children had previously had an inadequate response to PAH therapy or had refused IV prostanoid therapy and 9 of the children were switched to inhaled iloprost from IV or SC prostanoid therapy. Inhaled iloprost (median dose: 5 μg six times daily) was as effective as iNO in lowering mPAP and PVR index (PVRI). WHO functional class improved in 35% of the children, remained unchanged in 50%, and decreased in 15%. Sixty-four percent of patients continued to receive long-term inhaled iloprost, with the remainder stopping iloprost because of lower-airway reactivity, clinical deterioration, or death. Acute bronchoconstriction was a problem in some children, as well as poor compliance with the aerosolized iloprost delivery system and requirement for frequent administration (up to nine times daily). Nevertheless, the main utilization of inhaled iloprost in children has been in the critical care setting. When used for postoperative pulmonary hypertensive crisis, inhaled iloprost has been shown to lower mean PAP and improve systemic oxygen saturation (67). When iloprost is used together with iNO, there are no additive or synergistic effects. Acute administration of inhaled iloprost has been shown to lower mean PAP to the same extent as iNO with oxygen. Iloprost has a half-life of 20 to 25 minutes and therefore six to eight inhalations a day are required to be clinically effective.

H. Bosentan

Endothelin-1 (ET-1) is a potent vasoconstrictor peptide and has been implicated in the pathogenesis of PAH (68). In patients with PAH, ET-1 expression and plasma levels are increased and correlate inversely with prognosis. Two receptor subtypes, ETA and ETB, mediate the activity of ET-1. ETA receptors are located on vascular smooth muscle cells and mediate vasoconstriction, whereas ETB receptors are located on endothelial cells and causes endothelium-dependent vasodilation via the release of NO and prostacyclin (PGI2) and clearance of circulating ET-1 (69,70).

Bosentan is an oral dual endothelin receptor antagonist (71) that has been shown to improve exercise capacity, quality of life, and hemodynamics with lowering of PAH and PVR in adults (72,73) and in children with PAH (7,74). The largest cohort of children with PAH treated with bosentan was in an open-label, retrospective U.S. clinical trial (7). Eighty-six children were treated with bosentan either with or without IV epoprostenol or SC treprostinil. mPAP and PVRI were decreased after at least eight weeks of bosentan therapy. WHO functional status improved ($p < 0.001$), and Kaplan–Meier survival estimates at one and two years were 98% and 91%, respectively, which compares favorably with historical populations (9). Bosentan appeared to be well tolerated, with peripheral edema being the most frequent adverse event (8% of patients). However, this study is limited by its retrospective nature and lack of a control group.

Other less well-powered, open-label studies in smaller numbers of patients, often case series or retrospective studies, have been reported regarding the use of bosentan in children with PAH (74–78). In a study specifically in PAH patients with systemic to pulmonary shunt, bosentan therapy produced short-term improvement (4 months) with respect to WHO functional class and 6MWT distance in both children ($n = 10$) and adults ($n = 20$) (79). However, there was a progressive decline in the beneficial effect of bosentan after one year. The decline was most pronounced in the children, who tended to have more severe disease at baseline.

Bosentan is usually well tolerated in children in the dosing regimen of 31.25 mg b.i.d. for patients weighing 10 to 20 kg, 62.5 mg b.i.d. for those weighing 20 to 40 kg, and 125 mg b.i.d. for those weighing >40 kg. Bosentan has been successfully used in children receiving long-term IV epoprostenol therapy. Concomitant use of bosentan allowed for a decrease in epoprostenol dose and its associated side effects (77). Risk associated with endothelin receptor antagonists therapy include hepatotoxicity (dose related), teratogenicity, and possibly male infertility (27). Bosentan may also decrease the effectiveness of warfarin therapy because of induction of CYP3A4 and CYP2C9. The safety of bosentan therapy was recently reported from an Internet-based, postmarketing surveillance database, which compared pediatric patients aged 2 to 11 years ($n = 146$) with those aged ≥ 12 years ($n = 4443$) (27). Median bosentan exposure was 29 weeks in children. Elevated transaminase levels were reported in 2.7% of children aged 2 to 11 years compared with 7.8% of patients aged ≥ 12 years, and the overall discontinuation rate from bosentan was 14% in young children compared with 28% in patients aged ≥ 12 years, suggesting that bosentan may be better tolerated in children than in adults. Given its potential hepatotoxicity, liver function tests should be performed monthly in patients receiving bosentan (both children and adults). Currently, a specific pediatric formulation of bosentan is under investigation.

I. Sildenafil

PDE-5 inhibitors prevent the breakdown of cyclic GMP thereby raising cyclic GMP levels resulting in pulmonary vasodilation. Sildenafil was the first drug of this class and is still the most commonly used, particularly in young children with PAH (80). Sildenafil is as effective a pulmonary vasodilator as iNO, potentiates pulmonary vasodilation with NO (81,82), and may be particularly beneficial in conjunction with iNO where withdrawal of NO may lead to rebound PAH (83). In addition to NO, sildenafil has been shown to reduce significantly PAP with no significant effect on systemic arterial or central venous pressure in children with PAH following cardiac surgery. No significant dose effect was seen, a 0.5 mg/kg/dose every four hours being as efficacious compared with a 2 mg/kg/dose (84). In neonates with pulmonary hypertension associated with a congenital diaphragmatic hernia resistant to iNO, sildenafil was shown to improve cardiac output by reducing PAH (85). The effects of oral sildenafil (0.25–1 mg/kg four times daily) were investigated in a pilot study of 14 children aged 5.3 to 18 years with PAH (86). Mean 6MWT distance increased significantly from baseline (278 ± 114 m) to 432 ± 156 m at 12 months ($p = 0.005$); a plateau was reached between 6 and 12 months. Median mPAP and PVRI decreased significantly, and sildenafil was well tolerated. The results of this small study must be confirmed in a large, randomized, controlled clinical trial that will be completed soon. In children with PAH, sildenafil was shown to improve oxyhemoglobin saturation and exercise capacity without significant side effects (87). Moreover, PDE-5 appears to be highly expressed in the hypertrophied human right ventricle, and acute inhibition of PDE-5 with oral sildenafil was shown to improve RV contractility (88). The principle side effects include erections and systemic hypotension. The dose administered is 0.5 to 1 mg/kg/dose given three to four times a day. While sildenafil has been approved for the treatment of WHO functional class II to IV PAH in adults, data in children are limited.

Currently no data are available for children treated with other endothelin receptor antagonists (ambrisentan and sitaxentan) or other PDE inhibitors (tadalafil), but we may expect studies in the future.

J. Combination Therapy

There is an increased interest in the combined use of drugs that have different sites of action in PAH. As for patients with heart failure, combination therapy is an attractive option to address simultaneously the multiple pathophysiological pathways of PAH. Acting on many different pathways may be more efficacious than acting on a single one, by additive or synergistic effects. In adult patients with PAH, the initiation of combination therapy with epoprostenol and bosentan trended for a greater improvement in hemodynamics when compared with the initiation of epoprostenol alone (89). In adult patients with PAH who were deteriorating despite chronic treatment with prostanoids, addition of bosentan or sildenafil appeared to improve hemodynamics and exercise capacity (90–92). Addition of inhaled iloprost to existing bosentan therapy was shown to improve hemodynamics and delay clinical worsening (93). A therapeutic approach utilizing the combination of bosentan, sildenafil, and inhaled iloprost has been shown to improve survival, the need for lung transplantation and for IV iloprost therapy, and to provide acceptable results in patients with severe PAH (94).

These encouraging preliminary data for adults with PAH explain why we have included the potential for combination therapy in our proposed therapeutic algorithm.

More studies are needed to help establishing guidelines for combination therapy. Whether combination therapy should be used as a first step by simultaneous initiation of two or more drugs or by addition of a second treatment to a previous therapy once insufficient is still not known. Even if empiric combination of drugs is not uncommon in pediatric patients with PAH, there is a clear lack of studies in this area. Further studies are needed to determine the true combined effects of these drugs, particularly in the pediatric population.

K. Nonpharmacological Treatment Options

On the basis of the current adult algorithm, surgery may be considered when the patient deteriorates despite maximal pharmacological therapy. Atrial septostomy may benefit patients with severe PAH with recurrent syncope and intractable right-heart failure. Although this procedure is associated with a risk of worsening hypoxemia, it was shown to relieve symptoms in a case series (95). A case study suggested that Potts shunt (anastomosis between the descending aorta and the left pulmonary artery) may be an alternative surgical option for patients with suprasystemic PVR (96). Lung or heart-lung transplantation may also be offered to patients who do not respond to pharmacological therapy. The decision to refer a patient for transplantation and the timing of referral should be based on the prognosis of the patient, the local waiting time for transplantation, and the expected survival after transplantation (5,20). The three-year survival rate for pediatric patients undergoing lung transplantation is currently 68.7% (97).

VI. Future Aspects

A. PDGF Receptor Antagonists

Platelet-derived growth factor (PDGF) has been implicated in endothelial cell dysfunction and proliferation and migration of vascular smooth muscle cells. It is thought that altered PDGF signaling may be involved in the vascular remodeling observed in PAH (98,99) and that PDGF receptor antagonist such as imatinib could reverse pulmonary vascular disease (100). The result of a phase 2 adult trial will be available soon.

B. Tyrosine Kinase Inhibitors

Inhibition of tyrosine kinases, including PDGF receptor, can reduce PAP in experimental and clinical PAH. The multikinase inhibitor sorafenib (inhibits c-Raf and b-Raf and tyrosine kinase) prevents pulmonary remodeling and improves cardiac and pulmonary functions in experimental PAH. Sorafenib appears to exert direct myocardial antihypertrophic effects, mediated via inhibition of the Raf kinase pathway. The combined inhibition of tyrosine and serine/threonine kinases may provide an option to treat PAH and associated right-heart remodeling (101).

C. Soluble Guanylate Cyclase

Alterations of the NO receptor, soluble guanylate cyclase (sGC), may contribute to the pathophysiology of PAH. BAY 63-2521 is a novel, orally available compound that

directly stimulates sGC and sensitizes it to its physiological stimulator, NO. Upregulation of sGC in pulmonary arterial smooth muscle cells has been noted in human
idiopathic PAH lungs. Stimulation of sGC may reverse right-heart hypertrophy and
structural lung vascular remodeling. sGC may thus offer a new target for therapeutic
intervention in PAH (102). The result of a phase 2 adult trial will be available soon.

D.   Vasoactive Intestinal Peptide

Vasoactive intestinal polypeptide (VIP) has a potent vasodilatory effect on the pulmonary and systemic circulation. Continuous IV infusion of VIP appears to decrease the
PVR/SVR ratio in patients with PAH, suggesting an overall pulmonary vasodilatory
effect, and may become a new therapeutic agent in the future (103–105).

E.   HMG-CoA Reductase Inhibitors

The 3-hydroxy-3-methylglutaryl CoA (HMG-CoA) reductase inhibitor simvastatin has
been shown to attenuate and induce regression of chronic hypoxic PAH in animal
models. Statins are known to inhibit Rho kinase (ROCK). ROCK activity is thought to
be increased under hypoxic conditions and may be normalized with simvastatin treatment. Inhibition of ROCK expression and activity may be an important mechanism of
statin effect in PAH (106,107).

F.   Serotonin Inhibitors

Serotonin (5-hydroxytryptamine) is a pulmonary vasoconstrictor and smooth muscle cell
mitogen. Pulmonary hypertension is associated with a substantial increase in serotonin
(5-HT)2B receptor expression in pulmonary arteries, which leads to hyperplasia of the
pulmonary artery smooth muscle cells. Upregulation of lung 5-HT appears necessary to
initiate the development of pulmonary vascular remodeling, whereas a sustained
increase in 5-HT expression may underlie both the progression and the maintenance of
PAH. Activation of 5-HT(2B) receptors is a limiting step in the development of PAH
(108), and serotonin transporter polymorphism may explain the different clinical manifestations of familial and idiopathic PAH (109). Complete reversal of established PAH
by fluoxetine, a 5-HT inhibitor, may provide a rationale for new therapeutic strategies
(110).
    Several novel other therapies have been proposed and are currently under active
investigation either in animal models or in preliminary studies in adults (e.g., endothelial
cell progenitors, metalloproteinase inhibitors, potassium channel openers, etc.) and may
also be of interest for pediatric patients in the near future (111,112). Currently no data
are available in children regarding novel therapies currently being studied in adults [e.g.,
imatinib, vasoactive intestinal peptide (aviptadil), or sGC stimulators].

VII.   Outcome Measures

There is much ongoing debate concerning appropriate end points for determining
the prognosis and treatment response in adults with PAH (113–117). The accepted
outcome measures in clinical trials in adults, particularly 6MWT distance, functional

class, right-heart catheterization measures, and survival, have also been the most common outcome measures in studies of children with PAH. Additional outcome measures such as quality of life (118–120) and noninvasive end points such as biochemical markers (e.g., BNP) (121) and echocardiographic or magnetic resonance imaging have attracted increasing interest (122–124).

Six-minute walking distance remains the standard tool for testing exercise capacity in most clinical trials in adults with PAH (125). Six-minute walking distance is difficult to standardize in children, but the recent publication of reference values in healthy children according to age, height, and sex will assist in the future application of this end point and its interpretation in clinical trials in children with PAH (126–128).

Right-heart catheterization in children has a clear diagnostic role, but its prognostic utility is not proven and requires validation. Repeat cardiac catheterizations in children is not deemed reasonable due to the inherent risk associated with the procedure and the requirement for anesthesia in small children (129,130).

In adults with primary PAH, plasma BNP was shown to be a noninvasive prognostic indicator (121). A study in the United Kingdom investigated the relationship between plasma BNP level, functional status, and outcome in 50 children with PAH (21), and found a positive correlation between plasma BNP level and WHO functional class. However, plasma BNP had limited sensitivity for predicting death rates or need for transplantation in this study. A Dutch study also investigated the prognostic utility of NT-pro-BNP in 29 children with PAH (23). Higher NT-pro-BNP levels were associated with higher WHO functional class ($r = 0.34$, $p = 0.04$) and increased mortality rates ($\chi^2 = 9.93$, $p = 0.002$). Similarly, a U.S. prospective study of 78 children with PAH found that patients with a BNP concentration greater than 180 pg/mL had increased mortality rates (22). The latter study also monitored changes in BNP levels over time and assessed their correlation with hemodynamic and echocardiographic parameters. Although absolute BNP levels did not show a strong correlation with commonly used hemodynamic and echocardiographic data, temporal changes in BNP levels correlated significantly with temporal changes in hemodynamic and echocardiographic data. Thus, monitoring of changes in BNP concentrations over time may provide a useful noninvasive means to monitor disease severity and assess prognosis in pediatric patients with PAH.

VIII.   Outcome of Pediatric PAH

Historically, untreated PAH in children carried a poor prognosis with a median survival of less than one year (2,3). Although epidemiological data in children are scarce, some data on survival are available for children with PAH.

For children with idiopathic PAH responding to acute vasodilator testing and treated with CCBs, Yung et al. reported survival rates at 1, 5, and 10 years of 97%, 97%, and 81%, respectively, with treatment success rates of 84%, 68%, and 47%, respectively, but treatment success decreased significantly when acute responders became nonresponders (6). For nonresponders with idiopathic PAH treated with IV epoprostenol, survival at 1, 5, and 10 years was 94%, 81%, and 61%, respectively, with treatment success rates of 83%, 57%, and 37%, respectively. In the recent medical era (after 1995), survival was even better for children with IPAH treated with IV epoprostenol (i.e., survival rates of 97%, 97%, and 78% at 1, 5, and 10 years) (6). In children with severe primary PAH treated with continuous prostacyclin, Barst et al. reported survival rates of 86.9%,

72.4%, and 63.3% at one, two, and three-years, respectively (2). For children with idiopathic PAH, Haworth et al. reported survival rates of 85.6%, 79.9%, and 71.9% at one, three, and five years, respectively (8), for those treated with a combination of IV epoprostenol with either bosentan or sildenafil, or both. In associated PAH, survival rates were 92.3%, 83.8%, and 56.9% at one, three, and five years, respectively, with postoperative CHD-associated PAH having the worst outcome.

IX. Conclusions

Advances in the understanding of pulmonary vasculature have led to new therapeutic options and improved survival in children with severe PAH. The timely diagnosis of PAH is crucial as early treatment leads to improved outcome. In children with PAH, an extensive workup is necessary to determine the etiology, as the most successful strategy involves treatment of the underlying disorder. Initial evaluation includes acute vaso-dilator testing at cardiac catheterization, which determines initial and long-term therapy. To date, treatment of children with PAH has been somewhat pragmatic in the absence of approved medications and has generally paralleled recommendations for adults.

National registries have been established to yield information on the diagnosis, prognosis, and treatment outcome in children with PH, but patient numbers have been too low to provide definitive conclusions. The recently published U.K. national registry indicates that survival has improved with the use of adult PAH-specific therapies and suggests that combination therapy (epoprostenol with bosentan or sildenafil) may achieve the best outcomes (29). However, information concerning treatment of PAH in children remains scarce and there is a need for further, larger, controlled, longer-term studies. Clinical research is evolving and should better define in the future the role of new therapies for children with PAH. Appropriate end points, preferably noninvasive, should be identified for use in assessing treatment response.

References

1. Sitbon O, McLaughlin VV, Badesch DB, et al. Survival in patients with class III idiopathic pulmonary arterial hypertension treated with first line oral bosentan compared with an historical cohort of patients started on intravenous epoprostenol. Thorax 2005; 60(12): 1025–1030.
2. Barst RJ, Rubin LJ, McGoon MD, et al. Survival in primary pulmonary hypertension with long-term continuous intravenous prostacyclin. Ann Intern Med 1994; 121(6):409–415.
3. Barst RJ. Pharmacologically induced pulmonary vasodilatation in children and young adults with primary pulmonary hypertension. Chest 1986; 89(4):497–503.
4. Sandoval J, Bauerle O, Gomez A, et al. Primary pulmonary hypertension in children: clinical characterization and survival. J Am Coll Cardiol 1995; 25(2):466–474.
5. Widlitz A, Barst RJ. Pulmonary arterial hypertension in children. Eur Respir J 2003; 21(1): 155–176.
6. Yung D, Widlitz AC, Rosenzweig EB, et al. Outcomes in children with idiopathic pul-monary arterial hypertension. Circulation 2004; 110(6):660–665.
7. Rosenzweig EB, Ivy DD, Widlitz A, et al. Effects of long-term bosentan in children with pulmonary arterial hypertension. J Am Coll Cardiol 2005; 46(4):697–704.

8. Haworth SG, Hislop AA. Treatment and survival in children with pulmonary arterial hypertension: the UK Pulmonary Hypertension Service for Children 2001 to 2006. Heart 2009; 95(4):312–317.
9. Barst RJ, Maislin G, Fishman AP. Vasodilator therapy for primary pulmonary hypertension in children. Circulation 1999; 99(9):1197–1208.
10. Barst RJ. Recent advances in the treatment of pediatric pulmonary artery hypertension. Pediatr Clin North Am 1999; 46(2):331–345.
11. Rich S, ed. Executive summary from the World Symposium on Primary Pulmonary Hypertension 1998, Evian, France, September 6–10, 1998, cosponsored by the World Health Organization. Available at: http://www.who.int/ncd/cvd/pph.html. Retrieved April 14, 2000.
12. Galie N, Torbicki A, Barst R, et al. Guidelines on diagnosis and treatment of pulmonary arterial hypertension. The Task Force on Diagnosis and Treatment of Pulmonary Arterial Hypertension of the European Society of Cardiology. Eur Heart J 2004; 25(24):2243–2278.
13. Hatle L, Angelsen BA, Tromsdal A. Non-invasive estimation of pulmonary artery systolic pressure with Doppler ultrasound. Br Heart J 1981; 45(2):157–165.
14. Yock PG, Popp RL. Noninvasive estimation of right ventricular systolic pressure by Doppler ultrasound in patients with tricuspid regurgitation. Circulation 1984; 70(4):657–662.
15. Masuyama T, Uematsu M, Sato H, et al. [Pulmonary arterial end-diastolic pressure non-invasively estimated by continuous wave Doppler echocardiography.] J Cardiogr 1986; 16(3):669–675.
16. Masuyama T, Kodama K, Kitabatake A, et al. Continuous-wave Doppler echocardiographic detection of pulmonary regurgitation and its application to noninvasive estimation of pulmonary artery pressure. Circulation 1986; 74(3):484–492.
17. Lopez-Candales A, Rajagopalan N, Kochar M, et al. Systolic eccentricity index identifies right ventricular dysfunction in pulmonary hypertension. Int J Cardiol 2007; 129(3):424–426.
18. Lopez-Candales A, Dohi K, Rajagopalan N, et al. Defining normal variables of right ventricular size and function in pulmonary hypertension: an echocardiographic study. Postgrad Med J 2008; 84(987):40–45.
19. Forfia PR, Fisher MR, Mathai SC, et al. Tricuspid annular displacement predicts survival in pulmonary hypertension. Am J Respir Crit Care Med 2006; 174(9):1034–1041.
20. Rashid A, Ivy D. Severe paediatric pulmonary hypertension: new management strategies. Arch Dis Child 2005; 90(1):92–98.
21. Lammers AE, Hislop AA, Haworth SG. Prognostic value of B-type natriuretic peptide in children with pulmonary hypertension. Int J Cardiol 2008 (in press).
22. Bernus A, Wagner BD, Accurso F, et al. Brain natriuretic peptide levels in managing pediatric patients with pulmonary arterial hypertension. Chest 2009; 135(3):745–751.
23. Van Albada ME, Loot FG, Fokkema R, et al. Biological serum markers in the management of pediatric pulmonary arterial hypertension. Pediatr Res 2008; 63(3):321–327.
24. Badesch DB, Abman SH, Simonneau G, et al. Medical therapy for pulmonary arterial hypertension: updated ACCP evidence-based clinical practice guidelines. Chest 2007; 131(6):1917–1928.
25. Sitbon O, Humbert M, Jais X, et al. Long-term response to calcium channel blockers in idiopathic pulmonary arterial hypertension. Circulation 2005; 111(23):3105–3111.
26. Haworth SG. The management of pulmonary hypertension in children. Arch Dis Child 2008; 93(7):620–625.
27. Beghetti M, Hoeper MM, Kiely DG, et al. Safety experience with bosentan in 146 children 2-11 years old with pulmonary arterial hypertension: results from the European Post-marketing Surveillance program. Pediatr Res 2008; 64(2):200–204.
28. Fasnacht MS, Tolsa JF, Beghetti M. The Swiss registry for pulmonary arterial hypertension: the paediatric experience. Swiss Med Wkly 2007; 137(35–36):510–513.

29. Haworth SG, Hislop AA. Treatment and survival in children with pulmonary arterial hypertension: The UK Pulmonary Hypertension Service for Children 2001-2006. Heart 2009; 95(4):312–317.
30. Simonneau G, Galie N, Rubin LJ, et al. Clinical classification of pulmonary hypertension. J Am Coll Cardiol 2004; 43(12 suppl S):5S–12S.
31. Mourani PM, Sontag MK, Younoszai A, et al. Clinical utility of echocardiography for the diagnosis and management of pulmonary vascular disease in young children with chronic lung disease. Pediatrics 2008; 121(2):317–325.
32. Beghetti M, Berger RM, Schulze-Neick I, et al. TOPP: the first international registry in pediatric pulmonary hypertension. Eur Respir J 2008; 32(suppl 52):169s–170s.
33. Christman BW, McPherson CD, Newman JH, et al. An imbalance between the excretion of thromboxane and prostacyclin metabolites in pulmonary hypertension. N Engl J Med 1992; 327(2):70–75.
34. Yoshibayashi M, Nishioka K, Nakao K, et al. Plasma endothelin concentrations in patients with pulmonary hypertension associated with congenital heart defects. Evidence for increased production of endothelin in pulmonary circulation. Circulation 1991; 84(6):2280–2285.
35. Eddahibi S, Humbert M, Fadel E, et al. Serotonin transporter overexpression is responsible for pulmonary artery smooth muscle hyperplasia in primary pulmonary hypertension. J Clin Invest 2001; 108(8):1141–1150.
36. Gorenflo M, Bettendorf M, Brockmeier K, et al. Pulmonary vasoreactivity and vasoactive mediators in children with pulmonary hypertension. Z Kardiol 2000; 89(11):1000–1008.
37. Black SM, Kumar S, Wiseman D, et al. Pediatric pulmonary hypertension: Roles of endothelin-1 and nitric oxide. Clin Hemorheol Microcirc 2007; 37(1–2):111–120.
38. Hislop AA, Springall DR, Oliveira H, et al. Endothelial nitric oxide synthase in hypoxic newborn porcine pulmonary vessels. Arch Dis Child Fetal Neonatal Ed 1997; 77(1): F16–F22.
39. Barst RJ, Stalcup SA. Endothelial function in clinical pulmonary hypertension. Chest 1985; 88(4 suppl):216S–220S.
40. Hall SM, Haworth SG. Onset and evolution of pulmonary vascular disease in young children: abnormal postnatal remodelling studied in lung biopsies. J Pathol 1992; 166(2): 183–193.
41. Haworth SG. Pulmonary vascular remodeling in neonatal pulmonary hypertension. State of the art. Chest 1988; 93(3 suppl):133S–138S.
42. Haworth SG. Pulmonary hypertension in the young. Heart 2002; 88(6):658–664.
43. Rosenzweig EB, Widlitz AC, Barst RJ. Pulmonary arterial hypertension in children. Pediatr Pulmonol 2004; 38(1):2–22.
44. Haworth SG. Pathophysiological and metabolic manifestations of pulmonary vascular disease in children. Herz 1992; 17(4):254–261.
45. Wagenvoort CA. The pathology of primary pulmonary hypertension. J Pathol 1970; 101(4):Pi.
46. Allen KM, Haworth SG. Cytoskeletal features of immature pulmonary vascular smooth muscle cells: the influence of pulmonary hypertension on normal development. J Pathol 1989; 158(4):311–317.
47. Newman JH, Wheeler L, Lane KB, et al. Mutation in the gene for bone morphogenetic protein receptor II as a cause of primary pulmonary hypertension in a large kindred. N Engl J Med 2001; 345(5):319–324.
48. Thomson JR, Machado RD, Pauciulo MW, et al. Sporadic primary pulmonary hypertension is associated with germline mutations of the gene encoding BMPR-II, a receptor member of the TGF-beta family. J Med Genet 2000; 37(10):741–745.
49. Rosenzweig EB, Morse JH, Knowles JA, et al. Clinical implications of determining BMPR2 mutation status in a large cohort of children and adults with pulmonary arterial hypertension. J Heart Lung Transplant 2008; 27(6):668–674.

50. Harrison RE, Berger R, Haworth SG, et al. Transforming growth factor-beta receptor mutations and pulmonary arterial hypertension in childhood. Circulation 2005; 111(4):435–441.

51. Grunig E, Koehler R, Miltenberger-Miltenyi G, et al. Primary pulmonary hypertension in children may have a different genetic background than in adults. Pediatr Res 2004; 56(4): 571–578.

52. Loyd JE, Butler MG, Foroud TM, et al. Genetic anticipation and abnormal gender ratio at birth in familial primary pulmonary hypertension. Am J Respir Crit Care Med 1995; 152(1): 93–97.

53. Rich S, Seidlitz M, Dodin E, et al. The short-term effects of digoxin in patients with right ventricular dysfunction from pulmonary hypertension. Chest 1998; 114(3):787–792.

54. Fuster V, Steele PM, Edwards WD, et al. Primary pulmonary hypertension: natural history and the importance of thrombosis. Circulation 1984; 70(4):580–587.

55. Frank H, Mlczoch J, Huber K, et al. The effect of anticoagulant therapy in primary and anorectic drug-induced pulmonary hypertension. Chest 1997; 112(3):714–721.

56. Rich S, Kaufmann E, Levy PS. The effect of high doses of calcium-channel blockers on survival in primary pulmonary hypertension. N Engl J Med 1992; 327(2):76–81.

57. Sandoval J, Aguirre JS, Pulido T, et al. Nocturnal oxygen therapy in patients with the Eisenmenger syndrome. Am J Respir Crit Care Med 2001; 164(9):1682–1687.

58. Frostell C, Fratacci MD, Wain JC, et al. Inhaled nitric oxide. A selective pulmonary vasodilator reversing hypoxic pulmonary vasoconstriction. Circulation 1991; 83(6):2038–2047.

59. Frostell CG, Blomqvist H, Hedenstierna G, et al. Inhaled nitric oxide selectively reverses human hypoxic pulmonary vasoconstriction without causing systemic vasodilation. Anesthesiology 1993; 78(3):427–435.

60. Ghofrani HA, Pepke-Zaba J, Barbera JA, et al. Nitric oxide pathway and phosphodiesterase inhibitors in pulmonary arterial hypertension. J Am Coll Cardiol 2004; 43(12 suppl S): 68S–72S.

61. Yung GL, Kriett JM, Jamieson SW, et al. Outpatient inhaled nitric oxide in a patient with idiopathic pulmonary fibrosis: a bridge to lung transplantation. J Heart Lung Transplant 2001; 20(11):1224–1227.

62. Channick RN, Newhart JW, Johnson FW, et al. Pulsed delivery of inhaled nitric oxide to patients with primary pulmonary hypertension: an ambulatory delivery system and initial clinical tests. Chest 1996; 109(6):1545–1549.

63. Ivy DD, Parker D, Doran A, et al. Acute hemodynamic effects and home therapy using a novel pulsed nasal nitric oxide delivery system in children and young adults with pulmonary hypertension. Am J Cardiol 2003; 92(7):886–890.

64. Doran AK, Ivy DD, Barst RJ, et al. Guidelines for the prevention of central venous catheter-related blood stream infections with prostanoid therapy for pulmonary arterial hypertension. Int J Clin Pract Suppl 2008; 160:5–9.

65. Simonneau G, Barst RJ, Galie N, et al. Continuous subcutaneous infusion of treprostinil, a prostacyclin analogue, in patients with pulmonary arterial hypertension: a double-blind, randomized, placebo-controlled trial. Am J Respir Crit Care Med 2002; 165(6):800–804.

66. Ivy DD, Doran AK, Smith KJ, et al. Short- and long-term effects of inhaled iloprost therapy in children with pulmonary arterial hypertension. J Am Coll Cardiol 2008; 51(2):161–169.

67. Limsuwan A, Wanitkul S, Khosithset A, et al. Aerosolized iloprost for postoperative pulmonary hypertensive crisis in children with congenital heart disease. Int J Cardiol 2007 Dec 18 [Epub ahead of print].

68. Galie N, Manes A, Branzi A. The endothelin system in pulmonary arterial hypertension. Cardiovasc Res 2004; 61(2):227–237.

69. Ozaki S, Ohwaki K, Ihara M, et al. ETB-mediated regulation of extracellular levels of endothelin-1 in cultured human endothelial cells. Biochem Biophys Res Commun 1995; 209(2):483–489.

70. Fukuroda T, Fujikawa T, Ozaki S, et a. Clearance of circulating endothelin-1 by ETB receptors in rats. Biochem Biophys Res Commun 1994; 199(3):1461–1465.
71. Rubin LJ, Roux S. Bosentan: a dual endothelin receptor antagonist. Expert Opin Investig Drugs 2002; 11(7):991–1002.
72. Rubin LJ, Badesch DB, Barst RJ, et al. Bosentan therapy for pulmonary arterial hypertension. N Engl J Med 2002; 346(12):896–903.
73. Channick RN, Simonneau G, Sitbon O, et al. Effects of the dual endothelin-receptor antagonist bosentan in patients with pulmonary hypertension: a randomised placebo-controlled study. Lancet 2001; 358(9288):1119–1123.
74. Maiya S, Hislop AA, Flynn Y, et al. Response to bosentan in children with pulmonary hypertension. Heart 2006; 92(5):664–670.
75. Barst RJ, Ivy D, Dingemanse J, et al. Pharmacokinetics, safety, and efficacy of bosentan in pediatric patients with pulmonary arterial hypertension. Clin Pharmacol Ther 2003; 73(4): 372–382.
76. Gilbert N, Luther YC, Miera O, et al. Initial experience with bosentan (Tracleer) as treatment for pulmonary arterial hypertension (PAH) due to congenital heart disease in infants and young children. Z Kardiol 2005; 94(9):570–574.
77. Ivy DD, Doran A, Claussen L, et al. Weaning and discontinuation of epoprostenol in children with idiopathic pulmonary arterial hypertension receiving concomitant bosentan. Am J Cardiol 2004; 93(7):943–946.
78. Krishnan U, Krishnan S, Gewitz M. Treatment of pulmonary hypertension in children with chronic lung disease with newer oral therapies. Pediatr Cardiol 2008; 29(6):1082–1086.
79. van Loon RL, Hoendermis ES, Duffels MG, et al. Long-term effect of bosentan in adults versus children with pulmonary arterial hypertension associated with systemic-to-pulmonary shunt: does the beneficial effect persist? Am Heart J 2007; 154(4):776–782.
80. Galie N, Ghofrani HA, Torbicki A, et al. Sildenafil citrate therapy for pulmonary arterial hypertension. N Engl J Med 2005; 353(20):2148–2157.
81. Abrams D, Schulze-Neick I, Magee AG. Sildenafil as a selective pulmonary vasodilator in childhood primary pulmonary hypertension. Heart 2000; 84(2):E4.
82. Prasad S, Wilkinson J, Gatzoulis MA. Sildenafil in primary pulmonary hypertension. N Engl J Med 2000; 343(18):1342.
83. Atz AM, Wessel DL. Sildenafil ameliorates effects of inhaled nitric oxide withdrawal. Anesthesiology 1999; 91(1):307–310.
84. Raja SG, Danton MD, MacArthur KJ, et al. Effects of escalating doses of sildenafil on hemodynamics and gas exchange in children with pulmonary hypertension and congenital cardiac defects. J Cardiothorac Vasc Anesth 2007; 21(2):203–207.
85. Noori S, Friedlich P, Wong P, et al. Cardiovascular effects of sildenafil in neonates and infants with congenital diaphragmatic hernia and pulmonary hypertension. Neonatology 2007; 91(2):92–100.
86. Humpl T, Reyes JT, Holtby H, et al. Beneficial effect of oral sildenafil therapy on childhood pulmonary arterial hypertension: twelve-month clinical trial of a single-drug, open-label, pilot study. Circulation 2005; 111(24):3274–80.
87. Karatza AA, Bush A, Magee AG. Safety and efficacy of Sildenafil therapy in children with pulmonary hypertension. Int J Cardiol 2005; 100(2):267–273.
88. Nagendran J, Archer SL, Soliman D, et al. Phosphodiesterase type 5 is highly expressed in the hypertrophied human right ventricle, and acute inhibition of phosphodiesterase type 5 improves contractility. Circulation 2007; 116(3):238–248.
89. Humbert M, Barst RJ, Robbins IM, et al. Combination of bosentan with epoprostenol in pulmonary arterial hypertension: BREATHE-2. Eur Respir J 2004; 24(3):353–359.
90. Hoeper MM, Taha N, Bekjarova A, et al. Bosentan treatment in patients with primary pulmonary hypertension receiving nonparenteral prostanoids. Eur Respir J 2003; 22(2):330–334.

91. Ghofrani HA, Rose F, Schermuly RT, et al. Oral sildenafil as long-term adjunct therapy to inhaled iloprost in severe pulmonary arterial hypertension. J Am Coll Cardiol 2003; 42(1): 158–164.

92. Stiebellehner L, Petkov V, Vonbank K, et al. Long-term treatment with oral sildenafil in addition to continuous IV epoprostenol in patients with pulmonary arterial hypertension. Chest 2003; 123(4):1293–1295.

93. McLaughlin VV, Oudiz RJ, Frost A, et al. Randomized study of adding inhaled iloprost to existing bosentan in pulmonary arterial hypertension. Am J Respir Crit Care Med 2006; 174(11):1257–1263.

94. Hoeper MM, Markevych I, Spiekerkoetter E, et al. Goal-oriented treatment and combination therapy for pulmonary arterial hypertension. Eur Respir J 2005; 26(5):858–863.

95. Micheletti A, Hislop AA, Lammers A, et al. Role of atrial septostomy in the treatment of children with pulmonary arterial hypertension. Heart 2006; 92(7):969–972.

96. Blanc J, Vouhe P, Bonnet D. Potts shunt in patients with pulmonary hypertension. N Engl J Med 2004; 350(6):623.

97. ISHLT transplant registry quarterly reports for lung in Europe. The International Society for Heart & Lung Transplantation, 2008. Available at: https://www.ishlt.org/registries/quarterlyDataReportResults.asp?organ=LU&rptType=recip_p_surv&continent=3. Accessed December 15, 2008.

98. Ghofrani HA, Seeger W, Grimminger F. Imatinib for the treatment of pulmonary arterial hypertension. N Engl J Med 2005; 353(13):1412–1413.

99. Barst RJ. PDGF signaling in pulmonary arterial hypertension. J Clin Invest 2005; 115(10): 2691–2694.

100. Schermuly RT, Dony E, Ghofrani HA, et al. Reversal of experimental pulmonary hypertension by PDGF inhibition. J Clin Invest 2005; 115(10):2811–2821.

101. Klein M, Schermuly RT, Ellinghaus P, et al. Combined tyrosine and serine/threonine kinase inhibition by sorafenib prevents progression of experimental pulmonary hypertension and myocardial remodeling. Circulation 2008; 118(20):2081–2090.

102. Dumitrascu R, Weissmann N, Ghofrani HA, et al. Activation of soluble guanylate cyclase reverses experimental pulmonary hypertension and vascular remodeling. Circulation 2006; 113(2):286–295.

103. Rubinstein I. Human VIP-alpha: an emerging biologic response modifier to treat primary pulmonary hypertension. Expert Rev Cardiovasc Ther 2005; 3(4):565–569.

104. Janosi T, Petak F, Fontao F, et al. Differential roles of endothelin-1 ETA and ETB receptors and vasoactive intestinal polypeptide in regulation of the airways and the pulmonary vasculature in isolated rat lung. Exp Physiol 2008; 93(11):1210–1219.

105. Haydar S, Sarti JF, Grisoni ER. Intravenous vasoactive intestinal polypeptide lowers pulmonary-to-systemic vascular resistance ratio in a neonatal piglet model of pulmonary arterial hypertension. J Pediatr Surg 2007; 42(5):758–764.

106. Girgis RE, Mozammel S, Champion HC, et al. Regression of chronic hypoxic pulmonary hypertension by simvastatin. Am J Physiol Lung Cell Mol Physiol 2007; 292(5): L1105–L1110.

107. Badejo AM Jr., Dhaliwal JS, Casey DB, et al. Analysis of pulmonary vasodilator responses to the Rho-kinase inhibitor fasudil in the anesthetized rat. Am J Physiol Lung Cell Mol Physiol 2008; 295(5):L828–L836.

108. Launay JM, Herve P, Peoc'h K, et al. Function of the serotonin 5-hydroxytryptamine 2B receptor in pulmonary hypertension. Nat Med 2002; 8(10):1129–1135.

109. Willers ED, Newman JH, Loyd JE, et al. Serotonin transporter polymorphisms in familial and idiopathic pulmonary arterial hypertension. Am J Respir Crit Care Med 2006; 173(7): 798–802.

110. Guignabert C, Raffestin B, Benferhat R, et al. Serotonin transporter inhibition prevents and reverses monocrotaline-induced pulmonary hypertension in rats. Circulation 2005; 111(21): 2812–2819.

111. Rhodes CJ, Davidson A, Gibbs JS, et al. Therapeutic targets in pulmonary arterial hypertension. Pharmacol Ther 2009; 121(1):69–88.

112. Michelakis ED, Wilkins MR, Rabinovitch M. Emerging concepts and translational priorities in pulmonary arterial hypertension. Circulation 2008; 118(14):1486–1495.

113. Kawut SM, Palevsky HI. New answers raise new questions in pulmonary arterial hypertension. Eur Respir J 2004; 23(6):799–801.

114. Kawut SM, Palevsky HI. Surrogate end points for pulmonary arterial hypertension. Am Heart J 2004; 148(4):559–565.

115. Peacock A, Naeije R, Galie N, et al. End points in pulmonary arterial hypertension: the way forward. Eur Respir J 2004; 23(6):947–953.

116. Roberts K, Preston I, Hill NS. Pulmonary hypertension trials: current end points are flawed, but what are the alternatives? Chest 2006; 130(4):934–936.

117. Humbert M, Sitbon O, Simonneau G. Treatment of pulmonary arterial hypertension. N Engl J Med 2004; 351(14):1425–1436.

118. McKenna SP, Doughty N, Meads DM, et al. The Cambridge Pulmonary Hypertension Outcome Review (CAMPHOR): a measure of health-related quality of life and quality of life for patients with pulmonary hypertension. Qual Life Res 2006; 15(1):103–115.

119. Taichman D, Zlupko M, Harhay M, et al. Evaluation of disease-specific health-related quality of life in pulmonary arterial hypertension. Am J Respir Crit Care Med 2008; 177:A918.

120. Taichman DB, Shin J, Hud L, et al. Health-related quality of life in patients with pulmonary arterial hypertension. Respir Res 2005; 6:92.

121. Nagaya N, Nishikimi T, Uematsu M, et al. Plasma brain natriuretic peptide as a prognostic indicator in patients with primary pulmonary hypertension. Circulation 2000; 102(8):865–870.

122. McLure LER, Peacock AJ. Imaging of the heart in pulmonary hypertension. Int J Clin Pract 2007; 61(s156):15–26.

123. Sallach SM, Peshock RM, Reimold S. Noninvasive cardiac imaging in pulmonary hypertension. Cardiol Rev 2007; 15(2):97–101.

124. Sciomer S, Magri D, Badagliacca R. Non-invasive assessment of pulmonary hypertension: Doppler-echocardiography. Pulm Pharmacol Ther 2007; 20(2):135–140.

125. Miyamoto S, Nagaya N, Satoh T, et al. Clinical correlates and prognostic significance of six-minute walk test in patients with primary pulmonary hypertension. Comparison with cardiopulmonary exercise testing. Am J Respir Crit Care Med 2000; 161(2 pt 1):487–492.

126. Lammers AE, Hislop AA, Flynn Y, et al. The 6-minute walk test: normal values for children of 4-11 years of age. Arch Dis Child 2008; 93(6):464–468.

127. Geiger R, Strasak A, Treml B, et al. Six-minute walk test in children and adolescents. J Pediatr 2007; 150(4):395–399, 399.e1–399.e2.

128. Li AM, Yin J, Au JT, et al. Standard reference for the six-minute-walk test in healthy children aged 7 to 16 years. Am J Respir Crit Care Med 2007; 176(2):174–180.

129. Hoeper MM, Lee SH, Voswinckel R, et al. Complications of right heart catheterization procedures in patients with pulmonary hypertension in experienced centers. J Am Coll Cardiol 2006; 48(12):2546–2552.

130. Friesen RH, Williams GD. Anesthetic management of children with pulmonary arterial hypertension. Paediatr Anaesth 2008; 18(3):208–216.

33

Practical Management of Pulmonary Arterial Hypertension in the Intensive Care Unit

BENJAMIN SZTRYMF and MARC HUMBERT
Université Paris Sud 11, Service de Pneumologie et Réanimation Respiratoire, Hôpital Antoine Béclère, Assistance Publique Hôpitaux de Paris, Clamart, France

I. Introduction

Pulmonary arterial hypertension (PAH) is characterized by progressive remodeling of small pulmonary arteries leading to elevated pulmonary vascular resistance and right-heart failure. PAH patients may suffer from acute right-heart failure requiring management in the intensive care unit (ICU). These episodes of decompensated right ventricular failure necessitate close monitoring, and specialized management may include high-dose intravenous diuretics, as well as inotropic and vasoconstrictive drugs. Many studies have evaluated acute right-heart failure in the absence of preexisting pulmonary hypertension (mainly acute pulmonary embolism), and guidelines are available in this setting. By contrast, very few studies have investigated acute heart failure in PAH patients. Despite the apparent similarities with other causes of acute right-heart failure, the physiological mechanisms might be different in PAH, because of previous adaptation of the right ventricle to chronic elevation of pulmonary vascular resistance and that of the left ventricle to dilated and hypokinetic right ventricle. In the absence of comprehensive studies in PAH, precise therapeutic end points remain elusive. This chapter will focus on practical management and predictors of outcome of acute worsening of PAH.

II. Management in the ICU

In the absence of validated guidelines, decompensated right ventricular failure in patients with preexisting pulmonary hypertension can be managed by the following steps.

A. Identification and Treatment of a Possible Cause of the Acute Episode

Chronic diseases are characterized by a delicate balance between persistent functional impairment and adaptation factors. In most chronic diseases, identification of a triggering factor of an exacerbation is one of the mainstays of the therapeutic strategy. This is especially true when considering rapidly corrected triggering factors, such as fluid retention in left-heart disease. However, some triggers such as sepsis may induce major pathophysiological changes that cannot be corrected rapidly. Indeed, severe sepsis has been proven to alter myocardial function affecting both ventricles (1,2).

Few data exist on triggers of acute worsening of PAH. Recently, analysis of a retrospective cohort of PAH patients displaying decompensated right ventricular failure indicated that mortality was higher in case of an infectious cause as compared with what was observed in patients with other causes of worsening or without recognized triggering factors (3). Our recent experience is broadly similar, with sepsis being associated with more severe evolution despite adapted antibiotic therapy and management, suggesting poorer prognosis (4). Besides infections that are the most common causes of severe heart failure in PAH patients, arrhythmias are frequently involved, supporting the concept that maintenance of sinus rhythm is of crucial importance to avoid arrhythmias-induced decrease of cardiac output. In addition, PAH patients should be treated with anticoagulants to prevent venous thromboembolic disease, which may be the cause of acute heart failure in patients with preexisting pulmonary hypertension. Of note, acute pulmonary embolism is a relatively common mode of revelation of chronic thromboembolic pulmonary hypertension (CTEPH): it is widely accepted that one must suspect a diagnosis of CTEPH when estimated mean pulmonary artery pressure exceeds 40 mmHg at the time of acute pulmonary embolism in a patient without known preexisting chronic heart or lung disease. In PAH patients treated with intravenous epoprostenol, central line infection and pump failure are major causes of decompensated right ventricular failure. A rare cause of worsening, which should always be suggested in these patients, remains epoprostenol-induced pulmonary edema in patients with pulmonary veno-occlusive disease and/or pulmonary capillary hemangiomatosis (see chap. 17).

B.   Right Ventricular Preload Balance

Fluid retention is a common feature of right-heart failure. However, little clinical evidence is available regarding the preload balance, even in cases of acute right-heart failure without preexisting right-heart illness (5,6). The aim of preload balance is to avoid volume overload on a failing right ventricle, which could lead to distension and ischemia of the right-heart chambers and to decreased cardiac output, at least in part due to the ventricles' interdependence (7). Intravenous diuretics and even hemofiltration have been helpful in the setting of right-heart failure in PAH patients. In our practice, basic management of acute heart failure of PAH patients usually includes high doses of intravenous furosemide in ICU, together with continuous intravenous dobutamine and/or norepinephrine if needed (see the following text).

C.   Right Ventricular Afterload Reduction

The relevance of urgent initiation of PAH specific therapy in patients hospitalized in ICU for acute right-heart failure remains a matter of debate. Indeed, these agents are not considered as emergency medications, because they presumably act, at least in part, through long-term antiproliferative and vasodilatory properties (8). Furthermore, there is concern about possible systemic hypotensive effects in unstable patients with heart failure, low cardiac output, and hypotension. Nevertheless, recent experience has emphasized the safety and efficacy of vasodilator therapy in some patients (9–11). In our practice, the use of continuous inhaled nitric oxide (10 ppm) has been useful and safe in a series of PAH patients with decompensated right-heart failure. Indeed, this agent is a potent pulmonary vasodilator without systemic vasodilatory effects. Nevertheless, one must state that there is no randomized controlled study of this agent in decompensated PAH. One case report has suggested that inhaled iloprost might be safe and useful in the setting of acute circulatory shock due to PAH (12). It has also been used in a cohort of patients as a bridge to atrial septostomy (13). In addition, successful use of inhaled milrinone has been reported in acute PAH worsening of unknown origin (14). In our practice, some PAH patients experiencing acutely decompensated right ventricular failure have been treated with continuous intravenous epoprostenol and/or oral bosentan on the top of other supportive measures (oxygen, diuretics, dobutamine, and/or norepinephrine). No side effects, such as systemic hypotension, have been recorded in such patients managed carefully in the ICU. Of note, this therapeutic strategy proposed in the most severe cases allowed some dramatic improvement and could be used as a bridge to lung transplantation for some patients (Sztrymf et al., submitted). In summary, there is an urgent need for compiling more data to firmly conclude on the role of these specific therapies in acute worsening of PAH. While there are safety concerns about the use of vasodilators in such cases, the reduction of right ventricular afterload might be one key of therapeutic success. Lastly, right ventricular assistance device, in case of refractory heart failure, could be an interesting rescue therapy in this difficult-to-manage PAH population (see the following text) (15).

D. Right Ventricular Contractility Optimization

Inotropic and/or vasoconstrictive agents are of major interest in case of severe hemodynamic impairment. The main goals of such treatments are to enhance cardiac output without increasing pulmonary vascular resistance or decreasing systemic arterial pressure. There is no systematic clinical study of these agents in PAH patients with decompensated right ventricular failure. However, they are widely used in acute heart failure complicating the course of PAH, and data are now available. Dobutamine is a treatment of choice for the management of right-heart failure in PAH. This inotropic agent improves right ventricle–pulmonary artery coupling by increasing cardiac output and decreasing pulmonary vascular resistance at doses not exceeding 5 µg/kg/min (16). In theory, higher doses may induce systemic hypotension by peripheral β-adrenoreceptors stimulation. In our clinical practice, dobutamine at a dose ranging from 2.5 to 15 µg/kg/min has been helpful in the management of acute worsening of PAH, the higher doses often necessitating vasoconstrictive comedication such as norepinephrine. Dopamine has been proven to increase cardiac output and systemic pressure in acute pulmonary embolism (17). However, there is less experience with dopamine than with dobutamine in PAH, at least in part because tachycardia and arrhythmia are the main side effects of this drug, raising concern about its benefit:risk ratio in this indication. Norepinephrine also improves right ventricle–pulmonary artery coupling (16). There is consistent experimental information on the beneficial effects of norepinephrine on coronary artery blood flow and right ventricular performance (18). By contrast, one must bear in mind that the potent vasoconstrictive properties of this drug may be deleterious in patients with severe Raynaud's phenomenon, mainly in scleroderma-associated PAH. Norepinephrine has been studied in a cohort of pulmonary hypertensive patients experiencing anesthesia-induced systemic hypotension (19). In this setting, different from decompensated PAH, it induced an increase in systemic pressure but no change in pulmonary vascular resistance or cardiac output. In our practice, norepinephrine is a drug of choice in acute right-heart failure and persistent hypotension despite dobutamine therapy.

There are no available data to support the use of epinephrine in PAH patients. Phenylephrine and vasopressin have been shown to have potential paradoxical effects, with increase in pulmonary vascular resistance and decrease in cardiac output (20,21). Right ventricular assistance device, in case of severe refractory heart failure, seems to be a promising rescue therapy, especially in patients who are listed for urgent lung or heart-lung transplantation (15). The precise role of this device in the therapeutic algorithm has to be further investigated.

E. Other Therapies

Oxygen therapy is recommended in decompensated PAH patients who are usually characterized by significant hypoxemia and low mixed venous oxygen saturation, which may be aggravated by the possible opening of a patent foramen ovale. When considered in PAH patients, intubation and mechanical ventilation are always a matter of concern because of the risks of hemodynamic life-threatening worsening already documented in other types of right ventricular failure.

III. Prognostic Markers in ICU

A. Circulating Biomarkers

Serum levels of brain natriuretic peptide (BNP) and N-terminal fragment of pro–brain natriuretic peptide (NT-pro-BNP) are associated with long-term outcome in PAH (22,23). The prognostic value of these biomarkers has also been demonstrated in acute pulmonary embolism, a model of acute right ventricular pressure overload (24,25). BNP is secreted by cardiac ventricles through a constitutive pathway and is increased according to the degree of myocardial stretch, damage, and ischemia. An experimental study has indicated an increase in BNP mRNA expression as soon as the first day after main pulmonary artery coarctation in rats (26). Recent data suggest that BNP and NT-pro-BNP levels are reliable prognostic markers in acute worsening of PAH (3,4). Of note, the evolution of these biomarkers (when monitored daily for instance) may be a predictor of outcome in ICU (4). Troponin has been shown to be associated with prognosis in PAH when evaluated in stable patients (27). Short-term evolution and right ventricular dysfunction in acute pulmonary embolism are also associated with elevated serum level of troponin (28,29). Nevertheless, recent data do not plead in favor of a statistical link with survival in acutely worsened PAH, mainly because this biomarker is not commonly elevated in PAH, raising the issue of its sensitivity in severe PAH (3,4). Elevated C-reactive protein (CRP) plasma levels may be indicative of an infectious background in PAH patients displaying acute heart failure. In our experience, high CRP and BNP levels are indeed predictors of poor prognosis in acute worsening of PAH (4).

Renal impairment and water regulation imbalance have been extensively studied in left ventricular failure (30). By contrast, no study has addressed this question in acute right-heart failure complicating the course of PAH. However, recent data suggest that cardiac output and right atrial pressure in pulmonary hypertension might be part of a complex pathophysiological network including renin-angiotensin-aldosterone, natriuretic peptides, vasopressin, and sympathetic nervous system, resulting in metabolic abnormalities (31). In left-heart disease, data suggest that these abnormalities are associated to survival (32). In stable PAH patients, hyponatremia is predictive of survival (33). Recent preliminary data also suggest a link between survival and daily evolution of serum sodium level when monitored in the ICU (persistent hyponatremia being associated with increased mortality) (4). A recent study also provides evidence that serum creatinine was associated with survival in patients with stable PAH (34). Similarly, a link has been shown between serum creatinine levels and outcome of PAH patients in the ICU (4). These preliminary results have to be confirmed in a larger prospective cohort of PAH patients.

B. Echocardiographic Parameters

Several echocardiography measurements such as tricuspid annular displacement (tricuspid annular plane systolic excursion, TAPSE) or pericardial effusion have been correlated with right ventricular function and mortality in stable PAH patients (35). Whether these parameters are also relevant in acute worsening of PAH has to be further investigated. If validated, these parameters might allow a noninvasive monitoring of right ventricular function and could be helpful to guide management.

In conclusion, management of PAH patients in ICU remains a poorly studied but important area of care for this devastating condition. As in other chronic illnesses, triggers such as sepsis may destabilize the fragile balance between disease and adaptation factors. There is an urgent need for more data on this subgroup of PAH patients to better manage these acute life-threatening episodes.

References

1. Rudiger A, Singer M. Mechanisms of sepsis-induced cardiac dysfunction. Crit Care Med 2007; 35:1599–1608.
2. Parker MM, McCarthy KE, Oqnibene FP, et al. Right ventricular dysfunction and dilatation, similar to left ventricular changes, characterize the cardiac depression of septic shock in humans. Chest 1990; 97:126–131.
3. Kurzyna M, Zyłkowska J, Fijałkowska A, et al. Characteristics and prognosis of patients with decompensated right ventricular failure during the course of pulmonary hypertension. Kardiol Pol 2008; 66:1033–1039.
4. Sztrymf B, Bertoletti L, Hamid AM, et al. Survival and prognostic factors of acute exacerbations of pulmonary arterial hypertension. Eur Respir J 2007; 30 (suppl 51):342.
5. Mercat A, Diehl JL, Meyer G, et al. Hemodynamic effect of fluid loading in acute massive pulmonary embolism. Crit Care Med 1999; 27:540–544.
6. Ozier Y, Dubourg O, Farcot JC, et al. Circulatory failure in acute pulmonary embolism. Intensive Care Med 1984; 10:91–97.
7. Haddad F, Doyle R, Murphy DJ, et al. Right ventricular function in cardiovascular disease: pathophysiology, clinical importance, and management of right ventricular failure. Circulation 2008; 117:1717–1731.

8. Humbert M, Sitbon O, Simonneau G. Treatment of pulmonary arterial hypertension. N Engl J Med 2004; 351:1425–1436.

9. Bender KA, Alexander JA, Enos JM, et al. Effects of inhaled nitric oxide in patients with hypoxemia and pulmonary hypertension after cardiac surgery. Am J Crit Care 1997; 6:127–131.

10. Rex S, Schaelte G, Metzelder S, et al. Inhaled iloprost to control pulmonary artery hypertension in patients undergoing mitral valve surgery: a prospective, randomized-controlled trial. Acta Anaesthesiol Scand 2008; 52:65–72.

11. De Santo LS, Mastroianni C, Romano G, et al. Role of sildenafil in acute post-transplant right ventricular dysfunction: successful experience in 13 consecutive patients. Transplant Proc 2008; 40:2015–2018.

12. Olschewski H, Ghofrani HA, Walmrath D, et al. Recovery from circulatory shock in severe primary pulmonary hypertension with aerosolization of iloprost. Intensive Care Med 1998; 631–634.

13. Kurzyna M, Dąbrowski M, Bielecki D, et al. Atrial septostomy in treatment of end-stage right heart failure in patients with pulmonary hypertension. Chest 2007; 131:977–983.

14. Buckley MS, Feldman JP. Nebulized milrinone use in a pulmonary hypertensive crisis. Pharmacotherapy 2007; 1763–1766.

15. Kindo M, Radovancevic B, Gregoric ID, et al. Biventricular support with the Jarvik 2000 ventricular assist device in a calf model of pulmonary hypertension. ASAIO J 2004; 50:444–450.

16. Kerbaul F, Rondelet B, Motte S, et al. Effects of norepinephrine and dobutamine on pressure-load induced right ventricular failure. Crit Care Med 2004; 32:1035–1040.

17. Layish DT, Tapson VF. Pharmacologic hemodynamic support in massive pulmonary embolism. Chest 1997; 111:218–224.

18. Mebazaa A, Karpati P, Renaud E, et al. Right ventricular failure, from pathophysiology to new treatments. Intensive Care Med 2004; 30:185–196.

19. Kwak YL, Lee CS, Park YH, et al. The effect of phenylephrine and norepinephrine in patients with chronic pulmonary hypertension. Anesthesia 2002; 57:9–14.

20. Rich S, Gubin S, Hart K. The effects of phenylephrine on right ventricular performance in patients with pulmonary hypertension. Chest 1990; 98:1102–1106.

21. Leather HA, Segers P, Berends N, et al. Effects of vasopressin on right ventricular function in an experimental model of acute pulmonary hypertension. Crit Care Med 2002; 30:2548–2552.

22. Nagaya N, Nishikimi T, Uematsu M, et al. Plasma brain natriuretic peptide as a prognostic indicator in patients with primary pulmonary hypertension. Circulation 2000; 102:865–870.

23. Fijalkowska A, Kurzyna M, Torbicki A, et al. Serum N-terminal brain natriuretic peptide as a prognostic parameter in patients with pulmonary hypertension. Chest 2006; 129:1313–1321.

24. Kucher N, Printzen G, Goldhaber SZ. Prognostic role of brain natriuretic peptide in acute pulmonary embolism. Circulation 2003; 107:2545–2547.

25. Pieralli F, Olivotto I, Vanni S, et al. Usefulness of bedside testing for brain natriuretic peptide to identify right ventricular dysfunction and outcome in normotensive patients with acute pulmonary embolism. Am J Cardiol 2006; 97:1386–1390.

26. Adachi S, Ito H, Ohta Y, et al. Distribution of mRNAs natriuretic peptides in right ventricular hypertrophy after pulmonary arterial banding. Am J Physiol 1995; 268:H162–H169.

27. Torbicki A, Kurzyna M, Kuca P, et al. Detectable cardiac troponin T as a marker of poor prognosis among patients with chronic precapillary pulmonary hypertension. Circulation 2003; 108:844–848.

28. Meyer T, Binder L, Hruska N, et al. Cardiac troponin I elevation in acute pulmonary embolism is associated with right ventricular dysfunction. J Am Coll Cardiol 2000; 36:1632–1636.

29. Mehta NJ, Jani K, Khan IA. Clinical usefulness and prognostic value of elevated cardiac troponin I levels in acute pulmonary embolism. Am Heart J 2003; 145:821–825.

30. Schrier RW. Water and sodium retention in oedematous disorders: role of vasopressin and aldosterone. Am J Med 2006; 119:S47–S53.

31. Damman K, Navis G, Smilde T, et al. Decreased cardiac output, venous congestion and the association with renal impairment in patients with cardiac dysfunction. Eur J Heart Fail 2007; 9:872–878.
32. Gheorghiade M, Abraham WT, Albert NM, et al. Relationship between admission serum sodium and outcome in patients hospitalized for heart failure: an analysis from the OPTIMIZE-HF registry. Eur Heart J 2007; 28:980–988.
33. Forfia PR, Mathai SC, Fisher MR, et al. Hyponatremia predicts right heart failure and poor survival in pulmonary arterial hypertension. Am J Respir Crit Care Med 2008; 177:1364–1369.
34. Konstam MA, Gheorghiade M, Burnett JC Jr., et al. Effects of oral Tolvaptan in patients hospitalized for worsening heart failure: the EVEREST outcome trial. JAMA 2007; 297:1319–1331.
35. Forfia PR, Fisher MR, Mathai SC, et al. Tricuspid annular displacement predicts survival in pulmonary hypertension. Am J Respir Crit Care Med 2006; 174:1034–1041.

34

End Points and Clinical Trial Design in Pulmonary Arterial Hypertension: Clinical and Regulatory Perspectives

ANDREW J. PEACOCK
Golden Jubilee National Hospital, Glasgow, U.K.

I. Introduction

Between 2000 and 2007, more than 2000 patients with pulmonary arterial hypertension (PAH) were enrolled in placebo-controlled trials. At the time of writing, most of these trials have been published and seven therapies are now licensed for PAH. This is remarkable success by any medical standard and has led, in turn, to many more trials of new therapies, combinations of therapies, and therapies given at time points earlier in the course of the disease, but, rightly, there is concern that these trials are well *designed* and use *end points* that reflect adequately the success or failure of the new approaches. Given the interest in the treatment of PAH, it is appropriate to consider the *design of trials* of new therapies or combinations of therapy for PAH and also to consider the end points that will be measured when trying to decide whether a drug or combination of drugs is effective or not. Treatments for PAH are always expensive, sometimes invasive and carry significant side effects. In order to convince patients, treating physicians, funding agencies, and regulatory bodies of the value of treatments it is, therefore, extremely important to conduct trials of appropriate design using end points of appropriate quality.

In May 2003, the first meeting devoted solely to the discussion of End Points and Trial Design in Pulmonary Arterial Hypertension was held in Gleneagles, Scotland. The format of the meeting was a series of workshops for each of the end point areas. Their deliberations were subsequently published in the European Respiratory Journal (ERJ) (1). At that time, many of the randomized controlled trials (RCT) for PAH had used six-minute walk test (6MWT) and/or resting hemodynamics as their primary end points. In this chapter, the validity of these end points and *trial designs* and whether there are better end points and/or more appropriate trial designs is considered. These issues were considered at the Second End Points Conference at Turnberry, Scotland, in 2007 (2).

II. End Points in Trials of Therapy for Pulmonary Arterial Hypertension

A. Definitions

A primary end point is one that is clinically meaningful. In the context of PAH, the most clinically meaningful end point is survival, but in this treatment era, it is considered unethical to withhold treatment in a sick patient, so it is unlikely that we will see survival trials in the future. Another clinically meaningful end point is exercise tolerance. Most trials have measured exercise tolerance using the six-minute walk distance (6MWD). There are advantages and disadvantages of the six-minute walk (6MW) (see the following text).

- A secondary end point is also called a surrogate end point (3). These may be hemodynamic variables, blood biomarkers, imaging, quality of life (QoL), or others. Both the FDA and the European Medicines Agency (EMEA) permit the use of surrogate end points for the licensing of drugs for PAH, but they must be convinced that this end point will predict clinical benefit on the basis of epidemiological, therapeutic, or pathophysiological evidence.

Many clinicians feel that the current end points used in clinical trials of PAH are not as relevant as they might be. This frustration has been articulated recently (4).

What is clear, however, is that since the trials of currently licensed therapies mostly used combination of 6MW, functional class, and hemodynamics, all new studies will likely require significant improvement in one or more of these variables before they will be approved. Any new end point would probably need to be tested alongside traditional end points and shown to be demonstrably better if it is to be considered a primary or first-level secondary end point in the future. It is now worth considering the various end points that have been or could be used in the assessment of patients with PAH.

Exercise Testing

The most common symptoms for patients with PAH are shortness of breath and fatigue. These symptoms appear initially only on exercise, and it is only later that they are present at rest as the patient transitions from World Health Organization (WHO) class II through III to IV. The progressive nature of symptoms as a consequence of the hemodynamic derangement is shown in Figure 1. From this diagram, it is clear that in the initial stages, as the peripheral pulmonary arterial disease develops, pulmonary artery pressure (PAP) rises but cardiac output (CO) is maintained. At this point, there are no symptoms. Later, as pulmonary vascular resistance (PVR) increases, symptoms develop on exercise because the CO cannot rise with exercise. Finally, in the later stages, although the PAP may not rise further, there is a decline in CO because of the high outflow impedance and there are symptoms even at rest. At this point, the PAP may actually fall. This fall in PAP with advanced disease has confused the nonexpert who may feel that treatment has been effective because of the fall of pressure when, in reality, the fall in pressure is a consequence of the diminishing CO and cardiac reserve. Given that the CO is so critical to the maintenance of wellbeing and cardiac failure is the normal mode of death, end points need to reflect CO and in the absence of noninvasive measures of CO, the best measure has been some form of exercise testing.

A measure of exercise capacity (6MWT) has been used in nearly all clinical trials in PAH. A 6MWT is really just a measure of steady-state exercise capacity. Measuring the variables that are likely to be affected by PAH, namely physiological dead space, oxygen delivery to the tissues, arterial hypoxemia, and early anaerobic threshold, necessitates a full cardiopulmonary exercise test.

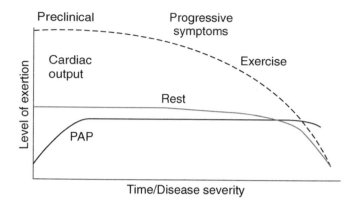

Figure 1 (*See color insert*) In the early phase of the disease, patients have an asymptomatic rise in PAP, with preservation of CO both at rest and on exertion. As the disease progresses, resting cardiac ouput remains stable, but the ability to raise stroke volume and CO on exercise is progressively impaired—resulting in progressive exertional symptoms. In the later stages of the disease, advanced right ventricular failure results in a fall in resting CO with fatigue and breathlessness at rest and right-heart failure. *Abbreviations*: PAP, pulmonary artery pressure; CO, cardiac output.

Six-Minute Walk Testing

The 6MWT is a measure of functional limitation and correlates loosely with peak aerobic capacity (5). The test was originally developed as a measure of functional capacity in patients with heart disease. The 6MWD has prognostic significance in PAH (6–8) and is a relatively simple and inexpensive test. In addition, 6MWD has been accepted by regulatory agencies as a primary end point for drug trials when secondary end points such as WHO functional class, cardiopulmonary hemodynamics, and/or time to clinical worsening (TtCW) are supportive of clinical improvement.

Advantages of 6MWD as an end point are as follows:

- Measure of function
- Simple and cheap
- Relates to prognosis
- Measures improvement in clinical trials

Disadvantages of 6MWD as an end point are as follows:

- "Ceiling effect" (9,10)
- Format not perfectly standardized (5,11)
- Format not modified for age, height, sex, weight, musculoskeletal differences, etc.

Cardiopulmonary Exercise Testing

Cardiopulmonary exercise testing (CPET) measures integrated cardiopulmonary performance at rest and during exercise (12).

Advantages of CPET as an end point are that it is comprehensive and several measures correlate function and/or survival, for example,

- ventilatory equivalents for O_2 and CO_2 (VEO_2 and $VECO_2$) correlate with disease severity (12),
- maximum O_2 consumption (VO_2 max) relates to cardiac function, and
- the same also tracks response to therapy (13,14).

The disadvantage of CPET as an end point is that it is

- technically demanding, limiting usefulness in multicenter clinical trials.

Other Measures of Exercise Capacity

Measurement of exercise duration at a constant work rate may amplify the changes in exercise capacity with drug therapy (13–15). Measurement of treadmill exercise time has been employed in smaller studies of PAH treatments as a primary (16–18) or secondary (19) end point with favorable results. In PAH, exercise time may be a more sensitive method for detecting clinically relevant changes in patients with impaired exercise capacity, however, the magnitude of the change likely overestimates the improvement relative to what would be seen using 6MWD as the measure of exercise capacity (20). Nevertheless, in patients with less severe disease or in those already treated with PAH drugs, measurement of exercise time may allow more sensitive tracking of exercise capacity (21).

Biological Markers

At present, the most useful markers have been those that monitor right ventricular (RV) dysfunction, in particular the natriuretic peptides. It is known that stretching of the atria or the ventricles releases natriuretic peptides, particularly brain natriuretic peptides (BNPs).

Advantages of biomarkers such as BNP as an end point are as follows:

- Easily measured in peripheral blood.
- N-terminal fragment of pro–brain natriuretic peptide (NT-pro-BNP) concentration in plasma does not change with posture, exercise, etc.
- Proportional to survival (22) as is troponin (23).
- Proportional to 6MWD and VO_2max (24).
- Has a threshold for RV function (25,26).
- Linearly related to RV [but not left ventricular (LV)] function in PAH (26).

The disadvantage of biomarkers such as BNP as an end point is that

- no proof yet that BNP tracks improvement or deterioration in RV function or clinical state.

Not surprisingly, BNP or NT-pro-BNP levels are now used routinely in nearly all expert centers around the world and in at least two clinical trials: the EARLY (Endothelial Antagonist tRial in mildLY symptomatic PAH patients) study of bosentan in functional class II (FCII) patients (10) and the ARIES (Ambrisentan in Pulmonary Arterial Hypertension: Randomized, Double-blind, Placebo-controlled Multicenter Efficacy Study) study of ambrisentan. We wait for further large-scale studies to see whether these promises are fulfilled.

Hemodynamics

Invasive catheterization of the right heart has been available for over 100 years (27) and is still considered essential for the proper diagnosis and staging of patients with PAH (28–30). Routinely, measurements of PAP and blood flow are made, allowing calculation of PVR.

Advantages of hemodynamics as an end point are as follows:

- Direct measure of intracardiac/pulmonary pressures and indirect measure of CO and LV function
- Essential for diagnosis of all new patients with PAH

Disadvantages of hemodynamics as an end point are as follows:

- The measurements are made in unfamiliar and possibly frightening circumstances (the cardiac catheterization laboratory).
- The measurements are made with the patient supine and at rest.
- Invasive.
- Poor correlation between PAP and 6MWD (6).
- Does not discriminate between different causes of PAH such as idiopathic pulmonary arterial hypertension (IPAH) versus connective tissue disease (CTD)-PAH (31).

A number of attempts have been made to try and improve the information available from invasive hemodynamics, which are as follows:

- Pressure-flow relationships: single-point measures of pressure and flow to calculate vascular resistance can either underestimate or overestimate because of assumptions that are made about the zero crossing of the pressure-flow relationship. Better are multipoint measurements (32) made at rest than that made on exercise. It has been shown that patients who have no change in PVR as measured by single-point estimation may actually have a change in the slope of the line describing pressure versus flow, indicating that there has been improvement (33,34).
- Measurement of vascular properties: In PAH there is change in the actual function of the vessel wall. Reeves et al. measured a distensibility quotient called alpha and showed that whereas in acute hypoxic pulmonary hypertension, there was no change in distensibility, in chronic hypoxia or in an ageing subject, this decreased (35). Blyth et al. found a relationship between alpha, pulse pressure, and survival in PAH (36). It appears also that the function of the major vessels can dictate prognosis. Mahapatra et al. showed in patients with IPAH that the pulmonary artery capacitance as measured by stroke volume divided by pulmonary artery pulse pressure was predictive of survival (37).

- Ambulatory PAP: Given the concerns about single measurements of PAP, it is tempting to try and measure PAP over a prolonged period, preferably during normal physical activity. Raeside showed that PAP can more than double on exercise in patients with PAH or during sleep in patients with chronic hypoxic lung disease (38–40). These measurements are, however, specialized, requiring a micromanometer-tipped pulmonary artery catheter, which is attached to an online processing system and does not provide concurrent measurements of flow. Clearly, these measurements will be used to validate other techniques rather than being used widely in the pulmonary hypertension community.

Ultimately, we will need noninvasive techniques, particularly for the measurement of CO, as this is so fundamental in the assessment of status in patients with PAH.

Imaging

Echocardiography

Echocardiography (ECG) was and is likely to remain, for some time, the most important screening tool for patients with suspected PAH (41,42).

Advantages of ECG as an end point are as follows:

- Noninvasive
- Cheap and widely available
- Relates to prognosis (43)
- Can estimate PAP (44–46)
- Correlates with improvement in RV indices (47)

The disadvantage of ECG as an end point is that

- because of complex geometry of RV, it cannot measure accurately RV size, shape mass, and function.

Newer techniques such as the systolic excursion of the tricuspid annulus (TAPSE), which is a measure of the longitudinal contraction (the dominant direction of contraction) of the right ventricle, amplification of echocardiograph signals by hypoxia, dobutamine or exercise, or the new technologies of three-dimensional (3D) ECG and tissue Doppler ECG (48–51) may alter our perception, but currently, the place of echo is largely for screening.

Magnetic Resonance Imaging

Magnetic resonance imaging (MRI) with a cardiac package allowing measurements throughout the cardiac cycle both at rest and on exercise is now held to be the "gold standard" in right-heart imaging in patients with PAH

Advantages of cardiac magnetic resonance (MR) as an end point is that it can make 3D measurements and hence can estimate with accuracy RV size, shape, mass, and function, for example,

- ventricular mass index, which correlates with PAP at cardiac catheterization (52);
- RV mass change with treatment of PAH (53–55);

- change in RV stroke volume with exercise (56);
- ventricular interdependence (57); and
- RV damage in PAH by gadolinium enhancement (58,59).

Disadvantages of cardiac MR as an end point are as follows:

- Expensive, so not widely available.
- Patient claustrophobia.
- Metallic objects cannot enter scanner.

We need longitudinal studies of RV mass and chamber size after prolonged therapy, and a large-scale European project is currently under way (the Euro MR project) to examine these changes. We will also need to validate MR-derived measures of CO and PA flow. At present, the expense and lack of availability of MR means that it cannot be used in large-scale clinical trials. In the future, availability of MR is likely to increase. In the meantime, there is evidence that MR variables in human PAH relate to NT-pro-BNP measurements (26), so BNP may be a surrogate for the abnormalities in RV function detected on MR.

CT Scanning

CT scanning is a rapid evolving technique in cardiovascular imaging. Recent technical advances such as the development of multislice- and multidetector-row CT make it possible to measure dynamic heart images in an acceptable period of time (60). Although the main role in phenotyping PAH is well established (61), the role of CT in longitudinal assessment of PAH is largely unexplored. However, it is reasonable to expect results similar to MRI on RV structure and function with the now widely available 64-slice ECG gated scanners.

Advantages of CT as an end point are as follows:

- Has an important role in finding cause of PAH [e.g., interstitial lung disease (ILD), pulmonary thromboembolic disease (PTE), etc.], so cardiac studies can be done at the same time
- Widely available and relatively inexpensive
- Can look at pulmonary arterial tree at the same time as RV (as can MRI) (62,63)

The disadvantage of CT as an end point is its

- high-radiation dose for which it cannot be repeated.

It is concluded that although it is too early to use an imaging end point as a primary study end point, there is a need to use these variables as secondary or additive end points in studies. In addition, imaging of the right ventricular structure and function during treatment might lead to a better understanding of the effects of therapy. RV end diastolic volume and stroke volume or CO seem to be the most sensitive variables to be monitored during treatment. Although it is recognized that imaging of the heart during exercise might provide more valuable information, these measurements are highly technically demanding, limiting their use as end points.

Clinical Variables Including Time to Clinical Worsening and Quality of Life

Quality of Life

It has been suggested, not least by the regulatory agencies, that QoL is the most important end point in measurements of efficacy of drug therapy. Unfortunately, it has always been very difficult to objectify QoL measurements, and until recently, there had been no specific health-related QoL measures in PAH.

Advantages of QoL as an end point are as follows:

- Easy, cheap, and quick
- Measures things of particular value to patients

Disadvantages of QoL as an end point are as follows:

- Until recently, tests were not specific to PAH (64–68).
- Specific test is now available Cambridge Pulmonary Hypertension Outcome Review (CAMPHOR) (69) but not yet has proven efficacy, and must be adapted for different countries and languages.

Time to Clinical Worsening

The most important end point for the evaluation of the efficacy of treatments in clinical medicine is mortality. Measurement of several individual variables constituting morbidity in rare and severe diseases such as PAH poses difficult challenges including large sample size for study populations and prolonged follow-up periods in multicenter cooperative trials. Therefore, a composite end point defined as TtCW has been developed and has been included among the secondary efficacy end points in recent trials. TtCW is defined as the time from the randomization to the first event, which usually includes

- all-cause mortality,
- hospitalization due to PAH,
- need for interventional procedures (listing for transplantation or atrial septostomy), and
- clinical progression of PAH.

Advantages of TtCW as an end point are as follows:

- Measures "real-life" clinical events
- More sensitive than noncomposite end points
- Useful where patients of better clinical state (e.g., FCII) are being studied

Disadvantages of TtCW as an end point are as follows:

- Prolongation of TtCW does not cotrack with improvement in 6MWT or QoL. This is not surprising in view of the fact that 6MWT is a measure of improvement, whereas TtCW is a measure of *absence* of deterioration. It seems likely that measures such as TtCW are more suitable for patients in FCII, whereas 6MWT is more suitable for patients in FCIII and FCIV. One solution might be to use both end points as coprimary end points or reserve each for appropriate groups of patients.

- Criteria for hospitalization for PAH are different for different units and different countries often depending on variables such as distance of patient from the center, availability of beds, etc.
- Availability of transplantation and atrial septostomy varies between countries depending on wealth of the country, availability of donors, etc.
- The definition of clinical progression of PAH is extremely heterogeneous and includes a variable combination of the following criteria: deterioration of 6MWD from baseline (usually from 10–20%), increases of one or more New York Heart Association (NYHA)/WHO functional class, signs and symptoms of right-heart failure, and escalation of medical treatments (usually the addition of targeted therapies such as prostanoids, endothelin receptor antagonists, and phosphodiesterase 5 inhibitors).

Because of the subjective nature of many of the criteria, it is advisable to appoint a blinded adjudication committee of PAH experts who have access to the patients' information and may confirm whether or not the event constitutes PAH progression. The analysis by the adjudication committee can be performed prospectively (in real time) or retrospectively after the end of the study.

If TtCW is chosen as primary end point in a randomized clinical trial, its components influence the sample size calculation according to the rate of events in the control group and to the expected improvement in the treatment arm. Obviously, the higher the number of events (and the larger the number of target events included in the option), the smaller the sample size and the observation period that will be needed.

III. Clinical Trial Design

In an era when placebo-controlled monotherapy studies in PAH are no longer acceptable, combination therapy is becoming the norm and we are studying patients with better functional class, *clinical trial design* has become increasingly important. Furthermore, though we have, in the past, "lumped" patients together with, for example, IPAH and CTD- and congenital heart disease (CHD)-PAH, it may not be appropriate as responses to therapy may differ a great deal.

A. Placebo-Controlled Studies (Superiority)

- All the current approved therapies for PAH—with the exception of epoprostenol, which was compared with conventional therapy—have been subjected to placebo-controlled studies to demonstrate superiority against placebo.

All these studies looked at morbidity in the form of exercise tolerance with various other secondary end points. Only epoprostenol has been shown to improve survival (compared with conventional therapy, i.e., not disease targeted) (70). Clearly, survival is an extremely important end point for these studies, and to try and get round the ethical problem, some authors (71) have recently compared survival of patients on therapy with survival based on data from the NIH registry, which was, of course, formulated in the pretreatment era (71,72). These are not true comparative survival studies because they were not designed so, however, given the ethical considerations, they are likely to be a best that we can achieve.

Since we now consider that placebo-controlled survival studies are not possible, we must also consider whether in the future placebo-controlled morbidity studies will be ethical. All the early trials were placebo controlled, and indeed, one or two of the studies being performed currently are also placebo controlled; but most studies that lasted between three and four months have shown a significant deterioration in the placebo-controlled group, and the current view is that if we are to do placebo-controlled studies in the future, these will need to be combination studies where the patients are always receiving an active agent even if the additional agent is a placebo. A possible exception to this rule is the patients with WHO class II function in whom it might be reasonable to plan a placebo-controlled study. This would need to be done with very tight control such that, if there is any deterioration, they can be put on treatment. We know that, for example, in the EARLY study (10) of Bosentan in FCII patients, there was deterioration in the placebo group. Another possibility is to do a placebo-controlled study of both morbidity and mortality in patients who are already on maximal combination therapy. Whether or not patients wish to be recruited to such a study is not known.

B. Noncomparative (Noninferiority) Studies

Clearly, it will not be possible to do comparative *superiority* studies between drugs because of the very large numbers of patients needed. An alternative approach is the comparative *noninferiority* study where drug A is compared with drug B and the sponsors need to show that it is not worse than the original therapy. Although the numbers needed are not as great as that needed for *superiority* studies, they are still considerable, and it is very unlikely that any company will wish to sponsor such a study, which will involve considerable expense with an indeterminate outcome (73,74).

IV. Conclusions

A. End Points

- **6MWT** will remain an important end point, particularly in the sicker patients, but there should be efforts to establish normal values depending on age, sex, body habitus, etc.
- **CPET** is safe even in the sicker patients, but the technical demands are such that it should only be used under stringent conditions.
- **Biomarkers** have been developed to assess the function of both the pulmonary vessels (largely endothelial markers) and the right heart. Only the markers of right-heart function/dysfunction have proven to be successful, particularly BNP and NT-pro-BNP, but we are not yet certain whether changes in the levels of these markers will track adequately the *changes* in cardiac function—either improvement or deterioration—with progression of disease.
- Resting **hemodynamics** are essential for the diagnosis of PAH, but the measurement of changes in resting hemodynamics in the assessment of response to therapy has proved to be disappointing. More interesting are the changes in *exercise* hemodynamics. These measurements are currently performed by

invasive catheterization, but in future there may be noninvasive techniques offering information of a similar value.

- **ECG** is likely to remain the screening tool of choice in the diagnosis of PAH and the exclusion of certain causes of PAH such as intracardiac shunt. Because of the difficulty of making 3D measurement with echo, it has not, in the past, been considered as a technique for the assessment of RV function. However, with the advent of 3D echo and also tissue Doppler, which can measure important variables such as RV strain, echo will play an increasing role.
- **Cardiac CT** is a valuable technique at present for diagnosis only, but newer cardiac function algorithms will allow measurement of RV function. The problem of the radiation dose, however, remains.
- **Cardiac MR** does not have the problem of radioactivity, and a number of studies have shown it to be useful in the measurement of RV mass, morphology, and function. Whether measurement of these variables will be useful as an end point must await the outcome of the large trials currently under way.
- **QoL** is an important component of patient assessment, and a new disease specific questionnaire (CAMPHOR) has been developed, but it needs to be translated and culturally adapted before it can used in large-scale multinational clinical trials.
- **TtCW** is valuable particularly in the fitter patients, but since it is a composite end point, we need a common definition of the adverse clinical events that comprise TtCW. These should include all-cause mortality, hospitalization for PAH, a measure of deterioration in exercise tolerance, and need for additional disease-targeted therapy, and an adjudication committee should be appointed to ensure consistency in the reporting of clinical events.

B. Clinical Trial Design

Most of the clinical trials have been blinded comparisons of the effects of the new drug against placebo on the morbidity of the disease. These have been done either in a monotherapy setting or in a combination setting. It is unlikely that we will see any of the following for reasons stated above.

- Survival trials
- Withdrawal trials
- Comparisons of one drug against another

Consideration should, however, be given to

- targeted trials where patients of a particular disease category, for example, CTD-associated PAH, are examined separately from those of the other types of PAH;
- crossover designs; and
- induction trials where aggressive early therapy with combinations of drugs is used to try and bring the disease under control before continuing with maintenance therapy.

V. Final Comment

Further clinical trials in PAH are going to be of combination therapies and will include patients at an earlier stage of disease (WHO class II). Clinical trial design will therefore be more difficult and crucial if we wish to be able to come to firm conclusions about the advisability or otherwise of combination therapy or early therapy with extremely expensive drugs. To convince patients, their doctors, the payers, and the regulators of the benefits of these therapies, our end points will need to be increasingly sophisticated and relevant to the condition we are—PAH.

Acknowledgments

The Scottish Pulmonary Vascular Unit is funded by the National Services Division of Scotland.

References

1. Peacock A, Naeije R, Galie N. End points in pulmonary arterial hypertension: the way forward. Eur Respir J 2004; 23(6):947–953.
2. Peacock A, Naeije R, Galie N, et al. End Points in pulmonary arterial hypertension: have we made progress. Eur Respir J 2009; 34:1–12.
3. Kawut SM, Palevsky HI. Surrogate end points for pulmonary arterial hypertension. Am Heart J 2004; 148(4):559–565.
4. Rich S. The current treatment of pulmonary arterial hypertension: time to redefine success. Chest 2006; 130(4):1198–1202.
5. Guyatt GH, Sullivan MJ, Thompson PJ, et al. The 6-minute walk: a new measure of exercise capacity in patients with chronic heart failure. Can Med Assoc J 1985; 132:919–923.
6. Miyamoto S, Nagaya N, Satoh T, et al. Clinical correlates and prognostic significance of six-minute walk test in patients with primary pulmonary hypertension: comparison with cardiopulmonary exercise testing. Am J Respir Crit Care Med 2000; 161:487–492.
7. Sitbon O, Humbert M, Nunes H, et al. Long-term intravenous epoprostenol infusion in primary pulmonary hypertension: prognostic factors and survival. J Am Coll Cardiol 2002; 40:780–788.
8. Paciocco G, Martinez FJ, Bossone E, et al. Oxygen desaturation on the six-minute walk test and mortality in untreated primary pulmonary hypertension. Eur Respir J 2001; 17:647–652.
9. Frost AE, Langleben D, Oudiz R, et al. The 6-min walk test (6MW) as an efficacy endpoint in pulmonary arterial hypertension clinical trials: demonstration of a ceiling effect. Vasc pharmacol 2005; 43:36–39.
10. Galie N, Rubin LJ, Hoeper MM, et al. Treatment of patients with mildly symptomatic pulmonary arterial hypertension with bosentan (EARLY study); a double-blind, randomised controlled trial. Lancet 2008; 371:2093–2100.
11. Oudiz RJ, Barst RJ, Hansen JE, et al. Cardiopulmonary exercise testing and six-minute walk correlations in pulmonary arterial hypertension. Am J Cardiol 2006; 97:123–126.
12. Sun X-G, Oudiz RJ, Hansen JE, et al. Exercise pathophysiology in primary pulmonary vascular hypertension. Circulation 2001; 104:429–435.
13. Oudiz RJ, Roveran G, Hansen JE, et al. Effect of sildenafil on ventilatory efficiency and exercise tolerance in pulmonary hypertension. Eur J Heart Fail 2007; 9(9):917–921.
14. Wax D, Garofano R, Barst RJ. Effects of long-term infusion of prostacyclin on exercise performance in patients with primary pulmonary hypertension. Chest 1999; 116:914–920.

15. Oga T, Nishimura K, Tsukino M, et al. The effects of oxitropium bromide on exercise performance in patients with stable chronic obstructive pulmonary disease. A comparison of three different exercise tests. Am J Respir Crit Care Med 2000; 161:1897–1901.
16. Sastry BK, Narasimhan C, Reddy NK, et al. Clinical efficacy of sildenafil in primary pulmonary hypertension: a randomized, placebo-controlled, double-blind, crossover study. J Am Coll Cardiol 2004; 43:1149–1153.
17. McLaughlin VV, Genthner DE, Panella MM, et al. Compassionate use of continuous prostacyclin in the management of secondary pulmonary hypertension: a case series. Ann Intern Med 1999; 130:740–743.
18. Gomberg-Maitland M, Tapson VF, Benza RL, et al. Transition from intravenous epoprostenol to intravenous treprostinil in pulmonary hypertension. Am J Respir Crit Care Med 2005; 172:1586–1589.
19. Tapson VF, Gomberg-Maitland M, McLaughlin VV, et al. Safety and efficacy of IV treprostinil for pulmonary arterial hypertension: a prospective, multicenter, open-label, 12-week trial. Chest 2006; 129:683–688.
20. Oudiz RJ, Wasserman K. Clinical efficacy of sildenafil in primary pulmonary hypertension. J Am Coll Cardiol 2004; 44:2256.
21. Gomberg-Maitland M, Huo D, Binca RL, et al. Creation of a model comparing 6-minute walk test to metabolic equivalents in evaluating the treatment effects in pulmonary arterial hypertension. J Heart Lung Transplant 2007; 26:732–738.
22. Nagaya N, Nishikimi T, Uematsu M, et al. Plasma brain natriuretic peptide as a prognostic indicator in patients with primary pulmonary hypertension. Circulation 2000; 102(8): 865–870.
23. Torbicki A, Kurzyna M, Kuca P, et al. Detectable serum cardiac troponin T as a marker of poor prognosis among patients with chronic precapillary pulmonary hypertension. Circulation 2003; 108(7):844–848.
24. Leuchte HH, Neurohr C, Baumgartner R, et al. Brain natriuretic peptide and exercise capacity in lung fibrosis and pulmonary hypertension. Am J Respir Crit Care Med 2004; 170(4): 360–365.
25. Fijalkowska A, Kurzyna M, Torbicki A, et al. Serum N-terminal brain natriuretic peptide as a prognostic parameter in patients with pulmonary hypertension. Chest 2006; 129(5): 1313–1321.
26. Blyth KG, Groenning BA, Mark PB, et al. NT-proBNP can be used to detect RV systolic dysfunction in pulmonary hypertension. Eur Respir J 2007; 69:737–744.
27. Fishman AP. A century of pulmonary hemodynamics. Am J Respir Crit Care Med 2004; 170(2): 109–113.
28. British Cardiac Society Guidelines and Medical Practice Committee, and approved by the British Thoracic Society and the British Society of Rheumatology. Recommendations on the management of pulmonary hypertension in clinical practice. Heart 2001; 86(suppl 1):I1–I13.
29. McGoon M, Gutterman D, Steen V, et al. Screening, early detection, and diagnosis of pulmonary arterial hypertension: ACCP evidence-based clinical practice guidelines. Chest 2004; 126(1 suppl):14S–34S.
30. Galie N, Torbicki A, Barst R, et al. Guidelines on diagnosis and treatment of pulmonary arterial hypertension. The Task Force on Diagnosis and Treatment of Pulmonary Arterial Hypertension of the European Society of Cardiology. Eur Heart J 2004; 25(24):2243–2278.
31. Kawut SM, Taichman DB, Archer-Chicko CL, et al. Hemodynamics and survival in patients with pulmonary arterial hypertension related to systemic sclerosis. Chest 2003; 123(2): 344–350.
32. McGregor M, Sniderman A. On pulmonary vascular resistance: the need for more precise definition. Am J Cardiol 1985; 55(1):217–221.

33. Castelain V, Chemla D, Humbert M, et al. Pulmonary artery pressure-flow relations after prostacyclin in primary pulmonary hypertension. Am J Respir Crit Care Med 2002; 165(3): 338–340.

34. Provencher R, Heave P, Sitbon O, et al. Changes in exercise haemodynamics during treatment in pulmonary arterial hypertension. Eur Respir J 2008; 32:393–398.

35. Reeves JT, Linehan JH, Stenmark KR. Distensibility of the normal human lung circulation during exercise. Am J Physiol Lung Cell Mol Physiol 2005; 288(3):L419–L425.

36. Blyth K, Syyed R, Chalmers J, et al. Pulmonary arterial pulse pressure and mortality in pulmonary arterial hypertension. Respir Med 2007; 101:2495–2501.

37. Mahapatra S, Nishimura RA, Sorajja P, et al. Relationship of pulmonary arterial capacitance and mortality in idiopathic pulmonary arterial hypertension. J Am Coll Cardiol 2006; 47(4): 799–803.

38. Raeside DA, Chalmers G, Clelland J, et al. Pulmonary artery pressure variation in patients with connective tissue disease: 24 hour ambulatory pulmonary artery pressure monitoring. Thorax 1998; 53(10):857–862.

39. Raeside DA, Smith A, Brown A, et al. Pulmonary artery pressure measurement during exercise testing in patients with suspected pulmonary hypertension. Eur Respir J 2000; 16(2): 282–287.

40. Raeside DA, Brown A, Patel KR, et al. Ambulatory pulmonary artery pressure monitoring during sleep and exercise in normal individuals and patients with COPD. Thorax 2002; 57(12): 1050–1053.

41. Mukerjee D, St George D, Knight C, et al. Echocardiography and pulmonary function as screening tests for pulmonary arterial hypertension in systemic sclerosis. Rheumatology (Oxford) 2004; 43(4):461–466.

42. Bossone E, Bodini BD, Mazza A, et al. Pulmonary arterial hypertension: the key role of echocardiography. Chest 2005; 127(5):1836–1843.

43. Raymond RJ, Hinderliter AL, Willis PW, et al. Echocardiographic predictors of adverse outcomes in primary pulmonary hypertension. J Am Coll Cardiol 2002; 39(7):1214–1219.

44. Abbas AE, Fortuin FD, Schiller NB, et al. Echocardiographic determination of mean pulmonary artery pressure. Am J Cardiol 2003; 92(11):1373–1376.

45. Syyed R, Reeves JT, Welsh D, et al. The relationship between the components of pulmonary artery pressure remains constant under all conditions in both health and disease. Chest 2008; 133:633–639.

46. Chemla D, Castelain V, Humbert M, et al. New formula for predicting mean pulmonary artery pressure using systolic pulmonary artery pressure. Chest 2004; 126(4):1313–1317.

47. Galie N, Hinderliter AL, Torbicki A, et al. Effects of the oral endothelin-receptor antagonist bosentan on echocardiographic and Doppler measures in patients with pulmonary arterial hypertension. J Am Coll Cardiol 2003; 41(8):1380–1386.

48. Pirat B, McCulloch ML, Zoghbi WA. Evaluation of global and regional right ventricular systolic function in patients with pulmonary hypertension using a novel speckle tracking method. Am J Cardiol 2006; 98:699–704.

49. Ruan Q, Nagueh SF. Clinical application of tissue Doppler imaging in patients with idiopathic pulmonary hypertension. Chest 2007; 131:395–401.

50. Sukmawan R, Watanabe N, Ogasawara Y, et al. Geometric changes of tricuspid valve tenting in tricuspid regurgitation secondary to pulmonary hypertension quantified by novel system with transthoracic real-time 3-dimensional echocardiography. J Am Soc Echocardiogr 2007; 20:470–476.

51. Forfia PR, Fisher MR, Mathai SC, et al. Tricuspid annular displacement predicts survival in pulmonary hypertension. Am J Respir Crit Care Med 2006; 174:1034–1041.

52. Saba TS, Foster J, Cockburn M, et al. Ventricular mass index using magnetic resonance imaging accurately estimates pulmonary artery pressure. Eur Respir J 2002; 20(6):1519–1524.

53. Roeleveld RJ, Vonk-Noordegraaf A, Marcus JT, et al. Effects of epoprostenol on right ventricular hypertrophy and dilatation in pulmonary hypertension. Chest 2004; 125(2):572–579.

54. Wilkins MR, Paul GA, Strange JW, et al. Sildenafil versus Endothelin Receptor Antagonist for Pulmonary Hypertension (SERAPH) study. Am J Respir Crit Care Med 2005; 26: 1993–1999.

55. van Wolferen SA, Boonstra A, Marcus JT, et al. Right ventricular reverse remodelling after sildenafil in pulmonary arterial hypertension. Heart 2006; 92(12):1860–1861.

56. Holverda S, Gan CT, Marcus JT, et al. Impaired stroke volume response to exercise in pulmonary arterial hypertension. J Am Coll Cardiol 2006; 47(8):1732–1733.

57. Roeleveld RJ, Marcus JT, Faes TJ, et al. Interventricular septal configuration at MR imaging and pulmonary arterial pressure in pulmonary hypertension. Radiology 2005; 234(3): 710–717.

58. Blyth KG, Groenning BA, Martin TN, et al. Contrast enhanced-cardiovascular magnetic resonance imaging in patients with pulmonary hypertension. Eur Heart J 2005; 19:1839–1845.

59. McKenzie JC, Kelley KB, Merisko-Liversidge EM, et al. Developmental pattern of ventricular atrial natriuretic peptide (ANP) expression in chronically hypoxic rats as an indicator of the hypertrophic process. J Mol Cell Cardiol 1994; 26(6):753–767.

60. Orakzai SH, Orakzai RH, Nasir K, et al. Assessment of cardiac function using multidetector row computed tomography. J Comput Assist Tomogr 2006; 30:555–563.

61. Ley S, Kreitner KF, Fink C, et al. Assessment of pulmonary hypertension by CT and MR imaging. Eur Radiol 2004; 14:359–368.

62. Hoffman EA, Simon BA, McLennan G. State of the Art. A structural and functional assessment of the lung via multidetector-row computed tomography: phenotyping chronic obstructive pulmonary disease. Proc Am Thorac Soc 2006; 3:519–532.

63. Nael K, Michaely HJ, Lee M, et al. Dynamic pulmonary perfusion and flow quantification with MR imaging. J Magn Reson Imaging 2006; 24:333–339.

64. Ware JE Jr., Sherbourne CD. The MOS 36-item short-form health survey (SF-36). I. Conceptual framework and item selection. Med Care 1992; 30(6):473–483.

65. Hunt S, McEwen J, McKenna S. Measuring Health Status. London: Croom Helm, 1986.

66. EuroQol—a new facility for the measurement of health-related quality of life. The EuroQol Group. Health Policy 1990; 16(3):199–208.

67. Rector TS, Cohn JN. Assessment of patient outcome with the Minnesota Living with Heart Failure questionnaire: reliability and validity during a randomized, double-blind, placebo-controlled trial of pimobendan. Pimobendan Multicenter Research Group. Am Heart J 1992; 124(4):1017–1025.

68. Shafazand S, Goldstein MK, Doyle RL, et al. Health-related quality of life in patients with pulmonary arterial hypertension. Chest 2004; 126(5):1452–1459.

69. McKenna SP, Doughty N, Meads DM, et al. The Cambridge Pulmonary Hypertension Outcome Review (CAMPHOR): a measure of health-related quality of life and quality of life for patients with pulmonary hypertension. Qual Life Res 2006; 15(1):103–115.

70. Barst RJ, Rubin LJ, Long WA, et al. A comparison of continuous intravenous epoprostenol (prostacyclin) with conventional therapy for primary pulmonary hypertension. The Primary Pulmonary Hypertension Study Group. N Engl J Med 1996; 334(5):296–302.

71. McLaughlin VV, Sitbon O, Badesch DB, et al. Survival with first-line bosentan in patients with primary pulmonary hypertension. Eur Respir J 2005; 25(2):244–249.

72. D'Alonzo GE, Barst RJ, Ayres SM, et al. Survival in patients with primary pulmonary hypertension. Results from a national prospective registry. Ann Intern Med 1991; 115(5): 343–349.

73. Galie N. Do we need controlled clinical trials in pulmonary arterial hypertension? Eur Respir J 2001; 17(1):1–3.

74. Galie N, Manes A, Branzi A. The new clinical trials on pharmacological treatment in pulmonary arterial hypertension. Eur Respir J 2002; 20(4):1037–1049.

Index

Abnormalities
  cardiopulmonary, 293
  intrinsic vascular, 267–268
ACBM. *See* Alveolarcapillary basement
    membrane (ACBM)
ACS. *See* Acute chest syndrome (ACS)
Activated partial thromboplastin time
    (aPTT), 309, 437
Activin receptor-like kinase 1 (ALK 1),
    1, 83, 163
  mutations, 153
Acute chest syndrome (ACS), 222,
    229–230
Acute episode, 452–453
Acute respiratory distress syndrome
    (ARDS), 222
Acute respiratory failure, 254
Acute vasodilator testing, in PAH patients
  agents for, 371–372
  responders to, 372
AD. *See* Aorta diameter (AD)
Adrenomedullin, 72, 370
Adventitial fibrosis, 23
aECA. *See* Antiendothelial antibodies (aECA)
Aerosolized inhalation, 342–343
Afterload balance
  in right ventricular, 453–454
Alanine aminotransferase (ALT), 355
Algorithms
  for treatment, 435–436
ALK1. *See* Activin-like kinase type 1
    (ALK1)
ALK 1. *See* Activin receptor-like kinase 1
    (ALK 1)
ALK1 gene, 163
ALT. *See* Alanine aminotransferase (ALT)

Altitude of residence
  hemodynamic studies of CMS, at,
    293–295
Alveolarcapillary basement membrane
    (ACBM), 268
Alveolar hypoxia, 252, 259
Alveolar macrophages, 275
Alveolar septa, 33
Ambrisentan, 189
  ARIES-1, 360, 361
  ARIES-2, 360, 361
American Association for the Study of Liver
    Disease (AASLD), 208
American College of Chest Physicians,
    372
21–Amino acid peptide, 352
Aminorex, 40
Anesthetic management, 426–427
Angiogenesis, 370
Angiogenic precursor cells, 48
Angiography, pulmonary, 156
Angioproliferation, 41–45
Angiosarcomas
  endarterectomy for, 406–407
  of the pulmonary artery, 111–112
Angioscope, 404
Anorexigen-associated PAH
  acute vasoreactivity testing, 155
  diagnosis, 154–157
  epidemiology, 151–152
  genetics, 152–153
  survival, prognosis factors, and impact
    of therapy, 157
Anti-α-actin staining, 31
Anticoagulation, 242
  for CTDs, 170

Antiendothelial antibodies (aECA), 162–163
Antifibrillarin antibodies (anti-U3 RNP), 162, 163
Anti-inflammatory drugs, for CTD, 167
Antiphospholipid antibodies syndrome, 306
Antiretroviral therapy
  effects of, on PAH-HIV, 200–202
Antitopoisomerase II-α antibodies, 163
Anti-U3 RNP. *See* Antifibrillarin antibodies (anti-U3 RNP)
Aorta diameter (AD), 278
aPTT. *See* Activated partial thromboplastin time (aPTT)
ARDS. *See* Acute respiratory distress syndrome (ARDS)
Arginase, 223
Arterial blood gases, evolution of, 258
AS. *See* Atrial septostomy (AS)
ASD. *See* Atrial septal defect (ASD)
Aspartate aminotransferase (AST), 355
AST. *See* Aspartate aminotransferase (AST)
Atrial septal defect (ASD), 126, 177, 179
Atrial septostomy (AS)
  echocardiography studies, 393
  hemodynamic effects, 391–392
  immediate outcome after, 388–391
  on long-term survival, 393–394
  overview, 385–386
  in PAH, 386
  for patients, 386–387
  procedure, 387–388
  rationale for, 386
  spontaneous closure of, 393
Auscultatory, crackles, 240
Autoimmune liver disease, 209

BAL. *See* Bronchoalveolar lavage (BAL)
Balloon dilation atrial septostomy (BDAS), 385, 387
  procedure-related mortality in, 390
Basic fibroblast growth factor (bFGF), 170, 181
BBAS. *See* Blade balloon atrial septostomy (BBAS)

BDAS. *See* Balloon dilation atrial septostomy (BDAS)
Benign tumors, 112
Beraprost
  dosage of, instructions for, 344
  double-blind placebo-controlled randomized study of, 343
Bernoulli's equation, 185, 255–256
β-adrenoreceptors, 454
β-blockers, 210
bFGF. *See* Basic fibroblast growth factor (bFGF)
Bilateral lung transplant (BLT), 413
Bilateral sequential lung transplantation (BSLT), 399
Biomarkers, 465
  circulating in, 455–456
  for comprehensive prognostic evaluation, 377
  end points trial in, 465
Blade balloon atrial septostomy (BBAS), 385
Blalock-Taussig shunt, 66, 179
Bleomycin-induced pulmonary fibrosis, 275
Blood stream infections, 340
BLT. *See* Bilateral lung transplant (BLT)
BMI. *See* Body mass index (BMI)
BMP. *See* Bone morphogenetic protein (BMP)
BMPR2. *See* Bone morphogenetic protein receptor 2 (BMPR2); Bone morphogenetic protein receptor type 2 (BMPR2) mutations
BNP. *See* Brain natriuretic peptides (BNP)
Body mass index (BMI), 411
Bone morphogenetic protein (BMP), 271
Bone morphogenetic protein receptor type 2 (BMPR2) mutations, 83, 152–153, 435
  and disease expression, 88–89
  and genetic modifiers, 89–90
  genetic testing for, 90–91
  HI and, 89
  HPAH and, 86–87
  in IPAH, 87–88
  prevalence of, in HPAH, 87

Bone morphogenetic protein type 2 receptor (BMPR2), 1, 47, 150, 152, 163, 240, 271, 273
heterozygous germline mutations in, 197
BOS. *See* Bronchiolitis obliterans syndrome (BOS)
Bosentan, 210, 211, 353, 354, 440, 445
BENEFIT, 358
BREATHE-1, 355–356
BREATHE-4, 357–358
BREATHE-5, 357
therapy, 168–169, 357
Brain natriuretic peptide (BNP), 135, 157, 256, 278, 356, 375, 432, 455, 465
in SCD, 227–228
BREATHE-5 trial, 189
Bronchial arteries, 105
Bronchiolitis obliterans syndrome (BOS), 401
Bronchoalveolar lavage (BAL), 275
BSLT. *See* Bilateral sequential lung transplantation (BSLT)

Caesarean section (CS), 426
Calcium channel blockers (CCB), 202, 240, 280, 325, 373, 424, 436, 438
Calcium-encrusting elastic fibers, 31–32
Cambridge Pulmonary Hypertension Outcome Review (CAMPHOR), 469
cAMP. *See* Cyclic adenosine monophosphate (cAMP)
CAMPHOR. *See* Cambridge Pulmonary Hypertension Outcome Review (CAMPHOR)
Cardiac catheterization, 293–294. *See also* Right-heart catheterization (RHC) *See also* Left-heart catheterization (LHC)
Cardiac index (CI), 278
Cardiac magnetic resonance (cMR), 127, 129
Cardiac output (CO), 385
Cardiomegaly, 96
Cardioplegia, 405
Cardiopulmonary abnormalities, 293
Cardiopulmonary bypass (CP), 315, 399

Cardiopulmonary exercise, 432
Cardiopulmonary exercise testing (CPET), 134–135, 156, 376, 464–465
Caveolin proteins, 46
CCB. *See* Calcium channel blockers (CCB)
CD68 stain, 27
Cell cultures for PAH, 72–73
The Center for Disease Control and Prevention, 214
Central venous catheter, cuffed, 342
Central venous pressure (CVP), 420
Cercariae, 215
Cerebral protection, 315
Cerro de Pasco, 294
cGMP. *See* Cyclic guanosine monophosphate (cGMP)
CHD. *See* Congenital heart disease (CHD)
CHD-associated PAH (CHD-PAH), 421
CHD-PAH. *See* CHD-associated PAH (CHD-PAH)
Chemla equation, 122
Chemokines, 30
Chemotherapy, 407
Chengdou, 294
Chest radiography, 96, 133, 154, 309
Chest tomography (CT) imaging, 133, 156
Chest X ray (CXR), 184
Children
diagnosis of PAH, 431–434
etiology of PAH, 434–435
future aspects, 442–443
outcome measures in PAH, 443–445
pathophysiology of PAH, 435
treatment of PAH, 435–442
Child-Turcotte-Pugh, 209
China
pulmonary hemodynamics in chronic high-altitude diseases in, 297
Chronic hemolytic anemia and PAH, 5
Chronic high-altitude diseases
ISMM consensus statement and, 300
pulmonary arterial pressure in, 294
pulmonary hemodynamics in, in China and Kyrgyzstan, 297

Chronic mountain sickness (CMS)
  in classification of HAPH, 299
  in classification of ISMM consensus
    statement, 298–299
  in classification of PH, 298
  as clinical complex syndrome, 293
  definition of, 293
  Hb threshold values, 301
  hemodynamic studies of
    at altitude of residence, 293–295
    with Doppler echocardiography, 296
    during recovery period at lower
      altitude, 296
  hemodynamic values in, 295
  history, 292–293
  limits of consensus statement on, 300
  management of, 301–302
  PAP in, 296
  prevention of, 301–302
  primary, 293
  scoring system for diagnosis of, 300
  secondary, 293
Chronic obstructive pulmonary disease
    (COPD), 59, 133, 250
  characteristics of PH in, 252–254
  comparison of three subgroups
    of, 255
  diagnosis of PH in, 255–256
  disproportionate PH in, 254–255
  evolution of PH in, 256–257
  PH mechanisms in, 251–252
  prevalence of, 251
  prognosis of PH in, 259
  resting and exercising PAPs in,
    253–254, 257
  right ventricular contractility in, 259
  treatment of PH in, 259–260
Chronic renal failure, 224
Chronic thromboembolic disease, 133
Chronic thromboembolic pulmonary
    hypertension (CTEPH), 6, 59,
    100, 103, 104, 106, 107, 108, 156,
    350–351, 403, 453
  chest radiography and, 309
  clinical presentation, 307–308
  endarterectomy surgery, patients
    selection for, 314–315

[Chronic thromboembolic pulmonary
    hypertension (CTEPH)]
  evaluation of patients with suspected,
    309–313
  history of, 307
  incidence of, 305–306
  MRA and, 313
  open-label study, 318
  PTE surgery and, 314–317
  pulmonary angiogram in patients, 312, 313
  pulmonary function testing and, 309
  right-heart catheterization and, 311
  risk factors of, 305–306
  use of PH-specific medical therapies,
    317–319
CI. *See* Cardiac index (CI); Confidence
    interval (CI)
Cine imaging, 313
Circulating biomarkers, 455–456
Circulatory arrest, 315–316
Cirrhosis, 210
Classical arteritis, 28
Clinical trial design
  noninferiority studies, 471
  placebo-controlled studies, 470–471
Clubbing, 240
cMR. *See* Cardiac magnetic resonance (cMR)
CMS. *See* Chronic mountain sickness (CMS)
"colander-like" lesions, 23, 31
Collagen, 65
Collateral systemic vessels, 113
Combination therapy, 441–442
  for CTDs, 169
  for PAH treatment, 367–368
  in patients with PAH, 379
  for vascular disease, 412
Comprehensive prognostic evaluation,
    376–378
  biomarkers, 377
  clinical signs, 376
  exercise performance, 376
  hemodynamics, 377–378
  RV function, 377–378
Computed tomographic (CT) scanning,
    310–311
  in cardiovascular imaging, 468
  of chest, 432

Computed tomography (CT), 267, 277
Confidence interval (CI), 196
Congenital heart disease (CHD), 4, 96, 340, 419, 434
   associated PAH, 178–181
      classification of, 178–181
      diagnosis and assessment, 183–187
      heart lesions and, 178–181
      pathophysiology of, 181–183
      persistent pulmonary hypertension of newborn (PPHN), 182–183
      therapies for, 189–192
   Eisenmenger syndrome, 178, 181, 188–189
   epidemiology, 176–178
   PH in, diagnosis and assessment, 183–187
Connective tissue diseases (CTD), 11, 33, 264, 341, 350, 412
   and PAH, 178
      mixed CTD (MCTD), 166
      primary Sjögren syndrome (pSS), 166–167
      rheumatoid arthritis (RA), 166
      systemic lupus erythematosus (SLE), 166
      systemic sclerosis (SSc), 161
         autoantibodies in, 162–163
         clinical features, 164
         detection of, algorithm for, 164–165
         genetic factors in, 163–164
         prognosis, 165–166
         vascular changes in, 162
      therapy
         anticoagulation, 170
         anti-inflammatory drugs, 167
         combination, 169–170
         endothelin receptor antagonists, 168–169
         lung transplantation (LT), 170
         phosphodiesterase inhibitors, 169
         prostaglandins, 167–168
         tyrosine kinase inhibitors, 170
   PAH associated with, 2–3
Connective tissue growth factor (CTGF), 268
Continuous intravenous epoprostenol therapy, 243

Contractility optimization
   in right ventricular, 454–455
Contradictions, general, 410–411
Contrast-enhanced MR angiography (ce-MRA), 108–109
Conventional medical therapy, 423–424
Conventional therapy, 437–438
   in children, 437–438
   for PAH
      general measures, to prevent clinical deterioration, 325
      physical activities, 326
   and PVOD, 242–243
COPD. *See* Chronic obstructive pulmonary disease (COPD)
cor pulmonale, 250
COX-2. *See* Cyclooxygenase 2 (COX-2)
CP. *See* Cardiopulmonary (CP)
CPET. *See* Cardiopulmonary exercise testing (CPET)
C-reactive protein (CRP), 455
CREST syndrome, 162
Crotalaria spectabilis, 63
CRP. *See* C-reactive protein (CRP)
CS. *See* Caesarean section (CS)
CT. *See* Computed tomographic (CT) scanning; Computed tomography (CT)
CTD. *See* Connective tissue diseases (CTD)
CTGF. *See* Connective tissue growth factor (CTGF)
CT imaging. *See* Chest tomography (CT) imaging
CVP. *See* Central venous pressure (CVP)
Cyanosis, 188, 189
Cyclic adenosine monophosphate (cAMP), 340
Cyclooxygenase 2 (COX-2), 72
CYP1B1. *See* Cytochrome P450 1B1 (CYP1B1)
Cytochrome P450 1B1 (CYP1B1), 86
Cytokines, 274

Dana Point meeting, 31
DE. *See* Doppler echocardiography (DE)
Dead-space ventilation, 309–310
Delayed transfusion reaction (DHTR), 229

DHTR. *See* Delayed transfusion reaction (DHTR)
Diastolic dysfunction
  left-sided heart disease and, 227
Diffusing capacity for carbon monoxide (D_LCO), 241, 254, 309
Digital substraction angiography (DSA), 101–102
Digoxin therapy
  children with frank right-heart failure, 437
Dilation lesions, 27–28
Diuretic therapy, 375
D_LCO. *See* Diffusing capacity for carbon monoxide (D_LCO)
DN. *See* Dominant negative (DN)
Dobutamine, 453
Dominant negative (DN) mutations, 72–73, 88–89
Dopamine, 454
Doppler echocardiographic PASP, 225–227
Doppler echocardiography (DE), 123, 125–126, 128, 133, 255–256, 277. *See also* Echocardiography, of PAH
  as effective screening tool, 136
  estimated PASP, 135–136
  hemodynamic studies of CMS with, 296
  transthoracic, 135–136
Double-blind placebo-controlled randomized study
  of beraprost, 343
Down syndrome, 177, 179
Drug-induced PAH, 2
Ductus arteriosus, 66
Dyspnea, 132, 198–199, 255, 277, 307

Early plexiform lesion, 41
Eccentricity index (EI), 432
ECE. *See* Endothelin-converting enzyme (ECE)
ECG. *See* Electrocardiogram (ECG)
Echocardiographic parameters, 456
Echocardiography
  to assess RV function, 377
  for pregnant patients, 422–423
  studies in SCD, 224–227

Echocardiography, of PAH, 185–186
  differential diagnosis of, 127
  Doppler and catheter diagnosis, 125
  Doppler-derived sPAP, upper normal limits of, 123–125
  follow-up of, 128–129
  latent pulmonary hypertension and, 125–127
  noninvasive estimation of, 122–123
  RV overload, consequences of
    fuctional, 128
    morphological, 127–128
ECMO. *See* Even circulatory support (ECMO); Extracorporeal membrane oxygenation (ECMO)
EI. *See* Eccentricity index (EI)
Eisenmenger syndromes, 4, 66, 178, 181, 188–189, 410. *See also* Congenital heart disease (CHD)
  in HLT, 400
  in PAH pregnancies, 421
Elastica van Gieson staining (EvG), 27
Electrocardiogram (ECG), 154, 184, 255, 296
  CPET and gas exchange, 134–135
  pulmonary function testing, 134, 154
EMEA. *See* European Medicines Agency (EMEA)
Endarterectomy surgery
  CTEPH patients selection for, 314–315
Endarteriectomy, 59
Endoglin *(ENG)*, 83, 87, 163, 164
Endothelial cell growth
  plexiform lesion, 45
Endothelial dysfunction
  hemolysis-associated, 223–224
  and HIV, 197
Endothelial progenitor cells (EPCs), 181
Endothelial prostacyclin synthase, 210
Endothelin antagonist trial, 378
Endothelin-converting enzyme (ECE), 183
Endothelin-1 (ET-1), 181, 183, 197, 268, 352, 440
  involvement in PH and ILD, 274
  plasma concentrations, 354
  schematic representation of, 353
Endothelin (ET) receptors, 353

Endothelin receptor antagonist (ERA), 325, 353–354, 373–374, 423, 425
  ambrisentan. *See* Ambrisentan
  bosentan. *See* Bosentan
  for CTDs, 168–169
  oral, 203
  sitaxsentan. *See* Sitaxsentan
Endothelin-1 receptor antagonists (ETRAs), 279
Endothelium, 268
End-stage renal disease (ESRD), 7
ENG. *See* Endoglin (ENG)
EPCs. *See* Endothelial progenitor cells (EPCs)
Epithelium, 268
Epoprostenol, 373, 439
  intravenous. *See* Intravenous epoprostenol
Epoprostenol, 33, 211
ERA. *See* Endothelin receptor antagonists (ERA)
ERJ. *See* European Respiratory Journal (ERJ)
ESRD. *See* End-stage renal disease (ESRD)
ET-1. *See* Endothelin-1 (ET-1)
ETRAs. *See* Endothelin-1 receptor antagonists (ETRAs)
ET receptors. *See* Endothelin (ET) receptors
European Medicines Agency (EMEA), 463
European Respiratory Journal (ERJ), 462
European Respiratory Society, 374
European Society of Cardiology, 372
Even circulatory support (ECMO), 412
Evian classification, of pulmonary hypertension, 218
Evidence-based treatment algorithm, 372, 373–374
Exercise
  capacity, 156
  right-heart catheterization and, 140–141
  testing for patients with PAH, 463–464
Extracorporeal membrane oxygenation (ECMO), 401

FAC. *See* Fractional area change (FAC)
Familial pulmonary arterial hypertension (FPAH), 83
  acute vasoreactivity testing, 155
  diagnosis, 154–157

[Familial pulmonary arterial hypertension (FPAH)]
  epidemiology, 151–152
  genetics, 152–153
  survival, prognosis factors, and impact of therapy, 157
Fenfluramine-associated PAH, 152
Fibroblastic foci, 26, 31
Fibronectin, 65
Fibrotic lesions, 23
Fibrotic process, 266–267
Fibrous, occlusion, 238
Fick's method, 138, 186–187
Flow and pressure relationship, in mitral stenosis
  Gorlin and Gorlin formulae of, 138–139
Forced vital capacity (FVC), 278
FPAH. *See* Familial pulmonary arterial hypertension (FPAH)
Fractional area change (FAC), 432
French PAH registry, 10–15
  anorexigen-associated with, 11, 12
  BMPR2 mutations, 12
  in CTD, 12–13
  overview, 10–11
  pulmonary hemodynamics in, 14
  regional prevalence of, 15
  in systemic sclerosis, 13
  in women, 11–12
French Registry, 151
Fulton index, 64
  in normoxia, 71
Fulvine, 64
Furosemide, 423, 453
FVC. *See* Forced vital capacity (FVC)

GA. *See* General anesthesia (GA)
GARD. *See* Global Alliance Against Chronic Respiratory Diseases (GARD)
Gaucher cells, 7
Gaussian distribution, 265
General anesthesia (GA), 422
Genetic manipulations
  in PAH, 70–73
Genetic modifiers
  BMPR2 mutations and, 89–90

GeoSentinel, 214
Global Alliance Against Chronic Respiratory Diseases (GARD), 17
GMP. *See* Guanosine monophosphate (GMP)
Goal-oriented therapy, 380–382
Golde score, 32
Gorlin and Gorlin formulae
  of flow and pressure relationship, in mitral stenosis, 138–139
Graham Steell murmur, of pulmonary regurgitation, 184
Granulomas, perivascular, 216
Guanosine monophosphate (GMP), 438

HAART. *See* Highly active antiretroviral therapy (HAART)
HACP. *See* High-altitude cor pulmonale (HACP)
HAHD. *See* Highaltitude heart disease (HAHD)
The Hallmarks of Cancer, 47
HAPH. *See* High-altitude pulmonary hypertension (HAPH)
Haploinsufficiency (HI), 84, 88–89
Hb. *See* Hemoglobin (Hb), threshold values
Hb S. *See* Hemoglobin S (Hb S)
Heart-lung transplantation (HLT), 399–400, 410
Hemangiomas, 46
Hemodynamic characteristics, of PCH, 244
Hemodynamics, 16, 466–467
  changes in pregnancy, 420–421
  for comprehensive prognostic evaluation, 377–378
  effects in AS, 391–392
Hemodynamic variables, evolution of, 258
Hemoglobin (Hb), threshold values, 301
Hemoglobin S (Hb S)
  polymerization, 222–223
Hemolysis, 223–224
Hemolytic anemia, 224, 225
Hemosiderin, 32
Hepatic aminotransferases, 360
Hepatic function, abnormal, 355
Hepatopulmonary syndrome, 207
Hepatosplenic disease, 216–219

Hereditable pulmonary arterial hypertension (HPAH), 83, 84
  BMPR2 mutations and, 86–87
Hereditary hemorrhagic telangiectasia (HHT), 1, 83, 87, 163
Heterozygous germline mutations in BMPR2, 197
HHT. *See* Hereditary hemorrhagic telangiectasia (HHT)
HHV-8. *See* Human herpesvirus 8 (HHV-8)
HI. *See* Haploinsufficiency (HI)
High-altitude cor pulmonale (HACP), 292
  studies on, in Kyrgyzstan, 297
High-altitude heart disease (HAHD), 292
  studies on, in China, 297
High-altitude pulmonary hypertension (HAPH), 298
  CMS in classification of, 299
High-resolution chest computed tomography (HRCT), 277
High-resolution computed tomography (HRCT), 95, 241
Highly active antiretroviral therapy (HAART), 50, 196, 197
HIV. *See* Human immunodeficiency virus (HIV)
HIV infection
  PAH associated with, 3–4
HIV nef gene, 50
HLT. *See* Heart-lung transplantation (HLT)
HMG-CoA. *See* 3-hydroxy-3-methylglutaryl CoA (HMG-CoA)
HMG-CoA reductase inhibitors, 443
Honeycomb lung, 266–267
HP. *See* Hypersensitivity pneumonitis (HP)
HPAH. *See* Hereditable pulmonary arterial hypertension (HPAH)
HRCT. *See* High-resolution chest computed tomography (HRCT); High-resolution computed tomography (HRCT)
Human herpesvirus 8 (HHV-8), 48, 198
Human immunodeficiency virus (HIV), 11, 432
  endothelial dysfunction and, 197
  HHV-8, 198
  nef protein, 198

[Human immunodeficiency virus (HIV)]
  patients, epidemiology of PAH in
    demographic features of, 196
    HIV infection. *See* Human
      immunodeficiency virus (HIV)
    incidence and prevalence of, 196–197
  portal hypertension and, 200
  pulmonary inflammation and, 198
Hydatic emboli, 407
Hydatid cysts, 112
3-Hydroxy-3-methylglutaryl CoA
  (HMG-CoA), 443
Hypercoagulability, hemolysis-associated,
  223–224
Hyperplasia, 276
Hypersensitivity pneumonitis (HP), 264
Hypertension pulmonary, schistosomiasis
  and, 216–217
Hypertensive pulmonary vascular disease
  histological classification of, 20–21
Hypoxemia, 265, 298, 310
  score system and, 301
Hypoxia-induced pulmonary hypertension,
  61–63
Hypoxia in PH, 6
Hypoxic pulmonary vasoconstriction, 252

ICU. *See* Intensive care unit (ICU)
Idiopathic pulmonary arterial hypertension
  (IPAH), 45, 83, 122, 126, 132,
    154–157, 238, 264, 367
  biomarkers, 135
  BMPR2 mutations in, 87–88
  chest X ray, 154
  CT imaging in, 133, 156
  ECG findings of, 154
    CPET and gas exchange, 134–135
    pulmonary function testing, 134, 154
  epidemiology, 151–152
  exercise and, 141, 156
  French Registry and, 151
  genetics, 152–153
  serological evaluations, 135
  survival, prognosis factors, and impact of
    therapy, 157
  symptoms, 132–133, 153

[Idiopathic pulmonary arterial hypertension
  (IPAH)]
  transthoracic echocardiography (TTE)
    for, 154
  vasodilator testing, 137, 155
  ventilation/perfusion lung scan, 156
Idiopathic pulmonary fibrosis (IPF), 26, 264
  CT angiogram of, 267
  MPAP in, 265
  pathogenesis of, 269
  prevalence of PH in, 265
Idiopathic spontaneous pneumothorax, 26
ILD. *See* Interstitial lung disease (ILD)
Iloprost, 342–343, 373, 424
  dosage of, instructions for, 343
IL-1ra. *See* Interleukin-1 receptor antagonist
  (IL-1ra)
Imatinib, 370
Immunohistochemical analysis, 23
Immunosuppressive therapy, in PVOD,
  242–243
Infections
  blood stream, 340
  HIV. *See* Human immunodeficiency virus
    (HIV)
Inferior vena cava (IVC), 400
Inflammation
  involvement in PH and ILD, 274–276
Inflammatory infiltrates, 35
Inhalation, aerosolized, 342
Inhaled iloprost, 434, 439
Inhaled nitric oxide (iNO), 372, 434
Inhibitors
  PDE-5. *See* Phosphodiesterase type 5
    (PDE-5), inhibitors
  phosphodiesterase, 374
  Rho kinase, 370
Initial therapy, PAH, 378–379
iNO. *See* Inhaled nitric oxide (iNO)
INR. *See* International normalized ratio
  (INR)
In situ thrombosis. *See* Thrombotic lesions
Intensive care unit (ICU)
  management in, 452–455
  prognostic markers in, 455–456
Interleukin-1 receptor antagonist (IL-1ra), 274
Internal elastica, 270

International normalized ratio (INR), 358, 437
International primary pulmonary hypertension study, 152
International Society for Heart and Lung Transplantation (ISHLT), 412
International Society of Mountain Medicine (ISMM), consensus statement
chronic high-altitude diseases and, 300
CMS in classification of, 298–299
limits of, on CMS, 300
International Society of Travel Medicine, 214
Interstitial lung disease (ILD)
clinical manifestations, 277
diagnosis of, 277–279
endothelin/receptors involvement in, 274
fibrotic process and, 266–267
inflammation and, 274–276
intrinsic vascular abnormalities, 267–268
pathogenesis of, 268–269
pathological changes, 276
prevalence of PH in, 264–266
prognosis of PH in, 266
RHC and, 277–279
TGF-β isoforms in, 271–273
Interstitial pulmonary fibrosis (IPF), 27
Interstitial smooth muscle, 31
Intima, 269
Intraluminal webs or bands, 104
Intrauterine device (IUD), 360
Intravenous epoprostenol, 338–340
dosage of, instructions for, 340
Intravenous prostanoids, 438–439
Intrinsic vascular abnormalities, 267–268
Intrinsic vascular disease, 277
IPAH. *See* Idiopathic pulmonary arterial hypertension (IPAH)
IPF. *See* Idiopathic pulmonary fibrosis (IPF)
ISHLT. *See* International Society for Heart and Lung Transplantation (ISHLT)
ISMM. *See* International Society of Mountain Medicine (ISMM), consensus statement
Isolated medial hypertrophy, 21–22

IUD. *See* Intrauterine device (IUD)
IVC. *See* Inferior vena cava (IVC)
IV epoprostenol, 434

Kaposi sarcoma, 47
Kerley B lines, 96, 241
Kyrgyzstan
pulmonary hemodynamics in chronic high-altitude diseases in, 297

Lactate dehydrogenase (LDH), 224
LAM. *See* Lymphangioleiomyomatosis (LAM)
LAP. *See* Left atrial pressure (LAP)
La Paz, Bolivia, 294
Latent pulmonary hypertension
echocardiographic tests for, 125–127
LDH. *See* Lactate dehydrogenase (LDH)
Left atrial pressure (LAP), 5
Left-heart catheterization (LHC), 138, 155
Left-sided heart disease
hemodynamic assessment of, 138–140
in PH, 5
in SCD, 227
Left ventricular end-diastolic pressure (LVEDP), 138, 139–140, 155, 180
Lesions
mechanism of, 217
plexiform, 197, 217
postcapillary, 238
Lhasa, Tibet, 294
LHC. *See* Left-heart catheterization (LHC)
Limbus, 45
5-Lipoxygenase adenovirus, 72
Liver transplantation (LT), 207
LMWH. *See* Low molecular weight heparin (LMWH)
Long-term oxygen therapy (LTOT), 257, 259–260
Low molecular weight heparin (LMWH), 423
LT. *See* Lung transplantation (LT)
LTOT. *See* Long-term oxygen therapy (LTOT)

Lungs
  biopsy, 21, 141
  honeycomb, 266
  metastasectomies, 407
  perfusion scanning, 98
  transplant, 192
  vascular pathology, 217
Lung transplantation (LT), 264,
        398–401, 409
  contradictions, 410–411
  CTDs and, 170
  indications to, 409–410
  and PVOD, 243
  referral for, 411
  timing of, 415–416
Lupus anticoagulant, 309
LVEDP. *See* Left ventricular end-diastolic
        pressure (LVEDP)
Lymphangioleiomyomatosis (LAM), 264

Macrophages, 31
Magnetic resonance angiography
        (MRA), 313
Magnetic resonance imaging (MRI),
        108–109, 133–134
  in right-heart imaging, 467–468
Main pulmonary artery diameter
        (MPAD), 277
Matrix metalloproteinases (MMPs), 269
Maximum oxygen capacity (max VO2), 432
max VO2. *See* Maximum oxygen capacity
        (max VO2)
MCTD. *See* Mixed connective tissue disease
        (MCTD)
MDCT angiography
  direct signs, 102–104
  indirect signs, 105
  pulmonary angiography, 105–108
MDCT angiography of the pulmonary
        arteries
  CT image postprocessing, 99
  CT signs of PH and RV dysfunction,
        99–100
  digital subtraction angiography (DSA),
        101–102
  technique, 98–99

Mean pulmonary arterial pressure (mPAP),
        100, 122, 264, 292, 357, 419, 431
  SaO_2 and, 294–295
Mean rightatrial pressures (mRAP), 385
Mediastinal fibrosis, 112
Mediastinum, 105
Medical Research Council (MRC), 259
Methemaglobin, 191
Microarray analysis, 268
Mitral stenosis, 64, 133
  flow and pressure relationship in, Gorlin
        and Gorlin formulae of, 138–139
Mitral valve stenosis, 21
Mixed connective tissue disease
        (MCTD), 166
MLPA. *See* Multiplex ligation-dependent
        probe amplification (MLPA)
MMPs. *See* Matrix metalloproteinases
        (MMPs)
Model for End-Stage Liver Disease (MELD)
        scoring systems, 209
Monocrotaline-induced pulmonary
        hypertension, 63–66
  intoxication with, 65
Monotherapy
  with endothelin receptor antagonist, 379
MPAD. *See* Main pulmonary artery
        diameter (MPAD)
mPAP. *See* Mean pulmonary arterial
        pressure (mPAP)
MRA. *See* Magnetic resonance angiography
        (MRA)
mRAP. *See* Mean rightatrial pressures
        (mRAP)
MRC. *See* Medical Research Council
        (MRC)
MRI. *See* Magnetic resonance imaging
        (MRI)
Multicenter Study of Hydroxyurea, 228
Multifactorial etiologies, 6–7
Multiplex ligation-dependent probe
        amplification (MLPA), 87
Multivariate analysis, 306
Muscularization, of pulmonary
        arterioles, 276
6MWD. *See* Six-minute walk distance
        (6MWD)

6MWT. *See* Six-minute walk test (6MWT)
Myocardial protection, 316

National Institutes of Health (NIH), 21,
 151, 381
 registry, 136
National Registry for Characterization of
 Primary Pulmonary Hypertension,
 151
Necrotizing arteritis, 20
nef antigen. *See* Negative factor (*nef*)
 antigen
Negative factor (*nef*) antigen, 198
Negative predictive value (NPV), 277
Neoplastic approach, 28, 30
Neuropsychic symptoms, 293
New York Heart Association (NYHA), 200,
 317, 351, 355, 470
NIH. *See* National Institutes of Health (NIH)
Nitric oxide (NO), 43, 260, 374, 425,
 435, 438
Nitric oxide synthetase (NOS), 182
NMD. *See* Nonsense-mediated decay
 (NMD)
NO. *See* Nitric oxide (NO)
Noctural oxygen therapy trial (NOTT), 259
Noninvasive tools
 BAL, 241
 HRCT of chest, 241–242
 oxygenation parameters, 241
 pulmonary function tests, 241
Nonpharmacological treatment, 442
Nonsense-mediated decay (NMD),
 84–85, 88
Nonspecific interstitial pneumonia
 (NSIP), 265
Norepinephrine, 453, 454
NOS. *See* Nitric oxide synthetase (NOS)
NOTT. *See* Noctural oxygen therapy trial
 (NOTT)
NPV. *See* Negative predictive value (NPV)
NSIP. *See* Nonspecific interstitial
 pneumonia (NSIP)
N-terminal fragment of pro-brain natriuretic
 peptide (NT-pro-BNP), 375,
 432, 455

N terminal (NT)-pro-BNP, 356
N-terminus fragment (NT)-proBNP,
 135, 157
NT-pro-BNP. *See* N-terminal fragment of
 pro-brain natriuretic peptide
 (NT-pro-BNP)
NYHA. *See* New York Heart Association
 (NYHA)

Obstructive PH
 endarterectomy for angiosarcomas,
 406–407
 hydatic emboli, 407
 tumor emboli, 407
Occlusion
 fibrous, 238
 thrombotic, 239
"Onion-skin" or "onion-bulb" lesion, 23, 25
Open-label study, 318
Oral endothelin antagonists, 210
Oral phosphodiesterase inhibitors, 210
Overcirculation-induced pulmonary
 hypertension, 66–69
 left to right shunt–induced, 66
 utero shunted lambs, 69
Oxygenation parameters, 241
Oxygen saturation (SaO$_2$), 294
 mPAP and, 295
Oxygen therapy
 in PAH, 455
Oxytocic drugs, 427

PA. *See* Pulmonary artery (PA)
PACES. *See* Pulmonary Arterial
 Hypertension Combination Study
 of Epoprostenol and Sildenafil
 (PACES)
PACES trial. *See* Pulmonary Arterial
 Hypertension Combination Study
 of Epoprostenol and Sildenafil
 (PACES) trial
PaCO$_2$. *See* Partial pressure of carbon
 dioxide (PaCO$_2$)
PAH. *See* Pulmonary arterial hypertension
 (PAH)

PAH associated with HIV infection
(PAH-HIV)
 demographic features of patients
  with, 196
 effects of antiretroviral therapy on,
  200–202
 incidence and prevalence of, 196–197
 oral ERAs, 203
 pathophysiology
  genetic predisposition in, 197
  pathology, 197
 prognostic factors for, 200
 prostacyclin and prostacyclin
  analogues, 202
 sildenafil, 202–203
PAH lesions
 complex, 26–27
 concentric and eccentric nonlaminar
  intimal fibrosis, 23
 concentric laminar intimal fibrosis, 23
 intimal fibrosis in idiopathic spontaneous
  pneumothorax and idiopathic
  pulmonary fibrosis, 23, 26
 medial hypertrophy, 22–23
 plexiform lesions, 28, 30
  inflammatory pattern in, 30–31
PAH-specific therapy, 424–425
 CCB, 424
 endothelin receptor antagonists, 425
 nitric oxide, 425
 phosphodiesterase type 5 inhibitors,
  424–425
 prostanoids, 424
Panlobular ground-glass opacities, 116
PaO$_2$. *See* Partial pressure of arterial
  oxygen (PaO$_2$)
PAOP. *See* Pulmonary artery occlusion
  pressure (PAOP)
PAP. *See* Pulmonary arterial pressure
  (PAP)
Parenchymal lung disease, 98
Parenchymal signs, 105
Park blade septostomy catheter, 387
Partial pressure of arterial oxygen (PaO$_2$),
  241, 309
Partial pressure of carbon dioxide
  (PaCO$_2$), 257

PASMC. *See* Pulmonary artery smooth
  muscle cell (PASMC)
PASP. *See* Pulmonary artery systolic
  pressure (PASP)
Patent ductus arteriosus (PDA), 177–178
Patient status
 defined, 374–375
PBF. *See* Pulmonary blood flow (PBF)
PCH. *See* Pulmonary capillary
  hemangiomatosis (PCH)
PCR. *See* Polymerase chain reaction (PCR)
PCWP. *See* Pulmonary capillary wedge
  pressure (PCWP)
PDA. *See* Patent ductus arteriosus (PDA)
PDE inhibitors. *See* Phosphodiesterase
  (PDE) inhibitors
PDE-5 inhibitors. *See* Phosphodiesterase 5
  (PDE-5) inhibitors
PDGF. *See* Platelet-derived growth factor
  (PDGF); Platelet-derived growth
  factor (PDGF) receptor
  antagonists
PEA. *See* Pulmonary endarterectomy (PEA)
Penetrance, 84
Perivascular granulomas, 216
Perls Prussian blue staining, 32
Persistent pulmonary hypertension (PPHN),
  306, 318
 of newborn, 69–70, 182–183
PGI$_2$. *See* Prostacyclin (PGI$_2$)
PH. *See* Pulmonary hypertension (PH)
Pharmacotherapy
 PAH specific, 394
Phenylephrine, 455
Phlebotomy, 188–189
Phosphodiesterase (PDE) inhibitors, 210,
  279, 374
 for CTDs, 169
Phosphodiesterase 5 (PDE-5) inhibitors,
  189, 424–425, 436
 sildenafil, 350–351
 tadalafil, 351–352
 vardenafil, 352
Plasma concentrations
 endothelin-1 (ET-1), 354
Plasminogen activator inhibitor (PAI-1)
 TPA *versus,* 307

Platelet-derived growth factor (PDGF), 41,
    63, 265, 268, 350, 442
  receptor antagonists, 63, 442
PLCH. *See* Pulmonary Langerhans cell
    histiocytosis (PLCH)
Pleural effusions, 96, 241
Plexiform lesions, 26–27, 45, 197, 217
  immunohistochemical characterization
    of, 46
Plexogenic arteriopathy, 210
Polycythemia, 298
Polymerase chain reaction (PCR), 86
Polymerization
  Hb S, 222–223
POPH. *See* Portopulmonary hypertension
    (POPH)
Portal hypertension
  HIV and, 200
Portopulmonary hypertension (POPH), 4
  clinical presentation, 207
  diagnosis, 207–208
  epidemiology, 209
  long-term survival, 210–211
  pathophysiology, 210
  screening, 208–209
  treatment, 210–211
Positive acute response, defined, 155
Positive predictive value (PPV), 277
Postcapillary lesions, 31, 238
Postpartum management
  for acute PH exacerbations, 427
Posttransplant lymphoproliferative disease
    (PTLD), 401
Potts procedure
  for transplantation, 402
Potts shunt, 179
PPH. *See* Primary pulmonary hypertension
    (PPH)
PPHN. *See* Persistent pulmonary hyperten-
    sion (PPHN)
PPV. *See* Positive predictive value (PPV)
Pregnancy
  clinical presentation of, 422
  epidemiology of, 421–422
  hemodynamic changes in, 420–421
  investigations for, 422–423
  IPAH in, 419

[Pregnancy]
  management of, 423–427
    algorithm for, 425
    anesthetic management, 426–427
    conventional medical therapy, 423–424
    PAH-specific therapy, 424–425
    postpartum management, 427
  prognosis of, 421–422
Preload balance
  in right ventricular, 453
Pre-LT prostacyclin therapy, 211
Preoperative imaging evaluation, 109–110
Primary pulmonary hypertension (PPH), 83,
    126, 152
Primary Sjögren syndrome (pSS), 166–167
Primum movens, 69
Procedure-related mortality
  in BDAS, 390
Prostacyclin (PGI$_2$), 43, 181, 210, 424, 438
  analogues, 202
  analogue therapy, 190
  beraprost, 343–344
  iloprost, 342–343
  intravenous epoprostenol, 338–340
  treprostinil, 340–342
Prostaglandins, 245
  CTDs, 167–168
Prostanoids, 373, 424
Prothrombin time (PT), 358
pSS. *See* Primary Sjögren syndrome (pSS)
PT. *See* Prothrombin time (PT)
PTE. *See* Pulmonary thromboendarterectomy
    (PTE)
PTLD. *See* Posttransplant lymphoproliferative
    disease (PTLD)
Pulmonary angiogram
  in CTEPH patients, 312, 313
Pulmonary angiography, 156
Pulmonary arterial adventitial thickening, 26
Pulmonary arterial hypertension, 97, 98
Pulmonary Arterial Hypertension and
    ReSponse to Tadalafil
    (PHIRST), 352
Pulmonary Arterial Hypertension Combina-
    tion Study of Epoprostenol and
    Sildenafil (PACES), 351
  trial, 169

Pulmonary arterial hypertension (PAH), 1–5,
216, 222, 237, 250, 264. *See also*
Conventional therapy, for PAH
acute vasodilator testing in. *See* Acute
vasodilator testing, in PAH patients
cell cultures, 72–73
CHD, 4
chronic hemolytic anemia, 5
clinical expression of, 84
female predominance, 86
genetic anticipation, 86
reduced penetrance, 85
variable expressivity, 85
connective tissue diseases (CTD), 2–3,
33, 35
complicating, 113–114
defined, 132, 161
diagnosis of, in HIV patients, 198–199
drug-induced, 2
end points in trials
biological markers, 465
CPET, 464–465
defined, 462–463
exercise testing, 463–464
hemodynamics, 466–467
imaging, 467–470
6MWT, 464
epidemiology of, 10–17
in developing countries, 17
French registry, 10–15
screening programme, 15–17
exercise capacity and, 156
familial, 1
genetic implications for clinical
evaluation, 90
genetic manipulations for, 70–73
hemodynamic definition of, 136–137
heritable, 1
with HIV infection, 3–4
hypoxia-induced, 61–63
measures, 371
monocrotaline-induced, 63–66
of newborn, 69–70
nonspecific supportive therapies in, 202
oral ERAs, 203
overcirculation-induced, 66–69
pathogenesis of, 40–52, 270, 272

[Pulmonary arterial hypertension (PAH)]
[pathogenesis of]
angioproliferation, 41–45
endocrine factors and, 50–51
endothelial cell growth, 45–48
immune system of, 48–50
overview, 40–41
pathophysiology of, 217
patient selections, 411–416
characteristics of, 412–413
comparative studies, 414–415
timing of transplantation, 415–416
transplant operation, 413
POPH, 4
prostacyclin and prostacyclin analogues, 202
recommendations, 371
RHC for. *See* Right-heart catheterization
(RHC)
right-heart catheterization and, 228
schistosomiasis, 4
schistosomiasis-associated, 218–219
sildenafil, 202–203
toxin-induced, 2
treatment of
cell-based therapy, 370–371
combination therapy, 367–368
evidence-based treatment algorithm,
372, 373–374
growth factor synthesis, inhibitors
of, 370
guanylate cyclase activators, 370
Rho kinase Inhibitors, 370
serotonin receptor and transporter
function, 368–369
VIP, 370
treatment of, in SCD, 230–231
Pulmonary arterial hypertension (PAH),
echocardiography of
differential diagnosis of, 127
Doppler and catheter diagnosis of, 125
Doppler-derived sPAP, upper normal
limits of, 123–125
echo-Doppler diagnosis, 126
follow-up of, 128–129
latent pulmonary hypertension and,
125–127
noninvasive estimation of, 122–123

[Pulmonary arterial hypertension (PAH), echocardiography of]
 RV overload, consequences of
  fuctional, 128
  morphological, 127–128
Pulmonary arterial obstruction, 208
Pulmonary arterial pressure (PAP)
 in chronic high-altitude diseases, 294
 in CMS, 296
 noninvasive estimation of, 122–123
Pulmonary arterioles
 muscularization of, 276
Pulmonary arteritis, 112–113
Pulmonary artery
 angiosarcoma of, 111–112
 occlusion pressure, 207
 trunk, 218
Pulmonary artery occlusion pressure
  (PAOP), 136–137, 138, 139–140
Pulmonary artery (PA), 269, 400
Pulmonary artery pressure (PAP), 5, 250, 463
 resting and exercising, in COPD,
  253–254, 257
Pulmonary artery sarcoma, 111
Pulmonary artery smooth muscle cell
  (PASMC), 89, 275
Pulmonary artery systolic pressure (PASP),
  135, 224
 DE-estimated, 135–136
Pulmonary blood flow (PBF), 385
Pulmonary capillary hemangiomatosis
  (PCH), 5, 20, 33, 114–116,
  115–116, 243–245, 409
 classification of, 237–238
 definition of, 237–238
 hemodynamic characteristics of, 244
 pathological assessment, 238–239
 specific therapy in PVOD, 243
Pulmonary capillary wedge pressure
  (PCWP), 240, 419
Pulmonary endarterectomy (PEA), 358
 contraindications for, 405–406
 in CTEPH, 403–404
 indications for, 405–406
 limits of, 405–406
 technique of, 404–405
Pulmonary function tests, 241, 309

Pulmonary hemodynamics
 in chronic high-altitude diseases, in China
  and Kyrgyzstan, 297
 studies of CMS, at altitude of residence,
  293–295
Pulmonary hemorrhage, 28, 32
Pulmonary hypertension (PH), 243
 characteristics of, in COPD, 252–254
 clinical manifestations, 277
 CMS and, 297–298
 definition of, 250
 development of RHF from, 257–259
 diagnosis of, 277–279
  in COPD, 255–256
 Doppler's echocardiography and, 255–256
 endothelin/receptors involvement in, 267
 evian classification of, 218
 evolution of, in COPD, 256–257
 exercise and, 140–141
 fibrotic process and, 266–267
 hemodynamic definition of, 136–137
 inflammation and, 274–276
 LTOT and, 259–260
 mechanisms, in COPD, 251–252
 pathogenesis of, during ILD, 269–271
 pathological changes, 276
 prevalence of, 251
  in ILD, 264–266
 prognosis of
  in COPD, 259
  in ILD, 266
 RHC and, 256, 277–279
 schistosomiasis and, 216–217
 score system and, 301
 severe or disproportionate of, in COPD,
  254–255
 specific medical therapies, use of,
  317–319
 TGF-β isoforms in, 271–273
 therapies targeting, 279–281
 vasodilator drugs and, 260
 Venice clinical classification of, 2
Pulmonary inflammation
 and HIV, 198
Pulmonary Langerhans cell histiocytosis
  (PLCH), 264
Pulmonary parenchymal disease, 96

Pulmonary regurgitation, Graham Steell
  murmur of, 184
Pulmonary thromboendarterectomy
  (PTE), 305
  CTEPH and, 314–315
  postoperative outcomes and, 315–317
Pulmonary vascular obstructive disease
  (PVOD), 182
Pulmonary vascular resistance (PVR), 59,
  134, 137, 139, 207, 251, 307, 339,
  352, 413, 419, 431
  calculating, 256
Pulmonary vasculature
  remodeling of, 252
Pulmonary vasculopathy, 26
Pulmonary veno-occlusive disease (PVOD),
  5, 20, 31–32, 114–116, 128, 197,
  200, 411, 432
  classification of, 237–238
  clinical features of, 240
  conventional therapy and, 242–243
  definition of, 237–238
  epidemiology of, 239
  genetic risk in, 240
  hemodynamic characteristics of,
    240–241
  HRCT of chest in, 242
  immunosuppressive therapy in, 242–243
  lung transplantation and, 243
  noninvasive tools. *See* Noninvasive tools
  pathological assessment, 238–239
  risk factors in, 240
  specific PAH therapy in, 243
Pulmonary venous hypertension, 33, 277
  right-heart catheterization and, 228
Pulmonary vessels, 105
Pulmonary wedge pressure (PWP), 4
Pulse oximeter oxygen saturation
  (SpO_2), 241
PVOD. *See* Pulmonary veno-occlusive
  disease (PVOD)
PVR. *See* Pulmonary vascular resistance
  (PVR)
PVRI. *See* PVR index (PVRI)
PVR index (PVRI), 439
PWP. *See* Pulmonary wedge pressure
  (PWP)

Qinghai score, 300
QoL. *See* Quality of life (QoL)
Quality of life (QoL), 463, 469

RA. *See* Regional anesthesia (RA);
    Rheumatoid arthritis (RA)
Randomized controlled trials (RCT), 462
Rashkind septostomy, 191
Raynaud's phenomenon, 240, 454
RCT. *See* Randomized controlled trials
    (RCT)
Receiver operating characteristic
    (ROC), 265
Receptors
  endothelin, 353
  involvement in PH and ILD, 274
Regional anesthesia (RA), 422
Rethrombosis, 405
REVEAL registry, 15, 50, 209
RHC. *See* Right-heart catheterization (RHC)
Rheumatoid arthritis (RA), 166
RHF. *See* Right-heart failure (RHF)
Rho kinase, inhibitors, 370
Rho kinase (ROCK), 443
Right-heart catheterization (RHC), 10, 123,
    125, 133, 134, 155, 228, 250,
    264, 311
  drawbacks of, 256
  and exercise, 140–141
  intracardiac shunt, evaluation of, 138
  left-heart disease, hemodynamic
    assessment of, 138–140
  PH and, 256
  PH and PAH, hemodynamic definition of,
    136–137
  for pregnant patients, 422–423
  pulmonary venous hypertension, evalua-
    tion of, 138
  role of, in diagnosis of PH and ILD,
    277–279
  in RV function, 377
  vasodilator testing, 137
Right-heart failure (RHF), 253
  development of, from PH, 257–259
right pulmonary artery (RPA), 100
Right ventricle (RV), 401, 421, 431

Right ventricular contractility, in
 COPD, 259
Right ventricular ejection fraction
 (RVEF), 259
Right ventricular failure (RVF), 385
Right ventricular hypertrophy (RVH),
 133, 292
Right ventricular outflow tract (RVOT), 100
Right ventricular pressure (RVP), 137
Right ventricular pressure systolic pressures
 (RVSP), 208
ROC. *See* Receiver operating characteristic
 (ROC)
ROCK. *See* Rho kinase (ROCK)
RV. *See* Right ventricle (RV)
RVEF. *See* Right ventricular ejection
 fraction (RVEF)
RVF. *See* Right ventricular failure (RVF)
RV function
 for comprehensive prognostic evaluation,
 377–378
RVH. *See* Right ventricular hypertrophy
 (RVH)
RV overload, consequences of
 fuctional, 128
 morphological, 127–128
RVP. *See* Right ventricular pressure
 (RVP)
RVSP. *See* RV systolic pressure (RVSP)
RV systolic pressure (RVSP), 432

SaO$_2$. *See* Oxygen saturation (SaO$_2$)
Sarcoidosis, 30–31
"Scarring" vasculitis-like lesions, 30–31
SCD. *See* Sickle cell disease (SCD)
Schistosoma haematobium, 214
Schistosoma intercalatum, 214
Schistosoma japonicum, 214, 215
Schistosoma mansoni, 214, 217
Schistosoma mekongi, 214
Schistosome
 life cycle of, 215–216
Schistosomiasis, 4
 classification of, 218
 diagnosis of, 218
 epidemiology of, 214

[Schistosomiasis]
 life cycle of, 215–216
 mechanism of lesion, 217
 PAH and, 218–219
 pulmonary hypertension and, 216–217
 treatment of, 219
 vascular lung pathology, 217
Schistosomiasis Control Initiative
 (SCI), 214
SCI. *See* Schistosomiasis Control Initiative
 (SCI)
Scimitar syndrome, 180
Scleroderma-related PAH. *See* Systemic
 sclerosis (SSc)
Selective serotonin reuptake inhibitor
 (SSRI), 369
Septal veins, 238
Septostomy, 454
Serology, 135, 219
Serotonin, 89
 inhibitors, 443
 transporter, 60
Serotonin transporter (SERT), 89–90,
 368–369
SERT. *See* Serotonin transporter (SERT)
sGC. *See* Soluble guanylate cyclase (sGC)
Shone's complex, 180
Sickle cell disease (SCD), 5
 BNP in, 227–228
 echocardiographic studies in, 224–227
 endothelial dysfunction, 223–224
 hemolysis, 223–224
 hypercoagulability, 223–224
 left-sided heart disease in, 227
 right-heart catheterization, 228
 treatment of PAH in, 230–231
 vasculopathy, 223–224
Sildenafil, 169, 189, 191, 202–203, 210,
 211, 350–351, 441, 445
Sildenafil Use in Pulmonary artERial
 hypertension (SUPER), 351
Simian immunodeficiency virus (SIV), 198
Simian immunoinsufficiency virus (SIV), 50
SIMS. *See* Subacute infantile mountain
 sickness (SIMS)
Single-lung transplantation (SLT), 399,
 400–401, 412

Sitaxsentan, 354
  STRIDE-1, 358
  STRIDE-2, 359
  STRIDE-2X, 359
SIV. *See* Simian immunodeficiency virus
  (SIV); Simian immunoinsuffi-
  ciency virus (SIV)
Six-minute walk distance (6MWD), 167,
  168, 169, 241, 278, 318, 338, 355
Six-minute walk test (6MWT), 135, 156,
  266, 374, 432, 462, 464
SLE. *See* Systemic lupus erythematosus
  (SLE)
SLT. *See* Single-lung transplantation
  (SLT)
SMC. *See* Smooth muscle cells (SMC)
Smooth muscle cells (SMC), 23, 27, 269
  hyperplasia, 27
  hypertrophy, 26
  in pulmonary arteries, 22
Soluble guanylate cyclase (sGC), 370,
  442–443
Soluble vascular cell adhesion molecule 1
  (sVCAM-1), 162
sPAP. *See* Systolic pulmonary arterial
  pressure (sPAP)
Splenectomy, 7
SpO₂. *See* Pulse oximeter oxygen saturation
  (SpO₂)
SSc. *See* Systemic sclerosis (SSc)
SSRI. *See* Selective serotonin reuptake
  inhibitor (SSRI)
Statins, 443
Steady-state exercise, PAP during, 253
Stromal cell gene expression, 49
Subacute infantile mountain sickness
  (SIMS), 298
SUPER. *See* Sildenafil Use in Pulmonary
  artERial hypertension (SUPER)
Supplemental oxygen therapy, 326
sVCAM-1. *See* Soluble vascular cell
  adhesion molecule 1 (sVCAM-1)
SVR. *See* Systemic vascular resistance
  (SVR)
Symptomatology, 132–133
Systemic lupus erythematosus (SLE), 33,
  113–114, 166, 244

Systemic sclerosis (SSc), 33, 161. *See also*
  Connective tissue diseases
  (CTDs), PAH and
  autoantibodies in, 162–163
  clinical features, 164
  detection of, algorithm for, 164–165
  genetic factors in, 163–164
  prognosis, 165–166
  vascular changes in, 162
Systemic vascular resistance (SVR), 420
Systolic pulmonary arterial pressure
  (sPAP), 122
  Doppler-derived, upper normal limits of,
  123–125

Tadalafil, 351–352
Takayasu's arteritis, 112–113, 244
Takayasu's disease, 156
TAPSE. *See* Tricuspid annular plane
  systolic excursion (TAPSE)
Tenascin-C, 65
Tetralogy of Fallot (TOF), 180, 184
TGF-β. *See* Transforming growth factor β
  (TGF-β)
TGF-β isoforms, in PH and ILD,
  271–273
Therapeutic modulation, of hemoglobin S
  polymerization, 223
Thromboembolic materials, 103
Thromboembolic PH
  differential diagnosis of chronic, 110
Thrombotic lesions, 23
  in pulmonary arteries, 437
Thrombotic materials
  organization and recanalization of, 23
Thrombotic occlusion, 31, 239
Thromboxane A2 (TxA2), 181
TIPG. *See* Tricuspid insufficiency peak
  gradient (TIPG)
Tissue plasminogen activator (TPA), 307
  versus PAI-1, 307
T lymphocytes, 31, 49
TOF. *See* Tetralogy of Fallot (TOF)
TOPP. *See* Tracking Outcomes and Practice
  in Pediatric PAH (TOPP) registry
Toxin-induced PAH, 2

TPA. *See* Tissue plasminogen activator (TPA)
TR. *See* Tricuspid regurgitation (TR)
Tracking Outcomes and Practice in Pediatric PAH (TOPP) registry, 434
Transforming growth factor β (TGF-β), 1, 83, 153, 181, 268
RII gene, 46
Transplantation
lungs and PVOD, 243
Potts procedure, 402
survival rate in, 401
types of, 399–401
Transplant operation, 413
Transthoracic Doppler echocardiography (TTE), 96, 135–136, 208
Transthoracic echocardiography (TTE), 154, 264–265, 277, 310
Trematode parasites, 214
Treprostinil, 167, 340–342, 373
dosage of, instructions for, 342
TREs. *See* Trinucleotide repeat expansions (TREs)
Tricuspid annular plane systolic excursion (TAPSE), 128, 375, 432
Tricuspid insufficiency peak gradient (TIPG), 124
Tricuspid jet method, 122, 123
echo-Doppler diagnosis. *See* Doppler echocardiography
Tricuspid regurgitant jet velocity (TRV), 225
Tricuspid regurgitation (TR), 255
Tricuspid valve regurgitation, 100
Tricyclic benzidene, 342
Trinucleotide repeat expansions (TREs), 86
Tropoelastin, 65
Troponin, 455
TRV. *See* Tricuspid regurgitant jet velocity (TRV)
TTE. *See* Transthoracic echocardiography (TTE)
Tumor emboli, 407
Tunica intima, 23–24
Tunica media, 31, 238
TxA2. *See* Thromboxane A2 (TxA2)
Tyrosine kinase inhibitors, 442
for CTDs, 170

Uterine leiomyomatosis, 112

Valsalva maneuvers, 437
Vardenafil, 352
Vascular ablation, 267
Vascular cell adhesion molecule 1 (VCAM-1), 223
Vascular endothelial growth factor (VEGF), 41, 162, 170, 183, 268
Vascular smooth muscle cell (VSMC), 48
Vasculopathy, hemolysis-associated, 223–224
Vasoactive intestinal peptide (VIP), 72, 89, 443
Vasoactive intestinal polypeptide (VIP), 370
Vasoconstriction, 23, 40
Vasoconstrictor, 352
Vasodilator drugs, and PH, 260
Vasodilators, 33
testing, 137
therapy, 41, 302, 453
VCAM-1. *See* Vascular cell adhesion molecule 1 (VCAM-1)
VCG. *See* Vectorcardiogram (VCG)
Vectorcardiogram (VCG), 297
VEGF. *See* Vascular endothelial growth factor (VEGF)
Veins, septal, 238
Venice and Dana Point classification, 28
Venice classification, 31
Veno-occlusive remodeling, 35
Venous lesions in IPAH lungs, 35–37
Ventilation-perfusion (V/Q) lung scan, 97–98, 156
Ventilation-perfusion (V/Q) mismatch, 400
Ventilation/perfusion (V/Q) scan, 98, 432
Ventilation-perfusion (V/Q) scintigraphy, 310
Ventricular septal defects (VSD), 176, 179, 413
Vessel restenosis, 271
Vessels, thin-walled, 266
VIP. *See* Vasoactive intestinal peptide (VIP); Vasoactive intestinal polypeptide (VIP)

Vitamin K antagonists (VKA), 423
VKA. *See* Vitamin K antagonists (VKA)
von Willebrand factor Antigen (vWF:Ag),
    135
V/Q. *See* Ventilation-perfusion (V/Q)
    mismatch
V/Q scan. *See* Ventilation/perfusion (V/Q)
    scan
V/Q scintigraphy. *See* Ventilation-perfusion
    (V/Q) scintigraphy
VSD. *See* Ventricular septal defects (VSD)
VSMC. *See* Vascular smooth muscle cell
    (VSMC)

vWF:Ag. *See* Von Willebrand factor
    Antigen (vWF:Ag)

Waterson shunt, 179
Wegener's granulomatosis, 30–31
Weigert-Hematoxylin-Phloxin-Saffron
    staining, 22
WHO. *See* World Health Organization (WHO)
WHPS staining, 22, 24, 29, 36
World Health Organization (WHO), 21,
    124, 214, 264, 318, 463
World Symposium in Dana Point, 33